Lippincott's
Illustrated Reviews:
Microbiology

Lippincott's Illustrated Reviews: Microbiology

William A. Strohl, Ph.D.

Department of Molecular Genetics and Microbiology
University of Medicine and Dentistry of New Jersey–
Robert Wood Johnson Medical School
Piscataway, New Jersey

Harriet Rouse, Ph.D.

Department of Molecular Genetics and Microbiology
University of Medicine and Dentistry of New Jersey–
Robert Wood Johnson Medical School
Piscataway, New Jersey

Bruce D. Fisher, M.D.

Department of Medical Education
Muhlenberg Regional Medical Center
Plainfield, New Jersey

Editors

Richard A. Harvey, Ph.D.

Department of Biochemistry
University of Medicine and Dentistry of New Jersey–
Robert Wood Johnson Medical School
Piscataway, New Jersey

Pamela C. Champe, Ph.D.

Department of Biochemistry
University of Medicine and Dentistry of New Jersey–
Robert Wood Johnson Medical School
Piscataway, New Jersey

Editor: Elizabeth A. Nieginski
Editorial Director: Julie P. Scardiglia
Managing Editor: Marette Magargle-Smith
Marketing Manager: Kelley Ray

351 West Camden Street
Baltimore, Maryland 21201-2436 USA

530 Walnut Street
Philadelphia, Pennsylvania 19106 USA

Printed in the United States of America

Library of Congress Cataloging-in-Publication Data

Strohl, William A.
    Microbiology/William A. Strohl, Harriet Rouse, Bruce D. Fisher; editors, Richard A. Harvey, Pamela C. Champe; contributors, Sewell P. Champe...[et al.].
    p.; cm. – (Lippincott's illustrated reviews)
    Includes index
    ISBN# 0-397-51568-5
        1.Microbiology—Outlines, syllabi, etc. I. Rouse, Harriet. II. Fisher, Bruce L., M.D. III. Harvey,
Richard A., Ph.D. IV. Champe, Pamela C.V. Champe, Sewell P., 1932-VI. Title. VII. Series.
        [DNLM: 1. Microbiology—Outlines. QW 18.2 S921m 2001]
    QR62.S775 2001
    579—dc21
                    2001029441

Contributors:

Sewell P. Champe, Ph.D.

Waksman Institute

Rutgers University

Piscataway, New Jersey

Donald Dubin, M.D.

Department of Molecular Genetics and Microbiology

University of Medicine and Dentistry of New Jersey–

Robert Wood Johnson Medical School

Piscataway, New Jersey

Florence Kimball, Ph.D.

Department of Molecular Genetics and Microbiology

University of Medicine and Dentistry of New Jersey–

Robert Wood Johnson Medical School

Piscataway, New Jersey

Victor Stollar, M.D.

Department of Molecular Genetics and Microbiology

University of Medicine and Dentistry of New Jersey–

Robert Wood Johnson Medical School

Piscataway, New Jersey

William E. Winter, M.D.

Department of Pathology

University of Florida College of Medicine

Gainesville, Florida

Computer graphics:
Michael Cooper

Cooper Graphics

www.cooper247.com

 LIPPINCOTT WILLIAMS & WILKINS

A **Wolters Kluwer** Company

Philadelphia · Baltimore · New York · London
Buenos Aires · Hong Kong · Sydney · Tokyo

This book is dedicated to the memory
of Sewell Preston Champe,
whose gentle spirit and intellectual
generosity made this work possible.

Acknowledgments

We are grateful to the many friends and colleagues who generously contributed their time and effort to help us make this book as accurate and as useful as possible. The support of our other colleagues at the University of Medicine and Dentistry of New Jersey–Robert Wood Johnson Medical School is highly valued. We (RAH and PCC) owe special thanks to our Chairman, Dr. Masayori Inouye, who has encouraged us over the years in this and other teaching projects. We are particularly indebted to Dr. Mary Mycek of the University of Medicine and Dentistry of New Jersey–New Jersey Medical School, who participated actively in this project from its inception, and whose insights into recent advances in antimicrobial therapy provided an invaluable contribution to the timeliness and accuracy of this volume.

Without talented artists, an Illustrated Review would be impossible, and we have been particularly fortunate in working with Michael Cooper throughout this project. His artistic sense and computer graphics expertise have greatly added to our ability to bring microbiology "stories" alive for our readers. We are also highly appreciative of Dr. Hae Sook Kim and Linda Duckenfield, SM/MT (ASCP), for assistance in preparing photomicrographs.

The editors and production staff of the Lippincott Williams & Wilkins were a constant source of encouragement and discipline. We particularly want to acknowledge the tremendously helpful, supportive, creative contributions of our editors, Richard Winters and Elizabeth Nieginski, whose imagination and positive attitude helped us bring this complex project to completion. Final editing and assembly of the book has been greatly enhanced through the efforts of Marette Magargle-Smith.

Brief Contents

Special Features of This Book

InfoLinks

Unique features of this volume are references to *Lippincott's Illustrated Reviews: Biochemistry* and *Lippincott's Illustrated Reviews: Pharmacology*, which are the biochemistry and pharmacology volumes in the Lippincott Illustrated Review series. Designated as InfoLink references, they are located at the bottom of the page where relevant material is discussed.

 [1]See p. 383 in **Lippincott's Illustrated Reviews: Biochemistry** (2nd ed.) for a discussion of RNA polymerase II.

This permits a reader with an interest in learning additional information related to a particular topic to readily locate relevant material covered in other books in the series. InfoLink also emphasizes the interrelationships between these biomedical disciplines—a skill that is increasingly being tested by the USMLE, Step I.

The Microbial World

Introduction to Microbiology

1

I. OVERVIEW

Microorganisms can be found in every ecosystem and in close association with every type of multicellular organism. They populate the healthy human body by the billions as benign passengers (**normal flora**, see p. 7) and even as participants in bodily functions, for example, bacteria play a role in the degradation of intestinal contents. Microorganisms also serve as useful tools in many areas of current technology. However, in this volume, we primarily consider the role of microorganisms—bacteria, fungi, protozoa, helminths, and viruses—in the initiation and spread of human diseases. Those relatively few species of microorganisms that are harmful to humans, either by production of toxic compounds or by direct infection, are characterized as **pathogens**.

Most infectious disease is initiated by **colonization** (that is, the establishment of proliferating microorganisms on the skin or mucous membranes, Figure 1.1). The major exceptions are diseases caused by introduction of organisms directly into the bloodstream or internal organs. Microbial colonization may result in 1) **elimination** of the microorganism without affecting the host, or 2) **infection** where the organisms multiply and cause the host to react by making an immune or other type of response. Infection, in turn, can have several consequences, including **infectious disease,** where the organism causes tissue damage and impairment of body function. Infection is therefore distinct from disease. The two terms are nonetheless often used interchangeably.

II. PROKARYOTIC PATHOGENS

All prokaryotic organisms are classified as bacteria, whereas eukaryotic organisms include fungi, protozoa, and helminths, as well as humans. Prokaryotic organisms are divided into two major groups: the **eubacteria,** which include all bacteria of medical importance, and the **archaebacteria**, a collection of evolutionarily distinct organisms. Cells of prokaryotic and eukaryotic organisms differ in several significant structural features as illustrated in Figure 1.2.

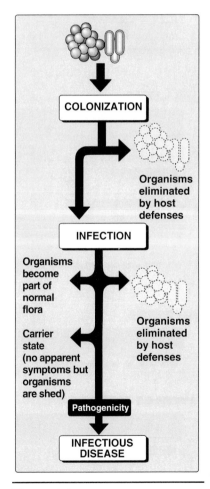

Figure 1.1
Some possible outcomes following exposure to microorganisms.

Lippincott's Illustrated Reviews: Microbiology,
by William A. Strohl, Harriet Rouse, Bruce D. Fisher.
Lippincott, Williams & Wilkins, Baltimore, MD © 2001

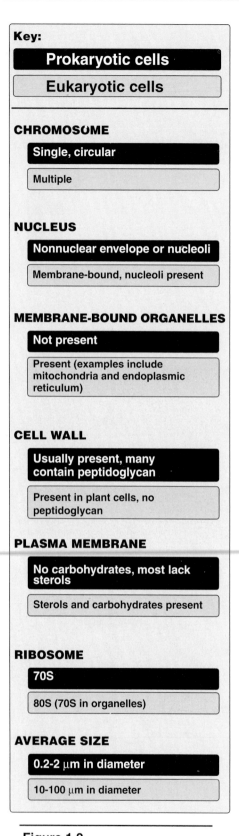

Key:

| Prokaryotic cells |
| Eukaryotic cells |

CHROMOSOME

| Single, circular |
| Multiple |

NUCLEUS

| Nonnuclear envelope or nucleoli |
| Membrane-bound, nucleoli present |

MEMBRANE-BOUND ORGANELLES

| Not present |
| Present (examples include mitochondria and endoplasmic reticulum) |

CELL WALL

| Usually present, many contain peptidoglycan |
| Present in plant cells, no peptidoglycan |

PLASMA MEMBRANE

| No carbohydrates, most lack sterols |
| Sterols and carbohydrates present |

RIBOSOME

| 70S |
| 80S (70S in organelles) |

AVERAGE SIZE

| 0.2-2 µm in diameter |
| 10-100 µm in diameter |

Figure 1.2
Comparison of prokaryotic and eukaryotic cells.

A. Typical bacteria

Most bacteria have shapes that can be described as either a rod, a sphere, or a corkscrew. Prokaryotic cells are smaller than eukaryotic cells (Figure 1.3). Nearly all bacteria, with the exception of the mycoplasma, have a rigid cell wall surrounding the cell membrane that determines the shape of the organism. The cell wall also determines whether the bacterium is classified as gram-positive or gram-negative (see p. 23). External to the cell wall may be flagella, pili, and/or a capsule. Bacterial cells divide by binary fusion. However, many bacteria exchange genetic information carried on plasmids—small, specialized genetic elements capable of self-replication—including the information necessary for establishment of antibiotic-resistance. Bacterial structure, metabolism, and genetics, and the wide variety of human diseases caused by bacteria, are described in detail in Unit III, beginning on p. 101.

B. Atypical bacteria

Atypical bacteria include groups of organisms such as mycoplasma, chlamydia, and rickettsia that, although prokaryotic, lack significant characteristic structural components or metabolic capabilities that separate them from the larger group of typical bacteria (see pp. 229, 235, and 259).

III. FUNGI

Fungi are nonphotosynthetic, generally saprophytic, eukaryotic organisms. Some fungi are filamentous, and are commonly called **molds**, whereas others—the **yeasts**—are unicellular (see p. 265). Fungal reproduction may be asexual, sexual, or both, and all fungi produce spores. Pathogenic fungi can cause diseases ranging from skin infections (**superficial mycoses**) to serious, systemic infections (**deep mycoses**).

IV. PROTOZOA

Protozoa are single-celled, nonphotosynthetic, eukaryotic organisms that come in a wide variety of shapes and sizes. Many protozoa are free-living, but others are among the most important parasites of humans. Members of this group infect all the major tissues and organs of the body. They can be intracellular parasites, or extracellular parasites in the blood, urogenital region, or the intestine. Transmission is generally by ingestion of an infective stage of the parasite, or by an insect bite. Protozoa cause a variety of diseases that are discussed in Chapter 24, p. 279.

V. HELMINTHS

Helminths are those groups of worms that live as parasites. These are multicellular eukaryotic organisms with complex body organization. They are divided into three main groups: tapeworms (cestodes), flukes (trematodes), and roundworms (nematodes). They are parasitic, receiving nutrients by ingesting or absorbing digestive contents, or ingesting or absorbing body fluids or tissues, and almost any organ in the body can be parasitized. All the major groups of helminths can cause disease in humans, as described in Chapter 25, p. 289.

VI. VIRUSES

Viruses are obligate intracellular parasites that do not have a cellular structure. Rather, a virus consists of molecule(s) of DNA ("DNA virus") or RNA ("RNA virus"), but not both, surrounded by a protein coat. A virus may also have an envelope derived from the plasma membrane of the host cell from which the virus is released. Viruses contain the genetic information necessary for directing their own replication, but require the host's cellular structures and enzymatic machinery in order to complete the process of their own reproduction. The fate of the host cell following viral infection ranges from rapid lysis releasing many progeny virions, to gradual, prolonged release of viral particles. Viruses cause a broad spectrum of diseases (see Unit V, beginning on p. 295).

VII. ORGANIZING THE MICROORGANISMS

Trying to assimilate the names and characteristics of pathogenic organisms can be an overwhelming experience unless the flood of information is organized into logical groupings. This is the basis for dividing the text into chapters that describe related organisms. In addition, the relationships between bacteria and between viruses have been visualized separately using two graphic formats throughout the book.

A. Hierarchical organization

The first is a hierarchical organization that resembles a family tree (Figures 1.4 and 1.5). These graphs provide a summary of the major characteristics of a particular microorganism. For example, tracing the lineage of staphylococci reveals that they have rigid cell walls, and are simple, unicellular, free-living organisms that are gram-positive cocci.

B. Pie chart organization

A second, simpler format represents selected groups of bacteria or viruses as wedges of a pie chart. These pie charts focus on the most important defining characteristics of a particular organism. For example, the bacteria are organized into eight groups according to Gram staining, morphology, and biochemical or other characteristics. The ninth section of the bacterial pie chart is labeled "Other", and is used to represent any organism not included in one of the other eight categories. In a similar way, viral pathogens are organized in into seven groups based on the nature of their genome, symmetry of organization, and the presence or absence of a lipid envelope. Figure 1.6 shows how the hierarchical classification is condensed to form pie charts.

C. Taxonomy

This book uses a taxonomic hierarchy for the classification of bacteria, fungi, protozoans, and helminths. [Note: The classification of viruses is described on p. 295.] Kingdoms are divided into evolutionarily related phyla, classes, orders, families, genera, and species. The first letter of the genus name is always capitalized, and the species name begins with a lower case letter. Both names are printed in italics.

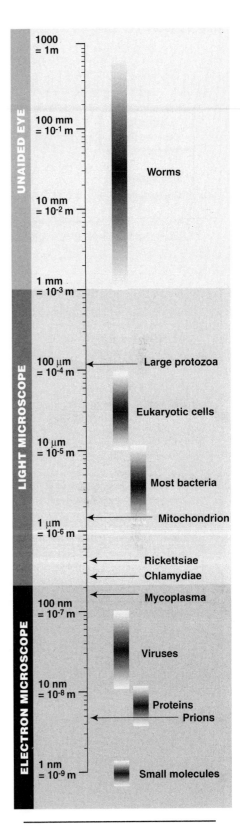

Figure 1.3
Relative size of organisms and molecules.

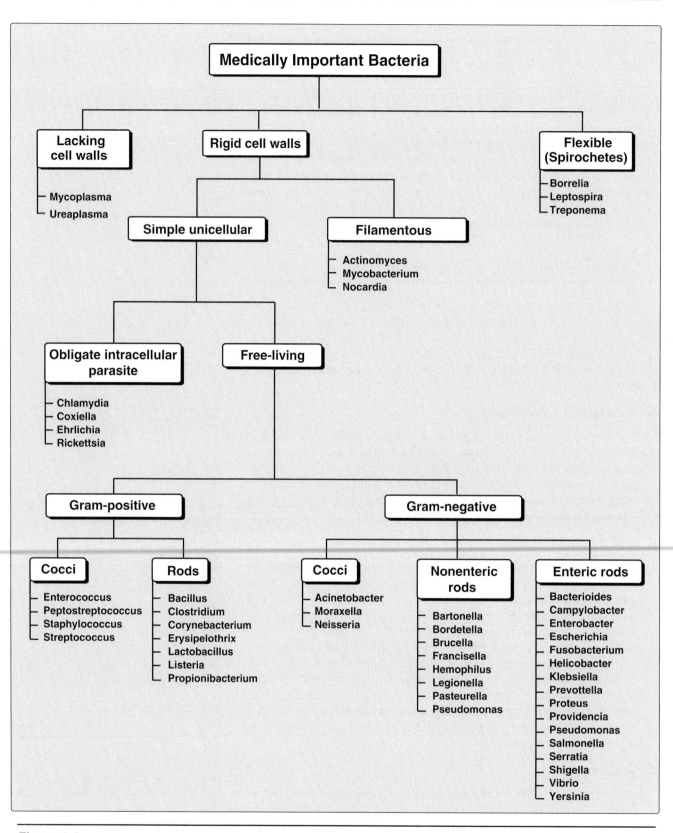

Figure 1.4
Classification of some medically important bacterial families.

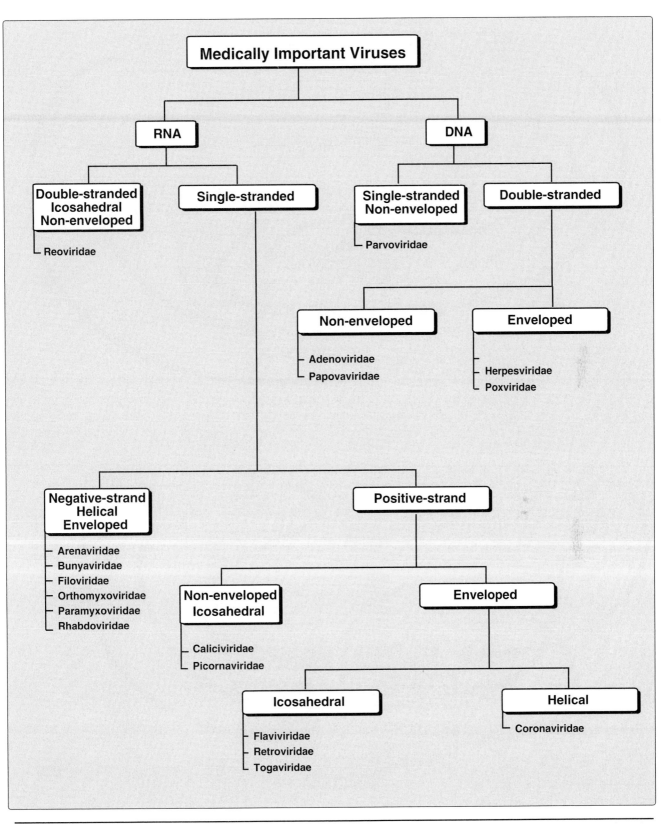

Figure 1.5
Classification of some medically important virus families.

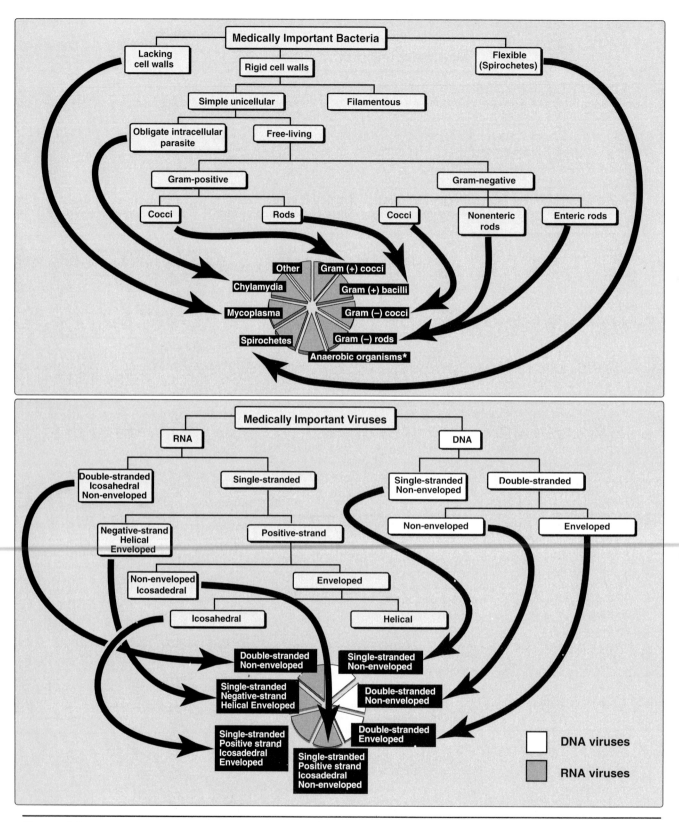

Figure 1.6
Condensation of hierarchical classification to pie chart representing the most important clinical groups of microorganisms. *Anaerobic bacteria are comprised of both gram-positive (for example, *Clostridial* species) and gram-negative rods (for example, *Bacteriodes* species).

Normal Flora

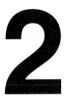

I. OVERVIEW

The human body is continuously inhabited by many different microorganisms—mostly bacteria, but also some fungi and other microorganisms—which, under normal circumstances in a healthy individual, are harmless, and may even be beneficial. These microorganisms are termed the **normal flora**. [Note: Although bacteria and other microorganisms have not been considered plants for many years, the term "flora" is still widely used to describe the microbial inhabitants of the human body.] The normal flora are also termed **commensals**, which literally means "organisms that dine together." Except for occasional transient invaders, the internal organs and systems are sterile, including the spleen, pancreas, liver, bladder, central nervous system, and blood. A healthy newborn enters the world in essentially sterile condition, but after birth it rapidly acquires normal flora from food and the environment, including other humans. The species contained in the "normal flora" cannot be rigidly defined for all humans, because those species present may vary from individual to individual, due to physiologic differences, diet, age, and geographic habitat. It is useful to be aware of the normal types and distribution of resident flora, because such knowledge helps provide an understanding of the possible infections that could result from injury to a particular body site, and also helps place in perspective the possible sources and significance of microorganisms isolated from the site of an infection.

II. DISTRIBUTION OF NORMAL FLORA IN THE BODY

The most common sites of the body inhabited by the normal flora are, as one might expect, those that are in contact or in communication with the outside world, namely the skin, eye, mouth, upper respiratory tract, gastrointestinal tract, and urogenital tract.

A. Skin

The skin can acquire any bacteria that happen to be in the immediate environment, but this **transient flora** either dies or is removable by washing. The skin surface does not provide a favorable environment for colonization by microorganisms. For example, it is generally dry (the moist regions of the skin are more conducive to bacterial growth than are the dry regions), it has a slightly acidic pH,

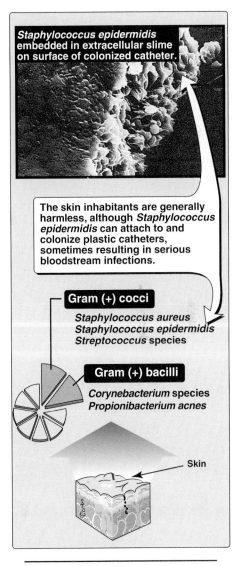

Figure 2.1
Some examples of bacteria that inhabit the skin. The fungi Candida and Pityrosporon are also part of the normal flora. *S. epidermidis* is shown in a scanning electron micrograph.

Lippincott's Illustrated Reviews: Microbiology, by William A. Strohl, Harriet Rouse, Bruce D. Fisher. Lippincott, Williams & Wilkins, Baltimore, MD © 2001

and the sweat glands produce a liquid containing a high concentration of sodium chloride that causes a hyperosmotic environment on the skin surface. Nevertheless, the skin supports a permanent bacterial population (**resident flora**), residing in multiple layers of the skin (Figure 2.1). The resident flora regenerate themselves even after vigorous scrubbing. Most common among the skin colonizers (10^3 to 10^4 per cm^2) are aerobic *Staphylococcus epidermidis* and other coagulase-negative staphylococci (see p. 143) that reside in the outer layers of the skin, and account for some ninety percent of the skin aerobes. Anaerobic organisms, such as *Propionibacterium acnes*, reside in the deeper skin layers, in hair follicles, and in sweat and sebaceous glands. The skin inhabitants are generally harmless, although *S. epidermidis* can attach to and colonize plastic catheters and medical devices that penetrate the skin, sometimes resulting in serious bloodstream infections.

B. Eye

The conjunctiva of the eye is colonized primarily by *S. epidermidis*, followed by *Staphylococcus aureus*, aerobic corynebacteria (diphtheroids), and *Streptococcus pneumoniae*. Other organisms that normally inhabit the skin are also present, but at a lower frequency (Figure 2.2). Tears, which contain the antimicrobial enzyme lysozyme, help limit the bacterial population of the conjunctiva.

C. Mouth and nose

The mouth and nose harbor many microorganisms, both aerobic and anaerobic (see Figure 2.3). Among the most common are diphtheroids (aerobic *Corynebacterium* species), *S. aureus*, and *S. epidermidis*. In addition, the teeth and surrounding gingival tissue are colonized by their own particular species, such as *Streptococcus mutans*. [Note: *S. mutans* can enter the bloodstream following dental surgery, and colonize damaged or prosthetic heart valves, leading to potentially fatal infective endocarditis.] Some normal residents of the nasopharynx can also cause disease. For example, *Streptococcus pneumoniae*, found in the nasopharynx of many healthy individuals, can cause acute bacterial pneumonia, especially in the aged and those whose resistance is

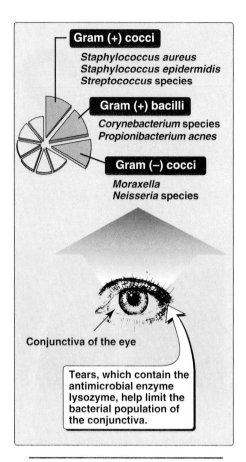

Figure 2.2
Some examples of bacteria that inhabit the conjunctival sac.

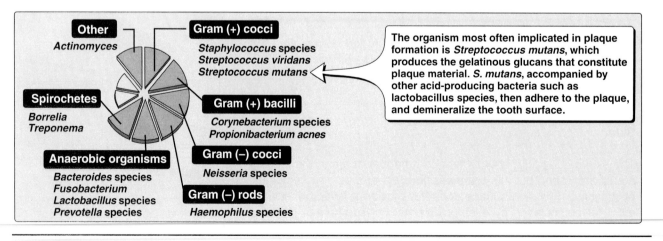

Figure 2.3
Some examples of bacteria that inhabit the mouth.

impaired. [Note: Pneumonia is frequently preceded by an upper or middle respiratory viral infection, which predisposes the individual to *S. pneumoniae* infection of the pulmonary parenchyma.]

D. Intestinal tract

In an adult, the density of microorganisms in the stomach is relatively low (10^3 to 10^5 per gram of contents) due to gastric enzymes and the acidic pH. The density of organisms increases along the alimentary canal, reaching 10^8 to 10^{10} bacteria per gram of contents in the ileum, and 10^{11} per gram of contents in the large intestine. Some twenty percent of the fecal mass consists of many different species of bacteria, over 99 percent of which are anaerobes (Figure 2.4). Bacterioides species constitute a significant percentage of bacteria in the large intestine. *Escherichia coli*, a facultatively anaerobic organism (see p. 26), constitutes less than 0.1 percent of the total population of bacteria in the intestinal tract. This endogenous *E. coli* is a major cause of urinary tract infections (see p. 178).

E. Urogenital tract

The low pH of the adult vagina is maintained by the presence of lactobacillus species, which are the primary components of the normal flora. If the lactobacillus population in the vagina is decreased, for example, by antibiotic therapy, the pH rises, and potential pathogens can overgrow. The most common example of such overgrowth is the yeast-like fungus, *Candida albicans* (see p. 274), which itself is a minor member of the normal flora of the vagina, mouth, and small intestine. The urine in the kidney and bladder is sterile, but can become contaminated in the lower urethra by the same organisms that inhabit the outer layer of the skin and the perineum (Figure 2.5).

III. BENEFICIAL FUNCTIONS OF NORMAL FLORA

The normal flora can provide some definite benefits to the host. First, the sheer number of harmless bacteria in the lower bowel and the mouth make it unlikely that in a healthy person, an invading pathogen could compete for nutrients and receptor sites. Second, some bacteria of the bowel produce antimicrobial substances to which the producers themselves are immune. Third, bacterial colonization of the newborn infant acts as a powerful stimulus for the development of the immune system (see p. 51). Fourth, bacteria of the gut provide some important nutrients, such as vitamin K, and also aid in the digestion and absorption of nutrients. [Note: Although humans can obtain vitamin K from food sources, if nutrition is impaired, bacteria can be an important supplemental source.]

IV. HARMFUL EFFECTS OF NORMAL FLORA

It is estimated that normal flora account for more clinical disease than that due to recognized pathogens. Clinical problems caused by the normal flora arise under the following conditions: 1) When the organisms are displaced from their normal site in the body to an abnormal site. An

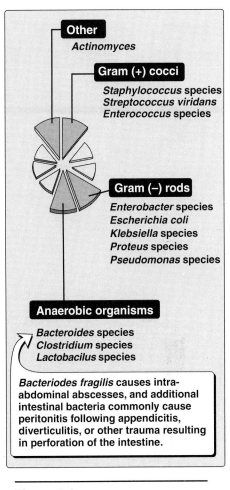

Other
Actinomyces

Gram (+) cocci
Staphylococcus species
Streptococcus viridans
Enterococcus species

Gram (−) rods
Enterobacter species
Escherichia coli
Klebsiella species
Proteus species
Pseudomonas species

Anaerobic organisms
Bacteroides species
Clostridium species
Lactobacilus species

Bacteriodes fragilis causes intra-abdominal abscesses, and additional intestinal bacteria commonly cause peritonitis following appendicitis, diverticulitis, or other trauma resulting in perforation of the intestine.

Figure 2.4
Some examples of bacteria that inhabit the gastrointestinal tract.

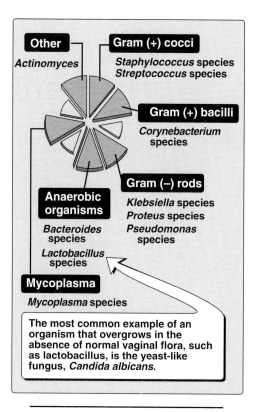

Gram (+) cocci
Staphylococcus species
Streptococcus species

Gram (+) bacilli
Corynebacterium species

Other
Actinomyces

Gram (–) rods
Klebsiella species
Proteus species
Pseudomonas species

Anaerobic organisms
Bacteroides species
Lactobacillus species

Mycoplasma
Mycoplasma species

The most common example of an organism that overgrows in the absence of normal vaginal flora, such as lactobacillus, is the yeast-like fungus, *Candida albicans.*

Figure 2.5
Some examples of bacteria that inhabit the vagina.

example already mentioned is the introduction of the normal skin bacterium, *Staphylococcus epidermidis*, into the bloodstream where it can colonize catheters and heart valves, resulting in bacterial endocarditis. 2) When potential pathogens gain a competitive advantage due to diminished populations of harmless competitor. For example, when normal bowel flora is depleted by antibiotic therapy leading to overgrowth by the resistant *Clostridium difficile*, which can cause a severe colitis (see p. 217). 3) When some harmless, commonly ingested food substances are converted into carcinogenic derivatives by bacteria in the colon. A well-known example is the conversion by bacterial sulfatases of the sweetener cyclamate into the bladder carcinogen cyclohexamine. 4) When individuals are immunocompromised, normal flora can overgrow and become pathogenic. [Note: **Colonization** by normal, but potentially harmful, flora should be distinguished from the **carrier state** in which a true pathogen is carried by a healthy (asymptomatic) individual and passed to other individuals where it results in disease. Typhoid fever is an example of a disease that can be acquired from a carrier (see p. 180).]

Study Questions

Choose the ONE correct answer

2.1 The primary effect of lactobacilli in the adult vagina is to

   A. maintain an alkaline environment.

   B. maintain an acidic environment.

   C. produce a protective mucus layer.

   D. increase fertility.

   E. keep the menstrual cycle regular.

Correct answer = B. Lactobacilli produce acid, which in turn inhibits the growth of potential pathogenic bacteria and fungi. Other possible effects are not known to be attributed to lactobacilli.

2.2 A patient presents with severe colitis associated with an overgrowth of *Clostridium difficile* in the lower bowel. The most likely cause of this condition was

   A. botulinum food poisoning.

   B. a stomach ulcer.

   C. compromised immune system.

   D. antibiotic therapy.

   E. mechanical blockage of the large intestine.

Correct answer = D. Antibiotic therapy can reduce the normal flora in the bowel thereby allowing pathogenic organisms normally present in low numbers to overgrow. None of the other answers explains the overgrowth of *C. difficile*.

2.3 The predominant bacterial species that colonizes the human skin is:

   A. *Lactobacillus.*

   B. *Candida albicans.*

   C. *Streptococcus pneumoniae.*

   D. *Staphylococcus epidermidis.*

   E. *Bacterioides fragilis.*

Correct answer = D. Human skin normally contains up to 10,000 *S. epidermidis* per cm^2. Other colonizing bacteria may be present, but in much lower numbers. *C. albicans* is a yeast-like fungus, not a bacterium.

Pathogenicity of Microorganisms

3

I. OVERVIEW

A pathogenic microorganism is defined as one that causes or is capable of causing disease. Some microorganisms are unequivocally pathogenic, whereas others (the vast majority) are generally harmless. Further, some pathogens cause disease only under certain conditions, examples of which include being introduced into a normally sterile body site, or infection of an immunocompromised host. This chapter considers the factors that influence whether or not a microorganism is a pathogen. Both bacterial and viral infections are discussed. Although the basic concepts of bacterial and viral pathogenesis are similar, a fundamental difference between bacterial and viral infections is that whereas most bacteria can reproduce both outside and (for some species) inside cells, viral reproduction is strictly and universally intracellular.

II. BACTERIAL PATHOGENESIS

The infectious process can, in general, be divided into several stages: 1) entry into the host with evasion of host primary defenses; 2) adhesion of the microorganism to host cells; 3) propagation of the organism; 4) damage to host cells by toxins or an inflammatory response; and 5) evasion of host secondary defenses. The pathogenicity of a microorganism depends on its success in completing some or all of these stages. The terms **virulence** and **pathogenicity** are often used interchangeably, although virulence has also come to denote the degree to which a given microbial isolate is pathogenic. For example, virulence can be quantified in terms of how many organisms are required to cause disease in fifty percent of those exposed to the pathogen (ID_{50}, where I = Infectious, and D = Dose), or to kill fifty percent of test animals (LD_{50}, where L = Lethal) (Figure 3.1). Such a definition is obviously subject to many conditions, for example, the site of inoculation, the immunocompetence of the host, and the kind of test animal.

A. Virulence factors

The factors that promote virulence have been studied extensively at both the cellular and, in some cases, the molecular level. Some of the more important classes of virulence factors are reviewed below.

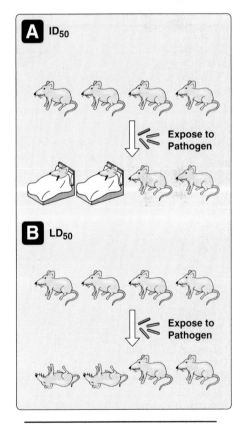

Figure 3.1
ID_{50} (I=infectious, D=dose) versus LD_{50} (L=lethal, D=dose).

Lippincott's Illustrated Reviews: Microbiology,
by William A. Strohl, Harriet Rouse, Bruce D. Fisher.
Lippincott, Williams & Wilkins, Baltimore, MD © 2001

A Fimbrial (Pilus) Adhesion

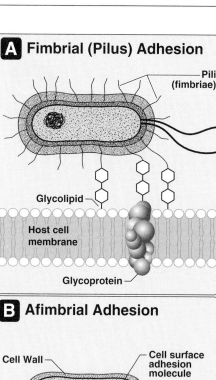

Pili (fimbriae)

Glycolipid

Host cell membrane

Glycoprotein

B Afimbrial Adhesion

Cell Wall

Cell surface adhesion molecule

C Hydrophobic Adhesion

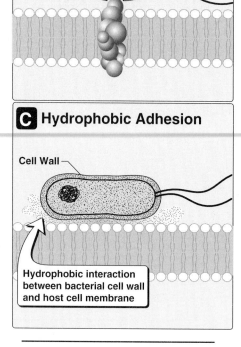

Cell Wall

Hydrophobic interaction between bacterial cell wall and host cell membrane

Figure 3.2
Bacterial adhesion to host cell membranes.

1. **Transmissibility:** The first step of the infectious process is the entry of the microorganism into the host by one of several ports: the respiratory tract, gastrointestinal tract, urogenital tract, or through skin that has been cut, punctured, or burned. Once entry is achieved, the pathogen must overcome a diversity of host defenses before it can establish itself. These include phagocytosis (see p. 56), the acidic environments of the stomach and urogenital tract, and various hydrolytic and proteolytic enzymes found in saliva, the stomach, and the small intestine. Bacteria that have an outer polysaccharide capsule [for example, *Streptococcus pneumoniae* (see p. 150), and *Neisseria meningitidis* (see p. 168)] have a better chance of surviving these host defenses.

2. **Adherence to host cells:** Some bacteria (for example, *Escherichia coli*, see p. 176) use their **pili** to adhere to the surface of host cells. Group A streptococci have similar structures (**fimbriae**, see p. 146). Other bacteria have cell surface adhesion molecules, or have particularly hydrophobic cell walls that allow them to adhere to the host cell membrane (Figure 3.2). In each case, adherence enhances virulence by preventing the bacteria from being carried away by mucus, or away from organs with significant fluid flow such as the urinary tract and the gastrointestinal tract. Adherence also allows each attached bacterial cell to form a microcolony. A striking example of the importance of adhesion is that of *Neisseria gonorrhoeae* in which strains that lack pili are not pathogenic (see p. 165).

3. **Invasiveness:** Invasive bacteria are those that can enter host cells or penetrate mucosal surfaces, thereby spreading from the initial site of infection. Invasiveness is facilitated by several bacterial enzymes, the most notable of which are **collagenase** and **hyaluronidase**. These enzymes degrade components of the extracellular matrix, thereby providing the bacteria with easier access to host cell surfaces. Entry into cells depends on specific bacterial surface proteins called **invasins**, which induce endocytosis by the host cells. Invasion is followed by inflammation, which can be either **pyogenic** (involving pus formation) or **granulomatous** (having nodular inflammatory lesions), depending on the organism. The pus of pyogenic inflammations contains mostly neutrophils, whereas granulomatous lesions contain fibroblasts, lymphocytes, and macrophages.

4. **Bacterial toxins:** Some bacteria cause disease by producing toxins, of which there are two general types: the exotoxins and the endotoxins. The **exotoxins**, which are proteins, are **secreted** by both gram-positive and gram-negative bacteria. In contrast, the **endotoxins**, which are lipopolysaccharides, are **not secreted**, but instead are integral components of the cell walls of gram-negative bacteria.

   a. **Exotoxins:** These include some of the most poisonous substances known. It is estimated that as little as one microgram of **tetanus exotoxin** can kill an adult human. The exotoxin proteins generally have two polypeptide components (Figure 3.3). One component is responsible for binding the protein to the host cell, whereas the second component is responsible for the toxic effect. In several cases, the precise target for the toxin has been identified. For example, **diphtheria toxin** is an enzyme that blocks protein synthesis. It does so by attaching an ADP-ribosyl group to the human protein elongation factor EF-2[1], thereby inactivating it (see p. 158). Most exotoxins are rapidly inactivated by moderate heating (60°C), notable exceptions being staphylococcal enterotoxin and *E. coli* heat-stable toxin (ST). In addition, treatment with dilute formaldehyde destroys the toxic activity of most exotoxins, but does not affect their antigenicity. Formaldehyde-inactivated toxins, called **toxoids**, are thus useful in preparing vaccines (see p. 37). Exotoxin proteins are in many cases encoded by genes carried on plasmids or temperate bacteriophage. An example is the diphtheria exotoxin that is encoded by the *Tox* gene of a temperate bacteriophage that can lysogenize *Corynebacterium diphtheriae*. Strains of *C. diphtheriae* that carry this phage are pathogenic, whereas those that lack the phage are non-pathogenic (see p. 158).

b. **Endotoxins:** These are heat-stable, **lipopolysaccharide** (LPS) components of the outer membranes of gram-negative—but not gram-positive—bacteria. They are released into the host's circulation following bacterial cell lysis. An LPS consists of polysaccharide O (somatic antigen) that protrudes from the exterior cell surface, a core polysaccharide, and a lipid component called lipid A that faces the cell interior. The lipid A moiety is responsible for the toxicity of this molecule. The main physiologic effects of LPS endotoxins are fever, shock, hypotension, and thrombosis, collectively referred to as **septic shock**. These effects are produced indirectly by activation of macrophages, with the release of cytokines, activation of complement, and activation of the coagulation cascade. Death can result from multiple organ failure. Elimination of the causative bacteria by antibiotics can initially exacerbate the symptoms by causing sudden massive release of the endotoxin into the circulation. Although gram-positive bacteria do not contain LPS, their cell wall peptidoglycan can elicit a shock syndrome similar to that caused by LPS, but usually not as severe. Because the peptidoglycan fragments of gram-positive bacteria are chemically so different from LPS, and are also less potent, they are generally not considered to be endotoxins.

B. Antigenic switching

A successful pathogen must somehow evade the host's immune system that recognizes bacterial surface antigens. One important evasive strategy for the pathogen is to change its surface antigens. This is accomplished by a number of mechanisms. One mechanism, called **phase variation**, is the genetically reversible ability of some bacteria to turn off and turn on the expression of genes coding for the surface antigens. A second mechanism, called **antigenic variation**, involves the modification of the gene for an expressed surface antigen by genetic recombination with one of many variable unexpressed DNA sequences. In this manner, the expressed surface antigen can assume many different antigenic structures (see Figure 14.3, p. 166).

[1]See p. 398 in *Lippincott's Illustrated Reviews: Biochemistry* (2nd ed.) for a discussion of elongation factors in protein synthesis.

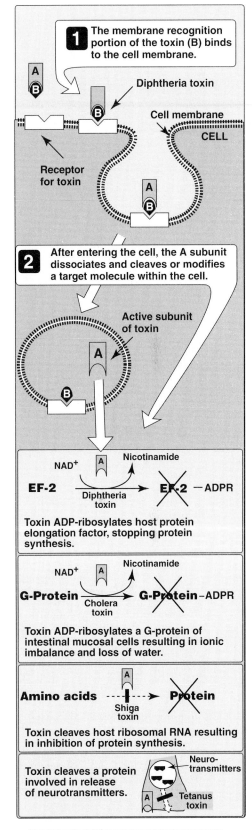

Figure 3.3
Action of exotoxins.

C. Which is the pathogen?

If a particular microorganism is isolated from an infected tissue, for example, from a necrotic skin lesion, one cannot conclude that the isolated organism caused the lesion. The organism could, for example, be a harmless member of the natural skin flora (see p. 7) that happened to be in the vicinity. Alternatively, the organism may not be a natural resident of the skin, but an opportunistic pathogen that secondarily infected the necrotic lesion. [Note: An **opportunistic pathogen** is an organism that is unable to cause disease in healthy, immunocompetent individuals, but can infect people whose specific or nonspecific defenses have been impaired.] A nineteenth century German microbiologist, Robert Koch, recognized this dilemma, and defined a series of criteria (called **Koch's postulates**) by which the identity of the causative microbial agent of a disease can be confirmed (Figure 3.4). [Note: Whereas this protocol has been successful in establishing the etiology of most infections, it fails if the causative organism cannot be cultured *in vitro*.]

D. Infections in human populations

Bacterial diseases may be **communicable** from person-to-person or **noncommunicable**. For example, cholera is highly communicable (the disease-causing organism, *Vibrio cholerae*, is easily spread), whereas botulism is noncommunicable because only those people who ingest the botulinum exotoxin are affected. Highly communicable diseases such as cholera are said to be **contagious**, and tend to occur as localized **epidemics** in which the disease frequency is higher than normal. When an epidemic becomes world-wide it is called a **pandemic**. Epidemics have many underlying causes. For example, sudden localized climatic changes can cause contamination of the water supply, increase the populations of disease-bearing insects, or make potential hosts more susceptible. Pandemics, such as the 1918 influenza pandemic, arise because the human population has never been exposed to, and thus has no immunity against, the specific strain of influenza virus.

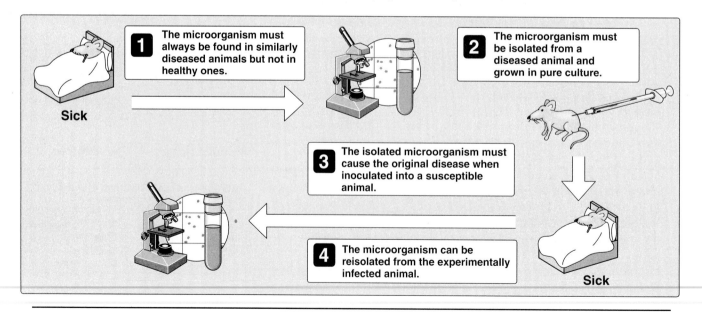

Figure 3.4
Koch's postulates.

III. VIRAL PATHOGENESIS

Viruses, by definition, can replicate only inside living cells. Consequently, the first pathogenic manifestations of viral infection are seen at the cellular level. The course of events following initial exposure to some viruses may include rapid onset of observable symptoms, which is referred to as an **acute infection**. Alternatively, the initial infection by other viruses may be mild or asymptomatic. Following the initial infection, the most common outcome is that the virus is cleared completely from the body by the immune system. However, the initial infection by certain viruses is followed by one of two alternative outcomes of medical significance: 1) establishment of a **persistent infection**, or 2) establishment of a **latent infection** (see p. 19).

A. Viral pathogenesis at the cellular level

Cells show a variety of different responses to viral infection depending on the cell type and the virus. Many viral infections cause no apparent morphologic or functional changes in the cell. When changes do occur, several (potentially overlapping) responses can be recognized (Figure 3.5).

1. **Cell death:** A cell can be directly killed by the virus. In most cases this is due to the inhibition of synthesis of cellular DNA, RNA, and protein. Some viruses have specific genes that are responsible for this inhibition. The dead or dying cells release a brood of progeny viruses that repeat the replication process. Examples of viruses that kill their host cells are adenovirus (see p. 312) and poliovirus (see p. 349).

2. **Transformation:** Some viruses can transform normal cells into malignant cells. In many ways, this is the opposite of cell death, because malignant cells have less fastidious growth requirements than do normal cells, and they have an indefinitely extended lifetime. Transformation is an irreversible genetic process caused by the integration of viral DNA into the host's DNA (see p. 305).

3. **Cell fusion:** Infection of cells with certain viruses causes the cells to fuse, producing giant, multinucleate cells—a specific kind of CPE. Viruses with this property include herpesviruses (see p. 319) and paramyxoviruses (see p. 382). The ability of infected cells to fuse is apparently due to virus-induced changes in the structure of the cell membrane.

4. **Cytopathic effect (CPE):** CPE is a catch-all term that refers to any visible change in appearance of an infected cell, for example, cell rounding, production of patches of stainable viral proteins inside the cell, and cell disintegration. Some viruses can be roughly identified by the time of onset and pattern of CPE in cell culture, as well as by the types of cells in which these viruses cause CPE.

B. Initial infections

Following initial multiplication at the primary site of entry, the viral infection may remain localized, or may become disseminated. The infection may be **asymptomatic (unapparent)**. Alternatively, typical symptoms of disease may occur, often in two temporally distinct

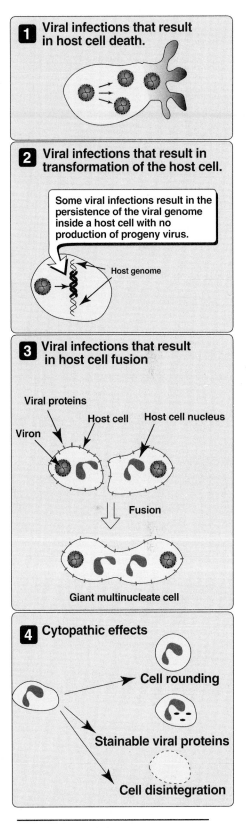

1 Viral infections that result in host cell death.

2 Viral infections that result in transformation of the host cell.

Some viral infections result in the persistence of the viral genome inside a host cell with no production of progeny virus.

Host genome

3 Viral infections that result in host cell fusion

Viral proteins
Host cell
Host cell nucleus
Viron

Fusion

Giant multinucleate cell

4 Cytopathic effects

Cell rounding

Stainable viral proteins

Cell disintegration

Figure 3.5
Types of viral pathogenesis at the cellular level.

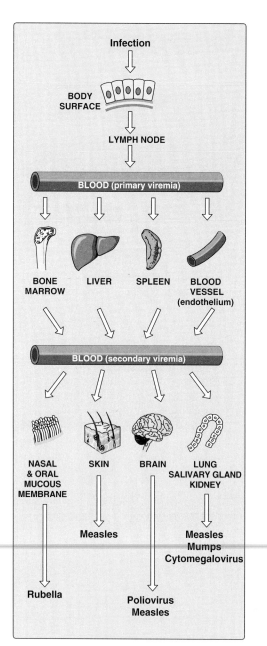

Figure 3.6
Examples of dissemination of virus to secondary sites in the body.

forms: 1) early symptoms at the primary site of infection, and 2) delayed symptoms due to dissemination from the primary site causing infection of secondary sites. The course of the acute infection (that is, the degree of dissemination, the severity of the disease, etc.) is not an absolute characteristic of a particular virus species. Instead, it is influenced primarily by the effectiveness and type of host defense mechanisms, and the virulence of the infecting virus.

1. **Routes of entry and dissemination to secondary sites:** Common routes by which viruses enter the body are essentially the same as for bacterial infections (that is, through the skin, the respiratory tract, the gastrointestinal tract, or the urogenital tract). In each case, some viruses remain localized and cause disease that is largely restricted to that primary site of infection. Other viruses undergo a round of multiplication in cells at the primary site, which may or may not be accompanied by symptoms, followed by invasion of the lymphatic system and the blood. [Note: The presence of virus in the blood is termed "**viremia**".] Virus is thereby disseminated throughout the body, and can infect cells at secondary sites characteristic for each specific virus type, thus causing the disease typically associated with that species (Figure 3.6).

   a. **Skin:** Introduction through the skin usually involves a break in the surface of the skin from an abrasion or cut, or by inoculation of the agent by an insect, animal bite, or a needle. The former is the typical route for virus infections that remain localized in the skin, for example, viruses that cause warts (see p. 307). Inoculation, on the other hand, usually leads to disseminated infections.

   b. **Respiratory tract:** Those viruses that enter the body via the respiratory tract and remain localized produce symptoms that are primarily in the respiratory passages (for example, rhinoviruses causing the common cold, see p. 352). Other inhaled viruses spread systemically after the primary infection, and produce a characteristic disease due to infection of cells at secondary sites, for example, measles (see p. 382) and chicken pox (see p. 324).

   c. **Gastrointestinal tract:** Viruses infecting via the GI tract follow a characteristic "**fecal-oral**" transmission pattern (that is, virus enters through the mouth via material contaminated with feces). Those viruses that remain localized in the cells of the GI tract may cause symptoms such as diarrheal disease, for example, enteric adenoviruses (see p. 313) or rotaviruses (see p. 393). However, many viral infections that remain localized in the GI tract are asymptomatic (that is, virus can be recovered from stool samples of individuals with no sign of disease). Some viruses that infect via the GI tract enter the lymphatic system and the blood, from which they spread to specific organ systems. There they can cause symptomatic disease unrelated to the GI tract, for example, in the liver (hepatitis A, see p. 352) or the central nervous system (poliovirus, see 349).

   d. **Genital tract:** Viruses infecting by this route are transmitted primarily during sexual contact. Such viruses (for example, herpes simplex virus, see p. 319) can cause local vesiculo-ulcerative lesions. Spread of the virus can affect nongenital tissues, such as the CNS, where herpesvirus may cause meningitis or encephalitis. [Note: Women who have a genital viral infection can pass the virus to a baby during its passage down the birth canal.]

2. **Typical secondary sites of localization:** The secondary sites of infection determine the nature of the delayed symptoms, and usually the major characteristics associated with the resulting disease. Viruses frequently exhibit tropism for specific cell types and tissues. This specificity is usually caused by the presence of specific host cell surface receptors recognized by particular viruses. Whereas any tissue or organ system is a potential target for virus infection, a few are of more general importance with respect to virus diseases.

   a. **Skin:** Viremia can result in a rash due to infection of cells in the epithelium. This type of rash contains infectious virus, and must be distinguished from those virus-associated rashes that have an immunologic basis and do not contain virus.

   b. **Central nervous system:** The most common route by which viruses infect the CNS is one whereby virus—carried by the blood—infects endothelial cells of the cerebral vessels, and ultimately is released into the brain itself. Alternatively, virus can be released from endothelial cells into the cerebrospinal fluid at the choroid plexus. A less common, but important route of viral spread is axonal migration of virus from peripheral nerve endings directly into the CNS. (For example, the latter route is employed by rabies virus, see 379.)

   c. **Fetus:** The fetus represents a special, but very important, site for secondary localization of virus infections. Virus from the maternal circulation infects cells of the placenta, thereby gaining access to the fetal circulation, and ultimately to all of the tissues of the developing fetus (Figure 3.7). Fetal death or developmental abnormalities are often the result, as cells participating in the growth and differentiation of organ systems are damaged or killed by the infection. Neonatal infection can also occur during birth when the fetus comes in contact with infected genital secretions of the mother.

3. **Virus shedding and mode of transmission:** The mode of transmission of a viral disease is largely determined by the tissues that produce progeny virus, and/or the fluids into which they are released. These are not necessarily the secondary sites of infection, but in fact are in many cases the site of primary infection at a time before symptoms are apparent.

   a. **Skin:** In only a few instances are skin lesions the major source of transmissible virus, warts (papilloma viruses, see p. 307) being the prime example. A number of diseases are characterized by virus-containing skin lesions, but are transmitted by virus shed from another site, for example, chicken pox, which is transmitted mainly by the respiratory route.

   b. **Respiratory tract:** Whereas the respiratory route is the obvious mode of transmission for viruses causing localized respiratory disease, it is also the major source for many viruses that cause

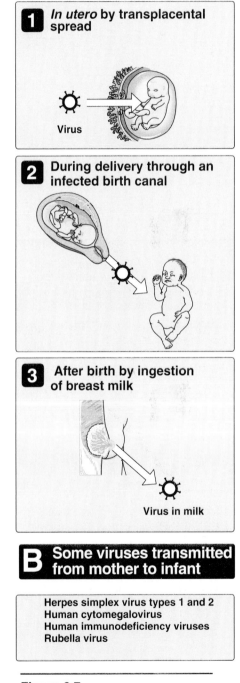

A Modes of virus transmission

Infected mothers can transmit viral infections to their offspring by three routes:

1 *In utero* by transplacental spread

Virus

2 During delivery through an infected birth canal

3 After birth by ingestion of breast milk

Virus in milk

B Some viruses transmitted from mother to infant

Herpes simplex virus types 1 and 2
Human cytomegalovirus
Human immunodeficiency viruses
Rubella virus

Figure 3.7
Mother-to-infant (vertical) transmission of viral infections.

systemic disease. In the latter case, it is the initial infection and shedding of virus from the respiratory tract that provides virus both for viremic spread to other organs and for transmission to other hosts. The fact that transmissible virus is present before symptoms of the generalized disease are apparent has important consequences in terms of attempts to control the spread of such diseases. For example, varicella (chicken pox, see p. 324) is transmissible one to two days before the characteristic rash appears.

c. **Gastrointestinal tract:** All those viruses whose portal of entry and primary site of replication are via the GI tract are shed from the infected host in the feces.

d. **Body fluids:** Some viruses are shed from the host in one or more body fluids, for example, urine, semen, milk, and obviously blood, although for many such viruses this does not constitute the major route of transmission. Milk has special epidemiologic significance in that it provides the means for efficient transmission of virus from an infected mother to her baby, thus maintaining a high level of chronic infection in a population (for example, with HIV, see p. 364).

4. **Factors involved in termination of the acute infection:** In a typical, uncomplicated, acute infection, virus is totally eliminated from the host in two to three weeks. This outcome is primarily a function of the host's immune system, with involvement of both cell-mediated and humoral responses. The relative importance of these two responses depends upon the virus and the nature of the disease.

a. **Cell-mediated responses:** The earliest immune system responses to virus infection are a generalized inflammatory response, accompanied by nonspecific killing of infected cells by **natural killer cells**. This latter activity is enhanced by interferon and other cytokines (see p. 55), and begins well before

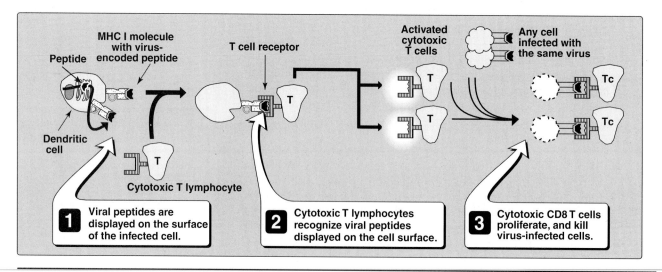

Figure 3.8
Activation and actions of cytotoxic T lymphocytes.

the virus-specific immune response. Later, cytolysis by virus-specific **cytotoxic T lymphocytes** that recognize virus peptides displayed on the cell surface, also eliminates infected cells (Figure 3.8, and see Figure 7.17, p. 74). These cellular responses are especially significant in that they help to limit the spread of the infection by killing infected cells before they have released progeny virus. [Note: The cell surface immunodeterminants recognized by the T cells are often derived from non-structural or internal proteins of the virus. Thus this response complements the inactivation of free virus by humoral antibody, which is directed against capsid or envelope proteins. In addition, the T cell response tends to be more group-specific, rather than strain- or species-specific, because the internal and non-structural proteins are more highly conserved among related viruses than are the capsid proteins.]

b. **Humoral response:** Whereas circulating antibodies may be directed against any of the virus proteins, those that are of greatest significance in controlling the infection react specifically with epitopes on the surface of the virion, and result in inactivation of the virus's infectivity (Figure 3.9). The process is called **neutralization**. This response is of primary importance in suppressing diseases that involve a viremic stage, but secretory antibodies (IgA) also play an important protective role in primary infections of the respiratory and GI tracts. Humoral antibodies also take part in killing infected cells by two mechanisms: 1) **antibody-dependent**, **cell-mediated cytotoxicity**, in which natural killer cells and other leukocytes bearing Fc receptors bind to the Fc portions of antibodies that are complexed to virus antigens on the surface of the infected cell and kill it; and 2) **complement-mediated lysis** of infected cells to which virus-specific antibody has bound.

C. Persistent infections

A **persistent** (**chronic**) infection is one in which virus is present continuously—usually at a low level—over an extended period of time after the acute infection and disease have ended (Figure 3.10). There may be no overt disease related to cell or tissue damage by virus replication itself, but there frequently is late development of an immunologically based disease due to, for example, immune complex deposition, or autoimmune cell-mediated cytotoxicity. Persistent infections have great epidemiologic significance because shedding of virus by asymptomatically infected individuals serves as a continual source of virus in the population. Hepatitis B virus is an important example of a human virus that can lead to persistent infections (see p. 342).

D. Latent infections

A latent infection is usually distinguished from a persistent infection by the fact that virus is not demonstrable continuously, but instead episodes of active virus replication and cell killing alternate with periods when no infectious virus or evidence of virus replication is present. Disease is usually manifest only during the recurrent episodes of virus replication. The human herpesviruses (see p. 322) are all capable of establishing latent infections.

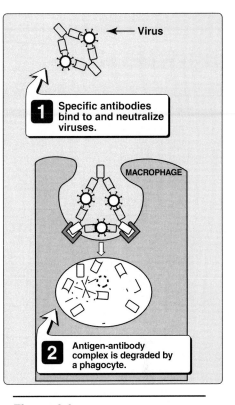

Figure 3.9
Neutralization of viruses. [Note: Antibodies may also prevent attachment of virus to the host cell.]

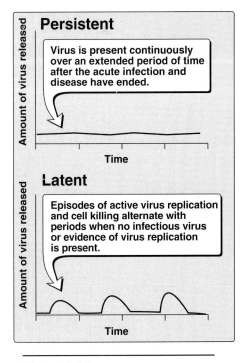

Figure 3.10
Persistent (chronic) and latent viral infections.

Study Questions

Choose the ONE correct answer.

3.1 Endotoxins belong to a class of biological molecules called

    A. mucopolysaccharides.

    B. lipopolysaccharides.

    C. nucleic acids.

    D. proteins.

    E. peptidoglycans.

> Correct answer = B. The endotoxins are integral lipopolysaccharide constituents of the outer membrane of gram-negative bacteria. The peptidoglycans, present in large amounts in gram-positive bacteria, can be toxic but are not considered to be endotoxins.

3.2 Exotoxins belong to a class of biological molecules called

    A. mucopolysaccharides.

    B. lipopolysaccharides.

    C. nucleic acids.

    D. proteins.

    E. peptidoglycans.

> Correct answer = D. The exotoxins are secreted toxic proteins that in many cases have a well-defined cellular site of action.

3.3 The mechanism of action of diphtheria toxin is to

    A. disrupt the cell membrane.

    B. block nucleic acid synthesis.

    C. block protein synthesis.

    D. interfere with neurotransmission.

    E. destroy the cell nucleus.

> Correct answer = C. Diphtheria toxin inactivates the polypeptide elongation factor EF-2 thereby blocking protein synthesis. Tetanus toxin interferes with neurotransmission.

3.4 An important defense function of cytotoxic T lymphocytes in viral infections is to

    A. lyse virus infected cells.

    B. fragment viral nucleic acids by nucleases.

    C. neutralize free virus particles.

    D. block cell respiration.

    E. lyse viral capsids.

> Correct answer = A. Cytotoxic T lymphocytes recognize viral peptides on the infected cell surface and lyse these cells. Often the recognized proteins are nonstructural or internal proteins of the virus, which tend to be more conserved than capsid structural proteins. This defense mechanism is thus directed against a broader range of virus variants than that of humoral antibodies, which are more often directed against species and strain-specific capsid proteins.

3.5 A 48-year-old woman presented at the emergency room complaining of urinary urgency and flank pain. Microscopic examination of a urine sample revealed gram-negative rods. Prior to initiation of antibiotic therapy, she abruptly developed fever, chills, and delirium. Hypotension and hyperventilation rapidly followed. These observations suggest that the patient is responding to the release of bacterial

    A. collagenase.

    B. exotoxin.

    C. hyaluronidase.

    D. lipopolysaccharide (LPS).

    E. peptidoglycan.

> Correct answer = D. The patient is most likely suffering from septic shock. In two thirds of patients, septic shock results from infection with gram-negative bacteria, such as *Escherichia coli*, *Klebsiella*, *Enterobacter*, *Proteus, Pseudomonas*, or *Bacteroides*. Septicemia is more common in persons whose resistance is already compromised by an existing condition. The gram-negative bacteria release endotoxins——heat-stable, lipopolysaccharide (LPD) components of the outer membranes. The main physiologic effects of LPS endotoxins are fever, hypotension, and thrombosis, collectively referred to as septic shock. These effects are produced by activation of macrophages with the release of cytokines, activation of complement, and activation of the coagulation cascade. Death can result from multiple organ failure. Gram-positive bacteria release exotoxins that can elicit a shock syndrome, but response is usually not as severe as that of gram-negative septic shock.

Diagnostic Microbiology

4

I. OVERVIEW

Identification of the organism causing an infectious process is frequently essential for effective antimicrobial and supportive therapy. Initial treatment may be empiric, based upon the microbiologic epidemiology of the infection and the patient's symptoms. However, definitive microbiologic diagnosis of an infectious disease usually involves one or more of the following five basic laboratory techniques, which guide the physician along a narrowing path of possible causative organisms: 1) direct microscopic visualization of the organism; 2) cultivation and identification of the organism; 3) detection of microbial antigens; 4) detection of microbial DNA or RNA; and 5) detection of an inflammatory or host immune response to the microorganism (Figure 4.1). All laboratory studies must first be directed by the patient's clinical information (that is, their history and physical examination), and then evaluated, taking into consideration the sensitivity and specificity of the test.

II. SENSITIVITY AND SPECIFICITY OF TEST RESULTS

The interpretation of laboratory tests is influenced by the reliability of the results. Ideally, a diagnostic test is positive in the presence of a pathogen (true-positive), and is negative in the absence of the pathogen (true-negative). However, in practice, no laboratory test is perfect. An assay may give negative results in the presence of the pathogen (false-negative) or positive results in the absence of pathogen (false-positive). Thus, it is useful to define the reliability of a diagnostic procedure in terms of its **sensitivity** and **specificity**. The sensitivity of a test is the probability that it will be positive in the presence of a pathogen:

$$\text{Sensitivity} = \frac{\text{True-positives}}{\text{True-positives} + \text{False-negatives}} \times 100 \text{ percent}$$

As the number of false-negatives approaches zero, the sensitivity approaches 100 percent (that is, all infected patients are detected). Specificity is the probability that a test will be negative if the pathogen is not present:

$$\text{Specificity} = \frac{\text{True-negatives}}{\text{True-negatives} + \text{False-positives}} \times 100 \text{ percent}$$

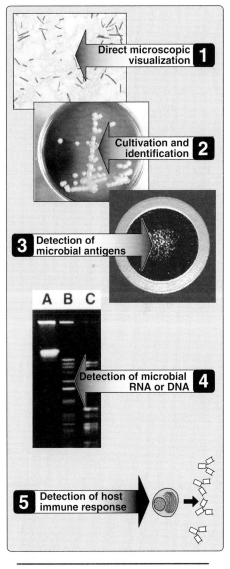

Figure 4.1
Some laboratory techniques that are useful in diagnosis of microbial diseases.

Lippincott's Illustrated Reviews: Microbiology, by William A. Strohl, Harriet Rouse, Bruce D. Fisher. Lippincott, Williams & Wilkins, Baltimore, MD © 2001

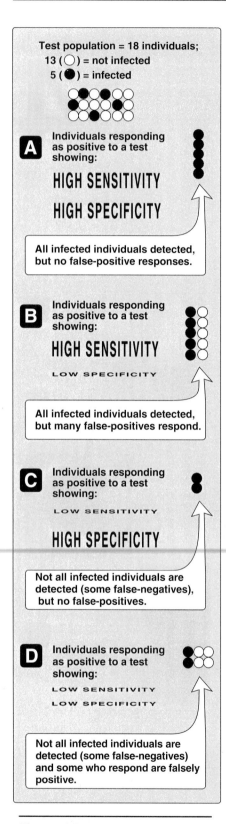

Figure 4.2
Effect of sensitivity and specificity of a test on the presence of false-positives and false-negatives.

As the number of false-positives approaches zero, the specificity approaches 100 percent (that is, all positive patients are actually infected). Figure 4.2 shows the results obtained with tests of high and low sensitivity/specificity. Clearly tests with both high sensitivity and specificity are desirable. However, a test with a high sensitivity but low specificity may be useful in screening programs. Such tests show few false-negatives and therefore can "rule out" the presence of a particular disease. Individuals that test positive may be among the many false-positives that are reported by tests with low specificity. Therefore disease in these individuals must be subsequently confirmed using a test of high specificity where false positives are infrequent.

III. PATIENT HISTORY AND PHYSICAL EXAMINATION

The **clinical history** is the single most important part of the evaluation of patients. For example, a history of cough points to the possibility of respiratory tract infection; dysuria suggests urinary tract infection. A history of travel to underdeveloped countries may implicate exotic organisms. For example, a patient who recently swam in the Nile has an increased risk of schistosomiasis. Patient occupations may suggest exposure to certain pathogens, such as brucellosis in a butcher, or anthrax in wool sorters. Even the age of the patient can sometimes guide the clinician in predicting the identity of pathogens. For example, a gram-positive coccus in the spinal fluid of a newborn infant is unlikely to be *Streptococcus pneumoniae* (pneumococcus), but most likely to be *Streptococcus agalactiae* (Group B). This organism is sensitive to penicillin G. By contrast, a gram-positive coccus in the spinal fluid of a forty-year-old is most likely to be *Streptococcus pneumoniae*. This organism is frequently resistant to penicillin G, and often requires treatment with a third generation cephalosporin (such as cefotaxime or ceftriaxone), or vancomycin. The etiology implied by the patient's age may thus guide initial therapy. A **physical examination** often provides confirmatory clues to the presence and extent (localized or disseminated) of disease. For example, erythema migrans (a large skin lesion with a bright red outer border and partial clear central area, see p. 439) indicates early localized Lyme disease. Clues to the presence of bacteremia (a disseminated infection) may include chills, fever (or sometimes hypothermia), or cardiovascular instability heralding septic shock. Physical signs of pulmonary consolidation suggest pneumonia. Nonmicrobiologic laboratory studies, such as the white blood cell count (WBC), may also help determine the general cause of illness. For example, a very high WBC may imply bacterial infection, whereas a very low WBC may be seen with overwhelming bacterial infection or with certain viral illnesses.

IV. DIRECT VISUALIZATION OF THE ORGANISM

In nonviral infectious diseases, pathogenic organisms can often be directly visualized by microscopic examination of patient specimens, such as sputum, urine, or cerebrospinal fluid. The organism's microscopic morphology and staining characteristics can provide the first screening step in arriving at a specific identification. The organisms to be examined need not be alive nor able to multiply. Microscopy gives rapid and inexpensive results, and may allow the clinician to initiate treatment without waiting for the results of a culture, as noted in the spinal fluid example in the previous paragraph.

A. Gram stain

Because unstained bacteria are difficult to detect with the light microscope, most patient material is stained prior to microscopic evaluation. The most common and useful staining procedure—the Gram stain—separates bacteria into two classifications according to the composition of their cell walls. If a clinical specimen on a microscope slide is treated with a solution of crystal violet and then iodine, the bacterial cells will stain purple. If the stained cells are then treated with a solvent such as alcohol or acetone, gram-positive organisms retain the stain, whereas gram-negative species lose the stain, becoming colorless (Figure 4.3). Addition of the counterstain safranin stains the clear, gram-negative bacteria pink or red. Most, but not all, bacteria are stainable, and fall into one of these two groups. [Note: Microorganisms that lack cell walls, such as the mycoplasma, cannot be identified using the Gram stain.]

1. **Applications of the Gram stain:** The Gram stain is important therapeutically because gram-positive and gram-negative bacteria have differing susceptibilities to a variety of antibiotics, and the Gram stain may therefore be used to guide initial therapy until definitive identification of the microorganism can be obtained. In addition, the morphology of the stained bacteria can sometimes be diagnostic. For example, gram-negative intracellular diplococci in urethral pus provides a presumptive diagnosis of gonorrhea. Gram stains of specimens submitted for culture are often invaluable aids in the interpretation of culture results. For example, a specimen may show organisms under the microscope, but appear sterile in culture media. This discrepancy may suggest 1) fastidious organisms (bacteria with complex nutrient requirements) that are unable to grow on the culture media employed; or 2) labile organisms, such as gonococcus or anaerobic organisms, that may not survive transport. In these cases, direct visualization with the Gram stain may provide the only clue to the nature, variety, and relative proportions of infecting organisms.

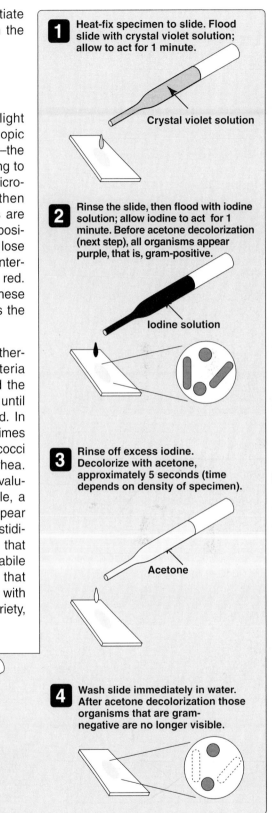

1 Heat-fix specimen to slide. Flood slide with crystal violet solution; allow to act for 1 minute.

Crystal violet solution

2 Rinse the slide, then flood with iodine solution; allow iodine to act for 1 minute. Before acetone decolorization (next step), all organisms appear purple, that is, gram-positive.

Iodine solution

3 Rinse off excess iodine. Decolorize with acetone, approximately 5 seconds (time depends on density of specimen).

Acetone

6 Wash in water, blot and dry in air. Gram-negative organisms are visualized after the application of the counterstain.

5 Apply safranin counterstain for 30 seconds.

Safranin

4 Wash slide immediately in water. After acetone decolorization those organisms that are gram-negative are no longer visible.

Figure 4.3
Steps in Gram stain method.
Key: ● = Gram-positive violet color. ⬭ = Gram-negative red color. ⬭ = Colorless.

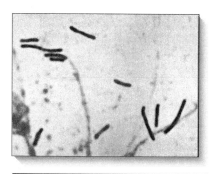

Figure 4.4
Mycobacterium tuberculosis stained with acid-fast stain.

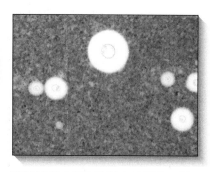

Figure 4.5
India ink preparation of *Cryptococcus neoformans* in cerebrospinal fluid. These yeast cells are identified by their large transparent capsules that exclude the India ink particles.

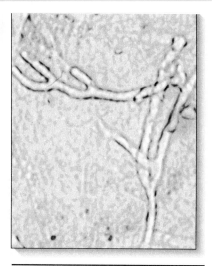

Figure 4.6
Fungi in unstained nasal sinus exudate, made distinct from other materials (such as cells) with potassium hydroxide.

2. **Limitations of the Gram stain:** The number of microorganisms required is relatively high—visualization with the Gram stain requires greater than 10^4 organisms per milliliter. Liquid samples with low numbers of microorganisms, for example in cerebrospinal fluid, require centrifugation to concentrate the pathogens. The pellet is then examined after staining.

B. **Acid-fast stain**

Stains such as Ziehl-Neelsen (the classic acid-fast stain) are used to identify organisms that have waxy material (mycolic acids) in their cell walls (Figure 4.4, and p. 448). Most bacteria that have been stained with carbolfuchsin can be decolorized by washing with acidic alcohol. However, certain bacteria, called acid-fast, retain the carbolfuchsin stain after being washed with an acidic solution. The most clinically important acid-fast bacteria is *Mycobacterium tuberculosis*, which appears pink, often beaded, and slightly curved. Acid-fast staining is reserved for clinical samples from patients suspected of having mycobacterial infection.

C. **India ink preparation**

This is one of the simplest microscopic methods. It is useful, for example, in detecting *Cryptococcus neoformans* in cerebrospinal fluid (Figure 4.5). A drop of centrifuged cerebrospinal fluid is mixed with a drop of India ink on a microscope slide beneath a glass cover slip. Cryptococci are identified by their large transparent capsules that displace the India ink particles.

D. **Potassium hydroxide (KOH) preparation**

Treatment with KOH dissolves host cells and bacteria, sparing fungi (Figure 4.6). A drop of sputum or skin scraping is treated with ten percent KOH, and the specimen is examined for fungal forms.

V. GROWING BACTERIA IN CULTURE

Although the Gram stain, or other direct microscopic observations, may be useful in guiding initial empiric therapy, definitive microbiologic diagnosis of an infectious disease usually involves identifying the organism in culture on artificial media. Culturing is routine for most bacterial and fungal infections, but is rarely used to identify helminths or protozoa. Culturing of many pathogens is straightforward, for example, streaking a throat swab onto a blood agar plate in search of group A β-hemolytic streptococcus. However, certain pathogens are very slow growing (for example *Mycobacterium tuberculosis*), or are cultured only with difficulty (for example, *Bartonella henselae*). Microorganisms isolated in culture are identified using such characteristics as colony size, shape, color, hemolytic reactions on solid media, as well as odor, and metabolic properties. In addition, pure cultures provide samples for antimicrobial susceptibility testing (see p. 33). The success of culturing depends on appropriate collection and transport techniques (see p. 25), and on selection of appropriate culture media, because some organisms may require special nutrients. Thus, when submitting samples for culture, the physician must alert the laboratory to likely pathogens whenever possible, especially when unusual organisms are suspected.

A. Collection of specimens

Many organisms are fragile, and must be transported to the laboratory with minimal delay. For example, gonococci and pneumococci are very sensitive to heating or drying. Samples must be cultured promptly, or if this is not possible, transport media must be used to extend the viability of the organism to be cultured. When anaerobic organisms are suspected, the patient's specimen must be protected from the toxic effect of oxygen. Liquid samples can be drawn into a syringe (expelling any air) and the syringe capped (carefully) before transport to the laboratory (Figure 4.7). Alternatively, clinical samples can be placed in a capped serum vial containing an oxygen-free atmosphere and a minimal volume of an anaerobic transport medium that supports the survival of suspected pathogens.

B. Media

Two general strategies are used to isolate pathogenic bacteria, depending on the nature of the clinical sample. The first method uses **enriched media** to promote the nonselective growth of any bacteria that may be present. The second approach employs **selective media** that only allow growth of specific bacterial species from specimens that normally contain large numbers of bacteria, for example stool, genital tract secretions, or sputum. [Note: Isolation of a bacterium is usually done only on **solid medium**. **Liquid medium** is used to grow larger quantities of a culture of bacteria that has already been isolated (that is, it is a **pure culture**).]

1. **Enriched media:** Media fortified with blood, yeast extracts, or brain or heart infusions are useful in growing fastidious organisms. For example, **sheep blood agar** contains protein sources, sodium chloride, and five percent sheep blood, and supports the growth of most gram-positive and gram-negative bacteria isolated from human sources (see p. 453). However, *Haemophilus influenzae* and *Neisseria gonorrhoeae*, among others, are highly fastidious organisms. They require **chocolate agar**, which contains red blood cells that have been lysed (see p. 445). This releases intracellular nutrients, such as hemoglobin, hemin ("X" factor), and NAD^+ ("V" factor), required by these organisms. Enriched media are useful for culturing normally sterile body fluids such as blood or cerebrospinal fluid, where the finding of any organisms provides reasonable evidence for infection due to that organism. On the other hand, the failure to culture an organism may indicate that the culture medium is inadequate, or the incubation conditions do not support bacterial growth. For example, anaerobic bacteria do not grow under the aerobic culture conditions most commonly utilized in routine culture methods.

2. **Selective media:** The most commonly used selective medium is **MacConkey agar** (see p. 444), which supports the growth of most gram-negative rods, especially the Enterobacteriaceae, but inhibits growth of gram-positive organisms and some fastidious gram-negative bacteria, such as haemophilus and neisseria species. Growth on blood agar and chocolate agar, but not MacConkey agar suggests a gram-positive isolate or a fastidious gram-negative species. In contrast, most gram-negative rods

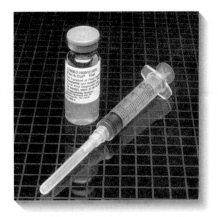

Figure 4.7
Anaerobic transport media containing a nonnutritive medium that retards diffusion of oxygen after addition of the specimen. Microorganisms may remain viable for up to 72 hours.

often form distinctive colonies on MacConkey agar. This agar is also used to detect organisms able to metabolize lactose (Figure 4.8). Clinical samples are routinely plated on blood agar, chocolate agar, and MacConkey agar. **Hektoen enteric agar** is also a selective medium that differentiates lactose/sucrose fermenters and nonfermenters, as well as H_2S producers and nonproducers. It is often used to culture *Salmonella* and *Shigella* species. **Thayer-Martin** agar is another selective medium composed of chocolate agar supplemented with several antibiotics that suppress the growth of nonpathogenic neisseria and other normal and abnormal flora. This medium is normally used to isolate gonococci (see p. 449).

C. Growth conditions

An optimal culture environment usually requires control of the oxygen and carbon dioxide concentrations. Most clinically relevant bacteria, for example, *Escherichia coli*, and the *Salmonella* and *Shigella* species, are **facultatively anaerobic** (that is, they are able to grow in the presence or absence of oxygen). However, some bacteria, such as *Pseudomonas*, *Neisseria*, *Brucella*, *Bordetella*, and *Francisella* species are strictly **aerobic** and cannot grow in the absence of oxygen. In contrast, **anaerobic bacteria**, such as *Bacteroides* and *Prevotella*, grow poorly in the presence of oxygen, whereas **strict anaerobes** are inhibited or killed by the presence of oxygen. In addition to oxygen, some bacteria require five percent to ten percent CO_2 for optimal growth. Automated systems are available that detect bacterial growth by sensing carbon dioxide released as a by-product of bacterial metabolism. Use of these sensitive techniques permits detection of bacterial multiplication before visible growth of the organisms is observed.

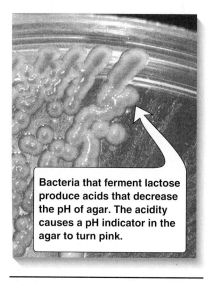

Bacteria that ferment lactose produce acids that decrease the pH of agar. The acidity causes a pH indicator in the agar to turn pink.

Figure 4.8
Lactose-fermenting, gram-negative rods produce pink colonies on MacConkey agar.

VI. IDENTIFICATION OF BACTERIA

The most widely used identification scheme involves determining the morphologic and metabolic properties of the unknown bacterium, and comparing these with properties of known microorganisms. Alternate identification schemes using nucleic acid–based methods are discussed on p. 31. Immunologic methods used in diagnosis are described on p. 28. [Note: It is important to start such investigations using pure bacterial isolates grown from a single colony.]

A. Single-enzyme tests

Different bacteria produce varying spectra of enzymes, for example, some of these enzymes are necessary for the bacterium's individual metabolism, and some facilitate the bacterium's ability to compete with other bacteria or establish an infection. Tests that measure single bacterial enzymes are simple, rapid, and generally easy to interpret. They can be performed on organisms already grown in culture, and often provide presumptive identification.

1. **Catalase test:** The enzyme catalase catalyzes the degradation of hydrogen peroxide to water and molecular oxygen ($H_2O_2 \rightarrow H_2O + O_2$). Catalase-positive organisms rapidly produce bubbles when

they are exposed to a solution containing hydrogen peroxide (Figure 4.9). The catalase test is key in differentiating between many gram-positive organisms. For example, staphylococci are catalase-positive, whereas streptococci and enterococci are catalase-negative.

2. **Oxidase test:** The enzyme cytochrome oxidase is part of electron transport and nitrate metabolism in some bacteria. The enzyme can accept electrons from artificial substrates, such as a phenylenediamine derivative, producing a dark, oxidized product (see Figure 4.9). This test assists in differentiating between groups of gram-negative bacteria.

3. **Urease:** The enzyme urease hydrolyzes urea to ammonia and carbon dioxide ($NH_2CONH_2 + H_2O \rightarrow 2NH_3 + CO_2$). The ammonia produced can be detected with pH indicators that change color in response to the increased alkalinity (see Figure 4.9). The test helps to identify certain species of enterobacteriaceae, *Corynebacterium urealyticum* and *Helicobacter pylori*.

4. **Pyrroglutamylaminopeptidase (PYR) test:** The enzyme pyrroglutamylaminopeptidase catalyzes a reaction that produces a bright red product in the presence of suitable reagents (see Figure 4.9). The PYR test can identify *S. pyogenes* and species of enterococci that are positive for the enzyme.

5. **Coagulase test:** Coagulase is an enzyme that causes a clot to form when bacteria are incubated with plasma. The test is used to differentiate *Staphylococcus aureus* (coagulase-positive) from coagulase-negative staphylococci.

B. Tests based on the presence of metabolic pathways

These tests measure the presence of a metabolic pathway in a bacterial isolate, rather than a single enzyme. Commonly used assays include those for oxidation and fermentation of different carbohydrates, the ability to degrade amino acids, and utilization of specific substrates. A widely used manual system for rapid identification of members of the family *Enterobacteriaceae* and other gram-negative bacteria makes use of twenty microtubes containing substrates for various biochemical pathways. The test substrates in the microtubes are inoculated with the bacterial isolate to be identified, and after five hours' incubation, the metabolic profile of the organism is constructed from color changes in the microtubes. These color changes indicate the presence or absence of the bacteria's ability to metabolize a particular substrate (Figure 4.10). The results are compared with a data bank containing test results from known bacteria. The probability of a match between the test organism and known pathogens is then calculated.

C. Automated systems

Microbiology laboratories are increasingly using automated methods to identify bacterial pathogens. For example, in the Vitek System, small plastic reagent cards containing microliter quantities of various biochemical test media in thirty wells provide a biochemical profile

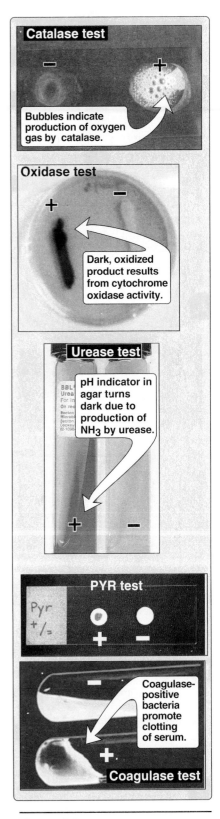

Catalase test

Bubbles indicate production of oxygen gas by catalase.

Oxidase test

Dark, oxidized product results from cytochrome oxidase activity.

Urease test

pH indicator in agar turns dark due to production of NH_3 by urease.

PYR test

Coagulase test

Coagulase-positive bacteria promote clotting of serum.

Figure 4.9
Some tests commonly used in identifying bacteria.

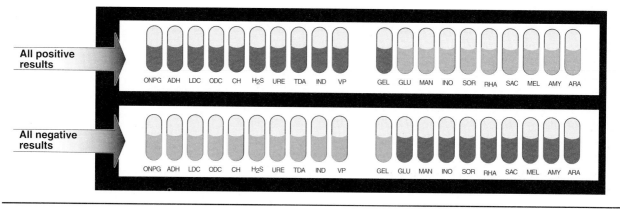

Figure 4.10
Rapid manual biochemical system for bacterial identification. Different appearances of the upper and lower pairs of wells indicate the positive or negative ability of a bacterium to utilize each substrate.

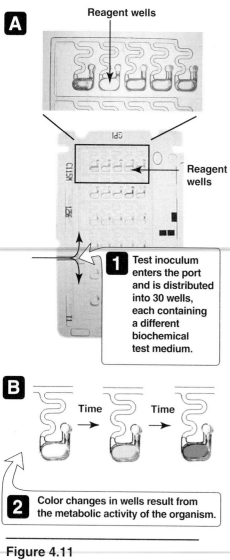

Figure 4.11
A. Vitek test card containing test wells.
B. Color of well changes with time.

that allows for organism identification (Figure 4.11). An inoculum derived from cultured samples is automatically transferred into the card, and a photometer intermittently measures color changes in the card that result from the metabolic activity of the organism. The data are analyzed, stored, and printed in a computerized data base.

VII. IMMUNOLOGIC DETECTION OF MICROORGANISMS

In the diagnosis of infectious diseases, immunologic methods take advantage of the specificity of antigen–antibody binding (see p. 79). For example, known antigens and antibodies are used as diagnostic tools in identifying microorganisms. In addition, serologic detection of a patient's immune response to infection, or antigenic or nucleic acid evidence of a pathogen in a patient's body fluids, is frequently useful. Examples of when this diagnostic approach is important include: 1) when the infecting microorganism is difficult or impossible to isolate (for example, in tularemia, or syphilis); 2) when a deep infection is difficult to culture (for example, in toxoplasmosis screening of pregnant patients); or 3) when a previous infection needs to be documented (for example, to establish prior streptococcal infection as the cause of rheumatic fever or acute glomerulonephritis). Most methods for determining whether antibodies or antigens are present in patients' sera or other body fluids require some type of **immunoassay** procedure, such as those described in this section.

A. Detection of microbial antigen with known antiserum

These methods of identification are often rapid, and show favorable sensitivity and specificity (see p. 21). However, unlike microbial culturing techniques, these immunologic methods do not permit further characterization of the microorganism, such as determining its antibiotic sensitivity, or characteristic metabolic patterns.

1. **Capsular swelling reaction:** Some bacteria having capsules can be identified directly in clinical specimens by a swelling reaction that occurs when the organisms are treated with serum containing specific antibodies (see p. 153). This method, sometimes called the **Quellung reaction**, can be used for all serotypes of *Streptococcus pneumoniae*, *Haemophilus influenzae* type b, and *Neisseria meningitidis* groups A and C.

2. **Slide agglutination test:** Some microorganisms, such as *Salmonella* and *Shigella* species, can be identified by agglutination (clumping) of a suspension of bacterial cells on a microscopic slide. Agglutination occurs when specific antibody directed against microbial antigen is added to the suspension, causing cross-linking of the bacteria.

3. **Counterimmunoelectrophoresis:** In this method, an unknown microbial antigen is placed in one circular well cut into a thin layer of agar. Antigen of known concentration is placed in an adjacent well to serve as a control. Antibodies of known specificity are placed in a well opposite the antigens. The conditions of the assay are such that the antigen and antibody have opposite charges. Both antigens and antibodies diffuse out of the wells, and eventually come into contact. The rate of their movement toward each other is accelerated by an electrical field placed across the agar gel. The maximum amount of antigen–antibody complex precipitation occurs when the total number of antigen binding sites on the antibodies equals the total number of epitopes on the antigens (the "equivalence point"). The precipitate forms an immobile, lattice-like structure that appears as an opaque band. This method is termed "counterimmunoelectrophoresis" because the antigen and antibody are migrating toward (that is, "counter" to) one another. Counterimmunoelectrophoresis has been used as a rapid, qualitative technique in determining the absence or presence of antigens in body fluids.

B. Identification of serum antibodies

Detection in a patient's serum of antibodies that are directed against microbial antigens provides evidence for a current or past infection with a specific pathogen. A discussion of the general interpretation of antibody responses includes the following rules: 1) antibody may not be detectable early in an infection; 2) the presence of antibodies in a patient's serum cannot differentiate between a present as opposed to a prior infection; and 3) a rise in antibody titer over a seven-to-ten day period does distinguish between a present and prior infection. Techniques such as complement fixation and agglutination can be used to quantitate antimicrobial antibodies. Using known antigens, methods such as agglutination reactions, immunofluorescence, and ELISA (see below), can also be used to detect antibodies (as well as antigens) in the patient's serum.

1. **Complement fixation:** One of the older but still useful methods for detecting serum antibody directed against a specific pathogen employs the ability of antibody to bind complement (Figure 4.12). A patient's serum is first incubated with antigen specific for the suspected infectious agent, followed by the addition of complement (see p. 90). If the patient's serum does contain IgG or IgM antibodies that target the specific antigen (indicating past or current infection), then the added complement will be sequestered in an antigen/antibody/complement complex ("complement fixation"). Next, sensitized (antibody-coated) indicator sheep red blood cells are added to the solution. If complement has been fixed (because the patient's serum contained antibodies against the added antigen), then little complement will be available to bind to the anti-

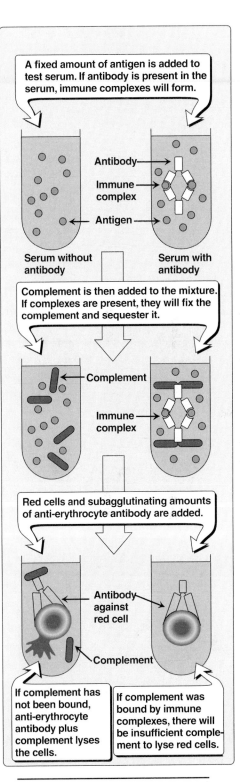

A fixed amount of antigen is added to test serum. If antibody is present in the serum, immune complexes will form.

Antibody
Immune complex
Antigen

Serum without antibody   Serum with antibody

Complement is then added to the mixture. If complexes are present, they will fix the complement and sequester it.

Complement
Immune complex

Red cells and subagglutinating amounts of anti-erythrocyte antibody are added.

Antibody against red cell
Complement

If complement has not been bound, anti-erythrocyte antibody plus complement lyses the cells.

If complement was bound by immune complexes, there will be insufficient complement to lyse red cells.

Figure 4.12
Complement fixation.

body–red blood cell complexes, and the cells will not lyse. If complement has not been depleted by initial antigen-antibody complexes (because the patient's serum does not contain antibodies to the specific antigen), the complement will bind to the antibody–red blood cell complexes, causing the cells to lyse. As hemolyzed red blood cells release hemoglobin, the reaction can be monitored with a spectrophotometer.

2. **Direct agglutination:** "**Febrile agglutinins**" is a test panel sometimes ordered to evaluate patients with fever of unknown origin, or when a suspected organism is difficult or dangerous to culture in the laboratory. This test measures the ability of a patient's serum antibody to directly agglutinate specific killed (yet intact) microorganisms. This test is used to evaluate patients suspected of being infected by *Brucella abortus* or *Francisella tularensis*, among others. The highest positive antibody titer is determined by performing serial dilutions of the patient's serum until reactivity is lost. For example, a titer of 1:320 (that is, detectable antibody to the organism at a serum dilution of 1:320) is a presumptive positive for brucellosis, and a titer of 1:40 to 1:80 is a presumptive positive for tularemia.

3. **Direct hemagglutination:** Antibodies directed against red blood cells can arise during the course of various infections. For example, such antibodies are typically found during infectious mononucleosis caused by Epstein-Barr virus (see p. 331) When uncoated (native) animal or human red blood cells are used in agglutination reactions with serum from a patient infected with such an organism, antibodies to red blood cell antigens can be detected (the patient's antibodies cause the red blood cells to clump). This test is therefore a direct hemagglutination reaction. In the case of some diseases, including pneumonia caused by *Mycoplasma pneumoniae*, IgM autoantibodies may develop that agglutinate human red blood cells at 4°C but not at 37°C. This is termed the "**cold agglutinins**" test.

C. **Other tests used to identify serum antigens or antibodies**

1. **Latex agglutination test:** Latex and other particles can be readily coated with either antibody (for antigen detection) or antigen (for antibody detection). Addition of antigen to antibody-coated latex beads causes agglutination that can be visually observed (Figure 4.13). For example, such methods are used to rapidly test CSF for antigens associated with common forms of bacterial or fungal meningitis. When antigen is coated onto the latex bead, antibody from a patient's serum can be detected.

2. **Enzyme-linked immunosorbent assay (ELISA):** In this diagnostic technique, antibody specific for an antigen of interest is bound to the walls of a plastic microtiter well (Figure 4.14). Patient serum is then incubated in the wells, and any antigen in the serum is bound by the antibody on the well walls. The wells are then washed, and a second antibody is added—this one also specific for the antigen, but recognizing epitopes different from those bound by the first antibody. After incubation, the wells are again

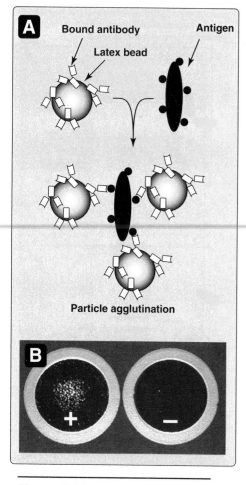

Figure 4.13
A. Schematic representation of antigens aggregating latex beads with bound antibody. B. Photograph of aggregation reaction.

washed, removing any unattached antibody. Attached to the second antibody is an enzyme, which, when presented with its substrate, produces a colored product, the intensity of the color produced being proportional to the amount of bound antigen. ELISAs can also be used to detect or quantitate antibody in a patient's serum. In this instance, the wells are coated with antigen specific for the antibody in question. The patient's serum is allowed to react with the bound antigen, the wells are washed, and a secondary antibody (that recognizes the initial antibody) conjugated to a color product-producing enzyme is added to the well. After a final washing, substrate for the bound enzyme is added to the well, and the intensity of the colored product can be measured. [Note: ELISA is used to detect the presence of serum antibodies against human immunodeficiency virus (HIV). Serum antibodies to HIV can generally be detected by an ELISA between five to seven weeks after infection.]

3. **Fluorescent-antibody tests:** Organisms in clinical samples can be detected directly by specific antibodies coupled to a fluorescent compound, such as fluorescein. In the **direct immunofluorescence antibody technique**, a sample of concentrated body fluid (for example, CSF or serum), tissue scraping (for example, skin), or cells in tissue culture is incubated with a fluorescein-labeled antibody directed against a specific pathogen. The labeled antibody bound to the microorganism absorbs ultraviolet light, and emits visible fluorescence that can be detected by the human eye, using a fluorescence microscope. A variation of the technique, the **indirect immunofluorescence antibody technique**, involves the use of two antibodies. The first, unlabeled antibody, called the target antibody, binds a specific microbial antigen in a sample such as those described above. This clinical sample is subsequently stained with a fluorescent antibody that recognizes the target antibody. Because a number of labeled antibodies can bind to each target antibody, the fluorescence from the stained microorganism is intensified. Both direct and indirect fluorescence methods can be used to detect viruses, such as cytomegalovirus and herpes simplex virus, within cultured cells. Bacteria that are difficult to grow, such as *Legionella pneumophila*, can also be directly identified in clinical samples.

VIII. DETECTION OF MICROBIAL DNA OR RNA

A highly specific method of pathogen detection involves identification of its DNA or RNA in a patient sample. The basic strategy is to detect a relatively short sequence of nucleotide bases of DNA or RNA (the target sequence) that is unique to the pathogen. This is done by hybridization with a complementary sequence of bases, referred to as the probe. [Note: In bacteria, DNA sequences coding for 16S ribosomal RNA sequences (rRNA) are commonly used targets, because each microorganism contains multiple copies of its specific rRNA gene, thus increasing the sensitivity of the assay.] The methods for detecting microbial DNA or RNA fall into two categories: direct hybridization, and amplification methods using the polymerase chain reaction[1] or one its variations.

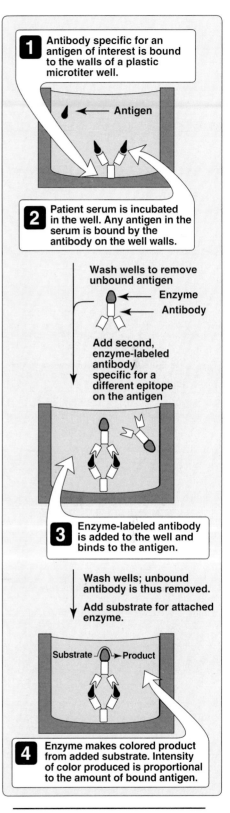

1 Antibody specific for an antigen of interest is bound to the walls of a plastic microtiter well.

← Antigen

2 Patient serum is incubated in the well. Any antigen in the serum is bound by the antibody on the well walls.

Wash wells to remove unbound antigen

← Enzyme
← Antibody

Add second, enzyme-labeled antibody specific for a different epitope on the antigen

3 Enzyme-labeled antibody is added to the well and binds to the antigen.

Wash wells; unbound antibody is thus removed.

Add substrate for attached enzyme.

Substrate → Product

4 Enzyme makes colored product from added substrate. Intensity of color produced is proportional to the amount of bound antigen.

Figure 4.14
Principle of enzyme-linked immunosorbent assay (ELISA).

 [1]See ***Lippincott's Illustrated Reviews: Biochemistry***, 2nd ed., Chapter 33 for a more detailed presentation of the techniques used in molecular biology.

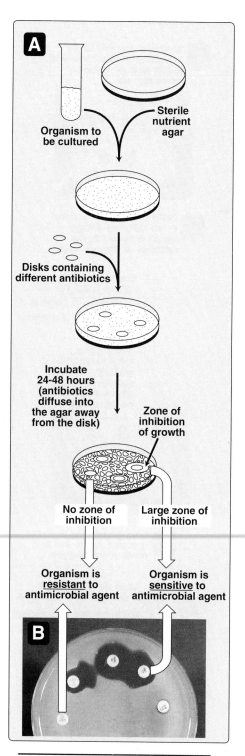

Figure 4.15
A. Outline of disk diffusion method for determining the sensitivity of bacteria to antimicrobial agents.
B. Photograph of culture plate with antibiotic-impregnated disks.

A. Direct hybridization methods

These methods use a **probe**—a single-stranded piece of DNA, usually labeled with an enzyme, a fluorescent molecule, a radioactive label, or with some other detectable molecule. The nucleotide sequence of the probe is complementary to the DNA of interest, called the **target DNA**. To obtain the target DNA, an appropriate sample from the patient is cultured to increase the number of the presumptive disease-causing microorganisms, and then treated, so that the microorganisms lyse, releasing their DNA. Single-stranded DNA, produced by alkaline denaturation of the double-stranded DNA, is first bound to a solid support such as a nitrocellulose membrane. The immobilized DNA strands are then available for hybridization to the microorganism-specific, labeled probe. Unbound probe is removed by washing the filter, and the extent of hybridization is then measured by the retention of the labeled probe on the filter. Direct use of nucleic acid probes generally requires a substantial amount of microbial DNA. For example, in the identification of *Mycobacterium tuberculosis* using direct hybridization, it generally takes a minimum of ten days of culturing a clinical sample to achieve growth sufficient for this test.

B. Amplification methods

Methods employing nucleic acid amplification techniques, such as the polymerase chain reaction (PCR), have a major advantage over direct detection with nucleic acid probes, because amplification methods allow specific DNA or RNA target sequences of the pathogen to be amplified millions of times without having to culture the microorganism itself for extended periods of time. Nucleic acid amplification methods are sensitive (often to fewer than ten organisms), very specific for the target organism, show positive results in the course of an infection, and are unaffected by the prior administration of antibiotics.

1. **Applications:** Nucleic acid amplification techniques are generally quick, easy, and accurate. A major use of these techniques is for the detection of organisms that cannot be grown *in vitro*, or for which current culture techniques are insensitive. Further, they are useful in the detection of organisms that require complex media or cell cultures and/or prolonged incubation times.

2. **Detection:** The amplified sequences are detected by a variety of methods, for example, by agarose gel electrophoresis, or by blotting the product onto a membrane such as a nitrocellulose filter, followed by probe hybridization (as described above). Newer detection methods capture the amplified target sequences in a well, using a complementary strand of DNA that has been fixed to the surface of the well.

3. **Limitations:** PCR amplification is limited by the occurrence of spurious false-positives due to cross contamination with other microorganisms' nucleic acid.

IX. SUSCEPTIBILITY TESTING

After a pathogen is cultured, its sensitivity to specific antibiotics serves as a guide in choosing antimicrobial therapy. Some pathogens, such as Streptococcus pyogenes and Neisseria meningitidis, usually have predictable sensitivity patterns to certain antibiotics. In contrast, most gram-negative bacilli, enterococci, and staphylococcal species often show unpredictable sensitivity patterns to various antibiotics, and require susceptibility testing to determine appropriate antimicrobial therapy.

A. Disk-diffusion method

The classic qualitative method to test susceptibility to antibiotics has been the Kirby Bauer disk-diffusion method, in which disks with exact amounts of different antimicrobial agents are placed on culture dishes inoculated with the microorganism to be tested. The organism's growth (resistance to the drug), or lack of growth (sensitivity to the drug) is then monitored (Figure 4.15). In addition, the size of the zone of growth inhibition is influenced by the concentration and rate of diffusion of the antibiotic on the disk. The disk-diffusion method is useful when susceptibility to an unusual antibiotic, not available in automated systems (see p. 28), is to be determined.

B. Minimal inhibitory concentration

Quantitative testing utilizes a dilution technique, in which tubes containing serial dilutions of an antibiotic are inoculated with the organism whose sensitivity to that antibiotic is to be tested. The tubes are incubated and later observed to determine the minimal inhibitory concentration (MIC) of the antibiotic necessary to prevent bacterial growth (Figure 4.16). In order to provide effective antimicrobial therapy, the clinically obtainable antibiotic concentration in body fluids should be greater than the MIC. Quantitative susceptibility testing may be necessary for patients who either fail to respond to antimicrobial therapy, or who relapse during therapy. [Note: In some clinical cases, the **minimum bactericidal concentration** may need to be determined. This is the lowest concentration of antibiotic (see next paragraph) that **kills** 100 percent of the bacteria, rather than simply inhibiting their growth.]

C. Bacteriostatic vs. bactericidal drugs

As noted above, antimicrobial drugs may be either bacteriostatic or bactericidal. **Bacteriostatic drugs** arrest the growth and replication of bacteria at serum levels achievable in the patient, thus limiting the spread of infection while the body's immune system attacks, immobilizes, and eliminates the pathogens. If the drug is removed before the immune system has scavenged the organisms, enough viable organisms may remain to begin a second cycle of infection. For example, Figure 4.17 shows a laboratory experiment in which the growth of bacteria is arrested by the addition of a bacteriostatic agent. Note that viable organisms remain, even in the presence of the bacteriostatic drug. By contrast, addition of a **bactericidal agent** kills bacteria, and the total number of viable organisms decreases. Though practical, this classification may be too simplistic because it is possible for an antibiotic to be bacteriostatic for one organism and cidal for another (for example, chloramphenicol is bacteriostatic against gram-negative rods, and bactericidal against pneumococci).

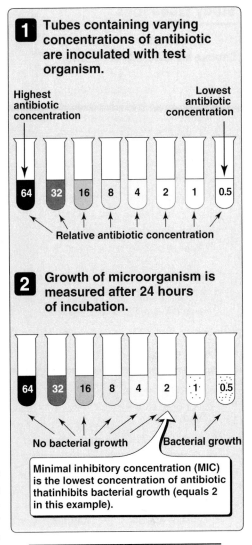

Figure 4.16
Determination of minimal inhibitory concentration (MIC) of an antibiotic.

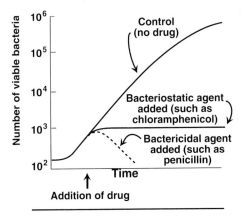

Figure 4.17
Effects of bactericidal and bacteriostatic drugs on the growth of bacteria *in vitro*.

Study Questions

Choose the ONE correct answer

4.1 Among 100 employees at a hospital, five were infected with a particular pathogen. When these people were tested for the presence of the pathogen, ten individuals gave a positive response. Subsequent evaluation by independent tests revealed that five of the ten were, in fact, infected and five were not. Which one of the following best describes the original test?

A. High sensitivity, high specificity

B. High sensitivity, low specificity

C. Low sensitivity, high specificity

D. Low sensitivity, Low specificity

E. Data do not allow a determination.

Correct answer = B. All infected individuals were detected, but many false positives occurred.

4.2 Chose the item that correctly matches the microorganism with an appropriate stain or preparation.

A. *Mycobacterium tuberculosis* — India ink

B. Fungi — KOH

C. *Cryptococcus neoformans* in cerebrospinal fluid — Zeehl-Nielsen (the classic acid-fast stain)

D. *Chlamydia* — Gram stain

E. *Escherichia coli* (a gram-negative bacterium)— Crystal violet followed by treatment with acetone.

Correct answer = B. Treatment with KOH dissolves host cells and bacteria, allowing fungi to be visualized. *Mycobacterium tuberculosis* is stained by the Zeehl-Nielsen stain (the classic acid-fast stain). *Cryptococcus neoformans* in cerebrospinal fluid is visualized with India ink. Organisms that are intracellular, such as chlamydia, or that lack a cell wall, such as mycoplasma or ureaplasma, are not readily detected by the Gram stain. Most bacteria stain purple with crystal violet and iodine. If the stained cells are then treated with acetone, gram-positive organisms retain the stain, whereas gram-negative species, such as *Escherichia coli*, lose the stain, becoming colorless. Visualization of *Escherichia coli* requires the addition of the counterstain safranin, which stains gram-negative bacteria pink or red.

4.3 Which one of the following media is most suitable for identifying *Neisseria gonorrhoeae* in a cervical swab?

A. Sheep blood agar

B. Chocolate agar

C. MacConkey agar

D. Thayer-Martin medium

E. Hektoen enteric agar

Correct answer = D. Sheep blood agar supports the growth of most bacteria, both gram-positive and gram-negative. Chocolate agar provides the growth requirements for fastidious organisms such as *Haemophilus influenzae* or *Neisseria gonorrhoeae*, as well as for most other less-fastidious bacteria. MacConkey agar supports most gram-negative rods, especially the *Enterobacteriaeceae*, but inhibits growth of gram-positive organisms and some fastidious gram-negative bacteria, such as haemophilus and neisseria species. Thayer-Martin medium, which is composed of chocolate agar supplemented with several antibiotics, suppresses the growth of nonpathogenic neisseria and other normal and abnormal flora, but permits the growth of gonococcus. Hektoen enteric agar is also a selective medium that is often used to culture *Salmonella* and *Shigella* species.

Vaccines and Antibiotics

5

I. OVERVIEW

The availability of vaccines has resulted in the global eradication of smallpox, and the virtual elimination of poliomyelitis, tetanus, and diphtheria in the United States (Figure 5.1). Protection of individuals from disease by vaccination can take two forms, passive and active immunization. **Passive immunization** is achieved by injecting a recipient with preformed immunoglobulins directed against an already present infection, whereas **active immunization** involves injection of modified or purified pathogens, or their products. Both provide protective immune responses. Active and passive immunization differ in significant ways, and the situations under which one or the other (or their combination, active-passive immunization) is preferred depends upon the type of infecting microorganism, the age of the patient, whether an individual anticipates imminent contact with a pathogen, or the time elapsed since contact with a pathogen. [Note: The reader is reminded of the common names for some childhood diseases discussed in this chapter: pertussis = whooping cough; rubella = german measles; rubeola = measles; varicella = chickenpox.]

II. PASSIVE IMMUNIZATION

Passive immunization is achieved by injecting a recipient with preformed immunoglobulins obtained from human (or occasionally equine) serum. Passive immunization is used to provide immediate protection to individuals who have been exposed to an infectious organism and lack active immunity to that pathogen. Because passive immunization does not activate the immune system, it generates no memory response. Passive immunity is not permanent, but dissipates after a few weeks to months, as the immunoglobulins are cleared from the recipient's serum.

A. Types of immunoglobulins used to give passive immunity

Two basic formulations of prepared immunoglobulins have been developed: one from the serum of pooled human donors, and one from serum obtained from hyperimmune donors (Figure 5.2).

1. **Nonspecific standard immune globulins:** This mixture of plasma proteins contains a broad spectrum of antibodies, with IgG predominating. These immunoglobulins (formerly known as **gamma globulins**) contain a mixture of antibodies reflecting the previous exposures of the plasma donors to various antigens, either by natural infection or by immunization. Standard immunoglobulin is

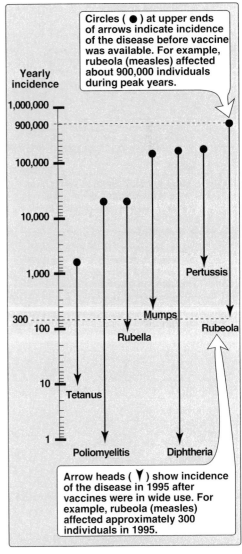

Figure 5.1
Incidence of vaccine-preventable diseases in the United States at their highest incidence and in 1995. [Note: Y-axis is a logarithmic scale.]

Lippincott's Illustrated Reviews: Microbiology, by William A. Strohl, Harriet Rouse, Bruce D. Fisher. Lippincott, Williams & Wilkins, Baltimore, MD © 2001

used for prevention or attenuation of illnesses for which there is no specific immunoglobulin preparation. This type of immunization is effective when given immediately before or after exposure to an infectious disease, such as hepatitis A.

2. **Hyperimmune human immunoglobulin:** This type of immunoglobulin contains high concentrations of antibodies directed against a specific pathogen or toxin (for example, varicella-zoster immunoglobulin, or diphtheria antitoxin). These may be given to patients who have recently been exposed to a specific pathogen.

B. Adverse effects

There are risks associated with the injection of preformed antibody. For example, the recipient can mount an adverse response to the antigenic determinants of the foreign antibody, potentially leading to systemic anaphylaxis. [Note: This is particularly true when the immunoglobulins are obtained from a nonhuman source, such as a horse.]

III. ACTIVE IMMUNIZATION

Active immunization is achieved by injection of viable or nonviable pathogens, or purified pathogen product, prompting the immune system to respond as if the body were being attacked by an intact infectious microorganism. Whereas passive immunization provides immediate protection, active immunization may require several days to months to become effective. Active immunization leads to prolonged immunity and is generally preferred over the short-term immunity provided by passive immunization with preformed immunoglobulins. Simultaneous administration of active and passive immunizations may be required after exposure to certain infections. For example, hepatitis B immunoglobulin, in combination with active immunization, provides post-exposure prophylaxis following accidental exposure to the pathogen.

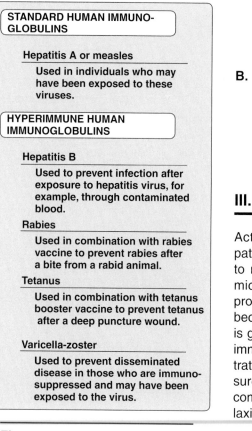

STANDARD HUMAN IMMUNO-GLOBULINS

Hepatitis A or measles

Used in individuals who may have been exposed to these viruses.

HYPERIMMUNE HUMAN IMMUNOGLOBULINS

Hepatitis B

Used to prevent infection after exposure to hepatitis virus, for example, through contaminated blood.

Rabies

Used in combination with rabies vaccine to prevent rabies after a bite from a rabid animal.

Tetanus

Used in combination with tetanus booster vaccine to prevent tetanus after a deep puncture wound.

Varicella-zoster

Used to prevent disseminated disease in those who are immuno-suppressed and may have been exposed to the virus.

Figure 5.2
Immunoglobulins used for passive immunization.

A. Formulations for active immunization

Vaccines are made with either 1) live, attenuated microorganisms; 2) killed microorganisms; 3) microbial extracts; 4) vaccine conjugates; or 5) inactivated toxins (toxoids). Both bacterial and viral pathogens are targeted by these diverse means.

1. **Live pathogens:** When live pathogens are used, they are **attenuated** (weakened) to preclude clinical consequences of infection. Attenuated microbes reproduce in the recipient, typically leading to a more robust and long-lasting immune response than can be obtained through vaccination with killed organisms. However, with live, attenuated vaccines there is a possibility that the attenuated vaccine strain will revert to an active pathogen after administration to the patient. For example, vaccine-associated poliomyelitis occurs following administration of approximately one out of every 2.4 million doses of live polio vaccine. All recent cases of polio in the United States are vaccine-associated. Also, live, attenuated vaccines should not be given to immunocompromised individuals because there is the potential for a disseminated infection.

2. Killed microorganisms: Killed vaccines have the advantage over attenuated microorganisms in that they pose no risk of vaccine-associated infection. As noted above, killed organisms often provide a weak or short-lived immune response. Some vaccines, such as polio and typhoid vaccines, are available both in live or killed versions.

3. Microbial extracts: Instead of using whole organisms, vaccines can be composed of antigen molecules (often those located on the surface of the microorganism) extracted from the pathogen or prepared by recombinant DNA techniques. The efficacy of these vaccines varies. In some instances, the vaccine antigen is present on all strains of the organism, and the vaccine thus protects against infection by all strains. With other pathogens such as the pneumococcus, protective antibody is produced against only a specific capsular polysaccharide—one among more than eighty distinct types. Immunity to one polysaccharide type does not confer immunity to any other type. For this reason, the pneumococcal vaccine is composed of 23 different polysaccharides, comprising the antigens produced by the most common types of disease-causing pneumococci. In the case of rhinovirus infections—the leading cause of the common cold—at least 100 types of the virus are known. It is not practical to develop a vaccine that confers protection to this large number of antigenic types. Some pathogens, such as influenza virus, frequently change their antigenic determinants. Therefore, influenza virus vaccines must also change regularly to counter the different antigens of the influenza A and B virus strains in circulation.

4. Vaccine conjugates: Vaccines can produce humoral immunity through B-cell proliferation leading to antibody production, which may or may not involve helper T cells (see p. 89). For example, pneumococcal polysaccharide and the polysaccharide of *Haemophilus influenzae* type b induce B-cell type-specific protective antibody without involvement of helper T cells. These T cell–independent responses are characterized by low antibody titers, particularly in children less than eighteen months of age. Thus, a conventional *H. influenzae* polysaccharide vaccine does not provide protection for children three to eighteen months. Consequently this organism has, in the past, produced severe infections in this age group. However, by covalently conjugating the *Haemophilus* polysaccharide to a protein antigen, such as diphtheria toxoid protein, *Haemophilus* vaccines produce a robust T cell–dependent antibody response even in three-month-old infants. Figure 5.3 shows the decreased incidence of *Haemophilus influenzae* disease following introduction of the conjugated vaccine. A conjugate vaccine for *Streptococcus pneumoniae,* and one for *Neisseria meningitidis*, are also currently available. The pneumococcal conjugate vaccine targets the seven strains of *Streptococcus pneumoniae* that are responsible for 85 percent of bacterial pneumonia in children. Clinical trials have shown that the conjugate vaccine substantially reduces childhood pneumonia. Figure 5.4 shows the favorable antibody response to conjugated polysaccharide obtained from *Neisseria meningitidis*.

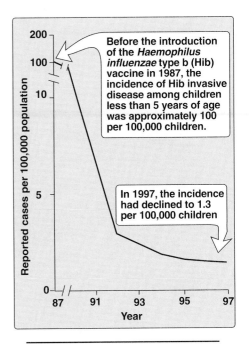

Figure 5.3
Incidence of infection in children due to *Haemophilus influenzae* type b (Hib) following introduction of a conjugate vaccine in 1987.

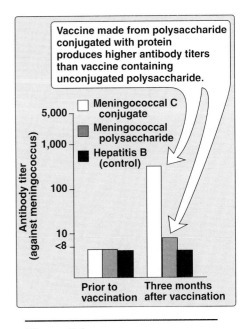

Figure 5.4
Serum bactericidal antibody response to vaccination with meningococcal C conjugate, meningococcal polysaccharide, and hepatitis B vaccine (control) in children, 15 to 23 months of age.

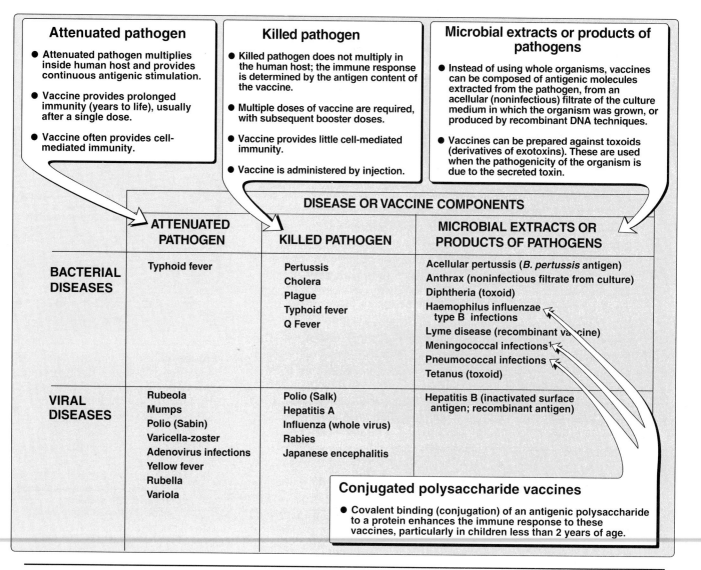

Attenuated pathogen

- Attenuated pathogen multiplies inside human host and provides continuous antigenic stimulation.
- Vaccine provides prolonged immunity (years to life), usually after a single dose.
- Vaccine often provides cell-mediated immunity.

Killed pathogen

- Killed pathogen does not multiply in the human host; the immune response is determined by the antigen content of the vaccine.
- Multiple doses of vaccine are required, with subsequent booster doses.
- Vaccine provides little cell-mediated immunity.
- Vaccine is administered by injection.

Microbial extracts or products of pathogens

- Instead of using whole organisms, vaccines can be composed of antigenic molecules extracted from the pathogen, from an acellular (noninfectious) filtrate of the culture medium in which the organism was grown, or produced by recombinant DNA techniques.
- Vaccines can be prepared against toxoids (derivatives of exotoxins). These are used when the pathogenicity of the organism is due to the secreted toxin.

DISEASE OR VACCINE COMPONENTS

	ATTENUATED PATHOGEN	KILLED PATHOGEN	MICROBIAL EXTRACTS OR PRODUCTS OF PATHOGENS
BACTERIAL DISEASES	Typhoid fever	Pertussis Cholera Plague Typhoid fever Q Fever	Acellular pertussis (*B. pertussis* antigen) Anthrax (noninfectious filtrate from culture) Diphtheria (toxoid) Haemophilus influenzae type B infections Lyme disease (recombinant vaccine) Meningococcal infections[1] Pneumococcal infections Tetanus (toxoid)
VIRAL DISEASES	Rubeola Mumps Polio (Sabin) Varicella-zoster Adenovirus infections Yellow fever Rubella Variola	Polio (Salk) Hepatitis A Influenza (whole virus) Rabies Japanese encephalitis	Hepatitis B (inactivated surface antigen; recombinant antigen)

Conjugated polysaccharide vaccines

- Covalent binding (conjugation) of an antigenic polysaccharide to a protein enhances the immune response to these vaccines, particularly in children less than 2 years of age.

Figure 5.5
Some diseases and their vaccines licensed for use in humans in the United States. [1]Meningococcal vaccine in development.

5. **Toxoids:** These are derivatives of bacterial exotoxins that can be produced by chemically altering the natural toxin, or by engineering bacteria to produce harmless variants of the toxin. Vaccines containing toxoid are used when the pathogenicity of the organism is due to the secreted toxin. Depending upon the specific vaccine, administration is generally via intramuscular or subcutaneous routes. Figure 5.5 shows the formulation of some of the vaccines currently licensed in the United States. Details of the various vaccines are presented in the chapters where the target microorganisms are discussed.

B. **Types of immune response to vaccines**

Vaccines containing killed pathogens (such as hepatitis A or Salk polio vaccine) or antigenic components of pathogens (such as hepatitis B subunit vaccine) do not enter host cells, and therefore they give rise to a primary B cell–mediated humoral response. These antibodies are ineffective in attacking intracellular organisms. By contrast, attenuated live vaccines (usually viruses) do penetrate into cells. This results in the production of intracellular antigens that are displayed on the surface of the infected cell, prompting a cytotoxic T cell response, which is effective in eliminating intracellular pathogens (see p. 74).

C. Effect of age on efficacy of immunization

1. **Passive immunity from mother:** Newborns receive serum IgG antibodies from their mothers, which gives them temporary protection against those diseases to which the mother was immune. In addition, maternal milk also contains secretory antibodies that provide some protection against intestinal and respiratory tract infections.

2. **Active immunization:** The infant's antibody-producing capacity develops slowly during the first year of life. Although the immune system is not fully developed, it is desirable to begin immunization at 2 months of age because diseases are common in this age group, and can be particularly severe (for example, whooping cough, *H. influenzae* meningitis). As with infants, the elderly have a reduced antibody response to vaccines.

D. Adverse reactions to active vaccination

The adverse consequences of vaccinations can range from very mild to severe and even life-threatening (Figure 5.6). Symptoms vary among individuals, and with the nature of the vaccination. Among the most common and mildest consequences of immunization are tenderness and swelling at the site of injection, and a mild fever (these complaints are occasionally more severe in neonates and young children). Symptoms vary with the nature of the vaccination. More severe consequences of vaccination, although rare, include cross-reactivity to host proteins, anaphylaxis, and the risks that derive either from contamination of a vaccine preparation with an unintended pathogen, or from reversion of the attenuated pathogen present in the vaccine. Reversion to pathogenicity represents a risk not just to the vaccine recipient but also to individuals the recipient comes in contact with and even to technicians working on vaccine manufacture and health care workers involved in administering vaccines.

IV. BACTERIAL VACCINES

Vaccines against commonly encountered bacterial pathogens are summarized in Figure 5.7. The recommended childhood immunization schedule is shown in Figure 5.8. Vaccines with more specialized indications are described below.

A. Less common bacterial pathogens

1. **Anthrax (Bacillus anthracis):** The anthrax vaccine consists of a noninfectious sterile filtrate from the culture of an attenuated strain of *Bacillus anthracis* that contains no dead or alive bacteria The filtrate is adsorbed to an adjuvant, aluminum hydroxide. [Note: **Adjuvants** are substances that when injected with an antigen, serve to enhance the immunogencity of that antigen.] The incidence of all forms of naturally occurring anthrax is low, particu-

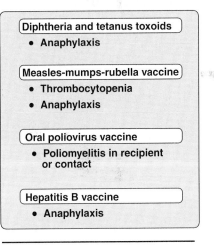

Figure 5.6
Rare adverse effects associated with childhood vaccines.

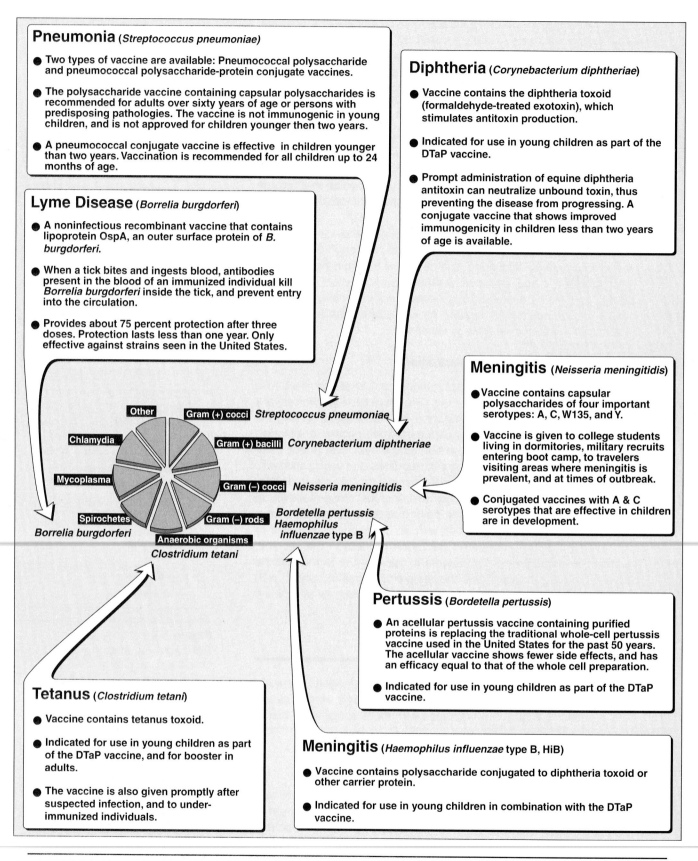

Pneumonia (*Streptococcus pneumoniae*)

● Two types of vaccine are available: Pneumococcal polysaccharide and pneumococcal polysaccharide-protein conjugate vaccines.

● The polysaccharide vaccine containing capsular polysaccharides is recommended for adults over sixty years of age or persons with predisposing pathologies. The vaccine is not immunogenic in young children, and is not approved for children younger then two years.

● A pneumococcal conjugate vaccine is effective in children younger than two years. Vaccination is recommended for all children up to 24 months of age.

Lyme Disease (*Borrelia burgdorferi*)

● A noninfectious recombinant vaccine that contains lipoprotein OspA, an outer surface protein of *B. burgdorferi*.

● When a tick bites and ingests blood, antibodies present in the blood of an immunized individual kill *Borrelia burgdorferi* inside the tick, and prevent entry into the circulation.

● Provides about 75 percent protection after three doses. Protection lasts less than one year. Only effective against strains seen in the United States.

Diphtheria (*Corynebacterium diphtheriae*)

● Vaccine contains the diphtheria toxoid (formaldehyde-treated exotoxin), which stimulates antitoxin production.

● Indicated for use in young children as part of the DTaP vaccine.

● Prompt administration of equine diphtheria antitoxin can neutralize unbound toxin, thus preventing the disease from progressing. A conjugate vaccine that shows improved immunogenicity in children less than two years of age is available.

Meningitis (*Neisseria meningitidis*)

● Vaccine contains capsular polysaccharides of four important serotypes: A, C, W135, and Y.

● Vaccine is given to college students living in dormitories, military recruits entering boot camp, to travelers visiting areas where meningitis is prevalent, and at times of outbreak.

● Conjugated vaccines with A & C serotypes that are effective in children are in development.

Other

Gram (+) cocci *Streptococcus pneumoniae*

Chlamydia

Gram (+) bacilli *Corynebacterium diphtheriae*

Mycoplasma

Gram (–) cocci *Neisseria meningitidis*

Spirochetes

Gram (–) rods *Bordetella pertussis*
Haemophilus influenzae type B

Borrelia burgdorferi

Anaerobic organisms

Clostridium tetani

Pertussis (*Bordetella pertussis*)

● An acellular pertussis vaccine containing purified proteins is replacing the traditional whole-cell pertussis vaccine used in the United States for the past 50 years. The acellular vaccine shows fewer side effects, and has an efficacy equal to that of the whole cell preparation.

● Indicated for use in young children as part of the DTaP vaccine.

Tetanus (*Clostridium tetani*)

● Vaccine contains tetanus toxoid.

● Indicated for use in young children as part of the DTaP vaccine, and for booster in adults.

● The vaccine is also given promptly after suspected infection, and to under-immunized individuals.

Meningitis (*Haemophilus influenzae* type B, HiB)

● Vaccine contains polysaccharide conjugated to diphtheria toxoid or other carrier protein.

● Indicated for use in young children in combination with the DTaP vaccine.

Figure 5.7
Summary of common vaccines against bacterial diseases. DTaP = diphtheria and tetanus toxoids and acellular pertussis vaccine.

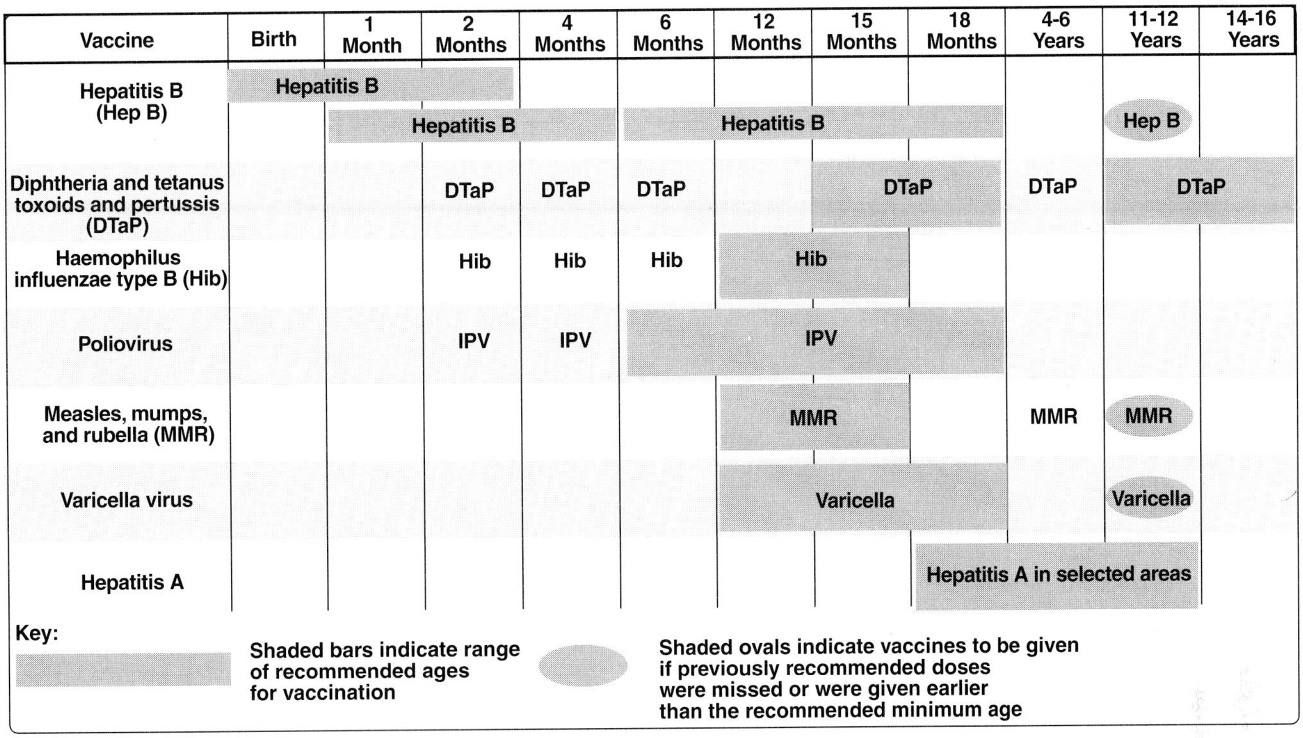

Vaccine	Birth	1 Month	2 Months	4 Months	6 Months	12 Months	15 Months	18 Months	4-6 Years	11-12 Years	14-16 Years
Hepatitis B (Hep B)	Hepatitis B	Hepatitis B			Hepatitis B					Hep B	
Diphtheria and tetanus toxoids and pertussis (DTaP)		DTaP	DTaP	DTaP		DTaP			DTaP	DTaP	
Haemophilus influenzae type B (Hib)		Hib	Hib	Hib	Hib						
Poliovirus		IPV	IPV		IPV						
Measles, mumps, and rubella (MMR)						MMR			MMR	MMR	
Varicella virus						Varicella				Varicella	
Hepatitis A									Hepatitis A in selected areas		

Key:

Shaded bars indicate range of recommended ages for vaccination

Shaded ovals indicate vaccines to be given if previously recommended doses were missed or were given earlier than the recommended minimum age

Figure 5.8
Recommended childhood immunization schedule for 2000. [Note: Immunization schedules may change each year, and clinicians should consult the Centers for Disease Control for details concerning current recommendations.] DTaP = diphtheria and tetanus toxoids and acellular pertussis vaccine. Hib = *Haemophilus influenzae* type B conjugate vaccine. MMR = measles-mumps-rubella vaccine. IPV = all-inactivate poliovirus vaccine.

larly the inhalation form of the disease. Thus, there is no opportunity to conduct field trials of the vaccine against inhalation anthrax, the form most likely to be used in a biological attack. Safety and efficacy of the vaccine are supported by studies in nonhuman primates where efficacy was close to 100 percent. The vaccine is recommended for goat hair and woolen mill workers, veterinarians, laboratory workers, and live-stock handlers who are at risk due to occupational exposure.

2. **Cholera (*Vibrio cholerae*):** Vaccine contains killed bacteria and is given to travelers.

3. **Typhoid fever (*Salmonella typhi*):** The most commonly used vaccine contains an attenuated recombinant strain of *S. typhi*. It is given to individuals living in or traveling to high-risk areas, and to the military.

4. **Plague (*Yersinia pestis*):** Vaccine that contains killed bacteria is given to high-risk individuals.

V. VIRAL VACCINES

Immunity to viral infection requires an immune response to antigens located on the surface of the viral particles, or on virus-infected cells. For enveloped viruses, these antigens are often surface glycoproteins.

The main limitation of viral vaccines occurs with viruses that show a genetically unstable antigenicity (that is, they exhibit antigenic determinants that continuously vary, such as with influenza viruses or the human immunodeficiency virus). Common viral pathogens for which there are vaccines include the following.

A. Hepatitis A

A formalin-inactivated whole virus vaccine produces antibody levels in adults similar to those observed following natural infection, and approximately fifteen times those achieved by passive injection of immunoglobulin. Projections indicate that immunity from hepatitis A virus will probably last for approximately ten years after two doses of vaccine. The vaccine is indicated for travelers to endemic areas, homosexual men, injecting drug users, and daycare workers. [Note: Currently in the United States, HAV vaccine is not recommended for children under the age of two years because residual anti-HAV passively acquired from the mother may interfere with vaccine immunogenicity.]

B. Hepatitis B

The currently used vaccine contains recombinant hepatitis surface antigen. Efficacy is 95 to 99 percent in healthy infants, children, and young adults. Its use is indicated for healthcare workers in contact with blood, and persons residing in an area with a high rate of endemic disease. Immunoglobulins obtained from hyperimmunized humans can provide passive immunity after accidental exposure (for example, a needle stick, or for the neonate of an infected mother). Active and passive treatments can be administered at the same time. However, the syringe with vaccine containing inactivated virus particles and one with anti-hepatitis B immunoglobulin must be injected into different sites on the body. (Obviously, if they are mixed together, the immunoglobulin will bind to the inactivated virus particles, rendering both inactive.) Recommended uses of hepatitis A and B vaccines are shown in Figure 5.9.

C. Varicella-zoster

This vaccine contains live, attenuated, temperature-sensitive varicella-zoster virus. Its efficacy in preventing chickenpox is approximately 85 to 100 percent in children, and this immunity is persistent. Most of the reported adverse events associated with varicella vaccine are minor, and serious risks appear to be rare. Anti–varicella-zoster immunoglobulin provides passive immunity for immunocompromised individuals at risk of infection.

D. Polio

Vaccination is the only effective method of preventing poliomyelitis. Both the inactivated polio vaccine and the live, attenuated, orally administered polio vaccine have established efficacy in preventing poliovirus infection and paralytic poliomyelitis (see p. 351).

1. **Inactivated poliovirus (Salk) vaccine:** The inactivated vaccine cannot cause poliomyelitis, and thus is safe for use in immunocompromised persons and their contacts. The disadvantages of this inactivated vaccine are: 1) administration is by injection only; 2) it

HEPATITIS A VACCINE

Routine immunization

Children living in communities with high hepatitis A rates and periodic disease outbreaks

Increased risk of hepatitis A

International travelers to regions of endemic disease
Homosexual men with multiple sexual partners
User of illicit injection drugs

HEPATITIS B VACCINE

Routine immunization

All infants and previously unvaccinated children by the age of 11 years

Increased risk of hepatitis B

People with multiple sexual partners
Sexual partner or household contacts of HBsAG-positive people
Homosexually active men
User of illicit injectable drug
Travelers to region of endemic disease
People occupationally exposed to blood or body fluids
Patients with renal failure
Patient receiving clotting-factor concentrates

Figure 5.9
Candidates for hepatitis immunization. HBsAg = hepatitis B surface antigen.

provides less gastrointestinal immunity, resulting in the possibility of asymptomatic infection of the gastrointestinal tract with wild poliovirus, which could be transmitted to other persons. To eliminate the risk for vaccine-associated paralytic poliomyelitis (see next section), an all-inactivated poliovirus vaccine schedule is recommended for routine childhood vaccinations in the United States.

2. **Attenuated live poliovirus (Sabin) vaccine:** Advantages of this vaccine include: 1) it can be administered orally; 2) it provides lifelong protection from poliovirus for more than 95 percent of recipients after the primary three-dose series; and 3) it provides early intestinal immunity. The main disadvantage of an attenuated live virus vaccine is the small risk of infection, estimated to be 1 per 2.4 million doses. The current recommendation for immunization against poliovirus is exclusive use of inactivated poliovirus vaccine. This eliminates the risk of contracting vaccine-associated paralytic poliomyelitis.

E. Influenza

The traditional "flu shot" vaccine contains formalin-inactivated virus. A newly-developed, live, attenuated influenza vaccine is administered intranasally. The vaccine provides peak protection about two weeks after its administration. Antigenic drift (see p. 388) requires that individuals be vaccinated annually prior to the winter flu season, which begins in November and lasts until the end of March. Vaccine efficacy of seventy to ninety percent is generally achieved in young adults. The vaccine is recommended for adults over the age of 65 years, high-risk persons six months of age or older, and those who might transmit the virus to persons at high risk.

F. Measles, mumps, and rubella (MMR)

This combination vaccine contains live, attenuated virus, and should be administered to young children prior to their entering school. Measles vaccine should also be administered to individuals traveling in endemic areas.

VI. DNA VACCINES

DNA vaccines represent a new approach to vaccination, and are currently under intense investigation. The proposed mechanism for these vaccines can be summarized as follows: The gene for the antigen of interest is cloned into a bacterial plasmid that is engineered to increase the expression of the inserted gene in mammalian cells (Figure 5.10). After being injected, the plasmid enters a host cell where it remains in the nucleus as an episome (that is, it is not integrated into the cell's DNA). Using the host cell's protein synthesis machinery, the plasmid DNA in the episome directs the synthesis of the protein it encodes. This antigenic microbial protein may leave the cells and interact with T helper and B cells, or it may be cleaved into fragments and presented as MHC I antigen complex on the cell surface, resulting in activation of killer T cells (see p. 74). This mechanism of action of DNA vaccines remains controversial, and many questions will have to be resolved before a clinically useful vaccine is available.

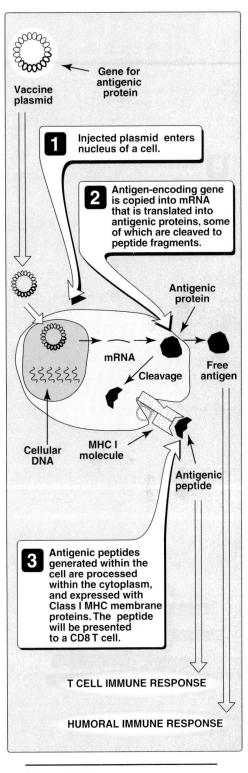

Figure 5.10
DNA vaccines produce antigen needed to generate immunity.

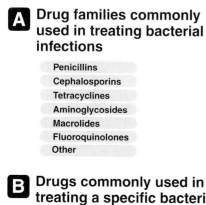

A. Drug families commonly used in treating bacterial infections

Penicillins
Cephalosporins
Tetracyclines
Aminoglycosides
Macrolides
Fluoroquinolones
Other

B. Drugs commonly used in treating a specific bacterial infection

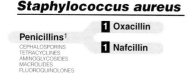

Staphylococcus aureus

Penicillins[1]   1 Oxacillin
CEPHALOSPORINS
TETRACYCLINES   1 Nafcillin
AMINOGLYCOSIDES
MACROLIDES
FLUOROQUINOLONES
Other   2 Vancomycin[2]

[1] Most isolates resistant to penicillin
[2] Vancomycin used when above drugs fail

Figure 5.11
A. Bar chart showing the six most commonly used drug families.
B. An example of the bar chart, with drugs of choice for the treatment of *Staphylococcus aureus* shown in bold print.

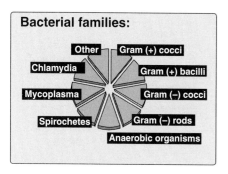

Figure 5.12
Organization of bacteria into nine families.

VII. OVERVIEW OF ANTIBIOTICS

Antimicrobial drugs are effective in the treatment of infections because of their selective toxicity (that is, they have the ability to kill or injure an invading microorganism without harming the cells of the host). In most instances, the selective toxicity is relative, rather than absolute, requiring that the concentration of the drug be carefully controlled to attack the microorganism while still being tolerated by the host. Selective antimicrobial therapy takes advantage of the biochemical differences that exist between microorganisms and human beings[1].

VIII. AGENTS USED IN BACTERIAL INFECTIONS

In this book, the clinically useful antibacterial drugs are organized into six families—the penicillins, cephalosporins, tetracyclines, aminoglycosides, macrolides, and fluoroquinolones, plus a seventh group labeled "Other" that is used to represent any drug not included in one of the other six drug families. Here and throughout the book, these seven groups are graphically presented as a bar chart (as a "drug stack", Figure 5.11A). The drug(s) of choice within each family that is/are used for treating a specific bacterial infection are shown in bold print, as illustrated for *S. aureus* in Figure 5.11B. [Note: As was introduced in Chapter 1 (see p. 3), the clinically important bacteria are also organized into groups based on Gram stain, morphology, and biochemical or other characteristics, and are represented as wedges of a "pie chart" (Figure 5.12). The ninth section of the bacterial pie chart is labeled "Other," and is used to represent any organism not included in one of the other eight categories. In this chapter, the pie chart is used to illustrate the spectra of bacteria for which a particular class of antibiotics is therapeutically effective.] The general mechanisms of action and antibacterial spectra of the major groups of antibiotics are presented below.

A. Penicillins

The penicillins are β-lactam antibiotics, named after the β-lactam ring that is essential to their activity. Penicillins selectively interfere with the synthesis of the bacterial cell wall (see p. 113)—a structure not found in mammalian cells. Penicillins are inactive against organisms devoid of a peptidoglycan cell wall, such as mycoplasma, protozoa, fungi, and viruses. To be maximally effective, penicillins require actively proliferating bacteria; they have little or no effect on bacteria that are not dividing. Their action is usually bactericidal (the bacteria die, see p. 33). The penicillins are the most widely effective antibiotics. For example, penicillin G is the cornerstone of therapy for infections caused by a number of gram-positive and gram-negative cocci, gram-positive bacilli, and spirochetes (Figure 5.13). Penicillins are also among the least toxic drugs known; the major adverse reaction to penicillins is hypersensitivity. Unfortunately, many bacteria have developed resistance to these drugs.

B. Cephalosporins

The cephalosporins are β-lactam antibiotics that are closely related both structurally and functionally to the penicillins, and are also

 [1] See ***Lippincott's Illustrated Reviews: Pharmacology*** (2nd ed.) for a more detailed discussion of antimicrobial drugs.

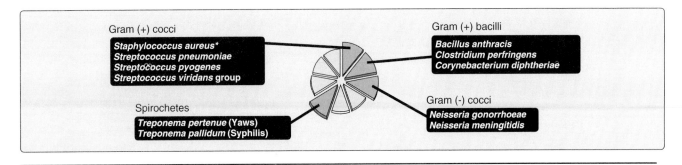

Figure 5.13
Summary of therapeutic applications of penicillin G. *Not producing β-lactamases or lacking penicillin-binding protein.

bactericidal. Cephalosporins have the same mode of action as the penicillins, but they tend to be more resistant than the penicillins to inactivation by β-lactamases produced by some bacteria. Cephalosporins are classified as first, second, third, or fourth generation, largely on the basis of bacterial susceptibility patterns and resistance to β-lactamases (see Figure 5.15). In this classification system, **first-generation** agents are active primarily against gram-positive organisms including methicillin-sensitive *Staphylococcus aureus*, and have limited activity against gram-negative bacilli. **Second-generation** agents have increased activity against gram-negative bacilli and variable activity against gram-positive cocci. **Third-generation** agents have significantly increased activity against gram-negative bacilli, with some of these agents active against *Pseudomonas aeruginosa*. [Note: Cefepime has been classified by some as **fourth-generation** because of its extended spectrum of activity against both gram-positive and gram-negative organisms that include *P. aeruginosa*.]

C. Tetracyclines

A number of antibiotics, including the tetracyclines, the aminoglycosides, and macrolides, exert their antimicrobial effects by targeting the **bacterial ribosome**, which has components that differ structurally from those of the mammalian cytoplasmic ribosomes. Binding of tetracyclines to the 30S subunit of the bacterial ribosome is believed to block access of the amino acyl-tRNA to the mRNA-ribosome complex at the acceptor site, thus inhibiting bacterial protein synthesis. Tetracyclines are **broad-spectrum antibiotics** (that is, many bacteria are sensitive to these drugs, Figure 5.14). Tetracyclines are generally **bacteriostatic** (the bacteria are prevented from multiplying, but are not killed by the drug, see p. 33).

D. Aminoglycosides

Aminoglycosides inhibit bacterial protein synthesis. Susceptible organisms have an oxygen-dependent system that transports the antibiotic across the cell membrane. All aminoglycosides are **bactericidal** (that is, the bacteria are killed). They are effective only against aerobic organisms, because anaerobes lack the oxygen-requiring transport system. Gentamicin is used to treat a variety of infectious diseases including those caused by many of the Enterobacteriaceae (see Figure 5.14), and in combination with penicillin, endocarditis caused by viridans group streptococci.

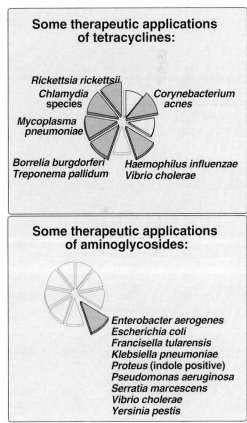

Figure 5.14
Summary of therapeutic applications of tetracyclines and aminoglycosides.

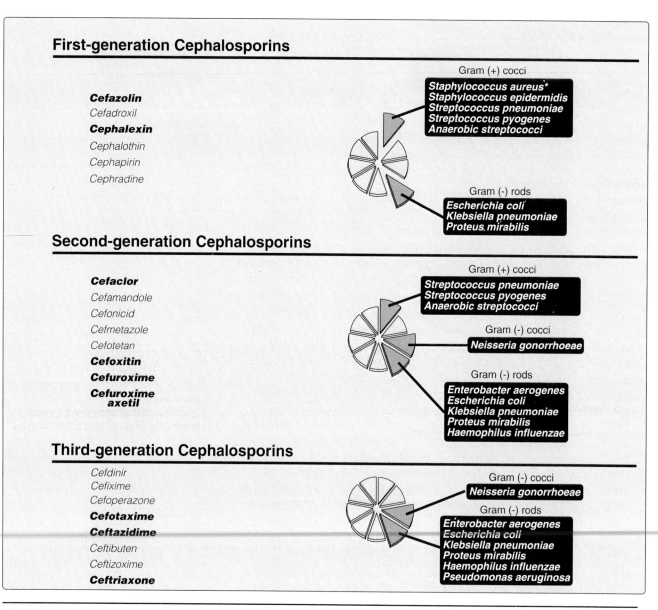

Figure 5.15
Summary of therapeutic applications of cephalosporins. The more useful drugs are shown in bold print. *Except methicillin-resistant *Staphylococcus aureus*.

E. Macrolides

The macrolides are a group of antibiotics with a macrocyclic lactone structure. Erythromycin was the first of these to find clinical application, both as the drug of first choice, and as an alternative to penicillin in individuals who are allergic to β-lactam antibiotics. Newer macrolides, such clarithromycin and azithromycin, offer extended activity against some organisms and less severe adverse reactions. The macrolides bind irreversibly to a site on the 50S subunit of the bacterial ribosome, thus inhibiting the translocation steps of protein synthesis. Generally considered to be **bacteriostatic** (see p. 33) they may be bactericidal at higher doses (Figure 5.16).

F. Fluoroquinolones

The fluoroquinolones uniquely inhibit the replication of bacterial DNA by interfering with the action of DNA gyrase (topoisomerase II[2]) during bacterial growth and reproduction. Binding of the quinolone to both the enzyme and the DNA to form a ternary complex inhibits the rejoining step, and thus can cause cell death by inducing cleavage of the DNA. Because DNA gyrase is a distinct target for antimicrobial therapy, cross-resistance with other more commonly used antimicrobial drugs is rare, but is increasing in the case of multi-drug–resistant organisms. All of the fluoroquinolones are **bactericidal**. Each quinolone drug is classified as belonging to one of four generations on the basis of its bacterial susceptibility patterns and pharmacodynamics. **First-generation** drugs (for example, nalidixic acid) are available for oral use only, and are characterized by a relatively narrow spectrum of antimicrobial activity. **Second-generation** fluoroquinolones (for example, ciprofloxacin, see Figure 5.16) can be used to treat systemic infections in addition to those localized within the urinary tract. These fluoroquinolones exhibit high intracellular penetration, allowing for the therapy of the so-called atypical organisms, such as *Chlamydia*, *Mycoplasma*, and *Legionella*. **Third-generation** drugs (for example, levofloxacin) have expanded activity against gram-positive bacteria and atypical pathogens. **Fourth-generation** quinolone drugs (such as moxifloxacin) have appreciable activity against anaerobes, such as *Bacteroides fragilis* and enhanced activity against gram-positive organisms

G. Other important antibacterial agents

1. **Vancomycin:** Vancomycin is a tricyclic glycopeptide that has become increasingly medically important because of its effectiveness against multiple drug-resistant organisms, such as methicillin-resistant staphylococci. Vancomycin inhibits synthesis of bacterial cell wall phospholipids as well as peptidoglycan polymerization at a site earlier than that inhibited by the β-lactam antibiotics. In order to curtail the increase in vancomycin-resistant bacteria (for example, *Enterococcus faecium* and *Enterococcus faecalis*), it is important to restrict its use to the treatment of serious infections caused by β-lactam–resistant gram-positive microorganisms, or for patients who have a serious allergy to the β-lactam antibiotics and who have gram-positive infections. Vancomycin is also used for potentially life-threatening antibiotic-associated colitis due to *Clostridium difficile* or staphylococci.

2. **Trimethoprim-sulfamethoxazole**, a combination called **co-trimoxazole**, shows greater antimicrobial activity than equivalent quantities of either drug used alone (Figure 5.17). The synergistic antimicrobial activity of co-trimoxazole results from its inhibition of two sequential steps in the synthesis of tetrahydrofolic acid: sulfamethoxazole inhibits the incorporation of PABA into folic acid, and trimethoprim prevents reduction of dihydrofolate to tetrahydrofolat.[3] A summary of clinically useful antimicrobial agents is found on pp. 460–464.

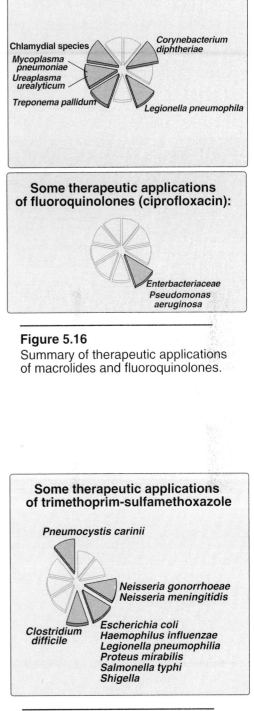

Figure 5.16
Summary of therapeutic applications of macrolides and fluoroquinolones.

Figure 5.17
Summary of therapeutic applications of trimethoprim-sulfamethoxazole.

[2]See pp. 323-324 in ***Lippincott's Illustrated Reviews: Pharmacology*** (2nd ed.) for a discussion of topoisomerases and the mechanism of action of fluoroquinolones.
[3]See p. 292 in ***Lippincott's Illustrated Reviews: Pharmacology*** (2nd ed.) for a discussion of tetrahydrofolate synthesis and co-trimoxazole.

IX. AGENTS USED IN VIRAL INFECTIONS

When viruses reproduce they utilize much of the host's own metabolic machinery. Therefore, few drugs are selective enough to prevent viral replication without injury to the host. Viruses are also not affected by antibacterial agents. Nevertheless, some drugs sufficiently discriminate between cellular and viral reactions to be effective and yet relatively nontoxic. For example, efficient management strategies are available for infections due to herpes simplex virus, varicella-zoster virus, cytomegalovirus, influenza A and B viruses, and chronic hepatitis B and C.

A. Organization of viruses

Trying to assimilate the names and characteristics of pathogenic viruses can be an overwhelming experience unless these agents are organized into logical groupings. Thus, the clinically important viruses can be conveniently divided into seven groups based on based on the nature of their genome, symmetry of organization, and the presence or absence of a lipid envelope (Figure 5.18; see also Figure 26.3, p. 296). This organization pie chart is presented throughout this book as a graphic aid in recalling the classification of the viruses. In Figure 5.19, the viral pie chart is used to summarize the therapeutic applications of selected antiviral agents, which are described below.

B. Treatment of herpesvirus infections

Most of the antiviral agents used in treating herpesvirus infections are nucleoside analogues that require conversion to mono-, di-, and triphosphate forms by either cellular kinases, viral kinases, or both to selectively inhibit viral DNA synthesis. This class of antiviral agents includes acyclovir, cidofovir, famciclovir, ganciclovir, penciclovir, valacyclovir, and vidarabine. A second class of antiviral drugs with action against herpesviruses is represented by the pyrophosphate analogue, foscarnet. Both groups of antiviral agents exert their actions during the acute phase of viral infections, and are without effect in the latent phase.

C. Treatment of acquired immunodeficiency syndrome (AIDS)

The antiretroviral drugs are divided into three main classes based on their mode of inhibition of viral replication. The first class represents the nucleoside analogues that inhibit the viral RNA-dependent DNA polymerase (reverse transcriptase) of HIV. A second class of reverse transcriptase inhibitors is non-nucleoside analogues. The third class is protease inhibitors. Therapy with these antiretroviral agents, usually in combinations (a "cocktail" of drugs referred to as **highly active anti-retroviral therapy**, or **HAART**, see p. 374), may be beneficial in prolonging survival, to reduce the incidence and severity of opportunistic infections in patients with advanced HIV disease, and to delay disease progression in asymptomatic HIV-infected patients.

D. Treatment of viral hepatitis

Prolonged (months) treatment with interferon-α has succeeded in reducing or eliminating indicators of hepatitis B virus replication in about one third of patients. However, recurrence of indications of the

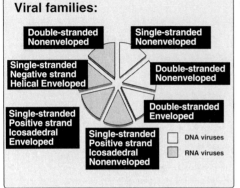

Figure 5.18
Organization of viruses into seven groups.

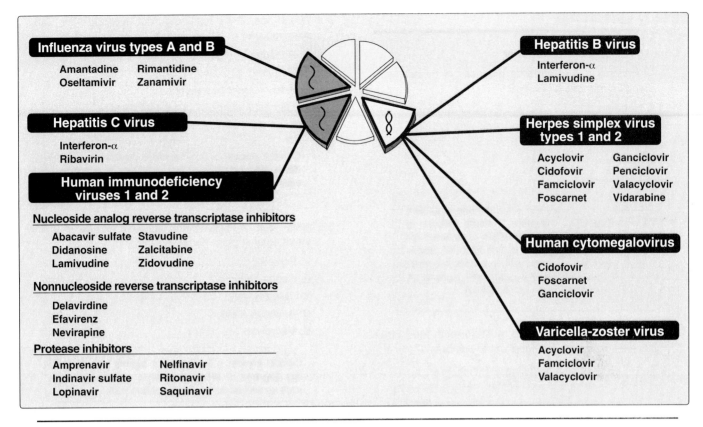

Figure 5.19
Summary of therapeutic applications of selected antiviral agents.

infection may occur after discontinuance of the therapy. Lamivudine, an oral nucleoside analogue, has been shown to be an effective treatment in patients with previously untreated chronic hepatitis B. However, only a minority of patients are cured or remain in remission after lamivudine therapy is withdrawn. Maintenance therapy may be indicated, but the long-term use of lamivudine is limited by the appearance of viral polymerase gene mutants, which leads to reemergence of disease. The therapy of choice for hepatitis C is interferon-α in combination with ribavirin. The overall rate of response to this drug combination is three times greater than that seen with interferon-α monotherapy. However, anemia is a common side-effect induced by ribavirin.

E. Treatment of influenza

First-generation antiviral agents effective against influenza A include two related drugs, amantadine and rimantidine. Both stop viral uncoating by inhibition of the viral M2 membrane protein (see p. 389). These agents reduce both the duration and the severity of flu symptoms, but only if given early in infection. Given before the onset of symptoms, these drugs can also prevent disease, and are useful for treating high-risk groups. Second-generation antiviral agents effective against influenza A and B include zanamivir and oseltamivir. They inhibit viral neuraminidase, thereby preventing the release of virus from infected cells.

Study Questions

Choose the ONE correct answer

5.1 Which one of the following diseases is treated with standard immune globulins?

A. Hepatitis B

B. Varicella

C. Rabies

D. Tetanus

E. Hepatitis A

Correct answer = E. Standard immune globlulins are not specific. Therefore, immune globulin is used for prevention or attenuation of illnesses for which there is no specific immunoglobulin preparation. This type of immunization is effective when given immediately before or after exposure to an infectious disease, such as hepatitis A.

5.2 Which one of the following most correctly describes vaccines containing live, attenuated pathogens?

A. Pathogen does not multiply in human host

B. Provides extended, sometimes life-long immunity

C. No possibility for reversion to pathogenic form

D. Provides little cell-mediated immunity

E. Administered by injection

Correct answer = B. Attenuated microbes reproduce in the recipient, typically leading to a more robust and longer-lasting immune response than can be obtained through vaccination with killed organisms.

5.3 Which one of the following best describes the components of vaccines against *Haemophilus influenzae* disease?

A. Live, attenuated *Haemophilus influenzae*

B. Killed *Haemophilus influenzae*

C. Toxoid derived from *Haemophilus influenzae*

D. Polysaccharide derived from *Haemophilus influenzae*

E. Polysaccharide derived from *Haemophilus influenzae* conjugated to a protein antigen

Correct answer = E. Covalent conjugates of capsular polysaccharide with diphtheria protein have been developed for *Haemophilus influenzae*. Unconjugated polysaccharide is weakly immunogenic in children under 2 year of age. However, the conjugated vaccine produces higher of titers of antibody, superior responsiveness in children under 2 years of age, and enhanced efficacy of booster administrations.

5.4 Which one of the following best describes the Sabin polio vaccine?

A. Provides little gastrointestinal immunity

B. Prepared with inactive virus

C. Administered by injection

D. Carries a small risk of causing disease

E. Is an example of passive immunity

Correct answer = D. The main disadvantage of attenuated live virus is the small risk of infection, estimated to be 1 per 2.4 million doses.

5.5 Which one of the following antibiotic groups is mainly active against gram-negative rods?

A. Penicillins

B. Cephalosporins

C. Tetracyclines

D. Aminoglycosides

E. Macrolides

Correct answer = D. The other agents have varying degrees of efficacy against gram-negative rods as well as some gram-positive rods.

5.6 A 25-year-old woman whose blood tested positive for hepatitis B surface antigen (HBsAg) gave birth to a full-term child. Which of the following therapies would be most likely to minimize the transmission of hepatitis B to the neonate?

A. Administer hepatitis B immunoglobulin

B. Administer hepatitis B vaccine

C. Administer hepatitis B immunoglobulin and hepatitis B vaccine.

D. Bottle-feed the neonate

E. Administer lamivudine, a drug used in the treatment of chronic hepatitis B.

Correct answer = C. Infants born to infected mothers are given hepatitis B immunoglobulin plus hepatitis B vaccine at birth, followed by additional doses of vaccine at one and six months. [Note: The two injections must be given at separate anatomical sites to prevent injected hepatitis B immunoglobulin from neutralizing the injected vaccine.] Perinatal infection of the neonate occurs at the time of delivery, and is not related to consumption of breast milk. Lamivudine is not indicated for prophylaxis in the neonate.

The Innate Immune System

6

I. OVERVIEW OF HOST DEFENSE MECHANISMS

The immune system is an interacting set of specialized cells and pro-teins designed to identify and destroy foreign invaders or abnormal substances before they can damage the body. Among the most com-monly encountered intruders are viruses, bacteria, fungi, and para-sites. For the immune system to mount a defense against foreign invaders, it must be able to tell the difference between material that is a normal component of the body ("self"), and material that is not native to the body ("nonself"). This is a remarkable achievement, because to differentiate between molecules that "belong" and those that are "for-eign," the immune system must be able to recognize billions of different structures on foreign antigens, including molecules that the body has never before encountered. The discrimination between self and non-self, and the subsequent destruction and removal of foreign material, is accomplished by the two arms of the immune system, the **innate** (or "**natural**") **immune system**, and the **adaptive** (or "**acquired**"), **specific immune system** (Figure 6.1). Some systems are fully operative the first time the body sees the foreign substance (innate immune system). Other systems require an initial exposure to the foreign substance in order to become fully active (adaptive immune system). Innate immu-nity is present in some form in all vertebrates and some invertebrates. Repeated exposure to a pathogen does not enhance the innate immune response. In contrast, the adaptive immune system (see p. 59), possessed only by vertebrates, utilizes a system of highly special-ized receptors for discriminating between self and nonself. Its response is enhanced with reexposure to the pathogen (for example, reinfection by a species of microorganism). Although it is convenient to define the immune system in terms of these two components, in reality their responsibilities overlap, and the innate and adaptive immune systems perform many of their functions by cooperative interactions. This Unit presents an overview of the immune response, containing information necessary for understanding the basic mechanisms by which the body wards off infectious pathogens.

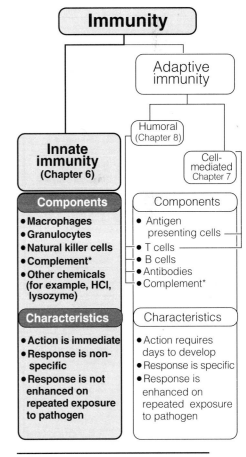

Figure 6.1
Components and characteristics of immune system. *Complement plays a role in both innate and acquired immunity; it is discussed in Chapter 8.

Lippincott's Illustrated Reviews: Microbiology,
by William A. Strohl, Harriet Rouse, Bruce D. Fisher.
Lippincott, Williams & Wilkins, Baltimore, MD © 2001

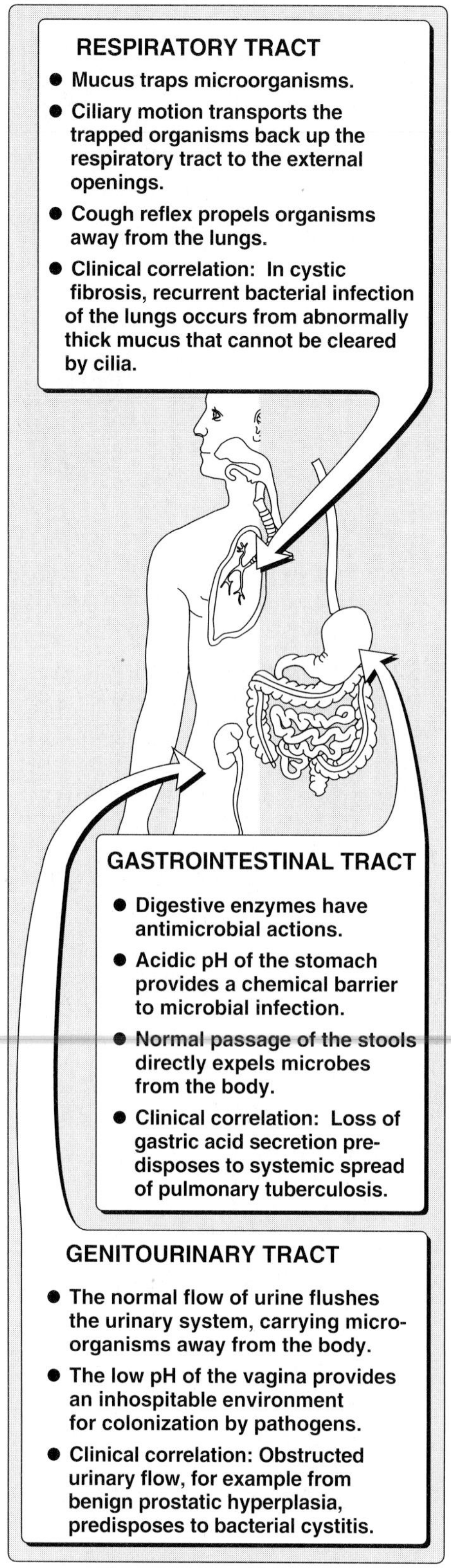

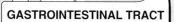

RESPIRATORY TRACT

- Mucus traps microorganisms.
- Ciliary motion transports the trapped organisms back up the respiratory tract to the external openings.
- Cough reflex propels organisms away from the lungs.
- Clinical correlation: In cystic fibrosis, recurrent bacterial infection of the lungs occurs from abnormally thick mucus that cannot be cleared by cilia.

GASTROINTESTINAL TRACT

- Digestive enzymes have antimicrobial actions.
- Acidic pH of the stomach provides a chemical barrier to microbial infection.
- Normal passage of the stools directly expels microbes from the body.
- Clinical correlation: Loss of gastric acid secretion predisposes to systemic spread of pulmonary tuberculosis.

GENITOURINARY TRACT

- The normal flow of urine flushes the urinary system, carrying microorganisms away from the body.
- The low pH of the vagina provides an inhospitable environment for colonization by pathogens.
- Clinical correlation: Obstructed urinary flow, for example from benign prostatic hyperplasia, predisposes to bacterial cystitis.

Figure 6.2
Protective components of internal body surfaces.

II. OVERVIEW OF THE INNATE IMMUNE SYSTEM

The body's first line of defense against invasion by microorganisms is the innate or "natural" immune system, which is essential for the health of an organism. Activation of the adaptive immune system following infection takes three to five days—an interval sufficient for most pathogens to damage the host. By contrast, the innate system is active at the time of infection, restraining the microorganism until the lymphocytes of the adaptive immune system can eliminate the pathogen. The innate immune system consists of protective cellular and chemical components found on the surfaces of the body, as well as a group of white blood cells and their derivatives, and plasma and interstitial proteins that offer subsurface protection. The response of the innate immune system can be divided into two stages. First, an initial, **noninflammatory reaction** occurs that depends on the body's static defenses, such as skin, gastric pH, or lysozyme in specialized body fluids such as tears, saliva, and mucus. Second, if pathogens breach these outer defenses, an **acute response** is triggered, in which local inflammation promotes the migration of phagocytes and plasma proteins into the infected tissues. The phagocytes respond to a few, highly conserved surface structures present in large groups of microorganisms, but not present in humans (such as unique lipopolysaccharides and peptidoglycans, lipoteichoic acids, and mannans). However, the phagocytes cannot always control the infection. Therefore, the continued presence of infective organisms triggers a second, more powerful line of defense, the adaptive immune system, described in Chapters 7 and 8.

III. ROLE OF EXTERNAL BODY SURFACES

The skin consists of sheets of dry, cornified epithelial cells. This barrier to bacteria and viruses is essentially impermeable unless damaged. The only portals of entry through intact skin are the hair follicles and sebaceous glands. These openings produce substances, such as fatty acids and enzymes, which have an antimicrobial effect. When combined with the acid pH of sebaceous secretions and sweat, these substances help prevent microbial infiltration. Tears, saliva, and mucus contain the enzyme **lysozyme**, which protects against infection by gram-positive (but not gram-negative) bacteria. **Commensal organisms**, the nonpathogenic microorganisms that constitute our normal microbial flora found on both external and internal body surfaces, are beneficial because they compete with potential pathogens. [Note: This balance is frequently upset during the prolonged administration of broad-spectrum antibiotics, resulting in elimination of normal flora, and subsequent overgrowth of pathogenic organisms, causing, for example, candidiasis (see p. 274) or *Clostridium difficile* infection (see p. 217).]

IV. ROLE OF INTERNAL BODY SURFACES

The normal movement of fluids and mucus is critical for clearing and cleaning the body surfaces, thus helping to prevent microbial invasion. Such mechanical factors are important in the respiratory, gastrointestinal, and genitourinary tracts (Figure 6.2). These mechanical defenses

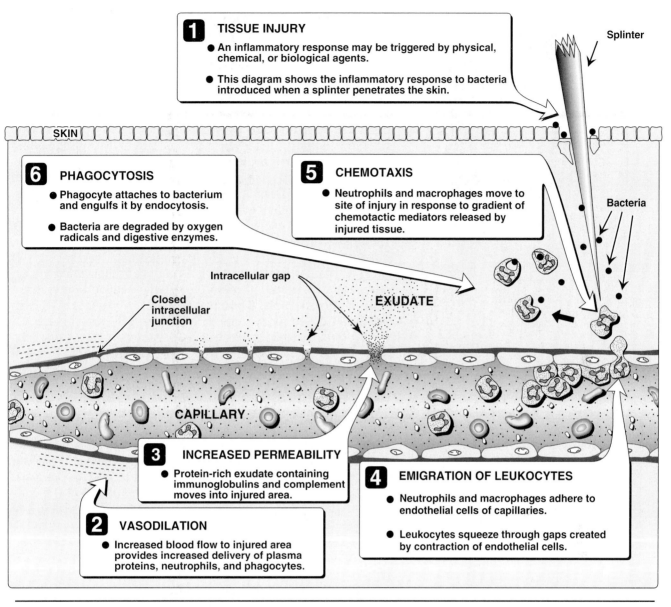

Figure 6.3
Sequence of events in acute inflammation in response to an injury, part of the innate immune response.

may be compromised by lifestyles in some individuals. For example, smoking, narcotics, and alcohol can impede the mechanisms that propel invading organisms from the lungs.

V. ACUTE INFLAMMATION RESULTING FROM INFECTION

If the surface chemical and physiologic defenses of the body are breached by a pathogen, inflammation can result. Inflammation is a local response of living tissue to injury—physical, chemical, or biological—in which the body attempts to localize and eliminate the injurious agent, eventually removing and repairing damaged tissue (Figure 6.3).

A. The inflammatory response

The inflammatory response causes the normally tight junctions between endothelial cells lining the capillaries, and between epithelial cells of the mucosal surface, to reversibly separate (see Figure 6.3). As a result, specialized cells and serum components can move from the plasma to the interstitial space to provide an immediate defense while the adaptive immune response is being mounted. Some of these cells (collectively called **phagocytes**) destroy the invading microorganism by phagocytosis followed by intracellular digestion, whereas others (**natural killer cells**) limit the infection by releasing compounds toxic to microorganisms. [Note: The inflammatory response is nonspecific, because it does not require a prior exposure to the pathogen; essentially the same response is triggered by a wide variety of agents, including microorganisms, chemicals, physical agents, or the presence of necrotic tissue.] Inflammation is also accompanied by an increased concentration of serum proteins called **acute-phase proteins**. For example, **C-reactive protein** is a major acute-phase protein produced by the liver in response to tissue damage. C-reactive protein binds to the cell walls of bacteria and fungi, and activates the **complement system**—a group of serum proteins that participate in an enzymatic cascade, resulting in the opsonization and lysis of pathogenic organisms (see p. 90).

B. Cell types active during acute inflammation

Innate immunity is mediated by a diverse group of cells. For example, in bacterial infections, **neutrophils** are the first line of cellular defense. They are the predominant cell to invade infected tissues in the first 24 to 48 hours, because neutrophils are abundant in the circulation, and are more mobile than monocytes. After one to two days, the neutrophils are replaced by **macrophages**. Cells participating in the inflammatory response include the following (Figure 6.4).

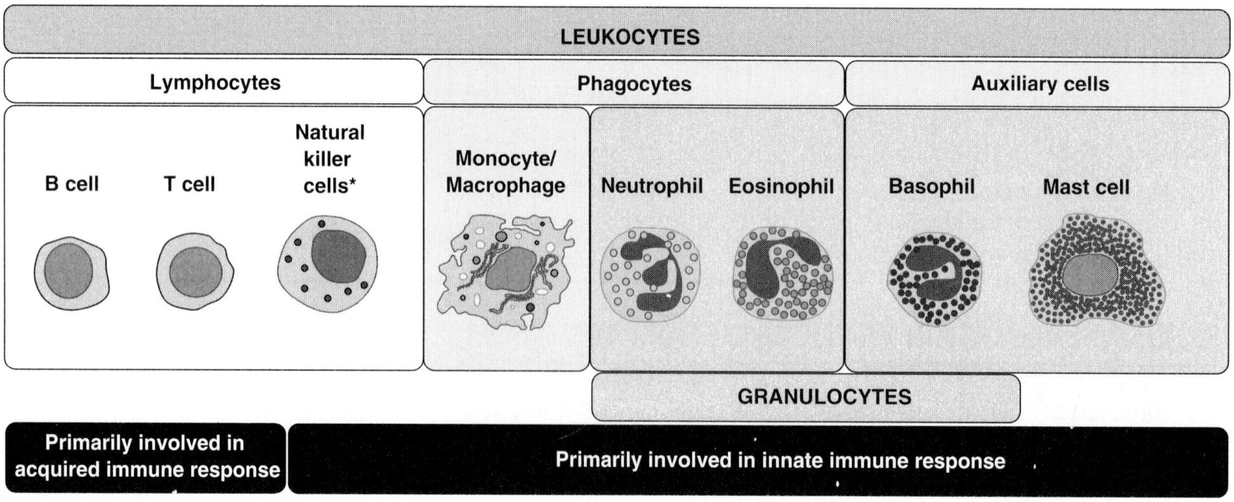

Figure 6.4
Major cell types involved in the immune response. *Natural killer cells are large, granular lymphocytes.

1. **Neutrophils:** Neutrophils, eosinophils, and basophils are **polymorphonuclear leukocytes** (also called **granulocytes**). Neutrophils (and monocytes) are armed with both oxygen-dependent and oxygen-independent mechanisms for killing bacteria. Neutrophils and macrophages have receptors for antibodies and complement so that microorganisms coated with these opsonins are more easily phagocytized.

2. **Macrophages:** Macrophages are large leukocytes that display receptors for molecules not normally exposed on the surfaces of vertebrate cells (for example, mannose). They thus have the ability (although very limited) to discriminate between "foreign" and "self" molecules. Macrophages also act as indiscriminate scavengers, engulfing and digesting broken pieces of the body's own cells, and even bits of dust and pollen that may enter the body through the lungs. They are produced from monocytes—phagocytic agranular leukocytes found in the peripheral blood. Macrophages enter the connective tissue spaces throughout the body, where they can differentiate and divide, creating the **monocyte/macrophage system** (formerly called the **reticuloendothelial system**). Unlike neutrophils, which live for only one to two days, mature macrophages live in the body's tissues for months. Figure 6.5 shows selected properties of neutrophils and macrophages.

3. **Eosinophils:** Although neutrophils are the key cells involved in most acute inflammatory reactions, there are some exceptions. For example, eosinophils are the dominant cells in allergic reactions, and reactions against invasive helminthic infections. [Note: **Eosinophilia** is a clinical characteristic of visceral larva migrans.]

4. **Basophils and mast cells:** These cells both have high-affinity receptors for IgE, and become coated with IgE antibodies. They are important in allergies in which allergens bind to surface-bound IgE molecules.

5. **Natural killer (NK) cells:** These cells are large, nonphagocytic, granular lymphocytes that destroy abnormal host cells, such as those that are virus-infected or neoplastic. [Note: Viral infection or neoplastic transformation of a cell can induce loss of class I major histocompatability molecule (MHC) expression (see p. 65). NK cells recognize and kill cells that appear to lack class I MHC molecules.] Target cell killing is accomplished by the NK cell release of compounds that have a variety of cytotoxic effects, including causing the formation of pores in the membrane of a target cell resulting in osmotic lysis, or triggering **apoptosis** (programmed cell death), leading to a more rapid cell death (see p, 75). NK cells can also induce apoptosis through surface contact with the target cell. The cytotoxic actions of natural killer cells are stimulated by interferons and interleukin-2 (IL-2). [Note: Cytotoxic T lymphocytes (see p. 63) that participate in the adaptive immune response are also characterized as killer cells. They appear later than the natural killer cells, at a time when the adaptive response has been mounted. Cytotoxic T lymphocytes kill target cells using mechanisms identical to those used by NK cells.]

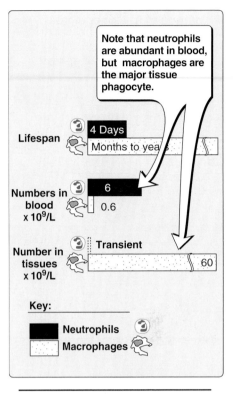

Figure 6.5
Comparison of neutrophils and macrophages.

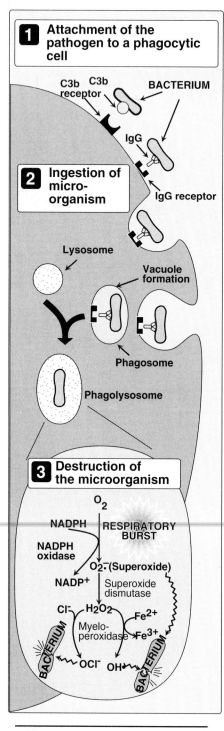

1 Attachment of the pathogen to a phagocytic cell

C3b receptor   C3b   BACTERIUM

IgG

2 Ingestion of micro-organism

IgG receptor

Lysosome

Vacuole formation

Phagosome

Phagolysosome

3 Destruction of the microorganism

O_2

NADPH   RESPIRATORY BURST

NADPH oxidase

O_2^- (Superoxide)

$NADP^+$ Superoxide dismutase

Cl^- H_2O_2 Fe^{2+}

Myelo-peroxidase Fe^{3+}

BACTERIUM

OCl^- $OH\cdot$ BACTERIUM

Figure 6.6
Neutrophil phagocytosis and the oxygen dependent myeloperoxidase system of killing.

VI. ROLE OF PHAGOCYTOSIS

Phagocytosis is part of the innate immune response, during which microorganisms, foreign particles, and cellular debris are engulfed by phagocytic cells such as neutrophils and monocytes in the circulation, and macrophages and neutrophils in interstitial spaces. It is an important defense mechanism, particularly during bacterial infections. Phagocytosis consists of three stages: 1) attachment of the microorganisms or foreign material to the phagocytic cell; 2) ingestion by the cell; and 3) degradation of the foreign material or microorganism within the phagocytic cells (Figure 6.6).

A. Attachment of the pathogen to a phagocytic cell

Phagocytosis is activated when a phagocyte attacks a target bacterium that has invaded the epithelial or mucosal layer. The binding process is enhanced when the invading organism is covered by IgG immunoglobulins, and/or the complement component C3b, a process called **opsonization** (see p. 94). [Note: Neutrophils and monocytes possess membrane receptors for these opsonizing agents, thus causing enhanced bacterial attachment to the phagocytes' cell membranes.]

B. Ingestion of foreign material or microorganisms

Following attachment to the cell membrane, a microorganism or foreign particle is engulfed by pseudopodia, and drawn into the cell by endocytosis. Once internalized, the bacteria are trapped within phagocytic vacuoles (**phagosomes**) in the cytoplasm. [Note: Phagosomes are visible as clear spaces within neutrophils and monocytes on Wright-Giemsa–stained peripheral smear, and provide direct evidence that phagocytosis has occurred.]

C. Destruction of the foreign material or microorganism

The phagosome containing the material to be destroyed fuses with a granule-containing lysosome, generating a **phagolysosome** (see Figure 6.6). Oxygen-dependent mechanisms for killing invading bacteria within the phagolysosome include 1) the formation of superoxide radicals ($O_2\cdot^-$) catalyzed by NADPH oxidase, 2) the formation of hypochlorite ion (OCl^-) catalyzed by myeloperoxidase (MPO)[1], and 3) spontaneous formation of hydroxyl radicals ($OH\cdot$). All of these compounds are highly toxic to most microorganisms. This process results in a transient increase in oxygen uptake, sometimes referred to as the **respiratory burst**. Oxygen-independent mechanisms destroy pathogens by pH changes in the phagolysosomes, and by digestion of the intruder using lysosomal enzymes (for example, proteases, hydrolases, and nucleases) obtained from the lysosomal granules. Also located in these granules are additional bactericidal proteins such as **bactericidal/permeability-increasing protein** (a cationic protein deposited onto bacterial surfaces). Overall, the MPO system is the most potent of these bactericidal mechanisms.

VII. THE MONOCYTE/MACROPHAGE SYSTEM

Monocytes enter the blood, and differentiate after they reach the capillaries of a particular tissue. These differentiated forms include **alveolar**

[1]See p. 115 in *Lippincott's Illustrated Reviews: Biochemistry* (2nd ed.) for a discussion of myeloperoxidase and phagocytosis.

macrophages in the lung, **Kupffer cells** in the liver, **microglial cells** in the CNS, **peritoneal macrophages** that float free in peritoneal fluid, and **splenic macrophages** in the spleen. Collectively, they are part of the widely-distributed **monocyte/ macrophage system** that is responsible for trapping and phagocytizing foreign substances (including microorganisms) in the bloodstream and tissues, thus serving an important function in the innate immune response. Macrophages continue to ingest foreign particles (Figure 6.7 shows a macrophage attacking a bacterium) until toxic substances from an ingested pathogen—or from the phagocytic process itself—kill the cells. [Note: Ingested bacteria, such as *Mycobacterium tuberculosis* (see p. 246), that resist attack may continue to live within the macrophage, which may travel by the lymphatic system to other tissues. Macrophages therefore can be an inadvertent vehicle for disseminating bacteria throughout the body.] Phagocytes act as effector cells for both the adaptive as well as the innate immune response systems. For example, the cells of the monocyte/macrophage system also function as antigen-presenting cells that display processed peptide fragments of antigens to specific T cells, thus causing T cell activation (see p. 63).

VIII. PHAGOCYTE DEFICIENCY OR DYSFUNCTION

Disorders of phagocytes involve an absolute decrease in granulocyte number (neutropenia), and/or decreased phagocyte (granulocyte and macrophage) function. Immunodeficiencies caused by primary (genetic) deficiencies or dysfunctions of phagocytes are rare. However, immunodeficiencies that occur secondary to another disease or physiologic insult are more common, for example, neutropenia caused by anti-cancer chemotherapeutic agents that suppress the bone marrow production of leukocytes, red blood cells, and platelets. Conditions that lead to phagocyte deficiency or dysfunction include the following.

A. Chronic granulomatous disease (CGD)

CGD is a group of disorders, most of which are X-linked recessive, with some that are autosomal recessive. They are characterized by a deficiency in the ability to mount an intracellular respiratory burst in phagocytes that have ingested bacteria. NADPH oxidase is the enzyme missing or defective in this disorder (Figure 6.8); this leads to decreased killing of phagocytized pathogens, especially catalase-positive bacteria (see p. 26). The intracellular survival of the bacterium results in the formation of a granuloma consisting of mononuclear cells. Symptoms occur by two years of age, with patients suffering from recurrent opportunistic infections, primarily involving bacteria and fungi. Treatment consists of broad-spectrum antibiotics and antifungal agents. Interferon-γ injections to activate phagocytes improve the clinical course of CGD.

B. Chediak-Higashi syndrome

In this autosomal recessive disorder, a defect of neutrophil lysosomes results in an inability to destroy invading pathogens. It is characterized by neutropenia and giant lysosomes located in granular inclusions. T cell and B cell functions are normal. Patients suffer from recurrent infections with pyogenic (pus-forming) bacteria such as staphylococci and streptococci.

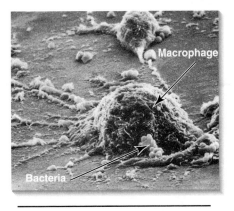

Figure 6.7
Scanning electron micrograph shows macrophages on the surface of peritoneal-dialysis catheters after the device was removed because of infectious complications.
A macrophage with pseudopodias is scavenging scattered clumps of bacteria.

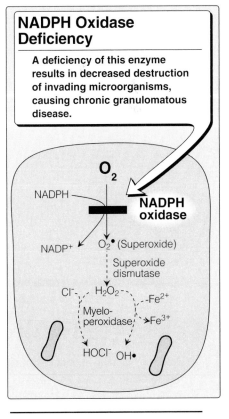

NADPH Oxidase Deficiency

A deficiency of this enzyme results in decreased destruction of invading microorganisms, causing chronic granulomatous disease.

Figure 6.8
NADPH oxidase deficiency.

Study Questions

Choose the ONE correct answer

6.1 Which one of the following is NOT a characteristic of the innate immune system?

A. It acts immediately or within hours of appropriate stimulus.

B. It involves granulocytes.

C. Its response is enhanced on repeated exposure to pathogen.

D. It involves one type of large, granular lymphocytes.

E. It involves macrophages.

> Correct answer = C. The response of the innate immune system is not enhanced on repeated exposure to pathogen (that is, it does not have a memory component). The innate immune system acts immediately (or within hours), and involves granulocytes, natural killer cells, and macrophages.

6.2 Which one of the following most correctly describes natural killer (NK) cells?

A. NK cells kill susceptible cells by phagocytosis and intracellular destruction.

B. NK cells target primarily extracellular bacteria.

C. NK cells are a subset of granulocytes.

D. NK cells are a subtype of lymphocytes.

E. The number of NK cells increases in response to specific antigen.

> Correct answer = D. NK cells are large, non-phagocytic, granular lymphocytes that destroy abnormal host cells, such as those that are virus-infected or neoplastic. Target cell killing is accomplished extracellularly by the NK cell's release of compounds that have a variety of cytotoxic effects. These effects include causing the formation of pores in the membrane of a target cell resulting in osmotic lysis, or triggering apoptosis.

6.3 Which one of the following statements concerning leukocytes is correct?

A. All phagocytes are granulocytes.

B. No cells of the innate immune system are lymphocytes.

C. Eosinophils are reactive against invasive helminthic infections.

D. Neutrophils have a longer lifespan than macrophages.

E. Macrophages are more abundant in the blood than tissue.

> Ccorrect answer = C. Eosinophils are the dominant cells in allergic reactions, and reactions against invasive helminthic infections. Phagocytes/monocytes are not granulocytes. The innate immune system involves natural killer cells, a large, granular lymphocyte. Neutrophils have a shorter lifespan than macrophages. Macrophages are more abundant in the tissues.

6.4 A one-year-baby is admitted to the hospital for evaluation of recurrent fungal diaper rash and staphylococcal furuncles. Physical examination revealed chronic lymphadenopathy, mild hepatomegaly, and splenomegaly. These clinical features suggested a tentative diagnosis of chronic granulomatous disease. Which of the following best describes the phagocytes of this patient?

A. Phagocytosis is accompanied by a respiratory burst.

B. NADPH oxidase activity is elevated

C. Phagocytosis produces reactive oxygen intermediates.

D. Ingested bacteria show increased intracellular survival.

E. Phagocytosis activates the hexose monophosphate shunt.

> Correct choice = D. Chronic granulomatous disease is characterized by a deficiency in the ability to mount an intracellular respiratory burst, and the decreased production of reactive oxygen intermediates in phagocytes that have ingested bacteria. NADPH oxidase is the enzyme missing or defective in this disorder. This leads to decreased killing of phagocytized pathogens, and to increased intracellular survival. Because NADPH is not consumed, the NADPH-generating hexose monophate shunt remains dormant.

T Cells and Cell-mediated Immunity

7

I. OVERVIEW

In many ways the immune system can be thought of as the body's security force. The innate immune system (see Chapter 6) is like the local police, providing immediate, nonspecific protection from all types of intruders. The local officer may not be able to fully restore order in all situations, but at least is immediately available, and can attempt to take charge until highly trained and specific reinforcements—provided by the adaptive immune system—can arrive. The adaptive immune system is more specific, dealing with unique invaders, much like a specialized force, such as a bomb squad or hostage rescue team. The specific security forces of the adaptive immune system are not immediately available, but can be summoned as needed. **Adaptive (acquired) immunity**, therefore, develops only after an individual has been exposed to a specific pathogen or other foreign material. The adaptive response is slower to develop than the innate response, but it is more powerful, because it targets specific pathogens and exhibits memory (that is, a subsequent confrontation with the same antigen produces a more rapid and intense immune response, often leading to life-long protection against many infectious agents). Adaptive immunity can be divided into humoral and cell-mediated responses (Figure 7.1). **Humoral immunity** results from the actions of soluble molecules, such as antibodies, in the body fluids. **Cell-mediated immunity**—the focus of this chapter—involves specialized lymphocytes and antigen presenting cells.

II. IMMUNOLOGY MAP

Before the details of cellular immunity are presented, it will be helpful to develop an overview of how humans identify and eliminate foreign (and potentially dangerous) molecules. The adaptive immune system can be described in terms of five fundamental processes: 1) cell maturation of participating lymphocytes; 2) processing of the nonself antigens; 3) recognition of antigenic epitopes; 4) clonal expansion of responding effector cells; and 5) elimination of foreign antigen by effector cells or molecules. These processes involve interactions between T cells, B cells, antigen-presenting cells, antibodies, and complement, as well as with the innate immune response, ultimately producing a complex web of interactions. As an aid to the reader, the authors have created a summary map that illustrates the interactions of the various components, and helps orient the reader as to where new information fits in the "big picture." Figure 7.2 previews the organization of the map, and the symbols used throughout the immunolgy unit.

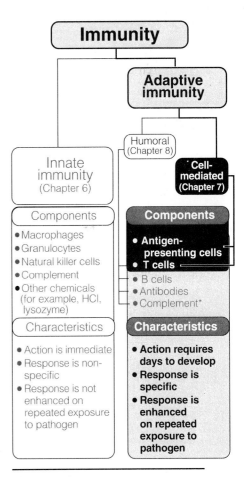

Figure 7.1
Components and characteristics of the immune system highlighting cell-mediated immunity featured in this chapter. *Complement plays a role in both innate and acquired immunity; it is discussed in Chapter 8.

Lippincott's Illustrated Reviews: Microbiology, by William A. Strohl, Harriet Rouse, Bruce D. Fisher. Lippincott, Williams & Wilkins, Baltimore, MD © 2001

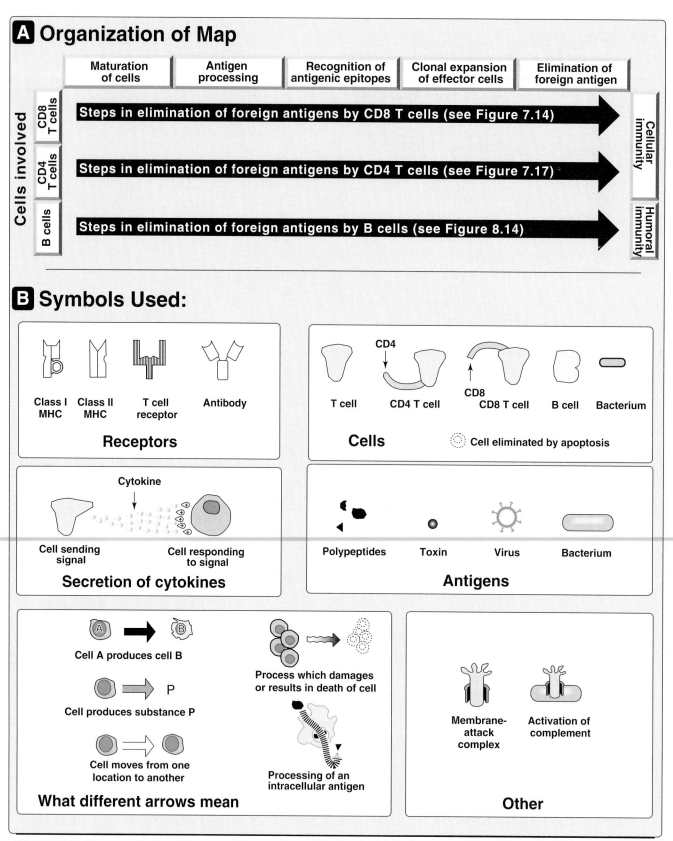

Figure 7.2
A. Organization of the Map. B. Symbols used in the Immunology Map. [Note: Relative size of cells and molecules are not drawn to scale.]

III. COMPONENTS OF THE ADAPTIVE IMMUNE SYSTEM

Generation of an immune response evolves from the actions of two major groups of cells: lymphocytes and antigen-presenting cells (Figure 7.1). Two types of lymphocytes, B cells and T cells, are the backbone of the adaptive immune system, acting as the body's sentries, and alerting the immune system when intruders invade the blood or tissues. Both T cells and B cells possess specialized receptors that are responsible for the antigen-specific responses and "**immunologic memory**" that are characteristic of the adaptive immune response. Transmembrane antibody oriented to the outside of the cell surface serves as the B cell receptor. T cells display on their surfaces T cell receptors (TCRs) that are analogous in structure to the B cell receptors, but are derived from unique sets of genes. [Note: Whereas antibodies are divalent (see p. 81), TCRs see only a single antigen peptide at a time.] The acquired immune response involves the proliferation of antigen-specific B and T cells, which occurs when the surface receptors of these cells bind to antigens. A brief overview of B and T cells and antigen-presenting cells follows. A more detailed description of the functions of these cells is provided later in this chapter, and in Chapter 8.

A. T cells

The first major group of lymphocytes, the T cells, plays a key role in **cell-mediated immunity**, by which **intracellular pathogens**, such as viruses or intracellular bacteria, are destroyed. T cells also activate phagocytes, causing them to efficiently degrade **phagocytized pathogens** such as fungi, obtained from the extracellular space. There are several different types of T cells, each performing a distinct function. These include **killer (cytotoxic) T cells** that specialize in identifying and killing cells infected with viruses, and **helper T**

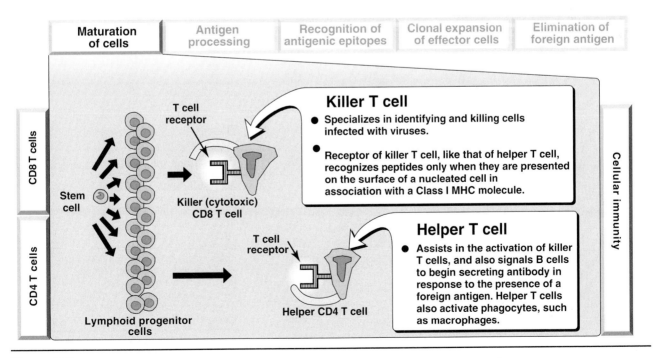

Figure 7.3
T cells with their antigen-recognizing receptors highlighted. The difference between CD4 and CD8 cells is presented on p. 68.

cells, which assist in the activation of killer T cells, and also signal B cells to begin secreting antibody in response to the presence of a foreign antigen. T cells do not secrete antibodies, but like B cells, they contain **cell surface receptors (TCRs,** Figure 7.3). Each receptor responds specifically to a unique peptide fragment of the pathogen. This antigen-derived peptide is not recognized free in solution, but rather is presented to the T cell in association with specialized proteins—major histocompatibility (MHC) molecules—contained on the surface of antigen-presenting cells such as activated macrophages. Each of the more than 10^{10} types of T cells and B cells has a unique receptor, thus making possible the extraordinary specificity and power of the adaptive immune response. T cell deficiency, such as is seen in AIDS patients, predisposes to infection with opportunistic pathogens such as cytomegalovirus, herpes virus, candida, and *Pneumocystis carinii.*

B. B cells

The second major group of lymphocytes, the B cells, mediate **humoral immunity,** by which **extracellular pathogens** (for example, bacteria, and viruses in their viremic phase) are eliminated. Each B cell produces antibody that is not secreted by the cell, but rather is a trans-membrane protein that functions as the B cell receptor (Figure 7.4). These receptors identify unique, antibody-binding motifs of antigens, called **epitopes** (or **antigenic determinants**). Epitopes can be thought of as the immunologically active region on a complex antigen—the part of the molecule that actually fits the B cell receptor, much as a lock does a key. Note that B cells bind unprocessed antigens (protein, carbohydrate, lipid, or nucleic acid) independent of antigen-presenting cells, whereas T cells recognize only peptides, and then only when they are presented on the surface of antigen-presenting cells in association with a MHC molecule. The recognition of a foreign antigen by the B cell receptor, coupled with a signal

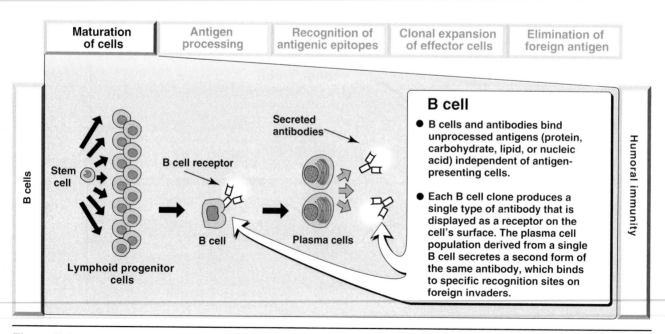

Figure 7.4
B cells and secreted antibodies with their antigen-recognizing receptors highlighted.

from helper T cells (see p.72), prompts the B cell to divide into many genetically identical **plasma cells**, called a **clone**. This plasma cell population, derived from a single B cell, produces antibodies with the same specificity as that of the B cell receptor. These antibodies bind to a specific recognition site on foreign invaders, resulting in 1) blocking the pathogen's binding to mucosa or target cells, 2) inactivating the virus, 3) direct opsonization of the pathogen, and/or 4) initiating complement activation and release of C3b (see p. 91) leading to opsonization, thus marking the pathogens for destruction by phagocytes. B cell deficiency predisposes to infection with encapsulated organisms like *Streptococcus pneumoniae* and *Haemophilus influenzae type b*.

C. Antigen-presenting cells

Antigen-presenting cells, which include macrophages, B cells, and dendritic cells (see p. 76), are equipped with specialized cell membrane proteins called the major histocompatibility complex (MHC, see p. 65). Antigen-presenting cells first phagocytize and partially degrade foreign molecules, then display a fragment of the peptide antigen in a cleft on the MHC molecules on their membrane. T cells recognize the antigen when it is bound by the MHC on the membrane of the antigen-presenting cell. This identification of a foreign antigen then triggers a cytotoxic or cytokine T cell response (see p. 74).

D. Cytokines

Information exchange between cells is afforded both by the direct interaction of molecules such as glycoproteins on cellular membranes of various immune cells, and by chemical signals or messengers called cytokines. Cytokines are soluble, antigen-nonspecific proteins that bind to cell surface receptors on a variety of cells (Figure 7.5). Cytokines usually function locally; thus, in some instances, the cell that secretes the cytokine also responds to that cytokine (**autocrine response**). In other cases, adjacent cells may respond to the cytokine (**paracrine response**). Cytokines are secreted by many different cell types, and affect not only the function of cells of the immune system, but also other systems in the body. The term cytokine includes the molecules known as **interleukins** (IL), **interferons** (IFN), **tumor necrosis factors** (TNF), **transforming growth factors** (TGF), and **colony-stimulating factors** (CSF). Cytokines and cytokine antagonists are being used in the treatment of immune deficiency disorders, cancer, and autoimmune diseases. Figure 7.5 summarizes the major functions of some of these compounds.

Cytokine	Actions
IL-1	• Enhances activity of NK cells • Attracts neutrophils and macrophages
IL-2	• Induces proliferation of antigen-primed T cells • Enhances activity of NK cells
IFN-γ	• Enhances activity of macrophages and NK cells • Increases expression of MHC molecules • Enhances production of IgG$_{2a}$
TNF-α	• Cytotoxic effect on tumor cells • Induces cytokine secretion in the inflammatory response

Figure 7.5
Summary of selected cytokines.

IV. LYMPHOID TISSUES AND ORGANS

Hematopoietic bone marrow stem cells give rise to all blood cells, including the lymphoid progenitor cells. Lymphocyte maturation, differentiation, and proliferation take place in the lymphatic organs. These include the primary lymphoid tissues and organs (the thymus gland in which T lymphocytes develop, and the bone marrow, in which B lymphocytes develop), and the secondary lymphoid tissues and organs (of which the spleen and lymph nodes are the most important), where mature lymphocytes encounter and respond to foreign antigens.

A. Primary lymphoid tissues and organs

Lymphoid tissues and organs are defined as primary because they include the sites where T and B lymphocyte production and initial maturation occur, prior to an encounter with an antigen.

1. **Thymus gland:** The bone marrow produces thymocyte precursors that travel to the thymus gland. The thymus gland consists of epithelial cells organized into a cortex and medulla, both of which are infiltrated with thymocytes. The conversion of thymocytes into mature lymphocytes occurs predominantly during fetal development until adolescence, when the thymus atrophies. [Note: Thymocyte development can still occur to a limited degree even after the thymus has atrophied.] Thymocytes differentiate in the cortex into subpopulations, characterized by specific surface glycoproteins (for example, CD3, plus CD4 and CD8, see p. 69). The T cells migrating to the medulla lose either CD4 or CD8 expression, thus becoming only singly CD4 or CD8 positive. They then enter the peripheral blood, which carries them to the secondary lymphoid organs, where antigen-driven T cell proliferation and further differentiation take place (see p. 67).

2. **Bone marrow:** B lymphocytes develop and mature in the bone marrow, and then travel by the blood stream to the secondary lymphoid organs. A mature B cell has cell-surface, antigen-specific receptors (antibodies) that have the same target specificity as do the antibodies that the cell will eventually secrete in response to a foreign antigen.

B. Secondary lymphoid tissues and organs

The secondary lymphoid tissues include the spleen, lymph nodes, and mucosa-associated lymphoid tissues. Within these tissues, mature T and B cells congregate, waiting for the appearance of nonself antigens. These antigens can be introduced by invading bacteria or other pathogens, or by modification of the surface of a host cell, for example, by infection with a virus.

1. **Spleen:** This organ is highly effective at removing foreign substances and damaged blood cell elements (for example, platelets and aged red blood cells) present in the circulation. The spleen thus serves as the "oil filter" of the circulation. It is also the site where many of the antibodies directed against foreign substances are synthesized. The spleen is organized into red pulp and white pulp, the latter being primarily found surrounding small arterioles (Figure 7.6). White pulp is very rich in lymphoid cells, approximately fifty percent of the lymphocytes consisting of mature B cells located in the follicles, and 35 percent consisting of mature T cells located in the periarteriolar sheet. Cells in the white pulp are ready to respond by differentiating and dividing when a foreign antigen is encountered. Splenectomy removes a large mass of otherewise antigen-responsive B cells, and thus makes containment and clearance of infections by certain encapsulated organisms like *Streptococcus pneumoniae*, and gram-negative organisms such as *Salmonella*, more difficult.

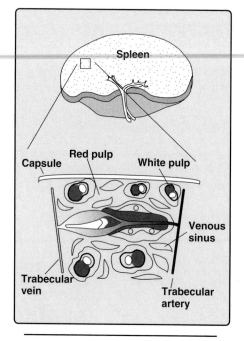

Figure 7.6
Schematic view of spleen.

2. **Lymph nodes:** These structures are located in numerous regions throughout the body. They are like "mini oil filters" that clear materials from the tissues that drain to the lymph nodes. A lymph node consists of a cortex and a medulla. The cortex contains primary lymphocytic follicles where B cells are located, and paracortical areas around the follicles where T cells are located (Figure 7.7). Following stimulation by antigen, the follicles form germinal centers containing large numbers of B cells undergoing cell division. [Note: Follicles lacking germinal centers are termed **"primary follicles"**, whereas follicles containing germinal centers are termed **"secondary" follicles**.] The medullary cords contain macrophages, and also **plasma cells** (the end-stage cell form of the B cell that migrated from the cortex, and, after contact with antigen and assistance from T cells, is able to produce antibodies). The macrophages (and other antigen-presenting cells) engulf and process the foreign antigens, and then present them to T cells. Those T cells that are specifically able to recognize the antigenic peptide undergo activation and subsequent cell division. Thus, exposure of B and T cells to a foreign antigen in the lymph node results in the release of antigen-specific antibodies and T cells into the lymphatic fluid. This fluid, carrying the antibodies and cells, exits the lymph node through the efferent lymphatic vessel, and proceeds to the systemic circulation through the thoracic duct.

3. **Mucosa-associated, secondary lymphoid tissues:** In addition to the spleen and lymph nodes, there are several other sites where lymphocytes interact with antigen and differentiate in order to produce antibodies, or become activated T cells. These secondary lymphoid tissues defend mucosal surfaces and are located at sites where the body is most likely to encounter pathogens, for example, the tonsils and adenoids. The largest percentage of lymphocytes in the body are located along the mucosal surfaces of the intestine in Peyer's patches.

V. THE MAJOR HISTOCOMPATIBILITY COMPLEX

As previously noted (see p. 62), the major histocompatibility complex (MHC) is a group of cell-surface proteins that are coded for by the MHC genes. MHC proteins play a pivotal role in "presenting" antigens to T cells. In fact, T cells do not respond to foreign peptides unless the antigen peptides are properly "presented" (that is, offered in combination with a MHC molecule). [Note: In humans, the MHC is called the **human leukocyte antigen (HLA) complex**.] Unlike most proteins that have a fixed, defined structure, key amino acid sequences in the MHC proteins vary widely from person to person, and thus they act as "identity markers" on the surface of cells. Interestingly, these proteins were first detected by their effect on transplant rejection (that is, tissue incompatibility).

A. Function of the MHCs

MHC molecules have the function of binding and forming a complex with small peptide fragments derived from cleavage of foreign antigens that contain a protein component. The MHC–peptide fragment complex is presented on the cell surface. There the complex can be

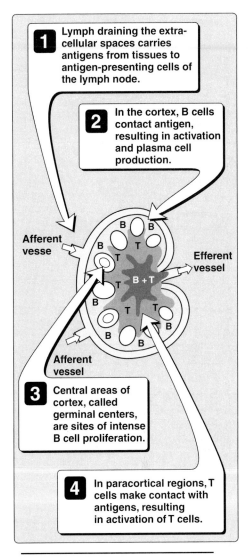

Figure 7.7
Schematic diagram of a lymph node.

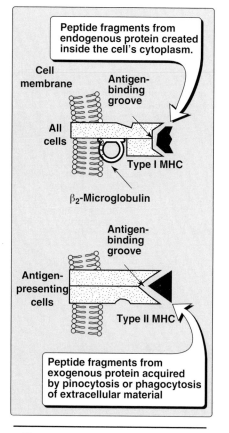

Figure 7.8
Schematic diagram of major histocompatability complex (MHC) molecules.

recognized by a T cell with the correct receptor, which identifies a composite of the foreign peptide and the MHC. This process is often referred to as "recognizing the antigen in the context of self". The presence of the MHC molecule, in effect, reassures the T cell that the antigen is being presented by a host (self) cell, whereas the foreign peptide acts as a marker alerting the T cell to the nature of the invader. Each MHC binds a collection of unique peptide sequences, each of which fits into the antigen-binding groove of the MHC molecule. This specificity is due to differences in the structure and charge of the MHC cleft. Thus it is highly probable that the degradation of a protein antigen will result in at least one peptide fragment that will bind to one of the available MHCs, and thereby stimulate a T cell response. Compounds that are not peptides, or peptides that cannot bind to any MHC, are only able to elicit an immune response with the assistance of a carrier (that is, they are haptens, see p. 79).

B. Classes of MHC molecules

There are two classes of MHC molecules that combine with peptides and present them to T cells: **class I**, which presents peptides from proteins made inside the cell, such as those produced during a viral infection, and **class II**, which presents peptides from extracellular and intravesicular proteins (including those derived from pathogenic organisms) that have entered a cell via phagocytosis or pinocytosis (Figure 7.8). [Note: Examples of extracellular pathogens include bacteria, fungi, and the non–cell-associated viremic phase of a viral infection. Pathogens that live in the intravesicular space include *Mycobacterium tuberculosis*.] Both class I and class II MHC molecules are two-chain, transmembrane proteins, each of which has a unique, extracellular cleft that serves as the peptide binding site (Figure 7.8). Unlike most proteins that have a single, defined amino acid sequence, the MHC molecules have a polymorphic region in which the amino acid sequence varies among the different

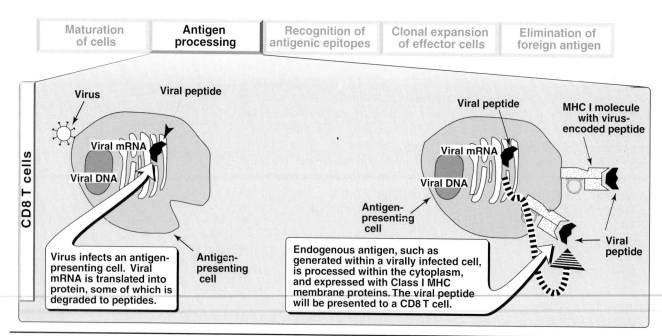

Figure 7.9
Antigen processing and presentation with Class I MHC proteins.

members of the MHC family of proteins. The extraordinary hetero-geneity of the MHCs is due to **genetic polymorphism** (having more than one stable form, or allele, of a gene at a single locus throughout the population). Within a single individual, the same class I MHC molecules are found on all nucleated cells of the body, but the same class II MHC molecules are found only on specialized cells called **antigen-presenting cells** (see p. 63). [Note: Antigen-presenting cells also express class I MHC molecules.] There are three different types of class I MHCs (HLA-A, HLA-B, and HLA-C), and three different types of class II MHCs in humans (HLA-DP, HLA-DQ, and HLA-DR).

1. **Class I MHCs:** All nucleated cells express class I MHC molecules. These compounds consist of two peptides. First, a single polypeptide chain is coded for by one of three genes (HLA-A, HLA-B, or HLA-C) located in the human leukocyte antigen (HLA) region of chromosome 6. On the surface of the cell, each of these transmembrane polypeptides is noncovalently associated with the second, small polypeptide, β_2-**microglobulin**, which is structurally homologous to a single immunoglobulin (Ig) domain, and is there-fore a member of the Ig supergene family (see p. 70). All three MHC class I molecules are expressed coordinately (at the same time). [Note: Interferon-γ increases the cell-surface concentration of class I and class II MHC molecules.] Class I MHCs bind small peptides produced in the cytoplasm by degradation of self-pro-teins, nonself proteins synthesized in bacteria- or virus-infected cells, or tumor cells (Figure 7.9). Specific T cell receptors of acti-vated CD8 T cells bind to class I MHC molecules complexed with the antigenic peptide fragment, resulting in the antigen-driven clonal expansion of the specific T cells, and ultimately the killing of the presenting (infected or tumor) cell. [Note: Viruses that escape class I MHC presentation can cause chronic viral infec-tions. For example, cytomegalovirus has the capacity to suppress class I MHC expression.]

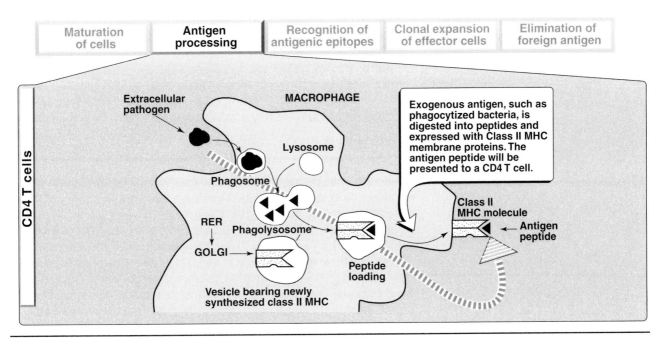

Figure 7.10
Antigen processing and presentation with Class II MHC proteins.

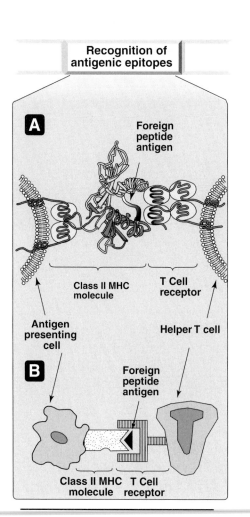

Figure 7.11
Two schematic representations of
a T cell recognizing a peptide antigen
presented by a Class II MHC molecule.
A. Peptide backbone represented
by ribbons; B. Symbols used in
this book. MHC = major histocompatibility complex.

2. Class II MHCs: These molecules are expressed by a select group of antigen-presenting cells, for example, macrophages, dendritic cells, and B cells (Figure 7.10). Class II MHCs are coded for by three sets of genes, DP, DQ, and DR, all located in the HLA region of chromosome 6. Each of these sets of genes codes for a cell-surface glycoprotein composed of two polypeptide chains that are called α and β. For example, the DPA1 gene encodes the DPα cell-surface chain, and the DPB1 gene encodes the DPβ cell-surface chain. Together, DPα and DPβ pair to produce the DP molecule. Class II MHCs bind peptides that are derived from antigens brought into antigen-presenting cells (APCs) by endocytosis or phagocytosis, and then degraded in vesicles by lysosomal acid hydrolases (Figure 7.10). As with the class I MHCs, the class II MHC-peptide fragment complex is presented on the surface of the APC (for example, macrophages, dendritic cells, and B cells), and this complex is recognized by the appropriate T cell receptor of CD4 T cells (Figure 7.11). Antigen-driven clonal expansion of the specific T cells occurs, resulting in cytokine-mediated helper T cells functions (see p. 72).

C. Non-MHC presentation of antigen

Class I and II MHC molecules present peptide antigens, but do not present carbohydrate or lipid antigens. However, the immune system recognizes self and nonself polysaccharides, for example, the blood group system.

D. Role of MHC diversity

What is the reason for the enormous diversity found in the MHCs? It is presumably a mechanism that is essential for protecting the species from the broadest possible number of pathogens. For example, if there were only one type of MHC on all human cells, the probability that all invading organisms have epitopes that could be recognized by the single MHC peptide binding cleft would presumably be small. Therefore, in the absence of a MHC-peptide complex no T cell response could be instituted, and a large segment of the human population could be killed by the resulting massive infection. [Note: B cells would still respond to the antigenic determinants on the invading organism, but would not receive T cell help. Therefore, B cells would only produce IgM (see p. 82), and could not undergo class switching or affinity maturation, etc.]

VI. T CELLS

During the immune response, T cells have the extremely important role of creating and directing cellular immunity. There are two important types of T cells: 1) **helper T cells** (**CD4 T cells**), which serve as helper cells for other lymphocytes (for example, B cells or CD8 T cells), phagocytes, and natural killer (NK) cells, and 2) the **cytotoxic T cells** (**CD8 T cells**, or **T "killer" cells**), which specialize in identifying and killing tumor cells, and cells infected with viruses or other microorganisms. [Note: CD4 and CD8 are membrane glycoproteins that are part of a group of surface antigens or "markers" that can be used to classify T and B cells, as well as other

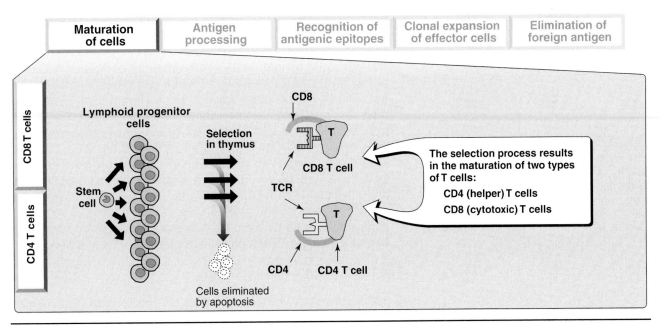

Figure 7.12
Maturation of T lymphocytes. TCR = T cell receptor.

cells in the body. Most of these markers serve as ligands, receptors, or co-receptors. These surface antigens are each assigned a CD number, where "CD" stands for "cluster of differentiation".]

A. Maturation of T cells

T cells arise from stem cells in the bone marrow. These nascent T cells migrate to the thymus gland where they mature, each cell acquiring a unique membrane receptor for antigen, the **T cell receptor (TCR)**. The immature T cell population in the thymus consists of millions of cells, each of which has a slightly different receptor that is specific for one particular peptide epitope ("**antigen peptide**") that is created by the degradation of a "foreign" protein. This diversity among the T cell receptors is generated through random combination of gene segments coding for the receptor.

1. **Testing for ability to recognize MHC molecules:** Each immature T cell is tested for its ability to recognize "self" major histocompatability complex (MHC) molecules. Those cells that fail to bind to MHC molecules undergo apoptosis (programmed cell death, Figure 7.12). Those cells whose receptors bind to an MHC-peptide complex are potentially useful, and are therefore selected for further maturation.

2. **Testing for ability to recognize MHC molecules:** The immature T cells undergo a further selection process that weeds out cells that react strongly to "self" peptides (Figure 7.12). [Note: In the thymus, it is believed that the only peptides bound by the MHC are self-peptides.] For example, if the receptor recognizes and binds to both MHC and self peptides too tightly, the cell is destroyed in

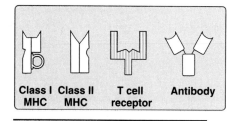

Figure 7.13
The immunoglobulin supergene family.

the thymus in order to prevent the autoimmune response that would occur if that T cell were released into the blood. When the selection process is complete, each T cell specifically recognizes one particular antigen peptide presented by one particular MHC molecule. [Note: Each MHC molecule can present thousands if not millions of peptides.] Thymocytes surviving thymic selection represent only about two percent of the starting population. When a T cell displays a CD8 marker on its surface, it recognizes peptides presented by the class I MHC, and functions as a cytotoxic killer T cell (see p. 73). When a T cell displays a CD4 marker on its surface, it recognizes peptides presented by the class II MHC, and functions as a helper T cell (see p. 72). Approximately two thirds of the peripheral blood T cells are CD4 T helper cells, and approxmately one third are CD8 cytotoxic cells. [Note: This is the basis for the CD4/CD8 ratio used to assess of HIV infection.]

B. The T cell receptor (TCR) complex

T cells express cell-surface receptors that allow them to recognize unique, antigen-derived peptide sequences. [Note: Remember that peptides derived from the extracellular space are offered by antigen-presenting cells, such as macrophages, in association with class II MHC molecules (see p. 68), whereas peptides derived from the intracytoplasmic space are offered by class I MHC molecules located on all nucleated cells (see p. 67).] These transmembrane receptors, found only on the surface of T cells, consist of two different polypeptide chains—either α plus β, or γ plus δ—that are attached to each other by disulfide bonds. [Note: Ninety-five of circulating T cells express the α/β T cell receptor. The role of the γ/δ T cell receptor is unclear.] The structure of these heterodimers is similar to those of the immunoglobulins (antibodies), and the TCRs are therefore referred to as members of the **immunoglobulin supergene family** (Figure 7.13). [Note: Whereas each circulating antibody can bind to two antigen epitopes (assuming there is no steric hinderance), TCRs bind to a single peptide–MHC complex.] A CD3 molecule is always associated with the TCR, and facilitates the transfer across the cell membrane of a signal that antigen peptide has been recognized. This results in the activation of intracellular kinases, causing a cascade of reactions that leads to alteration of transcription within the T cell, and T cell activation.

C. Activation of CD4 T cells

The activation of CD4 T cells occurs in the secondary lymphoid tissues. This is accomplished when a complex consisting of a **class II MHC** protein carrying a peptide fragment of a foreign antigen is transported to the surface of an **antigen-presenting cell** (**APC**, for example, a macrophage, dendritic cell, or B cell), and the complex is presented to an unprimed (naive) T cell (Figure 7.14).

1. **Generation of the antigen fragment–class II MHC complex:** Antigens, such as pathogenic microorganisms, enter the secondary lymphoid tissue by traveling free in the lymph, or are carried to the tissues after being phagocytized by macrophages or Langerhans cells (which become dendritic cells in the lymph

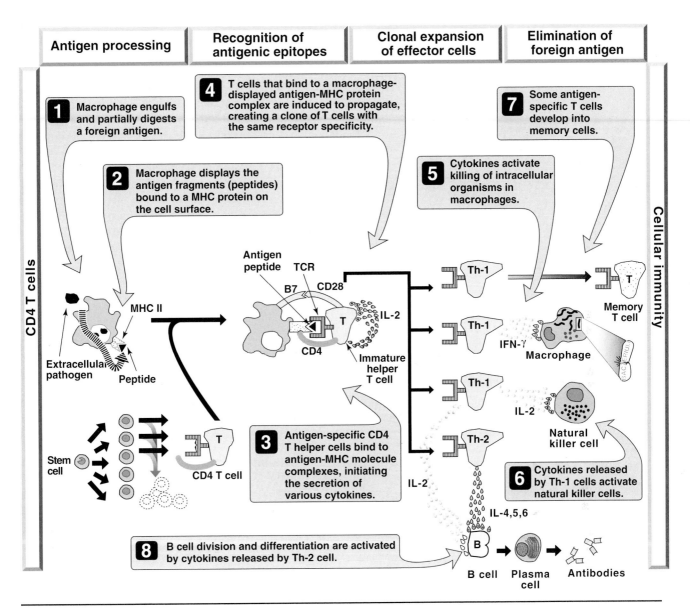

| Antigen processing | Recognition of antigenic epitopes | Clonal expansion of effector cells | Elimination of foreign antigen |

1 Macrophage engulfs and partially digests a foreign antigen.

2 Macrophage displays the antigen fragments (peptides) bound to a MHC protein on the cell surface.

4 T cells that bind to a macrophage-displayed antigen-MHC protein complex are induced to propagate, creating a clone of T cells with the same receptor specificity.

7 Some antigen-specific T cells develop into memory cells.

5 Cytokines activate killing of intracellular organisms in macrophages.

3 Antigen-specific CD4 T helper cells bind to antigen-MHC molecule complexes, initiating the secretion of various cytokines.

6 Cytokines released by Th-1 cells activate natural killer cells.

8 B cell division and differentiation are activated by cytokines released by Th-2 cell.

Figure 7.14
Summary of activation and actions of helper T cells. Th-1 and Th-2 are subpopulations of helper T cells.

nodes). [Note: Langerhans cells found in subcutaneous tissues should not be confused with the endocrine cells found in the pancreatic Islets of Langerhans.]. Peptide fragments approximately 12 to 25 amino acids in length are produced by the engulfing and digesting of extracellular, nonself material by cells such as macrophages. Each peptide fragment binds to a cleft in a class II MHC. [Note: Ingestion of microorganisms by macrophages triggers increased class II MHC and B7 expression. B7 is a cell membrane protein that is necessary for activation of naive CD4 and CD8 T cells.]

2. **Recognition of the antigen fragment–MHC complex by a CD4 T cell:** As recirculating CD4 and CD8 T cells leave the circulation

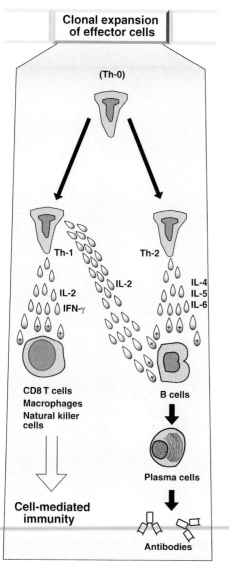

Figure 7.15
Differentiation of helper T cells
into subpopulations (Th-1 and Th-2).

and travel through the paracortical areas of the lymph node, APC–T cell interactions occur as the T cell passes through the cortex (Figure 7.14). The T cells explore the APCs to determine whether a particular APC is presenting a peptide that a specific T cell receptor can recognize. When the TCR recognizes the class II MHC–peptide complex, the CD4 molecule binds to a nonpolymorphic region of the class II MHC molecule. The CD4 molecule thus functions as a co-receptor. With the assistance of additional cell-surface proteins (**costimulatory signals**) provided by interaction of CD28 on the T cell and B7 on the APC, the CD4 T cell becomes activated. This process of T cell activation is referred to as "priming". It does not occur at the site of infection, but rather occurs in the lymph node paracortical regions that surround the follicles containing B cells. [Note: At the perimeter of the follicles, B cells can serve as APCs, presenting peptide fragments to T cells.] To facilitate the T cell TCR's inspection of the APCs for appropriate antigens, a series of cell membrane adhesion molecules (**adhesins**) are also required that allow transient, non-specific binding between the two cells.

D. Types of CD4 cells

CD4 cells can be divided into two major types: type 1 (Th-1) and type 2 (Th-2) helper cells. The production of cytokines by Th-1 cells facilitates cell-mediated immunity, particularly the activation of macrophages and T cell–mediated cytotoxicity. Th-1 and Th-2 cells also help B cells produce antibodies.

1. **Th-1 cells—a subpopulation of helper T cells:** When the APC antigen–class II MHC complex interacts with the TCR of the CD4 T cell, the CD3 protein complex transmits the signal that antigen peptide was recognized by the receptor. This turns on a complex series of intracellular pathways that result in the activation of the helper T cell. The naive CD4 T cell is initially termed a Th-0 cell, which has the potential to develop into a Th-1 cell or a Th-2 cell depending upon the cytokine milieu present in the paracortical space. For example, if a Th-0 cell is exposed to IFN-γ from NK cells, and to IL-12, produced by macrophages that have ingested or become infected by a foreign pathogen, then the Th-0 cell is induced to become a **Th-1** cell, the activator of **cell-mediated immunity**. The Th-1 cell stimulates itself to divide by beginning to secrete IL-2 (T cell growth factor), thus producing a clone of antigen-specific helper T cells. IL-2 can also activate the cytotoxic (CD8) T cells (Figure 7.15). In addition, Th-1 cells produce the cytokine, **IFN-γ**, which enhances the ability of APCs to increase the expression of their class II MHC and B7 proteins. This results in the presentation of increasing numbers of antigen peptides to CD4 T cells, thus enhancing the immune response. [Note: A subset of these antigen-specific helper T cells (along with some B cells, and cytotoxic T cells) become **memory cells**, which, when exposed to the same antigen peptide in the future, can be rapidly activated, thus leading to the anamnestic (secondary) immune response. For example, when antigens to which the Th-1 cells are reactive are injected intradermally, a local, cell-mediated immune

response known as a **delayed-type hypersensitivity (DTH) response** can develop. Pathogens such as viruses, mycobacteria, and some fungi are examples of organisms that induce a DTH response.]

2. **Th-2 cells—a subpopulation of helper T cells:** If Th-0 cells are exposed to IL-4 produced by a specialized subset of CD4 T cells, the Th-0 cells become Th-2 cells (see Figure 7.15). These cells express a cell-surface protein, CD40 ligand (CD40L), and secrete interleukins (for example, IL-4, IL-5, and IL-6). These proteins are required to activate B cells, which eventually become antibody-producing plasma cells (leading to **antibody-mediated**, or **humoral immunity**, see p. 79). Thus, *in vivo*, Th-1 and Th-2 cells represent the opposite ends of a continuum of CD4 T cells that vary in the types of cytokines secreted.

E. Mechanism of action of superantigens

Most antigens activate a limited number of helper T cells. Super-antigens, such as the staphylococcal toxic shock syndrome toxin (TSST-1), exfoliative dermatitis toxin (causing scalded skin syndrome, see p. 139), enterotoxins causing food poisoning and shock, and pyrogenic exotoxins (causing rheumatic and scarlet fevers, see pp. 148–149), are not processed by the APC, yet they bind both to class II MHC molecules (but not in the peptide cleft) and also to the TCR β chain (Figure 7.16). This leads to nonspecific activation of two to twenty percent of all T cells, and massive, unregulated cytokine release (for example, release of an endogenous pyrogen, IL-1). The high levels of circulating cytokines cause severe clinical problems, such as intravascular coagulation, hypotension, and shock.

F. Activation of CD8 T cells

The activation of CD8 T cells in the secondary lymphoid tissue results in the generation of **cytotoxic T cells** that constantly monitor nucleated cells for the possibility of intracellular infection by viruses or bacteria. Activated cytotoxic T cells can leave the lymph node, and travel to the site of inflammation, where virus-infected cells undergo a lethal response. Cytotoxic T cells also participate in killing foreign cells during rejection of transplanted tissue. Activated CD8 T cells produce IFN-γ, tumor necrosis factor-β (TNF-β), and additional cytokines.

1. **Creation of the antigen fragment–class I MHC complex:** Replicating intracellular pathogens produce proteins, some of which are degraded to peptides by the **proteasome** present in the cytoplasm of the infected cell (Figure 7.17). Proteasomes also degrade aged and denatured cytoplasmic self proteins. This mixture of self and nonself peptides is pumped into the lumen of the rough endoplasmic reticulum by TAP molecules (**t**ransporter of **a**ntigen **p**eptides). The peptides bind to class I MHC molecules in the lumen of the endoplasmic reticulum, and the peptide fragment–class I MHC complexes are transported to the cell surface of the infected cell (APC or "target" cell). [Note: Recall that all nucleated cells express class I MHC.]

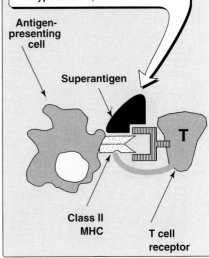

SUPERANTIGEN
- Binds to class II MHC molecules and the TCR (but not in the peptide cleft).
- Causes nonspecific activation of T cells.
- Massive, unregulated release of cytokines occurs.
- High levels of circulating cytokines cause severe clinical problems, such as intravascular coagulation, hypotension, and shock.

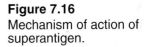

Figure 7.16
Mechanism of action of superantigen.

2. **Binding of the CD8 T cell to the antigen fragment–class I MHC complex:** A CD8 T cell with an appropriate TCR recognizes and binds to the antigen fragment–class I MHC complex on a cell surface, aided by adhesion molecules that stabilize the intercellular association. The costimulatory signal necessary for full activation of the cytotoxic T cell is either IL-2 secreted by Th-1 cells (see Figure 7.17), or the interaction of CD28 (present on the CD8 T cell) with B7 (present on the cell that is activating the CD8 T cell).

3. **Mechanisms of cell killing by activated cytotoxic T cells:** The two primary mechanisms by which cytotoxic T cells kill target cells are as follows (Figure 7.18).

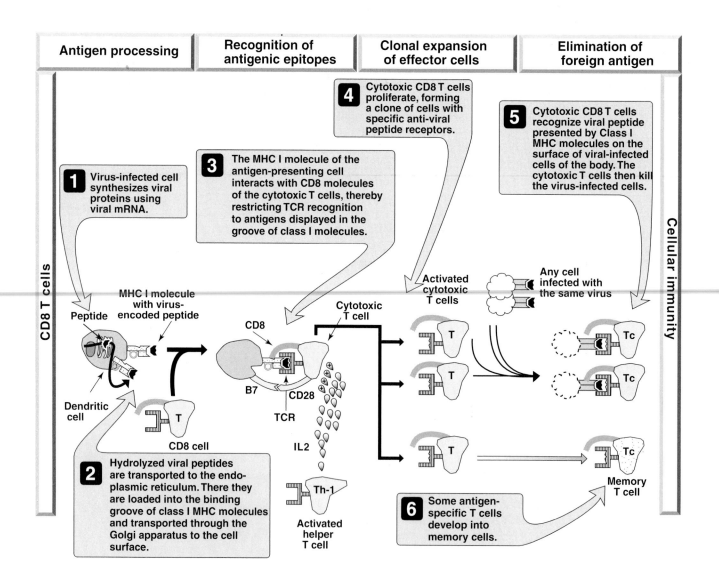

Figure 7.17
Summary of activation and actions of cytotoxic (CD8) T cells. [Note: Maturation of stem cells to T cells is not shown.]

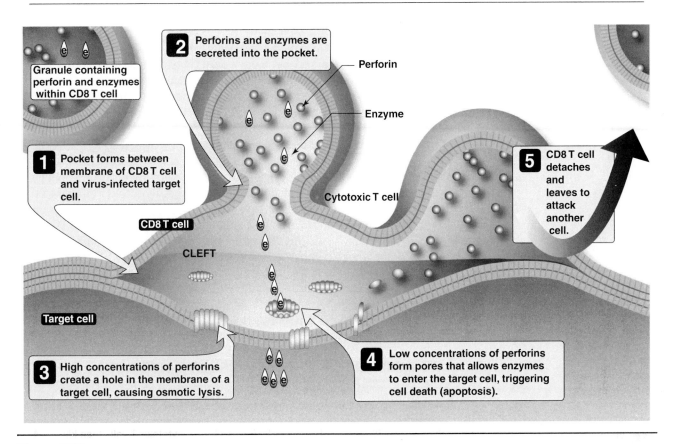

Figure 7.18
Cytotoxic actions of activated CD8 T cells.

a. **Induction of osmotic lysis:** Cytotoxic substances produced during CD8 T cell activation are released onto the surface of the target cell by exocytosis. These substances include **perforins**, which form channels through the target cell plasma membrane (similar to those formed by complement C9, see p. 92). If the perforin concentration is high, the channels cause an influx of water and leakage of cell contents, leading to death of the cell, with coincident death of any intracellular pathogens. However, the major role of perforins is to allow granzymes (see below) access to the interior of the target cell.

b. **Induction of apoptosis:** A second, and more significant, mechanism of cell killing utilizing perforins involves induction of **apoptosis** (programmed cell death), in which the cytotoxic T cell makes the target cell "commit suicide" by degrading its own DNA. This is accomplished by low concentrations of perforins that form a limited number of pores through which proteases (**granzymes**, sometimes called **fragmentins**) can pass. [Note: These proteases are located in granules in the activated cytotoxic T cell.] The enzymes induce the target cell's own apoptotic pathway. [Note: NK cells also use perforin, granzymes, among other mechanisms, to kill target cells.] The cytotoxic T cell can then detach from the dying target cell and attack additional infected cells. [Note: It is important to remember that CD8 T cells only attack cells in which pathogens such as viruses are replicating, or tumor antigens are being synthesized, and in which fragments of the resulting proteins are being presented by class I MHC molecules. Therefore killed viral vaccines (where no viral replication is occurring) do not elicit a cytotoxic CD8 T cell response, but only a CD4 T cell and antibody response.]

4. **Role of dendritic cells in the activation of CD8 T cells:** Dendritic cells (also referred to as interdigitating cells) are concentrated in the lymphoid tissues. In the skin, their precursors are the highly phagocytic Langerhans cells. When Langerhans cells have phagocytized pathogenic microorganisms, they move to the lymph node to become dendritic cells. Dendritic cells express high levels of both class I and class II MHC molecules, the costimulatory molecule B7, and the adhesion molecule ICAM. Unlike their parental Langerhans cells, dendritic cells are nonphagocytic, but they can be infected by many different viruses. As highly efficient APCs, dendritic cells are therefore able to activate both naive CD4 (which become functional helper cells), and naive CD8 T cells (which become functionally cytotoxic, and kill infected target cells).

VII. IMMUNODEFICIENCY DISORDERS INVOLVING T CELLS

Defects in components of the innate or adaptive immune systems that result in immunodeficiency predispose an individual to recurrent and potentially severe infections by a variety of pathogens. Even microorganisms that do not normally cause disease may act as pathogens in a compromised host, causing "**opportunistic**" infections (see p. 14). Serious immunodeficiency states are fatal if left untreated. This is graphically illustrated by the fact that since the appearance of widespread human immunodeficiency virus (HIV) infections in the early 1980s, acquired immunodeficiency syndrome (AIDS) has become the leading cause of death in American men and women between the ages of 25 and 44 years of age. Immune deficiency disorders can be described as **primary,** when the deficiency is genetic, or as **secondary,** when the immune deficiency is due to the presence of another disease (for example, malnutrition—the most common cause worldwide of immune deficiency). Primary immune deficiencies can be a result of an inherited or a somatic mutation. Immunodeficiency diseases in humans may result from 1) defects in B cell or antibody production (see p. 95); 2) defects of T cells with or without concurrent B cell defects (see p. 98); 3) phagocyte and/or natural killer cell defects (see p. 57); and 4) deficiencies in complement, cytokines, or other chemical mediators and receptors (see p. 99). [Note: **Chemotherapy** or **radiation therapy** for cancer, and **immunosuppression** as treatment for autoimmune disease or tissue transplantation, can also temporarily impair lymphocyte-mediated immune responses.] Defects in T cell development or function produce immunodeficiency disorders characterized predominantly by recurrent infections by **viruses, fungi,** or **protozoa.** These disorders result 1) because defective or inadequately activated CD8 T cells are unable to kill infected host cells ; 2) because CD4 T cells are unable to stimulate macrophages or other phagocytes to isolate or kill intra- or extracellular pathogens; and/or 3) because helper T cells are not present to stimulate B cells to produce IgG. They are therefore said to be **disorders of cell-mediated immunity**.

A. DiGeorge syndrome (congenital thymic aplasia or hypoplasia)

DiGeorge syndrome results from a defect in the embryonic development of the third and fourth pharyngeal pouches. Failure of proper development of the third pouch causes thymic aplasia or hypoplasia, whereas maldevelopment of the third and fourth pouches affects the parathyroid glands. The absence of a thymus causes a lack of T cell maturation, and the absence of a parathyroid results in hypocalcemia causing tetany (spasms or involuntary muscle contractions), and hyperphosphatemia. Congenital heart and kidney disorders are also observed in these infants. [Note: Although DiGeorge syndrome can result from small deletions in chromosome 22, it is generally not familial.] The absence of or reduction in T cells predisposes the patient to serious viral, fungal, and/or protozoal infections early in life. Antibody levels in the serum are low or normal. Treatment for this syndrome consists of transplantation of fetal thymus tissue.

B. Chronic mucocutaneous candidiasis

This disease involves an infection of the skin and mucous membranes by the yeast, *Candida albicans*, a normal resident of the skin (see p. 274). In this disorder, patients have a selective defect in the T cell response to *Candida*. However, they usually have a normal T cell response to pathogenic microorganisms other than *Candida*, and a normal B cell antibody response to pathogens including *Candida*. [Note: Antibody is generally not important in the body's response to fungal infections, including yeast.] Treatment involves administration of antifungal drugs. Patients with chronic mucocutaneous candidiasis may also suffer from a variety of endocrine dysfunctions, including adrenal and parathyroid gland hypofunction. Addison's disease (chronic adrenocortical insufficiency) is frequently the cause of death.

C. Acquired T cell immunodeficiency: Human immunodeficiency virus (HIV) infection

HIV binds to CD4 molecules, and thus infects and kills CD4 T cells and CD4-bearing cells of the monocyte/macrophage lineage, including CNS microglia (see p. 367). The loss of CD4 T cell function leads to impaired Th-1 activation of macrophages and NK cells, and decreased Th-1 activation of CD8 cytotoxic T cells, thus causing a devastating breakdown in the host immune response (Figure 7.19). In addition to recurrent, severe, opportunistic infections with organisms such as *Pneumocystis carinii* and cytomegalovirus (among others, see p. 368), unusual malignancies such as Kaposi's sarcoma are common. These clinical complications or sustained lymphopenia, when combined with confirmed HIV infection, constitute the **acquired immune deficiency syndrome** (**AIDS**, see p. 367).

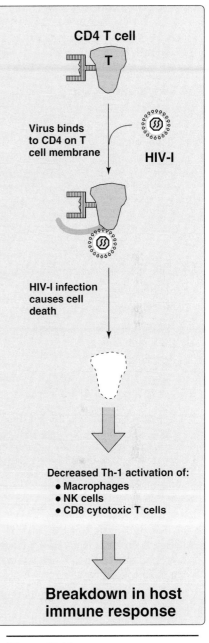

CD4 T cell

Virus binds to CD4 on T cell membrane

HIV-I

HIV-I infection causes cell death

Decreased Th-1 activation of:
- Macrophages
- NK cells
- CD8 cytotoxic T cells

Breakdown in host immune response

Figure 7.19
HIV infects and kills CD4 T cells.

Study Questions

Choose the ONE correct answer

7.1 T cell receptors recognize which type of molecule presented by MHC molecules?

    A. Oligonucleotides

    B. Oligosaccharides

    C. Glycoproteins

    D. Peptides

    E. Triglycerides

> Correct answer = D. T cell receptors only see peptides presented to them by MHC molecules. The other types of molecules are not bound or presented by MHC molecules. However, any molecule can theoretically be bound by antibodies.

7.2 The site of B cell development in mammals is:

    A. the bone marrow.

    B. the bursa of Fabricius.

    C. the thymus.

    D. the lymph nodes.

    E. the circulation.

> Correct answer = A. The bursa of Fabricius is in birds. The thymus is the site of T cell development. The lymph nodes are the sites where T and B cells see antigen and respond. The circulation is the "conduit" or "freeway" that connects the immune system together because lymphocytes and macrophages recirculate continuously through the body via the blood stream.

7.3 Developing T cells must be able to interact with self-MHC. If such a cell binds very tightly to a peptide–MHC complex presented by an antigen-presenting cell in the thymus, the result is:

    A. the thymocyte develops into a B cell.

    B. the thymocyte proliferates.

    C. the thymocyte undergoes apoptosis and dies.

    D. the thymocyte undergoes malignant transformation.

    E. the thymocyte leaves the thymus to enter the lymph node.

> Correct answer = C. If a positively selected T cell binds very tightly to a peptide–MHC complex presented by an antigen-presenting cell in the thymus, the thymocyte is triggered to undergo apoptosis and dies. This is called negative selection. Thymocytes never develop into B cells. Mature T cells proliferate outside the thymus in the lymph nodes when they encounter peptide–MHC complexes that they can respond to. Negative selection does not cause malignant transformation. Thymocytes only leave the thymus to enter the lymph nodes after they have survived both positive and negative selection and express a CD4 or CD8 molecule appropriate for the type of MHC that selected the T cell in the thymus (for example, T cells positively selected by their interaction with class I MHC must express CD8 to survive; T cells positively selected by their interaction with class II MHC must express CD4 to survive and exit the thymus).

7.4 Class I MHC molecules present peptides obtained from:

    A. phagolysosomes.

    B. the extracellular space.

    C. the interstitial fluid.

    D. the plasma.

    E. the cell cytoplasm.

> Correct answer = E. Class I MHC molecules present peptides obtained from the cell cytoplasm. Proteasomes break down foreign and aging cytoplasmic proteins into peptides. The TAP molecules pump these peptides into the lumen of the rough endoplasmic reticulum where the peptides bind to class I MHC molecules. Proteins in phagolysosomes, the extracellular space, the interstitial fluid, and the plasma all provide peptides potentially presented by class II MHC molecules.

7.5 The primary role of Th-2 cells is to:

    A. function as T killer cells.

    B. activate macrophages.

    C. activate NK cells.

    D. function as antigen-presenting cells.

    E. activate B cells.

> Correct answer = E. Th-2 cells function as helper cells for B cells. CD8 T cells function as T killer cells. Th-1 cells can help CD8 T cells, activate macrophages, and activate NK cells. Th-1 cells may also provide some cytokine help to B cells. Whereas B cells can function as antigen-presenting cells, T cells do not function in this role. Th-2 cells do play an important role in B cell activation.

B-Cells and Humoral Immunity

8

I. OVERVIEW

As noted previously (see p. 59), adaptive immunity can be divided into humoral and cell-mediated responses (Figure 8.1). Cell-mediated immunity involves specialized cells (Chapter 7), whereas humoral immunity—the focus of this chapter—results from the actions of soluble molecules, such as antibodies, and complement in the body fluids (Figure 8.1). Antibodies, the most important components of humoral immunity, are produced by B cells and their derivatives, the plasma cells. B cells can also serve as antigen-presenting cells to CD4 T cells. In turn, helper CD4 T cells provide assistance to B cells during their maturation and differentiation. In mammals, B cell development begins in the fetal liver, but before birth, this process moves to the bone marrow, which serves as the predominant, primary lymphoid organ for B cell differentiation. Further differentiation can also occur following migration of the B cells to the secondary lymphoid tissues, notably the white pulp of the spleen (see p. 64), germinal centers of lymph nodes (see p. 65), Peyer's patches in the intestine (see p. 65), and tonsils.

II. IMMUNOGENS AND ANTIGENS

An **immunogen** is defined as a substance that is capable of initiating an immune response (that is, it is immunogenic). An **antigen** is defined as a substance that can be bound by an antibody, or whose peptide fragment can be recognized by a T cell receptor via major histocompatability complex (MHC) molecule presentation (see p. 65). If a substance can react with an antibody (that is, it fits the definition of an antigen), but the substance cannot generate an immune response without the assistance of a carrier molecule, then that substance is called a **hapten**. [Note: Haptens are not immunogenic because they cannot bind to major histocompatability (MHC) proteins, and therefore are unable to activate helper T cells (see p. 71).] Thus, whereas all immunogens are antigens (that is, they can be bound by antibodies, or can be perceived by T cell receptors), not all antigens are immunogens. However, because almost all antigens are also immunogens, the term "antigen" is commonly employed as a single term to encompass both immunogen and antigen.

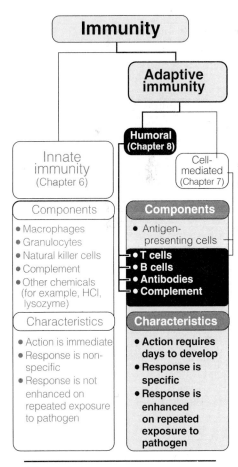

Figure 8.1
Components and characteristics of immune system highlighting the humoral immunity featured in this chapter.

Lippincott's Illustrated Reviews: Microbiology,
by William A. Strohl, Harriet Rouse, Bruce D. Fisher.
Lippincott, Williams & Wilkins, Baltimore, MD © 2001

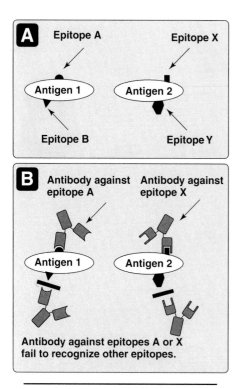

Figure 8.2
A. Antigens exhibiting epitopes.
B. Antibody specific for an epitope binds to antigen.

III. STRUCTURE AND FUNCTION OF ANTIBODIES

Antibodies are soluble, globular proteins that are important components of the acquired immune response. Originally called γ-globulins because they move more slowly in an electric field than do the α- and β-globulins (the name "globulin" comes from their globular shapes), antibodies are now referred to collectively as **immunoglobulins**. As a group, antibodies are able to recognize a great variety of epitopes (this spectrum of antibody specificities is referred to as a **repertoire**). However, each individual antibody recognizes only one antigenic epitope (see p. 62) or determinant of an antigen (Figure 8.2). They are therefore said to be highly **specific**. Antibodies have many functions, including neutralization of toxins, and activation of complement, which results in improved opsonization (see p. 94), and lysis of invading microorganisms. In humans, there are five classes (**isotypes**) of antibodies: IgM, IgD, IgG, IgA, and IgE. Each has unique structural and functional characteristics that are summarized below.

A. Antibody structure

All immunoglobulins are composed of the same basic units, consisting of four chains: two identical light (L) and two identical heavy (H) chains (Figure 8.3A). Each light chain is linked to a heavy chain by a disulfide bond, and the two heavy chains are similarly linked to each other. Treatment of an immunoglobulin with the enzyme papain produces three fragments (Figure 8.4). Two of the fragments are identical, and are referred to as **Fab** (fragment–antigen binding) because they retain the immunoglobulin's ability to bind specifically to an antigen. The third fragment does not bind antigen, but contributes to the

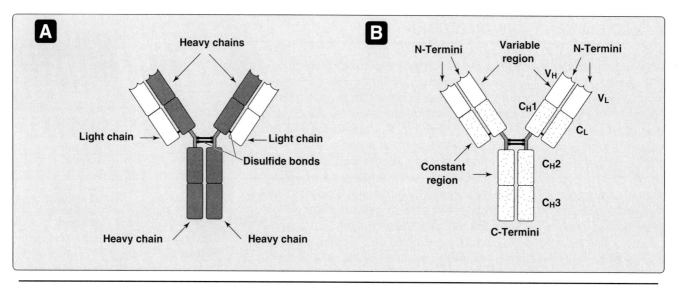

Figure 8.3
A. Immunoglobulin molecule with light chains shown in white, and heavy chains shown in gray.
B. Immunoglobulin molecule with variable region shown in white, and constant regions shown in textured gray.

antibody's biologic activity, such as binding complement, transplacental passage, or binding to mast cells. It can be crystallized, and is therefore called **Fc** (fragment–crystallizable). [Note: The Fc fragment is composed solely of portions of the H chains. Each Fab fragment is composed of the entire L chain plus a portion of the H chain.]

1. **Classes of L chains:** There are two classes of L chains, designated kappa (κ) and lambda (λ). Both are normally expressed in every individual. However, each B cell expresses (and each antibody contains) only one type of L chain—either κ or λ but not both.

2. **Classes of H chains:** Each person has five different H chains that help determine the biologic function of each of the five isotypes (classes) of immunoglobulins made by that individual (see Figure 8.5). For example, heavy chain μ is found in the isotype IgM, δ is found in IgD, γ is found in IgG, α is found in IgA, and ε is found in IgE. In a single antibody molecule, both L chains are identical and both H chains are identical. For example, IgA molecules can be $\alpha_2\kappa_2$ or $\alpha_2\lambda_2$.

3. **Constant and variable regions:** All immunoglobulin chains possess a constant ("C") region that determines the biologic action of an antibody, and a variable ("V") region that binds a unique epitope (Figure 8.3B). In a single individual, all members of a particular immunoglobulin isotype have an identical constant region, whereas every antibody molecule within that isotype has its own unique epitope-recognizing variable region. The V region of one H chain and one L chain are involved in antigen binding. Therefore, with two H–L pairs per antibody molecule, each four-chain antibody has two antigen-binding, or recognition, sites, and is said to be "**divalent**" or "**bivalent**" (see Figure 8.4).

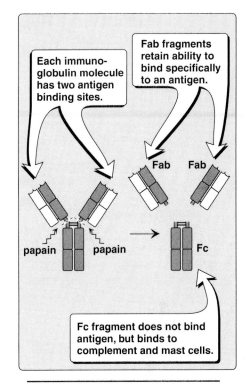

Figure 8.4
Y-shaped immunoglobulin molecule can be dissected by partial digestion with proteases, such as papain.

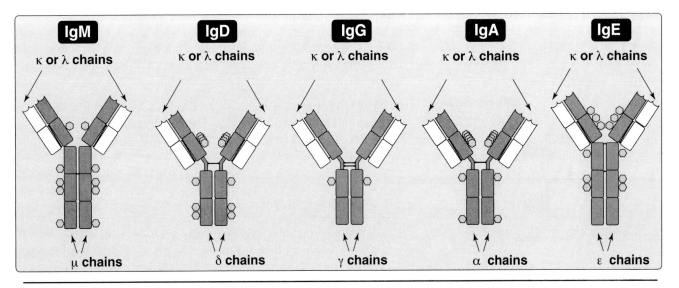

Figure 8.5
Structural organization of the monomers comprising the five major human immunoglobulin isotypes.
Note: ⬡ = carbohydrate.

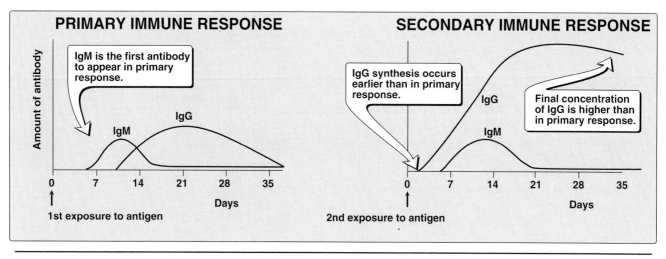

Figure 8.6
Synthesis of antibodies in the primary and secondary immune responses.

B. IgM

IgM is the first immunoglobulin to appear after exposure to an antigen (Figure 8.6). In the circulation, IgM exists as a pentamer of five four-chain units, with each monomer consisting of either two κ or two λ light chains plus two μ heavy chains (Figure 8.7). Each four-chain unit can be termed an IgM monomer. Monomeric IgM (noncirculating IgM) and IgD (see below) are present on the surface of mature, naive B cells. The five identical IgM monomers are connected to each other by a polypeptide joining (J) chain, and disulfide bonds between their Fc regions (Figure 8.7). IgM is the first class of antibody produced during the **primary immune response** (to either infection or immunization), and has a half-life of about ten days. Therefore, elevated IgM levels suggest recent exposure to antigen, such as an infection. Because of its high molecular weight, IgM is normally restricted to the intravascular space. However, when inflammation causes increased capillary permeability, plasma proteins, including IgM, can enter the interstitial space. IgM cannot neutralize toxins or viruses as efficiently as can IgG, because IgG usually has a higher affinity for antigens than does IgM. However, IgM is an efficient activator of complement.

1. **Natural isohemagglutinins:** Among the IgM antibodies are a group referred to as isohemagglutinins. These "natural" IgM antibodies are produced against bacterial antigens that structurally resemble the oligosaccharides that determine the ABO blood group types. Therefore, although individuals with type A blood group do not normally make antibodies against the bacterial type A oligosaccharide (because it is perceived as "self"), they do have isohemagglutinins against type B, and vice versa. Type O individuals produce isohemagglutinins against both type A and type B antigens, whereas type AB individuals do not make isohemagglutinins. These normally occurring IgM antibodies produce a **hemolytic transfusion reaction** when type B individuals receive type A blood, type A individuals receive type B blood, or type O individuals receive type A and/or B blood.

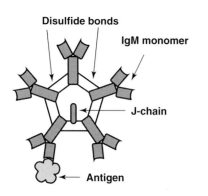

Figure 8.7
Pentameric IgM molecule, composed of five identical monomers.

2. Synthesis of IgM by the fetus: Although IgM cannot cross the placenta, fetuses over the age of five months can synthesize IgM. If elevated levels of fetal IgM are observed, congenital or perinatal infection may have occurred.

C. IgD

This immunoglobulin consists of two light chains (either two κ or two λ chains) plus two δ (heavy) chains (see Figure 8.5). It is present, with IgM, as a major surface component of mature, naive B cells (see p. 87). However, IgD is also present in very low amounts in serum where its function, if any, is unknown.

D. IgG

This immunoglobulin consists of two light chains (either two κ or two λ chains) plus two γ (heavy) chains. There are four subclasses in the IgG class of human immunoglobulins: IgG_1, IgG_2, IgG_3, and IgG_4. IgG is the predominant immunoglobulin in blood, lymph, peritoneal fluid, and cerebrospinal fluid, and it is distributed nearly equally between extra- and intravascular spaces. [Note: Most IgG subclasses have a half-life in serum of more than twenty days—the longest of all of the immunoglobulin isotypes. Therefore, IgG is particularly suitable for passive immunization done by the transfer of serum containing antibodies (**antiserum**).]

1. Time of production: IgG is formed late in the primary immune response to antigen. However, it is the predominant class of antibody produced when the body is subsequently exposed to the same antigen (the secondary immune response, see Figure 8.6).

2. Functions of IgG: IgG is a very versatile molecule. Examples of its functions include the following.

   a. Transfer from mother to fetus: IgG is the only class of immunoglobulin that can cross the placenta, thus conferring the mother's humoral immunity to infection to the fetus and neonate (see Figure 8.11). However, on the negative side, if the mother produces IgG against fetal red blood cell antigens, such as the Rh antigen, the fetal cells will be attacked, causing **erythroblastosis fetalis**—a hemolytic disease of the newborn. [Note: Congestive heart failure *in utero* from chronic anemia can cause severe edema of the newborn. This condition is termed **hydrops fetalis**.] The persistence of maternal IgG in the blood of a newborn can also make it difficult to use the presence of antibodies as an indicator of infection in the baby. For example, an HIV-positive mother's anti-HIV antibodies can still be present in her baby's blood up to 18 months after birth. Therefore, their presence is not clearly diagnostic for the status of the baby's potential infection. Instead, it is necessary to use highly sensitive tests on the baby's blood to identify viral proteins (such as p24) or viral RNA (see p. 360), because these compounds will be present at very low levels.

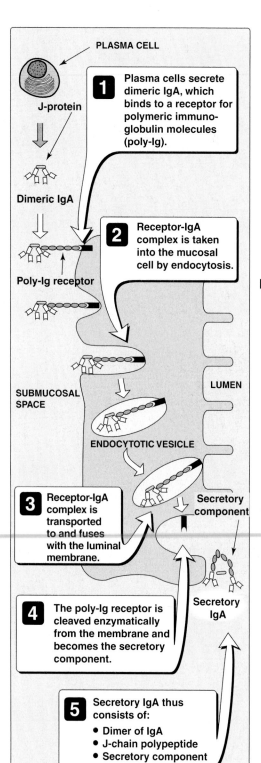

PLASMA CELL

J-protein

1 Plasma cells secrete dimeric IgA, which binds to a receptor for polymeric immuno-globulin molecules (poly-Ig).

Dimeric IgA

Poly-Ig receptor

2 Receptor-IgA complex is taken into the mucosal cell by endocytosis.

SUBMUCOSAL SPACE

LUMEN

ENDOCYTOTIC VESICLE

3 Receptor-IgA complex is transported to and fuses with the luminal membrane.

Secretory component

4 The poly-Ig receptor is cleaved enzymatically from the membrane and becomes the secretory component.

Secretory IgA

5 Secretory IgA thus consists of:
● Dimer of IgA
● J-chain polypeptide
● Secretory component

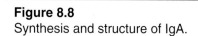

Figure 8.8
Synthesis and structure of IgA.

b. Opsonization: IgG can aid natural killer (NK) cells (see p. 55) in finding their targets. This is accomplished by the immunoglobulin binding through its Fab to an antigen such as a tumor cell or microorganism, and then binding through its Fc to the NK cell. The killer cell then destroys the pathogen by releasing lethal substances as previously discussed (see p. 55). This process is known as **antibody-dependent, cell-mediated cytotoxicity** (ADCC). Phagocytes can also be assisted in their killing function when antigens are coated with IgG, because phagocytes have Fc receptors. This opsonization function of IgG is more important than is ADCC.

c. Additional functions: IgG can also **immobilize bacteria** by binding to their cilia or flagella, **activate complement** (see p. 91), and **neutralize toxins** and some **viruses** by binding to them, and thus preventing them from reaching their receptors.

E. IgA

This immunoglobulin consists of two light chains (either two κ or two λ chains) plus two α (heavy) chains (Figure 8.5). The IgA class of immunoglobulins contains two subclasses, IgA_1 and IgA_2, present in a ratio of up to nine to one. IgA is the primary immunoglobulin found in external secretions, such as mucus, tears, saliva, gastric fluid, colostrum, and sweat, and it exists in different forms in these various solutions. For example, in serum, the IgA is monomeric (one four-chain unit). Because IgA does not fix complement, IgA is not very helpful in clearing infections in the blood stream or interstitial tissue. In contrast, IgA found in mucus secretions is present as a dimer, with the two four-chain units held together by a joining (J) peptide chain, which is also synthesized in the plasma cell (Figure 8.8). [Note: J chains are also found in IgM molecules as described on p. 82.]

1. **Synthesis of functional dimeric IgA:** The dimeric IgA molecules are released by plasma cells (mature B cells, see p. 88), and then bind to a receptor on the basal membranes of adjacent epithelial cells. This receptor is called the **poly-Ig receptor**. This receptor binds tightly to the IgA dimers, and transports them through the epithelial cells to extracellular fluids such as the mucus of the respiratory and digestive tracts. When the poly-Ig receptor–IgA dimer complex arrives on the exterior surface of the mucosal cell, the poly-Ig receptor is cleaved. The portion of the receptor that stays attached to the IgA dimer is called the **secretory piece** or **secretory (S) component**. The S component is resistant to degradation by digestive enzymes (see Figure 8.8).

2. **Functions of IgA:** The role of IgA in external secretions (secretory IgA) is to prevent microbial pathogens from attaching to and penetrating epithelial surfaces. In fact, IgA can be thought of as antibody "paint" on mucosal surfaces. It is particularly important in defending against local infections in the gastrointestinal and respiratory tracts. IgA present in breast milk provides the newborn with protection against infection. Although IgA does not activate complement, it can cause agglutination, and can also prevent viruses from entering cells.

F. IgE

This immunoglobulin consists of two light chains (either two κ or two λ chains) plus two ε (heavy) chains (see Figure 8.5). IgE is present in extremely low amounts in serum, due in part to its short half-life of two days, its slow rate of synthesis, and its rapid binding to cell surfaces that express Fc ε receptors (for example, mast cells and basophils). IgE does not activate complement nor agglutinate antigens. Nevertheless, it plays an important role in the immune response, because the Fc portion of the IgE ε chain has a high affinity for specific receptors on mast cells and basophils, to which the IgE binds for periods as long as months. If the antigen recognized by the IgE reappears during that period, it is bound by the immunoglobulin, cross-linking the Fc ε receptors. As a consequence, the mast cell or basophil is triggered to degranulate, releasing compounds such as histamine, leukotrienes, and heparin, which stimulate increased blood flow and vascular permeability leading to the symptoms of a hypersensitivity response (Figure 8.9). IgE may be elevated in allergic (**atopic**) individuals, and is responsible for many of the symptoms of allergies, bronchial asthma, and even systemic anaphylaxis. Allergy mediated by IgE is termed a **type I hypersensitivity response**. Eosinophils have receptors for IgE, and are attracted to sites where IgE has bound to a microorganism, for example, a parasite. IgE levels in serum rise particularly in response to infection with some parasites such as roundworms (*Ascaris*, see p. 293). A summary of the characteristics and functions of antibodies is presented in Figures 8.10 and 8.11.

IV. ANTIGEN-INDEPENDENT PHASE OF B CELL DEVELOPMENT

The maturation of B cells into antibody-producing plasma cells can be divided into two phases: an antigen-independent phase, followed by an antigen-dependent phase. During the antigen-independent phase, stem

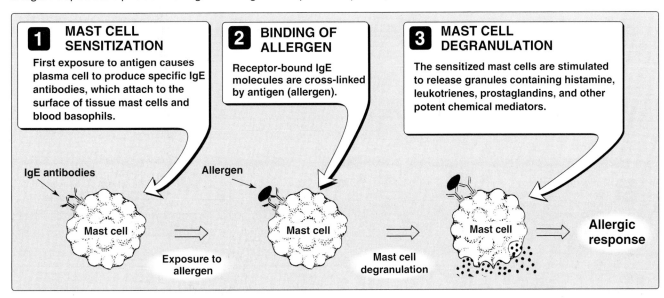

Figure 8.9
Hypersensitivity reactions mediated by IgE molecules.

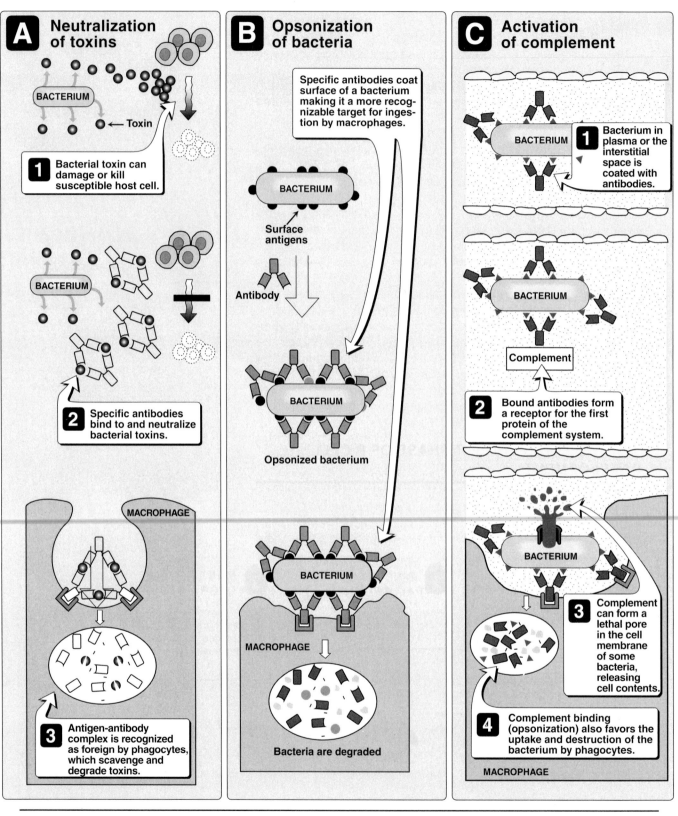

Figure 8.10
Some actions of antibodies.

	IgM	IgD	IgG	IgA	IgE
SERUM CONCENTRATION (mg/dl)	50 – 190	0.3 – 0.40	800 – 1700	140 – 420	<0.001
MAJOR CHARACTERISTICS	Very efficient against bacteraemia	Mainly lymphocyte receptor; major surface component of B cells	Most abundant internal Ig; longest half-life; crosses placenta; opsonizes antigen	Protects mucosal surfaces	Initiates inflammation; raised in helminthic infections; causes allergy symptoms
COMPLEMENT FIXATION (classic)	+++	–	++	–	–

Figure 8.11
Biological properties of major immunoglobin classes in humans.

cells in the bone marrow differentiate into pre-B cells that synthesize μ heavy chains. Without concurrent light chain production, these μ chains are located in the cytoplasm of the pre-B cell. Pre-B cells are converted to naive, immature B cells by the synthesis of either κ or λ light chains, which, when combined with μ heavy chains, result in the assembly of monomeric IgM molecules that are expressed on the B cell surface. These naive, immature B cells next undergo a period of selection, during which those cells that recognize self as antigen are eliminated (Figure 8.12A). These normal, developmental steps do not require exposure of the B cell to foreign antigen. With coexpression of monomeric IgM and IgD, the cell becomes a naive, mature B cell that is able to bind and respond to antigen (Figure 8.12B). Immature and mature naive B cells leave the bone marrow to seed lymph node follicles throughout the body. [Note: During the antigen-independent phase of development, the repertoire of B cell receptor specificities numbers more than 10^9, with each immunologically responsive B cell able to recognize a unique epitope.]

V. ANTIGEN-DEPENDENT ACTIVATION OF B CELLS

During the second phase of development, antigen is required for the activation of B cells, and their differentiation into antibody-producing plasma cells (Figure 8.13).

A. B cell function as an antigen-presenting cell (APC)

When a foreign antigen enters the body it eventually encounters a B cell with a receptor specificity that matches that particular antigen. The monomeric IgM and IgD on the surface of the naive, mature B cell binds the antigen, and the antigen–immunoglobulin complex is internalized. The antigen is degraded, producing a peptide that binds to a class II MHC protein (see p. 68). The antigen fragment–class II MHC protein complex appears on the surface of the cell, where it is recognized by a helper T cell with a receptor specific for the antigen fragment (see p. 71). [Note: Although Th-2 T cells are the most common helpers in B cell activation, some Th-1 cells also perform this function.]

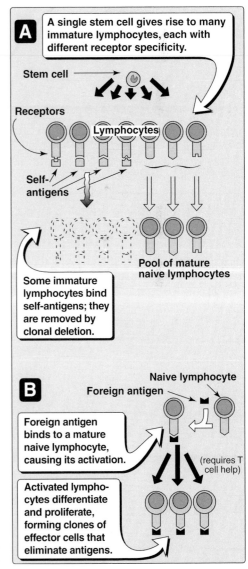

A A single stem cell gives rise to many immature lymphocytes, each with different receptor specificity.

Stem cell

Receptors

Lymphocytes

Self-antigens

Some immature lymphocytes bind self-antigens; they are removed by clonal deletion.

Pool of mature naive lymphocytes

B

Naive lymphocyte

Foreign antigen

Foreign antigen binds to a mature naive lymphocyte, causing its activation.

(requires T cell help)

Activated lymphocytes differentiate and proliferate, forming clones of effector cells that eliminate antigens.

Figure 8.12
A. B cell selection; B. B cell proliferation.

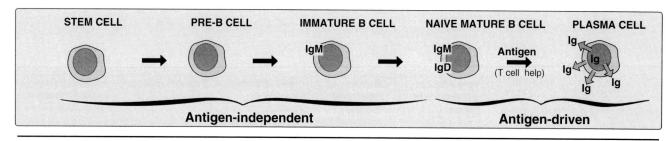

Figure 8.13
B cell differentiation from bone marrow stem cell to immunoglobulin-secreting plasma cell. [Note: Ig represents IgM, IgD, IgG, IgA, or IgE.]

B. Conversion of the activated B cell into a plasma cell

When the antigen-specific Th-2 (or Th-1) cell binds to the antigen fragment–class II MHC protein complex on the B cell, the Th-2 cell begins to secrete additional cytokines, including IL-4 and IL-5 (see p. 63). This cytokine secretion, and cell-to-cell contact [CD40L (L = ligand) on T cells and CD40 on B cells], act as costimulatory signals, causing the B cell to undergo antigen-dependent proliferation and differentiation. The eventual result of this sequence of events is the production of a clone of plasma cells producing large numbers of immunoglobulins specific for the initial antigen (Figure 8.14).

C. Immunoglobulin class switching

During the **primary immune response** (when an antigen enters the body for the first time), plasma cells secrete primarily IgM. However, immunoglobulin class switching does occur, for example, from IgM synthesis to IgG (predominantly), IgA, or IgE synthesis. This process is controlled by a specific set of cytokines released by the Th-1 and Th-2 cells. (Figure 8.6 illustrates the kinetics of an antibody response to a primary and secondary immunogenic stimulus.)

D. Somatic hypermutation of the B cell variable regions

During the primary and subsequent immune responses, somatic hypermutation in the antibody variable regions also occurs, primarily in the germinal centers of the spleen and lymph nodes. These mutations can result in the production of antibodies with a higher affinity for the antigen. The newly formed clones bearing receptors with the highest affinity for antigen are selected to proliferate, leading to an ever-increasing affinity of antibody for antigen. This process is called **somatic hypermutation**, and results in **affinity maturation** of B cell clones that respond to antigens with the highest affinity. The selected clones then proliferate more than other clones with lower affinities for the antigen.

E. Conversion of B cells to memory cells

During a normal immune response, some B cells become memory cells (see Figure 8.14). These remain temporarily quiescent, but retain the ability to become reactivated—if future reexposure

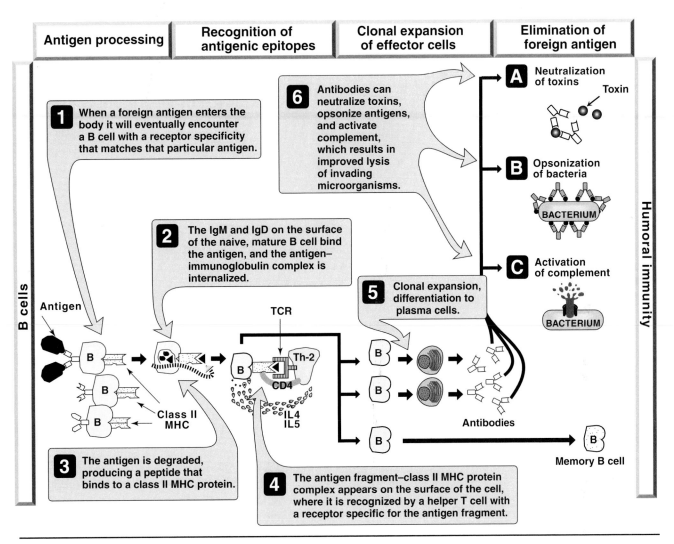

Figure 8.14
Summary of activation and actions of B cells. [Note: Maturation of stem cell to B cells is shown in Figure 8.12].
TCR = T cell receptor; MHC = major histocompatibility complex; Th = helper T cell (Th-1 or Th-2).

occurs—when the IgG, IgA, or IgE molecules on their surfaces recognize the specific antigen. Antibody production by these memory B cells is activated in part through interleukin release by memory T cells.

VI. T CELL–INDEPENDENT ACTIVATION OF B CELLS

For some types of antigens termed **T cell– (or thymus–) independent antigens (TI antigens)**, the costimulatory signal for the B cell can be supplied by the antigen itself. TI antigens are generally large molecules, such as polysaccharides, with several repeating antigenic determinants. These multivalent antigens cross-link B cell surface receptors, which results in activation of B cell clones (Figure 8.15). This leads to antibody production and cell proliferation. The lipopolysaccharide found in gram-negative bacterial cell walls is an example of a TI antigen, which explains why such bacterial infections are not as great a problem as viral or fungal infections in patients with defects in cellular immunity, for

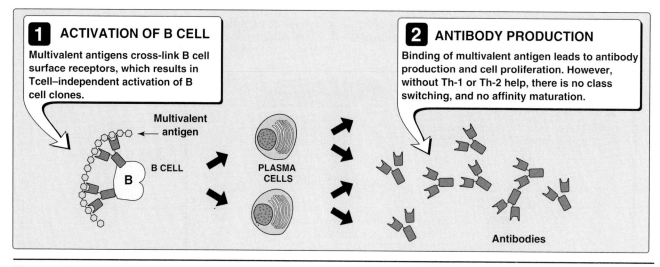

Figure 8.15
T cell–independent activation of B cells.

example, those with AIDS. [Note: Despite an IgM response to TI antigens, without Th-1 or Th-2 help, there is no class switching and no affinity maturation.]

VII. COMPLEMENT

Several circulating factors are involved in the immune response, including antibodies, complement proteins, inflammatory mediators, and acute phase reactants. Because in ancient times, body fluids were termed "humors," protection from infection supplied by plasma is referred to as **humoral immunity**. [Note: This is in contrast to **cell-mediated immunity**, which results from activation of phagocytes (a Th-1 cell activity, see p. 71), and target cell cytolysis (a function of CD8 T cells and natural killer cells, see p. 74).] Complement proteins are synthesized by hepatocytes, blood monocytes, epithelial cells of the gastrointestinal tract, and tissue macrophages. As part of the normal immune response, complement proteins are participants in the **classic complement pathway**, initiated by antigen-antibody complexes, and in the **alternative complement pathway**, in which an antigen is recognized by particular characteristics of its surface. The two arms of the complement system share opsonic and cytolytic (effector) pathways (Figure 8.16). A series of circulating and self-cell surface regulatory proteins keep the complement system in check. Plasma protein components of the complement system interact with specific cell membrane receptors (complement receptors, CRs) to effect many of the complement functions.

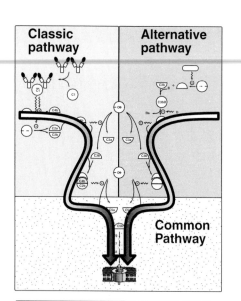

Figure 8.16
An overview of the merging of the classic complement system and the alternate pathway into a common pathway. See Figure 8.19 for details of these pathways.

A. Overview of complement functions

The approximately twenty plasma proteins that constitute this system were collectively named "complement" because they facilitate the actions of antibodies. The four major functions of complement include opsonization, target cytolysis, inflammation, and immune complex clearance (Figure 8.17). During an immune response, a cascade of complement proteins may be enzymatically activated to mark (**opsonize**) a foreign invader for phagocytosis by macrophages or neutrophils. This targeting enhances phagocytic removal of circulating antigen from the blood stream or other tissues. **Target cytolysis** can result when the **membrane attack complex** (**MAC**) of complement proteins pierces the plasma membrane of an infected cell or pathogenic invader. Complement can thus work in concert with antibodies to literally explode pathogens via osmotic lysis. [Note: The MAC is particularly important in the clearance of gram-negative organisms, such as *Neisseria meningiditis*, and *N. gonorrhoeae*.] Smaller molecular weight complement fragments generated during complement activation serve as important **inflammatory mediators** of the immune response (Figure 8.17).

B. Complement nomenclature

The complement system utilizes a unique nomenclature. Most complement plasma proteins are named with a capital "C," followed by a number (for example, C3). C′ is an abbreviation for the complement system. [Note: The complement proteins are numbered 1 through 9, although they do not function in numerical order.] When complement proteins are cleaved, the fragments are identified by small letters (for example, C3 is cleaved into C3a and C3b), where the "a" fragment usually has a lower molecular weight than the "b" fragment. Complement proteins can acquire enzymatic activity or assemble into multimolecular catalytic complexes. Those with enzymatic activity are indicated by a line drawn above the active protein or complex (for example, $\overline{C4b2b}$= C3 convertase, an enzyme able to cleave C3 into C3a and C3b). [Note: Proteins unique to the alternative pathway are identified by capital letters other than "C" (for example, B, D, and P).]

C. Classic complement pathway

Initiation of this pathway requires the formation of antigen–antibody complexes (Figure 8.18). The pathway involves the activation of nine major proteins (C1 through C9) plus several regulated steps that prevent inappropriate activation of the pathway. Because several of the activated intermediates in the pathway have enzymat ic activity, they serve to amplify the small, initial signal generated when antigen is bound by antibody. The details of this pathway are illustrated in Figure 8.19.

1. **Antibodies IgG and IgM bind C1:** When antigen is bound by antibody, the antibody Fc regions are "opened up", and are thus made available for binding circulating or interstitial fluid C1. This initiates the complement cascade (Figure 8.19). Two IgG$_1$, IgG$_2$, or IgG$_3$ molecules are required for C1 binding, whereas a single IgM is able to bind C1. IgG$_3$ activates complement more strongly than does IgG$_1$ or IgG$_2$. In contrast, IgG$_4$, IgA, IgD, and IgE do not bind C1, and therefore do not activate the classic pathway. [Note: The classic pathway can also be activated to a lesser degree by heparin, DNA, certain retroviruses, mycoplasma, C-reactive protein (CRP), mannose binding protein (MBP), and certain "trypsin-like" proteases.]

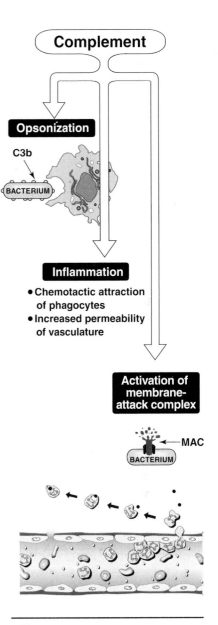

Figure 8.17
Major functions of complement. [Note: MAC = membrane attack complex; C3b = component of complement system.]

2. **Production of C3 convertase:** Activated C1 cleaves both C4 and C2 into two pieces (C4 → C4a + C4b; C2 → C2a + C2b). The pieces recombine, forming C4b2b (C3 convertase) on the target pathogen cell surface. [Note: The older nomenclature designated C2a as the larger and C2b as the smaller fragments. Current nomenclature conforms to the rule described on p. 91).]

3. **Production of C5 convertase:** C3 convertase cleaves C3 (C3 → C3a + C3b). Adding a C3b fragment to C4b2b creates the C5 convertase (C4b2b3b) of the classic pathway. [Note: C3b that attaches to the target surface serves as a powerful opsonin. C3a is soluble, and is an **anaphylatoxin** (that is, it induces mast cell degranulation and histamine release).]

4. **Formation of the membrane attack complex (MAC):** Cleavage of C5 by C5 convertase (C5 → C5a+C5b) produces C5b, which binds with C6 and C7. This complex (C5b67) inserts itself into the plasma membrane of the target cell. C8 binds to the complex (C5b678), forming small pores in the membrane. Finally, C9 polymerizes around the C5b678 complex, causing holes in the membrane that lead to osmotic lysis. [Note: The C5a that is released serves as the most potent anaphylatoxin in the body.]

D. **Alternative complement pathway**

This pathway does not require the formation of antigen–antibody complexes for activation (see Figure 8.18). Instead, it is activated by a group of unrelated substances found in the cell walls of some yeasts and bacteria (including lipopolysaccharide endotoxin found in the cell walls of gram-negative bacteria (see p. 13). It can also be activated by aggregated IgA, and by a substance found in cobra venom.

1. **Production of alternative pathway C3 convertase:** C3 is cleaved in three ways—either by C3 convertase in the classic pathway (see p. 91), by C3 convertase of the alternative pathway (see below), or by C3 spontaneously breaking down at a low rate to C3a and C3b. If the C3b that is spontaneously and continuously produced subsequently lands on a non-self surface, the alternative pathway is activated, in which C3b combines with serum factor B, forming a C3bB complex. Factor B in the complex is cleaved by serum factor D, producing C3bBb. C3bBb acts as the alternate pathway C3 convertase, capable of producing more C3b. [Note: C3bBb is prevented from dissociating by **properdin** (**Factor P**), a serum protein that stabilizes the C3bBb complex.]

2. **Production of alternative pathway C5 convertase and MAC:** C3b produced by C3 convertase binds to C3bBb, producing the alternative C5 convertase (C3bBb3b). [Note: C5 convertase may or may not still have factor P attached.] This C5 convertase enzyme complex produces the C5b that is necessary for formation of the membrane attack complex and cell lysis (see Figure 8.19).

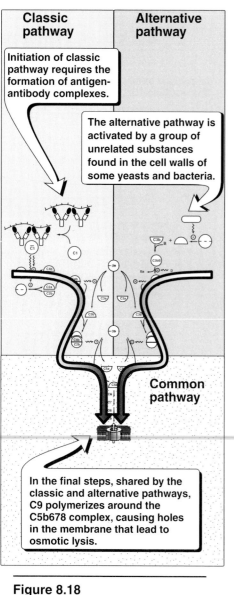

Classic pathway	Alternative pathway

Initiation of classic pathway requires the formation of antigen-antibody complexes.

The alternative pathway is activated by a group of unrelated substances found in the cell walls of some yeasts and bacteria.

Common pathway

In the final steps, shared by the classic and alternative pathways, C9 polymerizes around the C5b678 complex, causing holes in the membrane that lead to osmotic lysis.

Figure 8.18
An overview of the activation of the classic complement system and the alternate pathway. See Figure 8.19 for details of these pathways.

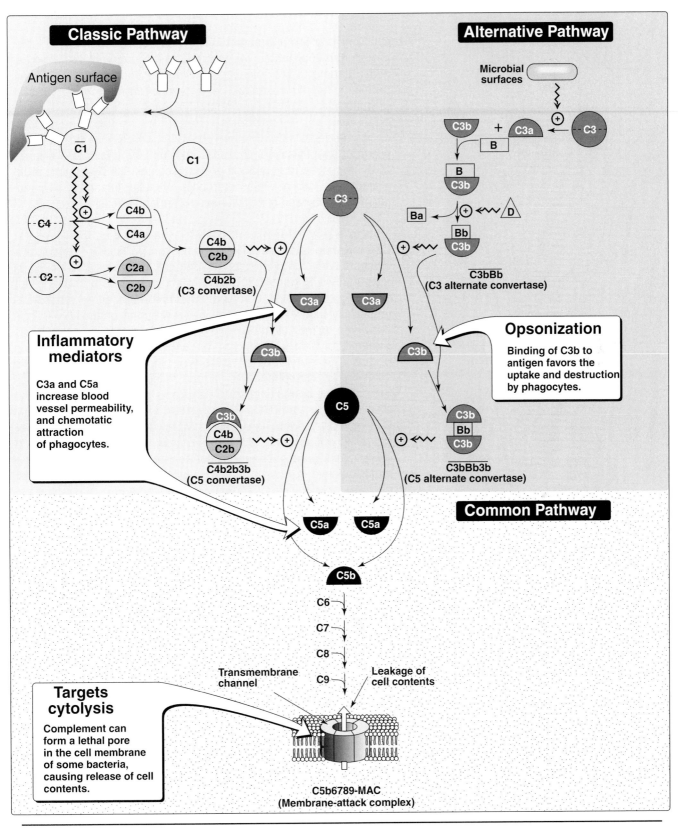

Figure 8.19
The complement system. See text for a detailed description of the process.

E. Additional roles of complement fragments in the immune response

1. **C3a and C5a are anaphylatoxins:** These compounds are soluble, proinflammatory molecules that cause the degranulation of mast cells, leading to the release of histamine and other active compounds. These substances cause contraction of smooth muscle and increase capillary permeability, leading particularly to bronchospasm and local edema. Present in the fluid phase, C3a enhances local inflammation. However, C5a is the body's most powerful anaphylatoxin. It passes into the fluid phase and diffuses away from the site of antigen-antibody contact. Its chemotatic properties attract and activate neutrophils, stimulate mast cell degranulation, and increase oxidative metabolism and adhesiveness.

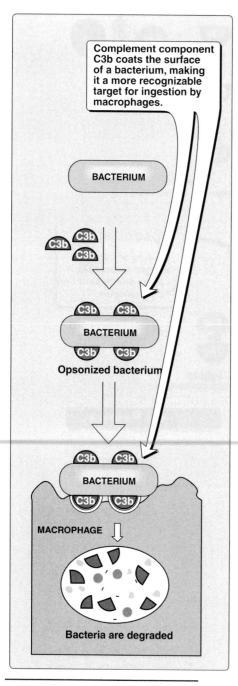

2. **C3b is a powerful opsonin and enhancer of phagocytosis:** Opsonization is the process of making a particulate antigen (for example, a microorganism or infected cell) more easily identified by a phagocyte (Figure 8.20). This is accomplished by coating the antigenic particle with complement components and/or antibodies (especially IgG) that can be recognized by the phagocyte. C3b is deposited on the cell membrane of microorganisms or infected cells targeted for destruction, thus marking the pathogen for removal (that is, C3b serves as an **opsonin**). Once the non-self target is coated with C3b, phagocyte surface receptors are readily able to recognize the bound C3b, which facilitates **immune adherence**, and thus enhances removal of the invader by phagocytosis. Multiple C3b molecules on the target surface provide a stronger stimulus for triggering phagocytosis than does a single opsonin molecule. C3b opsonization and subsequent enhancement of phagocytosis are major defense mechanisms, particularly against bacterial invaders, because phagocytized bacteria are digested and destroyed by the phagocyte. [Note: C3b also plays a role in the elimination of large immune complexes circulating in the blood by precipitating on their surfaces. Red blood cells, which express complement receptors on their surfaces, bind to the C3b, and thus ferry the attached immune complexes to the liver or spleen for removal.]

F. Regulation of complement activation

The pathways of complement activation are examples of the power of **molecular amplification**. At each step where an enzyme is activated (for example, in the activation of C1, and formation of C3 or C5 convertase), amplification occurs, thus increasing the efficiency whereby complement carries out its functions. However, these are powerful compounds, and in order to prevent an over-accumulation or unwanted expression of this pathway's components, there are **inactivators** of some complement components. For example, **C1 esterase inhibitor (C1INH)** prevents the activation of C1, thus halting the initiation of the classic pathway. [Note: C1INH deficiency causes **hereditary angioedema**.] Another inhibitor of the complement pathway is **decay accelerating factor**, expressed on the surface of self-cells, which inhibits C3 convertase, and thus protects cells from lysis by MAC (see p. 91). [Note: A deficiency of decay

Figure 8.20
Opsonization of bacterium by complement component C3b.

accelerating factor and homologous restriction factor increases red blood cells' susceptibility to spontaneous lysis by C′, producing paroxysmal nocturnal hemoglobinuria.]

VIII. IMMUNOLOGY MAP

Interactions between T cells, B cells, antigen-presenting cells, antibodies, and complement, as well as with the innate immune response, ultimately produce a complex web of interactions. As an aid to the reader, the authors have created a summary map (Figure 8.21) that visualizes the interactions of the various components, and helps orient the reader as to where new information fits in the "big picture."

IX. IMMUNODEFICIENCY DISORDERS DUE TO ANTIBODY OR B CELL DEFECTS

Defects in B cell production or development can lead to an absence of from one to all five classes of antibodies. These deficiencies therefore lead to **defects in humoral immunity**. The effect of such a deficiency is an inability to destroy extracellular pathogens, especially bacteria. For example, without adequate concentrations of antibody, complement activation and opsonization are deficient. Because pyogenic (pus-forming) bacteria have polysaccharide capsules or other surface structures that are antiphagocytic, the absence of opsonization makes it difficult for phagocytes to ingest and destroy them. Without antibodies available to neutralize infectious viruses, individuals with B cell defects are also particularly more susceptible to several types of viral infections (for example, poliovirus infections). Examples of disorders involving B cell or antibody defects include the following.

A. Bruton's X-linked infantile agammaglobulinemia (XLA)

XLA is an X-linked recessive disorder, and therefore is seen only in males. At about six months of age, when the titers of antibodies obtained transplacentally from the mother during gestation are significantly lower, the infant begins to suffer from a variety of bacterial infections. Typical pathogens include *Haemophilus influenzae*, *Streptococcus pneumoniae*, *Streptococcus pyogenes*, and *Staphylococcus aureus*, which cause otitis media, conjunctivitis, pharyngitis, abscesses, bronchitis, pneumonia, skin infections, and meningitis. XLA patients are also susceptible to certain viral and parasitic infections, including *Giardia lamblia* (see p. 281), which causes diarrhea and malabsorption. XLA patients commonly develop autoimmune connective tissue disorders, and a chronic, indolent, rheumatoid-like arthritis. The defective gene in XLA codes for a tyrosine kinase, and is named btk for "Bruton's tyrosine kinase." Immunoglobulin levels are very low (or undetectable), and B cells are essentially absent, although cytoplasmic μ+ pre-B cells (see p. 87) are present. Treatment consists of regular injections of intravenous immunoglobulin (IVIG).

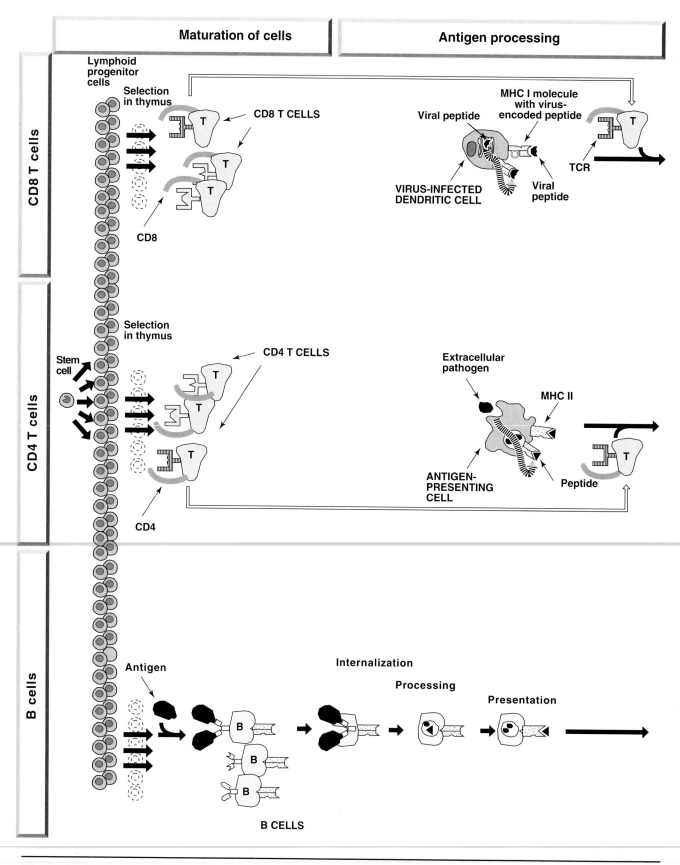

Figure 8.21
Summary of adaptive immune response. TCR = T cell receptor, MHC = major histocompatibility complex; TNF = tissue necrosis factor; INF = interferon.

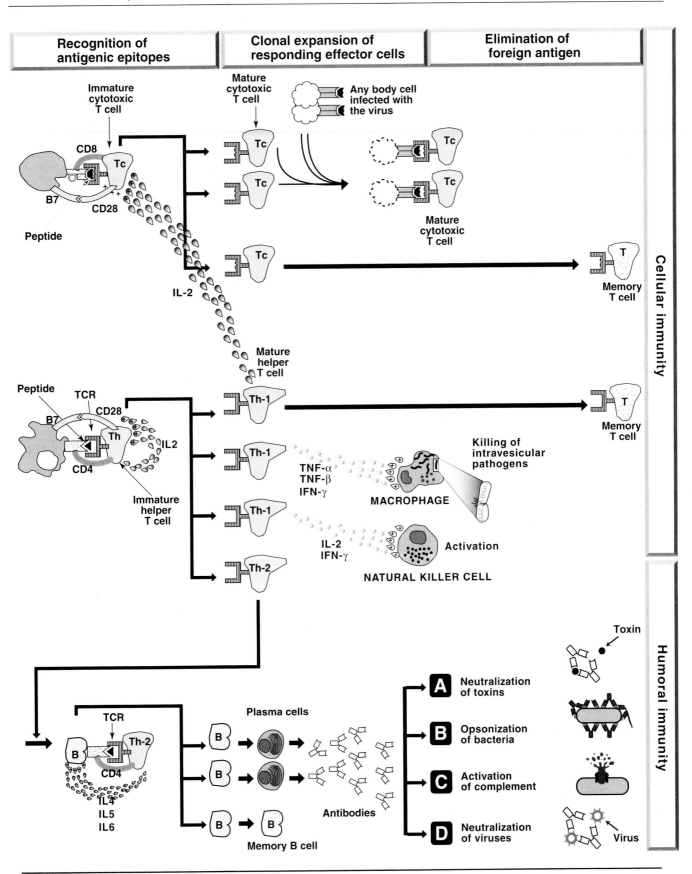

Figure 8.21 (continued)

B. IgA deficiency

This is the most common immune deficiency, affecting up to 1 in 800 individuals in the general population. Interestingly, most patients are asymptomatic, but a minority of patients develop severe, recurrent bacterial or viral sinopulmonary infections, and diarrhea. Allergies, autoimmune disorders, and pulmonary and gastrointestinal tumors may also develop. IgG subclass deficiency (for example, of IgG_2) may occur concurrently, and such patients are more likely to suffer recurrent infections than patients with isolated IgA deficiency. Treatment involves administration of broad-spectrum antibiotics as needed.

X. IMMUNODEFICIENCY DISORDERS DUE TO COMBINED T AND B CELL DEFECTS

Immunodeficiency disorders characterized by recurrent, often severe viral, fungal, and/or protozoal infections result predominantly from T cell deficiency, with variable degrees of B cell and antibody deficiency. The joint T and B cell defects may involve decreased lymphocyte number and/or impaired function. Because helper T cells are required for B cells to mount a normal antibody response, T cell deficiency can lead to defects in antibody-mediated (humoral) immunity. Defects in both T cell– and B cell–mediated immunity lead to "combined immunodeficiency (CID)." **Severe combined immunodeficiency (SCID)** implies the most serious forms of CID, with death frequently occurring early in infancy because of recurrent or persistent infections.

A. Overview of severe combined immunodeficiency (SCID)

This is a group of genetic diseases in which patients are susceptible to infection by all types of microorganisms, some of the most frequent being *Pneumocystis carinii*, cytomegalovirus, herpes virus, varicella virus, and *Candida*. Infants with SCID are born with a genetic defect that is either an X-linked or an autosomal recessive mutation, which affects production of T cells and may affect B cells. Without treatment, these babies rarely survive beyond one year, succumbing rapidly to massive infections. The classic triad of SCID symptoms includes persistent oral thrush, diarrhea, and pneumonia. [Note: In contrast to lobar bacterial pneumonias, the SCID pneumonia is often interstitial, resulting from *Pneumocystis carinii* infection.] Children with SCID do not tolerate live virus immunization. For example, an attempt to immunize using live polio virus may lead to progressive paralytic poliomyelitis, retardation, and death. Profound lymphopenia is characteristic of these diseases. Therapy for these disorders is generally bone marrow transplantation. Genetic defects that cause SCID include the following.

1. **Interleukin 2 receptor (IL-2R) gamma chain deficiency:** This X-linked, recessive disorder causes between fifty to sixty percent of all cases of SCID. (The remaining genetic mutations causing SCID are autosomal recessive.) The IL-2R gamma chain is a component of several additional interleukin receptors: IL-4R, IL-

7R, IL-11R, and IL-15R. Therefore, defects in the IL-2R γ chain result in defective development and differentiation of T cells. Defects in IL-4R also lead to poor B cell responses to IL-4, secreted by Th-2 helper cells, that is necessary for B cell proliferation, differentiation, and immunoglobulin synthesis.

2. **Adenosine deaminase (ADA) deficiency:** At least half of the autosomal recessive cases of SCID result from defects in adenosine deaminase[1] or purine nucleoside phosphorylase[2] in lymphoid stem cells. A deficiency of ADA causes the overproduction of dATP, an inhibitor of the enzyme ribonucleotide reductase[3] that is responsible for providing the cell with deoxyribonucleotides—the building blocks for DNA. Therefore, the stem cells cannot divide, and no T or B cells are produced. Clinically, this disorder cannot be differentiated from X-linked SCID. Experimental gene replacement therapy has been introduced as a potential cure for ADA deficiency.

B. Wiskott-Aldrich syndrome (WAS)

The hallmark of this X-linked, recessive disorder is a lack of IgM production in response to capsular polysaccharide antigens of bacteria. IgA and IgE are frequently increased, and IgG levels are within the normal range. Patients exhibit a characteristic eczema. Thrombocytopenia (low platelet count), and small platelets in a male with petechiae and immunodeficiency, are suggestive of this disorder.

C. Ataxia telangiectasia (AT)

This is an autosomal recessive condition, characterized by gait disturbance (ataxia), and dilated cutaneous and conjunctival capillaries (telangiectasia). AT is associated with T cell deficiency and depressed immunoglobulin levels (for example, IgA, IgG2, IgG4, and/or IgE). An ill-defined chromosome repair defect appears to lead to an increased incidence of lymphoreticular malignancies.

XI. IMMUNODEFICIENCY DISORDERS DUE TO DEFECTIVE OR DEFICIENT COMPLEMENT

Complement components play an important role in opsonization, chemotaxis, and the killing of bacteria, as well as facilitating removal of antigen-antibody complexes from the circulation. Because complement deficiency can lead to the decreased clearance of antigen-antibody immune complexes, patients with defects in C1 through C5 can suffer from imune complex glomerulonephritis. Complement deficiency can also cause systemic autoimmune diseases, including some collagen diseases such as lupus or lupus-like conditions.

[1]See p. 350 in **Lippincott's Illustrated Reviews: Biochemistry** (2nd ed.) for a discussion of adenosine deaminase deficiency.
[2]See p. 350 in **Lippincott's Illustrated Reviews: Biochemistry** (2nd ed.) for a discussion of purine nucleoside phosphorylase deficiency.
[3]See p. 353 in **Lippincott's Illustrated Reviews: Biochemistry** (2nd ed.) for a discussion of ribonucleotide reductase.

Study Questions

Choose the ONE correct answer

8.1 The portion of the antibody molecule that binds antigenic epitopes is

    A. termed the determinant.

    B. composed of a variable and a constant region of IgH and IgL.

    C. composed of the variable regions of IgH and IgL chains.

    D. the Fc fragment.

    E. two IgL chains.

> Correct answer = C. Determinants are synonymous with antigenic epitopes. Only the IgH and IgL variable regions bind antigens. Constant regions do not bind antigens. The Fc fragment is the major portion of the IgH constant region, and this fragment does not bind antigen. Two IgL chains together do not bind antigen.

8.2 IgM that is present on the naive mature B cell is

    A. a monomer.

    B. a dimer.

    C. a trimer.

    D. a pentamer.

    E. IgM is never expressed on naive mature B cells.

> Correct answer = A. Surface antibody is always present as a monomer on any type of B cell. IgA circulates in mucus as a dimer. Normally there are no circulating antibody trimers. IgM normally circulates as a pentamer. IgM is always present on naive mature and naive immature B cells.

8.3 IgE binds to

    A. T cells.

    B. B cells.

    C. macrophages.

    D. dendritic cells.

    E. mast cells.

> Correct answer = E. IgE binds to mast cells. When surface IgE is crosslinked on mast cells, the mast cells degranulate, releasing histamine as well as other vasoactive substances. The other cells lack Fc ε receptors.

8.4 Pre-B cells express

    A. TCR α chains.

    B. IgM.

    C. IgD.

    D. cytoplasmic κ or λ chains.

    E. cytoplasmic μ chains.

> Correct answer = E. Only T cells express TCRs. 95 percent of T cells express α/β TCRs. IgM is expressed on naive immature B cells. IgM and IgD are coexpressed on naive mature B cells. Once the pre-B cell expresses an IgL chain, surface IgM is expressed changing the pre-B cell into the naive immature B cell.

8.5 Naive mature B cells do not require which one of the following factors for activation?

    A. Surface antibody contact with antigen

    B. T cell cytokine stimulation

    C. B cell CD40 interaction with T cell CD40L

    D. Expression of IgM and IgD

    E. Antigen presentation to T cell via class I MHC

> Correct answer = E. All other factors are required. B cells do function as APCs. However, B cells present extracellular antigen peptides to T cells via class II MHC molecules.

8.6 In the alternative complement pathway, foreign antigen is recognized by

    A. circulating immunoglobulin IgM.

    B. circulating immunoglobulin IgG.

    C. the characteristics of the antigenic surface.

    D. CD40L.

    E. FAS ligand.

> Correct answer = C. IgM and IgG binding of an antigen can initiate the classic pathway of complement activation. CD40L is expressed by T cells that activate naive mature B cells. FAS ligand is expressed by NK and CD8 T cells.

Bacterial Structure, Growth, and Metabolism

9

I. OVERVIEW

The cellular world is divided into two major groups, based on whether or not the cells have a nucleus (that is, an internal membrane-enclosed region that contains the genetic material). Cells that have a well-defined nucleus are called **eukaryotic**, whereas cells that lack a nucleus are called **prokaryotic**. All bacteria are prokaryotes. In addition, bacterial DNA is not organized into the elaborate multi-chromosomal structures of the eukaryotes. Prokaryotes and eukaryotes employ very similar metabolic pathways to achieve cell growth and to maintain viability. Important differences exist, however, that distinguish prokaryotes from each other, and from eukaryotes. Central among these are mechanisms of energy generation, and the synthesis of substances and structures that are unique to bacteria, for example, the bacterial cell wall. A generalized prokaryotic cell is shown in Figure 9.1.

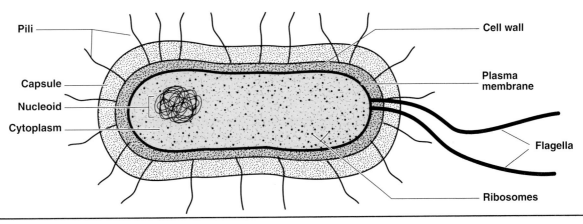

Figure 9.1
Generalized structure of a bacterial cell.

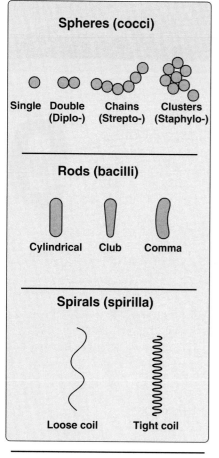

Figure 9.2
Typical shapes and aggregation
states of common bacterial species.

II. MORPHOLOGY

A primary means of identifying bacteria is by their morphology (for example, their shape, size, and aggregation properties) when viewed in the light microscope. Further identification is accomplished through their staining properties.

A. Cell shape

Bacteria exhibit three main shapes, which are determined by the molecular properties of the cell wall (Figure 9.2). These include **spherical forms** (the cocci, singular: coccus), **rod-like forms** (the bacilli, singular: bacillus)**,** and **spiral and curved forms** (the spirilla, singular: spirillum). In addition, a few species, termed **pleomorphic**, (for example, *Haemophilus influenzae*) lack a rigid cell wall, and thus have no defined shape. [Note: Variation of size and shape within a population may also result from asymmetric growth of the cell wall.]

B. Size

Most bacteria are one to five microns in length. Thread-like species (for example, spirilla) can be many times longer than their cross-sectional diameter. Typically, a bacterium is some hundred-fold larger than a virus, and ten-fold smaller than a eukaryotic cell (Figure 9.3).

C. Aggregation properties

Whereas the single isolated cell is the fundamental bacterial unit, many species exhibit distinctive aggregation states, for example, long chains, irregular clusters (see Figure 9.2), or regular clusters resembling crystals. These aggregation states are determined by the orientation of the cell division plane to the axis of the cell, and also the tendency of progeny cells to adhere to each other. The aggregates, although relatively stable and characteristic of the species, can be disrupted mechanically without loss of cell viability.

D. Staining properties

Bacteria can be divided into groups, depending on the structure of their cell walls as reflected in their staining characteristics. The most universally applied stain is the **Gram stain**. Bacteria with waxy mycolic acids in their cell walls can also be distinguished from other bacteria, using an **acid-fast stain**.

1. **The Gram stain:** If bacteria (for example, in a smear of a clinical sample on a microscope slide) are treated with a solution of crystal violet and then iodine, the cells stain purple. If the stained cells are then treated with a solvent such as alcohol or acetone, or a mixture of the two, some species (called **gram-positive**) retain the stain, whereas other species (called **gram-negative**) lose the stain, becoming colorless (see p. 23). The latter can subsequently be made visible using a counterstain such as safranin. Most, but not all, bacteria fall rather clearly into one of these two groups. This differential staining is attributable to the quite different molecular architecture of gram-positive and gram-

negative cell walls (see p. 105). A Gram stain can be rapidly and easily performed. It is important therapeutically because gram-positive and gram-negative bacteria have differing susceptibilities to a variety of antibiotics. Therefore the Gram stain may be used to guide therapy until definitive identification of the microorganism can be obtained (see p. 23).

2. **Acid-fast stain:** Most bacteria that have been stained with carbol-fuchsin can be decolorized by washing with acidic alcohol. Certain bacteria, however, retain the carbolfuschin stain after being washed with an acidic solution. Such bacteria, called acid-fast, typically have waxy material (**mycolic acids**) in their cell walls. The most clinically important of the acid-fast bacteria are *Mycobacterium tuberculosis* (see p. 246) and *Mycobacterium leprae* (see p. 255).

3. **Counterstains:** In the Gram and acid-fast staining procedures, the bacterial cells may be rendered invisible by the decolorization step. Visibility can be restored by using a counterstain that has a color distinctly different from the primary stain. For example, in the Gram staining procedure, the pink dye, safranin, is used as the counterstain. Therefore, gram-positive cells are purple (having retained the crystal violet) whereas gram-negative cells are pink (having been counterstained with safranin).

E. Imaging methods

Standard light or phase-contrast microscopy, combined with specific staining techniques (such as the Gram stain), is the most rapid method of establishing the presence and making the initial identification of most bacteria. Discernment of subcellular structure, however, requires the use of electron microscopy. **Transmission electron microscopy**, in which electrons pass through ultrathin sections of the specimen, is used to observe internal structures, such as ribosomes, and layers of the cell envelope (see Figure 1.3, p. 3). **Scanning electron microscopy** (SEM), in which electrons are scattered off the surface of metal-coated specimens, is used to observe details of the cell surface. Because the depth of field is so great in SEM, objects appear three-dimensional.

III. THE CELL ENVELOPE

The bacterial "cell envelope" is a term applied to all of the material external to and enclosing the cytoplasm. It consists of several chemically and functionally distinct layers, the most prominent of which are the **cell wall** and the **cell membrane**.

A. The cell wall

The bacterial cell wall determines the shape of the cell. It is composed of a cross-linked polymeric mesh called **peptidoglycan** (Figure 9.4). The glycan portion is a linear polymer of alternating monosaccharide subunits—**N-acetylglucosamine** (**NAG**) and **N-acetylmuramic acid** (**NAM**). This polymer is the carbohydrate "back-

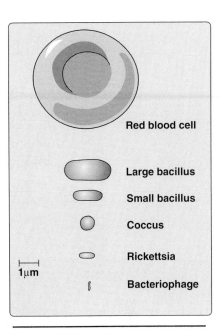

Figure 9.3
Relative sizes of a red blood cell, bacteria, and a bacterial virus.

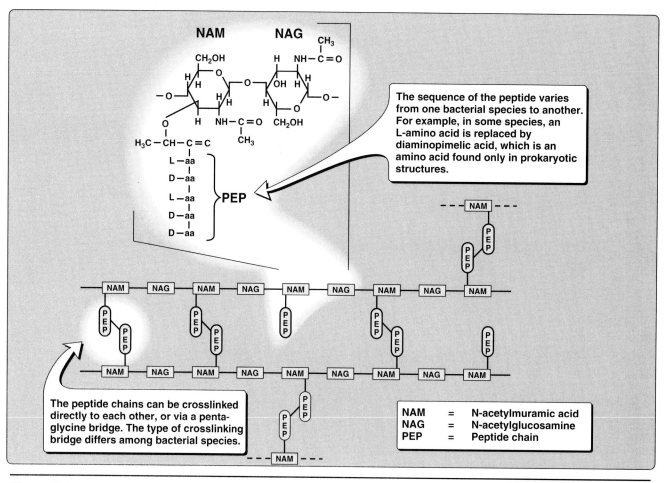

Figure 9.4
Structure of peptidoglycan, the major polymer of bacterial cell walls.

bone" of the mesh. The "peptido" portion of the polymer is a short string of amino acids that serves to cross-link polysaccharide adjacent strands at the NAM subunits of the backbone, thus forming a network with high tensile strength (Figure 9.4). [Note: The presence of D-amino acids helps to render the bacterial wall resistant to host peptidases, such as those in the intestine.] A primary function of the cell wall is to prevent the cell from exploding in hypotonic solutions due to its high internal osmotic pressure. In fact, the antibiotic penicillin causes bacteria to rupture, in part, because it interferes with the cross-linking of the peptidoglycan, thus weakening the cell wall. [Note: Penicillin also appears to activate endogenous lytic enzymes (**autolysins**) that contribute to the disruption.] A discussion of cell wall synthesis is presented on p. 111.

B. The cell membrane

The cell membrane is composed of phospholipid, the molecules of which form two parallel surfaces (called a lipid bilayer) such that the polar phosphate groups are on the outside of the bilayer and the nonpolar lipid chains are on the inside (Figure 9.5). [Note: This structure does not differ significantly from the typical eukaryotic plasma membrane.] The membrane acts as a permeability barrier,

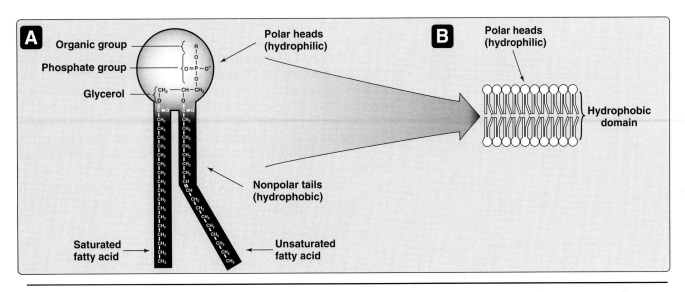

Figure 9.5
Structure of the lipid bilayer that constitutes the major portion of the bacterial cell membrane.
A. Phospholipid molecules. B. Lipid bilayer containing phospholipids.

restricting the kind and amount of molecules that enter and leave the cell. The permeability of the membrane is also selective. For example, lipid-soluble, small molecules such as molecular oxygen and carbon dioxide easily traverse the membrane, whereas charged molecules, and macromolecules in general, cannot pass through. The permeability of the membrane is selective also because of the presence of specific proteins embedded in the membrane that form channels (**porins**) and carriers (**permeases**) that facilitate the crossing of specific substances.

C. Differences between gram-positive and gram-negative species

The molecular details of the cell wall and membrane structures of gram-positive and gram-negative bacteria are shown in Figure 9.6. Additional surface layers such as a capsule or glycocalyx can be found in some species of gram-positive and gram-negative bacteria.

1. **Gram-positive organisms:** Gram-positive bacteria have a thick, multilayered, peptidoglycan cell wall that is exterior to the membrane. The peptidoglycan in most gram-positive species is covalently linked to teichoic acid, which is essentially a polymer of substituted glycerol units linked by phosphodiester bonds. [Note: For some teichoic acid variants, other alcohols, such as ribitol, may substitute for glycerol.] All gram-positive species also have teichoic acid in their membranes, where it is covalently linked to glycolipid. The teichoic acids are major cell surface antigens.

2. **Gram-negative organisms:** Gram-negative bacteria have two membranes—an outer membrane and an inner (cytoplasmic) membrane. Their peptidoglycan layer is located between the two membranes (analogous to a slice of bread with butter on both sides) in what is called the **periplasmic space**. The periplasmic space also contains enzymes and various other substances. In contrast to gram-positive cells, the peptidoglycan layer of gram-

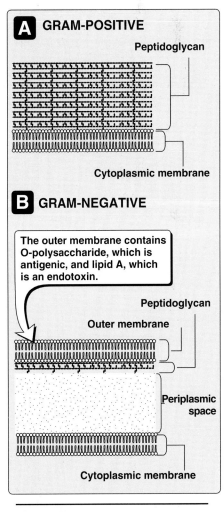

Figure 9.6
Comparison of gram-positive and gram-negative bacterial cell walls.

negative cells is thin, and the cells are consequently more susceptible to physical damage. The outer membrane is distinguished by the presence of various embedded lipopolysaccharides. The polysaccharide portion (**O-polysaccharide**) is antigenic, and can therefore be used to identify different strains and species. The lipid portion (called lipid A) is toxic to humans and animals. Lipid A, because it is an integral part of the membrane, is called an **endotoxin,** as opposed to **exotoxins**, which are secreted substances. [Note: Do not confuse either endo- or exotoxins with **enterotoxins**, which are exotoxins that are toxic for the mucosal membrane of the intestine. The word "enterotoxin" denotes the site of action, rather than its origin.]

D. The external capsule and glycocalyx

Many bacteria secrete a sticky, viscous material that forms an extracellular coating around the cell. The material is usually a polysaccharide, but in the case of pathogenic *Bacillus anthracis*, is poly-D-glutamic acid. If the material is tightly bound to the cell, and has an organized structure, it is called a **capsule** (see Figure 9.1, p. 101); if the material is loosely bound and amorphous, it is called a **slime layer** or **glycocalyx.** The capsule and glycocalyx allow cells to adhere to surfaces, protect bacteria from antibodies and phagocytosis, and act as diffusion barriers against some antibiotics, thus contributing to the organisms' pathogenicity.

E. Appendages

Many bacteria have hair-like appendages that project from the cell wall. These appendages are of two kinds, called **flagella** (singular: flagellum) and **pili** (singular: pilus).

1. **Flagella:** Prokaryotic flagella are long, semi-rigid, helical, hollow tubular structures composed of several thousand molecules of the protein, flagellin. They enable bacteria to propel themselves, for example, in response to a chemotactic stimulus. A flagellum is attached to the cell wall, the cell membrane, or both by a basal body, which is a complex molecular machine that rotates the flagellum like the screw propeller of a ship (Figure 9.7). Cells may have one or many flagella. Bacteria that have flagella often do not form compact colonies on an agar surface, but instead swarm over the surface of the agar if it is sufficiently wet, producing a scum-like mat. Flagella are highly antigenic.

2. **Pili:** Pili (also called **fimbriae**),which are shorter and thinner than flagella, function as attachment organs that promote specific cell-to-cell contact (see Figure 9.1, p. 101). The attachment can be between the bacterial cell and the host eukaryotic cell, or between one bacterial cell and another. An example of bacterium–to–eukaryotic cell interaction is the adherence of *Neisseria gonorrhoeae* to human mucosal cells (see p. 166). Strains of *N. gonorrhoeae* that lack pili are not pathogenic. An example of bacterium–to–bacterium attachment is the conjugal contact between mating cells of *Escherichia coli*, which is facilitated by the sex pili of the member of the mating pair that donates the DNA (see p. 121).

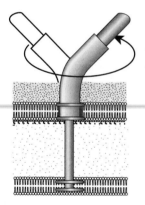

Figure 9.7
The flagellum rotator machine.

IV. THE CYTOPLASM

The cytoplasm is the complex mixture of substances enclosed by the envelope (see Figure 9.1, p. 101). It consists of an amorphous aqueous fluid in which are dissolved or suspended a myriad of metabolites, enzymes, ions, ribosomes, plasmids, and storage granules. Embedded in this fluid is a fibrous mass, called the nucleoid, which is composed of densely packed DNA, associated with RNA and proteins.

A. The nucleoid

The bacterial nucleoid is the equivalent of the nucleus of a eukaryotic cell in that it contains the preponderance of the cell's double-stranded DNA—the single circular chromosome of the bacterial cell. When stained with DNA-binding dyes, the nucleoid is visible in the light microscope. When thin sections are viewed in the electron microscope, the nucleoid appears as a mass of fibers, but it is not surrounded by any discernable membrane.

B. Ribosomes

In all organisms, prokaryotic and eukaryotic, ribosomes are the organelles that bring about the polymerization of amino acids to form polypeptide chains (proteins). These organelles may number as many as 70,000 in a rapidly growing bacterial cell. Bacterial ribosomes differ in composition and size from eukaryotic ribosomes (Figure 9.9). This explains the differential action of some antibiotics, such as streptomycin, which blocks protein synthesis by binding to the small ribosomal subunit in bacterial but not in eukaryotic cells.

C. Plasmids

A small fraction of the bacterial double-stranded DNA can exist as autonomously replicating circular molecules termed plasmids. Plasmids carry genes for a variety of functions that are generally not essential for the viability of the cell. However, plasmids can enhance bacterial survival by conveying antibiotic resistance, enhancing mating ability, and making possible toxin production.

V. SPORES AND SPORULATION

In order to enhance their survival during periods of environmental hostility (such as nutritional deprivation), some gram-positive rods undergo profound structural and metabolic changes. These result in the formation of a dormant cell called an **endospore** inside of the original cell. These endospores can be released from the original cell as free **spores** (Figure 9.8). [Note: The terms "endospore" and "spore" are often used interchangeably.] Spores are the most resistant life forms known. They are remarkably resistant to heat (they survive boiling), desiccation, ultraviolet light, and bacteriocidal chemical agents. In fact, sterilization procedures are assessed in terms of their ability to kill spores.

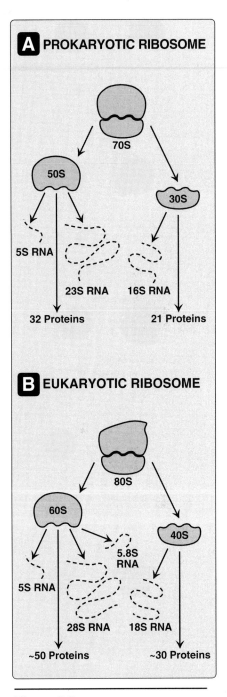

Figure 9.8
Ribosomal composition. (The number of proteins in the eukaryotic ribosomal subunits varies somewhat from species to species.)

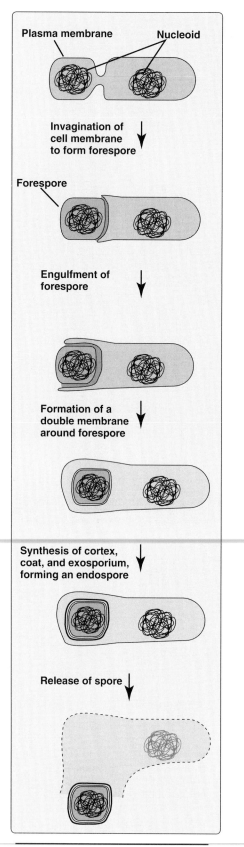

A. Sporulation

Sporulation can be thought of as a repackaging of a copy of bacterial DNA in a new form that contains very little water, has greatly reduced metabolic activity, does not divide, and has a restructured, highly impermeable, multi-layered envelope.

1. **The sporulation process:** Spore formation begins with the invagination of the parent cell membrane, producing a double membrane that encapsulates and isolates a copy of the bacterial DNA in what will become the **core** of the spore. In the space between the two membranes, two new peptidoglycan layers form. The innermost layer (the **wall**) is composed of the same type of peptidoglycan found in the envelope of the growing cell, whereas the thicker outer layer (the **cortex**) consists of a peptidoglycan with fewer cross-links. A keratin-like, highly impermeable shell (the **coat**) forms outside of both membranes, and, in turn, is covered by a lipoprotein layer (the **exosporium**) (Figure 9.9). The mature spore retains the complete machinery for protein synthesis, and in the core of the spore, new spore-specific enzymes are synthesized. At the same time, many of the enzymes of the original vegetative (nondividing) cell are degraded. One of the spore-specific enzymes is dipicolinic acid synthetase, which causes the accumulation of **calcium dipicolinate** to high levels (as much as ten percent of the cell's dry weight). When the endospore is completed, the parent cell lyses, releasing the spore.

2. **Spore germination:** To return to the vegetative state, spores must first be subjected to a treatment that weakens the spore coat (such as heat or extremes of pH), thus allowing germination to occur. If the activated spore is in a nutritious environment, which it senses by monitoring various key metabolites, it will begin to germinate. This process involves destruction of the cortex by lytic enzymes, followed by uptake of water, and release of dipicolinate from the cell.

B. Medical significance of sporulation

Some of the most notorious pathogens are spore-formers (Figure 9.10). These include *Bacillus anthracis* (anthrax, see p. 160), *Bacillus cereus* (gastroenteritis, see p. 162), *Clostridium tetani* (tetanus, see p. 215), *Clostridium botulinum* (botulism, see p. 213), and *Clostridium perfringens* (gas gangrene, see p. 210) (Figure 9.10). Spores of these organisms can remain viable for many years, and are generally not killed by boiling, but can be killed by autoclaving (that is, subjecting the spores to temperatures above 120°C at elevated pressure). [Note: In the absence of an autoclave, spores can largely be eliminated by a primary boiling to activate germination and, after a short period of vegetative growth, a second boiling.]

Figure 9.9
The formation of an endospore.

VI. GROWTH AND METABOLISM

All cells must accomplish certain metabolic tasks in order to maintain life. These tasks include uptake of nutrients, extraction of energy from the imported nutrients, synthesis or salvage of the building blocks of proteins, nucleic acids, polysaccharides, and lipids, and polymerization of these building blocks into macromolecules. All cells, whether they are bacteria or human, accomplish these metabolic tasks by very similar pathways. There are, however, some important differences that set bacteria apart metabolically from eukaryotic cells, and these differences can often be exploited in the development of antibacterial therapies.

A. Characteristics of bacterial growth

If bacterial cells are suspended in a liquid nutrient medium, the increase in cell number or mass can be measured in several ways. Techniques include microscopically counting the cells in a given volume using a ruled slide, by counting the number of appropriately diluted cells that are able to form colonies following transfer to a solid nutrient (agar) surface, or by quantitating the turbidity—which is proportional to cell mass—of a culture in liquid medium.

1. **Stages of the bacterial growth cycle:** Because bacteria reproduce by binary fission (one becomes two, two become four, four become eight, etc.), the number of cells increases exponentially with time (the **exponential** or **log phase** of growth). Depending on the species, the minimum doubling time can be as short as twenty minutes or as long as several days. For example, for a rapidly growing species such as *E. coli* in nutritionally complete medium, a single cell can give rise to some ten million cells in just eight hours. Eventually, growth slows and ceases entirely (**stationary phase**) as nutrients are depleted and toxic waste products accumulate. Most of the cells in stationary phase are not dead, however, because if they are diluted into fresh growth medium exponential growth will resume after a **lag phase**. [Note: If held in stationary phase for an extended period the cells will eventually die.] The phases of the growth cycle are illustrated in Figure 9.11.

2. **Surface growth:** If a single bacterial cell is placed on a solid nutrient agar surface, the progeny of this cell remain close to the site of deposition, and eventually form a compact macroscopic mass of cells (**colony**, Figure 9.12). For rapidly growing species, overnight incubation at 30° to 37°C is sufficient to produce visible colonies, each containing millions of cells. The gross characteristics of colonies (for example, color, shape, adherence, smell, and surface texture) can be useful guides for identification of the species of bacterium. [Note: Some species do not form compact circular colonies because the cells are capable of movement, and swarm over the agar surface, especially if the surface is moist. Other

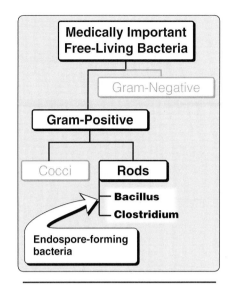

Figure 9.10
Medically important spore formers.

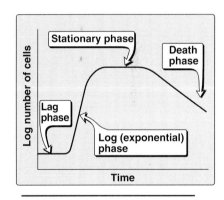

Figure 9.11
Kinetics of bacterial growth in liquid medium.

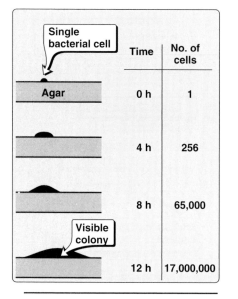

Figure 9.12
Growth of bacterial colonies on a solid, nutrient surface, for example, nutrient agar. [Note: The doubling time of the bacteria is assumed to be 0.5 hr.]

species, particularly the actinomycetes, grow as long filaments of cells (mycelial growth). The cells of such species may form compact colonies, but these have a fuzzy appearance due to the filaments advancing vertically and outward at the colony edge.]

B. Growth requirements

In order for bacteria to grow and divide, a variety of nutrition and growth requirements must be met. Different species of bacteria can vary widely in their needs for specific growth conditions, including such physical factors as appropriate temperature and pH. This must be taken into consideration when an attempt is made to culture an organism, because all growth requirements must be met in order for the organism to multiply.

1. **Nutrients:** All clinically important bacteria are **heterotrophs** (that is, they require organic carbon for growth). Heterotrophs may have very complex or very simple requirements for organic molecules. [Note: Organisms that can reduce carbon dioxide, and thus do not require organic compounds for cell growth, are called **autotrophs**.] Bacteria must also have access to the major elements nitrogen, sulfur, phosphorus, potassium, calcium, magnesium, and iron, plus some minor elements. Most bacteria require varying numbers of **growth factors**, which are organic compounds required by the cell in order to grow, but which the organism cannot itself synthesize (for example, vitamins). [Note: Organisms that require either a large number of growth factors or must be supplied with very specific ones are referred to as **fastidious**.]

2. **Oxygen requirement:** Bacteria can be categorized according to their growth responses in the presence and absence of oxygen. **Aerobic bacteria** (**aerobes**) such as *Mycobacterium tuberculosis* grow in the presence of oxygen, and can use oxygen as the terminal electron acceptor in energy production (see below). **Obligate aerobes** have an absolute requirement for oxygen. **Facultative** organisms such as *Escherichia coli* grow in the presence or absence of oxygen. Some of these, the "true" facultatives, use oxygen preferentially as the terminal electron acceptor when it is present, whereas **microaerophilic** organisms such as *Campylobacter jejuni*, require or tolerate oxygen, but at an oxygen pressure lower than that of the atmosphere. **Anaerobic bacteria** such as *Clostridium botulinum* can grow in the absence of oxygen, producing energy by fermentation (see below), whereas **obligate anaerobes** grow only in the absence of oxygen, and may in fact be killed by small amounts of oxygen. [Note: Obligate anaerobes lack the enzymes peroxidase and superoxide dismutase that are required for the elimination of the highly toxic peroxides and superoxide radicals that are by-products of metabolism in the presence of oxygen.]

C. Energy production

A distinctive feature of bacterial metabolism is the variety of mechanisms used to generate energy from these carbon sources. According to the biochemical mechanism used, bacterial metabolism can be categorized into three types: **aerobic respiration**, **anaerobic respiration**, and **fermentation** (Figure 9.13).

1. **Aerobic respiration** (or simply, respiration) is the metabolic process in which **molecular oxygen** serves as the final electron acceptor of the electron transport chain. In this process, oxygen is reduced to water. Respiration is the energy-generating mode used by all aerobic bacteria.

2. **Anaerobic respiration** is the metabolic process in which **inorganic compounds** other than molecular oxygen serve as the final electron acceptors. Depending on the species, the acceptors can be molecules such as nitrate or sulfate. Anaerobic respiration can be used as an alternative to aerobic respiration in some species (facultative organisms), but is obligatory in other species (some obligate anaerobes). [Note: Other obligate anaerobes use fermentation as their main mode of energy metabolism. This is particularly true among the anaerobic bacteria of medical importance.]

3. **Fermentation** is an alternative anaerobic process exhibited by some species. It is the metabolic process by which an **organic metabolic intermediate** derived from a "fermentable" substrate serves as the final electron acceptor. The substrates that can be fermented, and the final products, depend on the species. Sugars are excellent fermentable substrates because they yield reducible intermediates. In the fermentation of glucose to lactic acid, for example, the intermediate pyruvic acid is the final electron acceptor. Similarly, in the fermentation of glucose to ethanol, acetaldehyde (a derivative of pyruvic acid) is the final electron acceptor.

D. Cell wall synthesis

The bacterial cell wall, constructed on the surface of the cell membrane, is composed of a peptidoglycan polymer in which the repeating carbohydrate backbone subunit is NAG–NAM (see p. 103). These backbone chains are cross-linked by short peptides (PEP) to form a rigid meshwork (Figure 9.14).

1. **Activation of carbohydrate subunits:** As in all biological polymerizations, the NAM and NAG subunits are activated by attachment to a carrier, in this case, the nucleotide UDP.

2. **Synthesis of the linking peptide:** A pentapeptide is added to UDP–NAM by sequential transfer of amino acids, with the two terminal alanine residues added as a dipeptide. This pentapeptide may contain some nonstandard amino acids, for example, diaminopimelic acid (DAP, a metabolic precursor of lysine), and D-amino acids. As would be expected, the sequence is not dictated by an RNA template, but instead, by the specificity of the enzymes that form the peptide bonds.

3. **Transfer of the cell wall unit to bactoprenol phosphate:** The NAM–PEP moiety is transferred from the UDP carrier to a new carrier, bactoprenol phosphate (BPP), located on the inner surface of the cell membrane. At this point, UDP–NAG transfers NAG

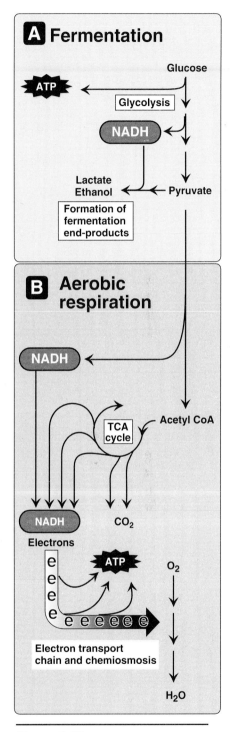

Figure 9.13
Overview of respiration, fermentation, and energy production in bacteria. [Note: Compounds other than oxygen, such as nitrate and sulfate, can be used as terminal electron acceptors in anaerobic respiration.]

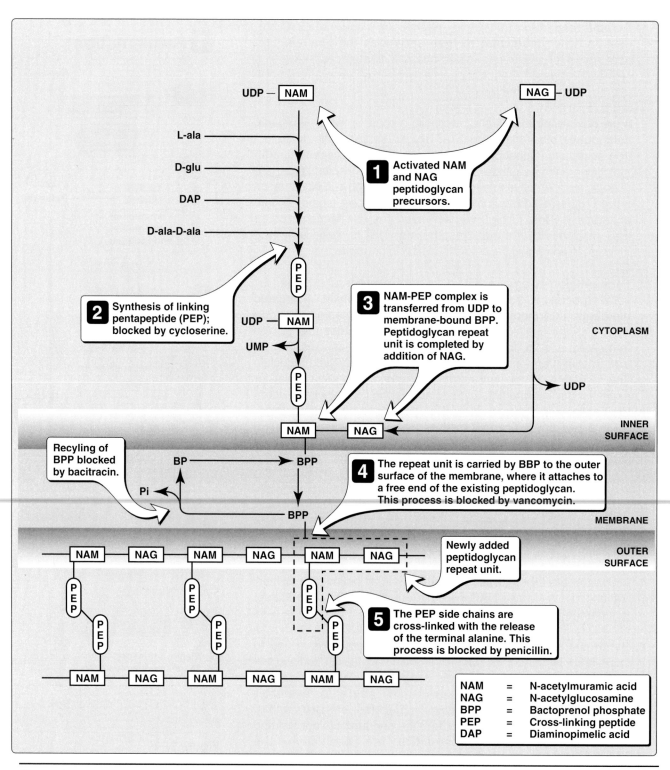

Figure 9.14
Synthesis of a bacterial cell wall.

to NAM–PEP, thereby completing the peptidoglycan repeat unit now attached to the carrier BPP.

4. **Addition of the repeat unit to the existing peptidoglycan:** BPP carries the NAG–NAM–PEP repeat unit through the cell membrane to the outside surface where the peptidoglycan of the existing cell wall is located. The repeat unit is added to a free end of the existing peptidoglycan, thereby increasing the length of the polymer by one repeat unit. Presumably, free ends are created by a limited hydrolytic loosening of the preexisting peptidoglycan.

5. **Cross-linking of the pentapeptide to the peptidoglycan backbone:** Although the N–terminal end of the pentapeptide is attached to the NAM moieties of the backbone, the C–terminal end is dangling free. Cross-linking is brought about by a transpeptidation reaction that bonds DAP of the peptide in one chain to the alanine (ala) at position four of the peptide in an adjacent chain, causing the release of the terminal ala. This mode of **direct** crosslinking is characteristic of *E. coli*, and many other gram-negative species. [Note: In gram-positive bacteria such as *Staphylococcus aureus*, a glycine pentapeptide is usually interposed between lysine (lys) at position three of one PEP, and ala at position four of the PEP to which the linkage is to be made (Figure 9.15).]

6. **Cell wall synthesis as a target of antibacterial agents:** Because many of the reactions involved in the synthesis of the bacterial cell wall do not occur in mammalian cells, bacterial cell wall synthesis is an ideal target for some highly specific antibacterial agents, particularly the β–lactam antibiotics.

   a. **β-Lactam antibiotics:** The penicillins and cephalosporins inhibit the enzymes that catalyze transpeptidation and carboxypeptidation reactions of cell wall assembly. These enzymes are called penicillin-binding proteins (PBPs) because they all have active sites that bind β-lactam antibiotics. No single PBP species is the target of β-lactam antibiotics; rather their lethal effect on bacteria is the result of inactivation of multiple species of PBPs. Most PBPs are involved in bacterial cell wall synthesis. However, β-lactamases—enzymes that catalyze hydrolysis of the β-lactam ring—bind penicillin, and are therefore also classified as PBPs. Most PBPs are membrane-bound except for β-lactamases, which may be either secreted or membrane-associated. Acquired resistance to β-lactam antibiotics may result from genetic modifications resulting in production of modified PBPs that have a lower affinity for β-lactam antibiotics (see p. 133).

   b. **Bacitracin, cyclosersine and vancomycin:** Other antibiotics that interfere with cell wall synthesis include bacitracin, which inhibits the recycling of bactoprenol phosphate; cycloserine, which inhibits synthesis of the D–ala–D–ala dipeptide that provides the two terminal residues of the pentapeptide; and vancomycin, which blocks incorporation of the NAG–NAM–PEP repeat unit into the growing peptidoglycan chain.

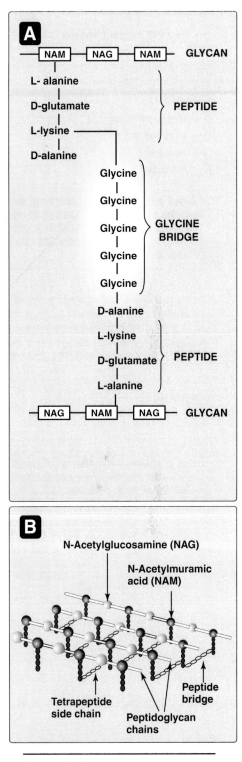

Figure 9.15
A. Glycine bridge in the peptidoglycan of *Staphylococcus aureus*.
B. Organization of peptidoglycan layer in gram-positive cells.

Study Questions

Choose the ONE correct answer

9.1 Bacteria whose cell walls retain crystal violet after decolorization are classified as

A. acid-fast.

B. potential pathogens.

C. gram-positive.

D. anaerobes.

E. mycobacteria.

> Correct answer = C. Mycobacteria are acid-fast, and owe their staining properties to mycolic acid. The binding of crystal violet (that is, gram-positive staining) is not related to pathogenicity or manner of respiration.

9.2 A bacterial culture with a starting density of 10^3 cells/ml is incubated in liquid nutrient broth. If the bacteria have both a lag time and a generation time of ten minutes, what will the cell density be at thirty minutes?

A. 1.0×10^3

B. 2.0×10^3

C. 3.0×10^3

D. 4.0×10^3

E. 6.0×10^3

> Correct answer = D. After a 10 minute lag, the bacteria with double in number at 20 minutes, and double again by 30 minutes.

9.3 Which of the following components are found in the cell walls of gram-positive bacteria, but not gram-negative bacteria?

A. Cytoplasmic membrane

B. Lipopolysaccharide

C. Outer membrane

D. Peptidoglycan

E. Teichoic acid

> Correct answer = E. Gram-positive bacteria have a thick, multilayered, peptidoglycan cell wall that is exterior to the membrane. The peptidoglycan in most gram-positive species is covalently linked to teichoic acid, which is essentially a polymer of substituted glycerol units linked by phosphodiester bonds. All gram-positive species also have teichoic acid in their membranes, where it is covalently linked to glycolipid. The teichoic acids are major cell surface antigens. Gram-negative bacteria have two membranes—an outer membrane and an inner (cytoplasmic) membrane. Their peptidoglycan layer is located between the two membranes in the periplasmic space. The periplasmic space also contains enzymes and various other substances. The outer membrane is distinguished by the presence of various embedded lipopolysaccharides.

9.4 In 1998, a large botulism outbreak occurred in El Paso, Texas. The foodborne illness was shown to be due to foil-wrapped baked potatoes that were held at room temperature for several days before use in dips at a Greek restaurant. The dip yielded botulinum toxin type A, as did stool (and in some cases serum) samples from 18 of the 30 affected patients. Four patients required mechanical ventilation; none died. What would be the expected outcome if the potatoes had be reheated to 100°C for 10 minutes before being served? [Hint: See p. 213 for properties of *Clostridium botulinum* toxin].

A. Heat would kill the spores of *Clostridium botulinum*.

B. Heat would promote the vegetative state.

C. Heat would inactivate the toxin in the potato dip.

D. Heat would increase the number of toxin-producing bacteria.

E. Heat would not alter the outcome.

> Correct answer = C. Clostridium botulinum spores are commonly found on raw potatoes and generally are not killed if the potatoes are baked in foil, which holds in moisture and thus keeps the potatoes' surface temperature at 100°C (below the temperature required for spore killing of >120°C). During storage at room temperature in the anaerobic environment provided by the foil, spores germinate and toxin forms. Heating at 100°C would kill most the Clostridium botulinum because the bacterium is large in its vulnerable, vegative state. The heat would also inactivate toxin produced. durng the room-temperature storage.However, any remaining spores would not be killed.

Bacterial Genetics

10

I. OVERVIEW

Because a single kind of molecule, DNA, is the genetic material of all cellular organisms, from bacteria to humans, basic genetic phenomena—gene mutation, gene replication, and gene recombination—are much the same for all life forms. The prototypic organism used in microbial genetic studies for the past fifty years is the enteric, gramnegative *Escherichia coli* (see p. 175). Indeed, much of what we know about the molecular basis of human heredity was first discovered from studies with *E. coli* and its viruses. An aspect of microbial genetics of great clinical importance is the ability of bacteria to transfer genes, especially genes for antibiotic resistance, to other bacteria both within and between species. Such transfer allows the flow of antibiotic resistance genes from nonpathogenic bacterial populations to pathogenic populations, with potentially dire consequences for public health.

II. THE BACTERIAL GENOME

The **genome** of an organism is defined as the totality of its genetic material. For bacteria, the genome consists of a single chromosome that carries all of the essential genes, and of one or more varieties of plasmid that generally carry nonessential genes (Figure 10.1).

A. The chromosome

All of the essential genes, and many nonessential genes, of the bacterium are carried on a single, long piece of circular doublestranded DNA. This molecular structure is called the "chromosome" by analogy with the heredity-carriers of eukaryotic cells. Most bacteria have chromosomes that contain 2000 to 4000 genes. The relatively small chromosome of the bacterium *Haemophilus influenzae* was the first cellular chromosome to be totally sequenced (1995). It has 1,830,137 base pairs, representing 1,743 genes. From this landmark achievement one can begin to understand what it takes to make a living cell. For example, the

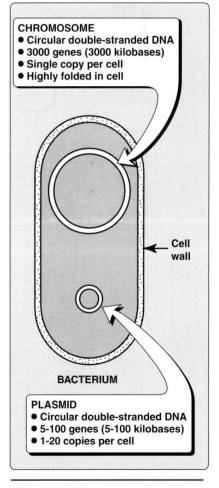

CHROMOSOME
- Circular double-stranded DNA
- 3000 genes (3000 kilobases)
- Single copy per cell
- Highly folded in cell

Cell wall

BACTERIUM

PLASMID
- Circular double-stranded DNA
- 5-100 genes (5-100 kilobases)
- 1-20 copies per cell

Figure 10.1
The bacterial genome. [Note: Helical double-stranded DNA shown as two concentric circles.]

Lippincott's Illustrated Reviews: Microbiology,
by William A. Strohl, Harriet Rouse, Bruce D. Fisher.
Lippincott, Williams & Wilkins, Baltimore, MD © 2001

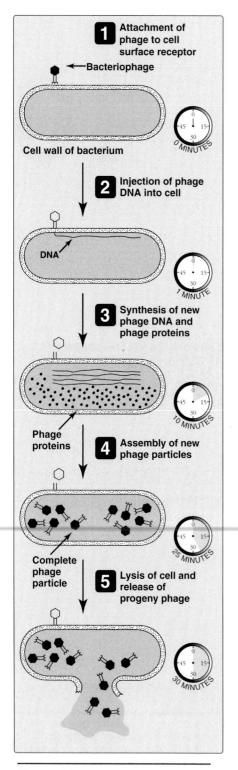

Figure 10.2
Bacteriophage replication. Clock indicates total elapsed time starting with attachment at t=0. [Note: Bacterial chromosome and plasmid are not shown.]

gene catalog of *H. influenzae* indicates that 141 genes participate in protein synthesis, 87 function in DNA synthesis, 105 are involved in energy metabolism, 123 function to regulate passage of materials across the cell membrane, etc.

B. Plasmids

Typically, bacteria contain small DNA circles called **plasmids**, which range in size from 1.5 kilobase (kb) pairs to 120 kb pairs (less than one-tenth the size of the bacterial chromosome). Plasmids replicate independently of the chromosome, and can exist in the cell as one copy or as many copies. Plasmids can carry genes for toxins, and for proteins that promote the transfer of the plasmid to other cells, but usually do not include genes that are essential for growth or replication of the cell. Many plasmids contain mobile DNA sequences (**transposons**) that can move between plasmids, and between plasmids and the chromosome. Transposons are in fact the repository for many antibiotic resistance genes, and are responsible for the ability of some plasmids to integrate into the chromosome.

III. BACTERIOPHAGE

A bacteriophage (**phage**) is a virus that replicates inside of a bacterial cell, and consists of nothing more than a piece of nucleic acid encapsulated in a protective protein coat. Depending on the phage, the nucleic acid can be DNA or RNA, double-stranded or single-stranded, and can have a size from about 3,000 bases (3 genes) to about 200,000 bases (200 genes). The typical replicative cycle (Figure 10.2) begins with attachment of the phage to receptors on the cell surface, followed by injection of the nucleic acid into the bacterial cell, leaving all or most of the protein outside the cell. [Note: This is in contrast to viral infection of vertebrate cells, where the entire virus is taken up by the cell, and its nucleic acid released intracellularly (see p. 299).] The phage nucleic acid takes over the cell's biosynthetic machinery to replicate its own genetic material, and to synthesize phage-specific proteins. These proteins consist of phage-specific enzymes and proteins of the phage coat. When sufficient coat proteins and new phage DNA have accumulated, these components self-assemble into mature phage particles with the DNA encapsulated by the phage coat. Release of the new phage particles is accomplished by a phage-specific enzyme (a lysozyme) that dissolves the bacterial cell wall. The number of phage particles in a sample can be determined by a simple and rapid plaque assay. If a single phage particle is immobilized in a confluent bacterial lawn growing on a nutrient agar surface this phage, within a few hours, will produce millions of progeny at the expense of neighboring bacterial cells, leaving a visible "hole" or plaque in the otherwise opaque lawn (Figure 10.3A).

A. Virulent phage

Phage are classified as virulent or temperate depending on the nature of their relationship to the host bacterium. Infection of a bacterium with a virulent phage inevitably results in the death of the cell by lysis, with release of newly replicated phage particles. Under optimal conditions, a bacterial cell infected with only one phage par-

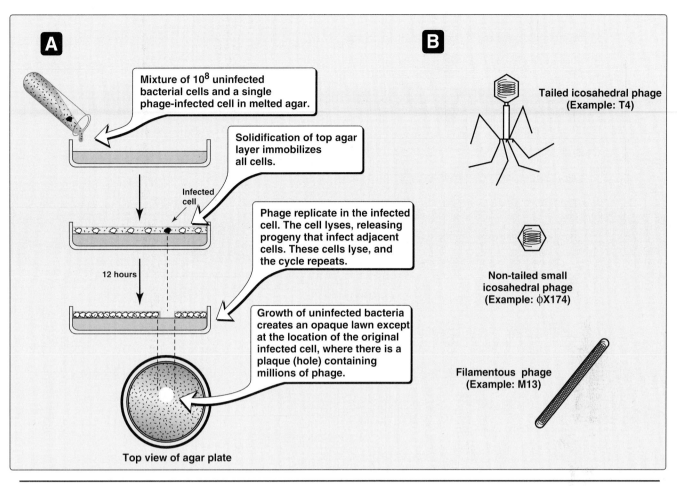

Figure 10.3
A. Visual detection of bacteriophage by the plaque method. B: Structures of representative bacteriophage.

ticle can produce hundreds of progeny phage in twenty minutes. Examples of extensively studied virulent phage, all of which are able to replicate in *E. coli*, are T2, T4, T7 (all double-stranded DNA), φX174 and MS-13 (both single-stranded DNA), and MS-2 (single-stranded RNA, Figure 10.3B). Generally, phage that attack one bacterial species do not attack other bacterial species.

B. Temperate phage

A bacterium infected with a temperate phage can have the same fate as a bacterium infected with a virulent phage (lysis rapidly following infection). However, an alternative outcome is also possible, namely, after entering the cell, the phage DNA, rather than replicating autonomously, can fuse or integrate with the chromosome of the host cell. In this state (the **prophage** state), the expression of phage genes is repressed indefinitely by a protein, termed the **repressor**, encoded within the phage genome. No new phage particles are produced, the host cell survives, and the phage DNA replicates as part of the host chromosome (Figure 10.4). [Note: The temperate bacteriophage lambda is the most thoroughly understood of all complex viruses.]

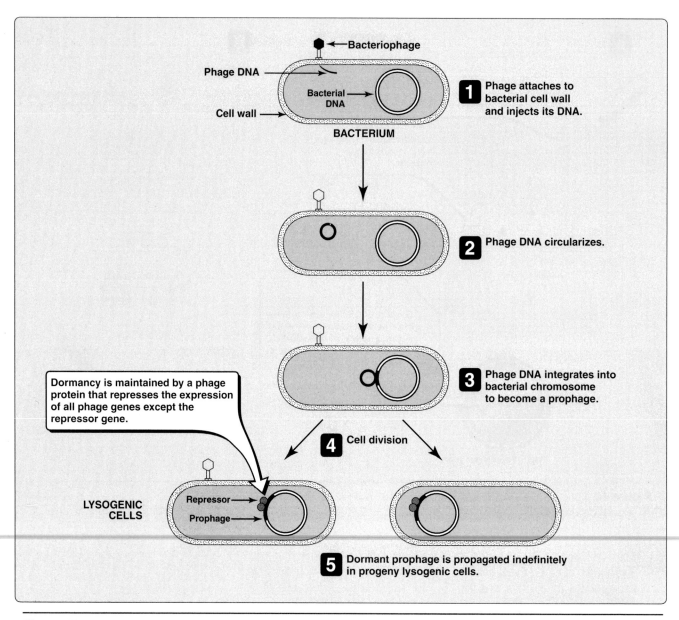

Figure 10.4
The integration of temperate phage DNA into the bacterial chromosome generates a lysogenic bacterium.

C. Lysogenic bacteria

Lysogenic bacteria are bacteria that carry a prophage; the phenomenon is termed **lysogeny**, and the bacterial cell is said to be **lysogenized**. Nonlysogenic bacteria can be made lysogenic by infection with a temperate phage. The association of prophage and bacterial cell is highly stable, but can be destabilized by various treatments, such as exposure to ultraviolet light, that damage the host DNA. When DNA damage occurs, repression of phage genes is lifted, the prophage excises from the host chromosome, replicates autonomously, and produces progeny phage particles. The host cell is lysed just as with a virulent phage. The emergence of the virus from its latent prophage state is called **induction** (Figure 10.5). Lysogenic bacteria sometimes have properties strikingly different from their nonlysogenic counterparts, for example, *Corynebacterium diphtheriae* is pathogenic because it carries a prophage that possesses a gene (the *tox* gene) that encodes the diphtheria toxin (see p. 158). Strains of *C. diphtheriae* that lack the prophage are nonpathogenic. Similarly, lysogenic strains of group A streptococcus (*Streptococcus pyogenes*) produce pyrogenic exotoxins (erythrogenic toxins, see p. 147). The acquisition by bacteria of properties due to the presence of a prophage is called **lysogenic conversion**.

IV. DNA REPLICATION

The replication of bacterial DNA is brought about by several multienzyme complexes. Most of our knowledge of the process derives from studies with *E. coli* and its phages.

A. Replicons and replication origins

In order to replicate in a prokaryotic cell, a piece of DNA must have a special sequence called a **replication origin**, which is recognized by the enzyme complex (**primasome**) that initiates DNA replication. DNA that possesses such an origin is called a **replicon** (Figure 10.6A). In general, DNA fragments transferred from one bacterial cell to another by conjugation, generalized transduction, or transformation (see below) are not replicons, and thus are not propagated unless they become integrated into a replicon such as a chromosome or a plasmid.

B. Circular versus linear replication

Because DNA polymerases proceed only in the 5' to 3' direction along the DNA template, the replication of linear DNA in all organisms requires special mechanisms to ensure that the ends of the molecules are completed. Bacteria, in general, do not have this problem because the chromosome and plasmids are in a circular configuration, and replicate as illustrated in Figure 10.6B. Replication of a circular molecule can generate either more circles or long chains (**concatenates**) composed of multiple repeats of the circular sequence. The concatenates are subsequently cut into chromosome-sized pieces. The linear DNA of some phages invariably has a short sequence at one end of the molecule that is repeated at the other end (direct **terminal repeats**). These terminal repeats allow the DNA to form either circles or chains.

V. GENE TRANSFER

Genes can be transferred from one bacterial cell to another by means of three distinct mechanisms: conjugation, transduction, and transformation. Because the transferred DNA usually does not contain an origin of replication, these genes will be passed on to succeeding generations only if the transferred DNA becomes incorporated into the recipient chromosome, which has an origin of replication.

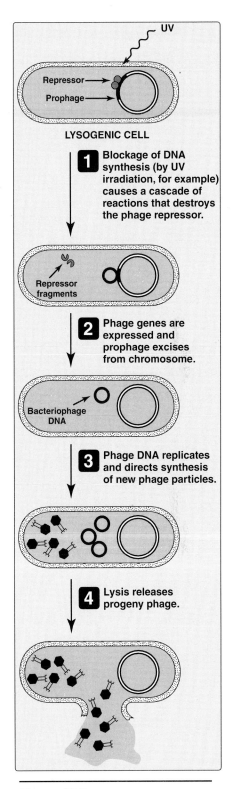

Figure 10.5
Induction of a lysogenic bacterium generates new phage particles.

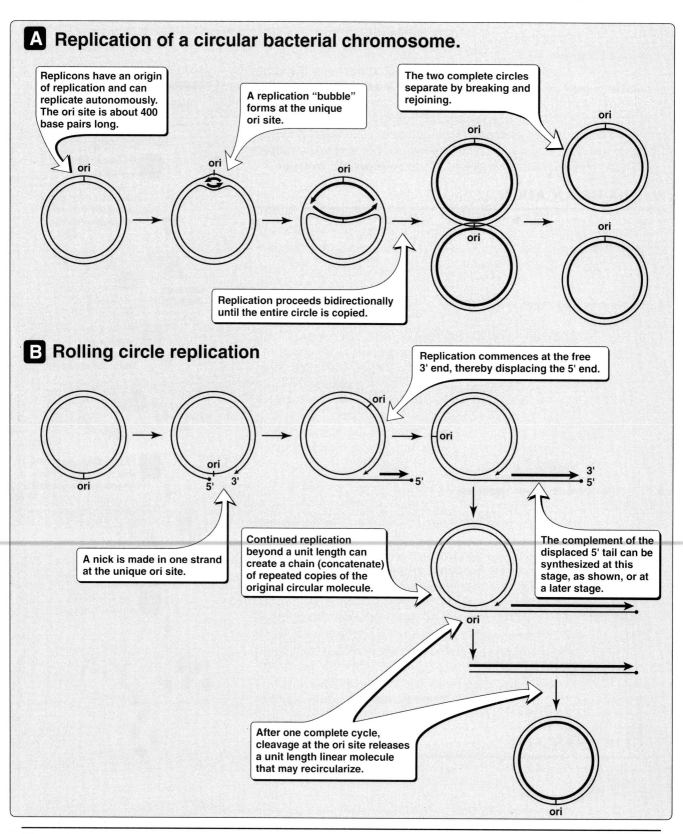

Figure 10.6
Replication of circular DNA. A: Bacterial chromosome; B: Mechanism used by some bacterial viruses, plasmids, and in chromosomal transfer.

A. Conjugation

Conjugation refers to the process by which bacteria transfer genes from one cell to another by means of cell-to-cell contact. The donor (male) and recipient (female) cells must have the proper genetic constitution in order to adhere to each other, and to form a cytoplasmic bridge between the cells through which DNA can pass. Specifically, the process requires the presence on the donor cell of hair-like projections called **sex pili** that make contact with specific receptor sites on the surface of the recipient cell. This contact results in the formation of a relatively stable cell pair, and the initiation of DNA transfer. Although the sex pilus is a hollow tube, there is no evidence that DNA passes through this tube. Rather, it is thought that after attachment to the potential recipient cell, the pilus retracts into the donor cell, thus bringing the donor and recipient cells into close contact.

1. **Conjugative plasmids:** Certain large plasmids (conjugative plasmids) carry genes that function to promote their own transfer to other cells, including genes that direct the synthesis of the sex pili. The **F** (for **fertility**) plasmid of *E. coli* is the prototype. If cells that carry the F plasmid (called F⁺) are mixed with a large excess of cells that lack the F plasmid (called F⁻), the F plasmid rapidly spreads, and the population will eventually become all F⁺ (Figure 10.7). The F plasmid carries some fourteen genes, including the structural gene for the pilus protein (**pilin**), that function in sex pilus (in this case called the **F pilus**) formation. The F plasmid can carry additional genes, such as genes for antibiotic resistance, and these genes are also transferred to recipient cells.

2. **Chromosomal mobilization:** The F plasmid can integrate into the chromosome in a manner similar to the integration of a prophage, thereby conferring on the chromosome the ability to transfer itself to other cells (Figure 10.8A). Strains of bacteria in which this fusion has occurred are called **Hfr**'s (for **h**igh-**f**requency **r**ecombination). The F plasmid can integrate at many different locations on the chromosome (although the process is not random, and specific sites are preferred), but each independently arising Hfr strain represents the integration at a single site. The transfer of the chromosome to a recipient cell occurs in a sequential manner, starting at the site of fusion of F with the chromosome, and proceeding at a rate of about forty kilobases (forty genes) per minute. The order of genes on the bacterial chromosome can be determined experimentally by noting the sequence in which the genes appear in recipient cells in a mating between an Hfr strain and a genetically marked recipient strain (Figure 10.8B). A conjugating pair is usually disrupted by viscous shear forces and Brownian motion before the entire chromosome enters the recipient. Although an average of only ten to twenty percent of the chromosome is transferred, nevertheless the entire chromosome can be mapped by using a number of different Hfrs whose transferred segments overlap. Conjugative transfer occurs concomitantly with DNA replication, so that the donor cell does not lose genetic information, but merely transfers the newly replicated copy of the information to the recipient.

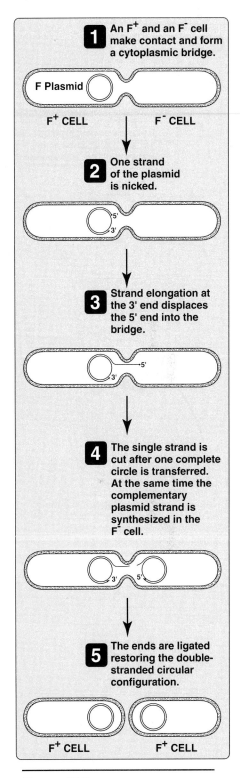

1 An F⁺ and an F⁻ cell make contact and form a cytoplasmic bridge.

F Plasmid

F⁺ CELL   F⁻ CELL

2 One strand of the plasmid is nicked.

3 Strand elongation at the 3' end displaces the 5' end into the bridge.

4 The single strand is cut after one complete circle is transferred. At the same time the complementary plasmid strand is synthesized in the F⁻ cell.

5 The ends are ligated restoring the double-stranded circular configuration.

F⁺ CELL   F⁺ CELL

Figure 10.7
Cell-to-cell transfer of a conjugative plasmid. (Chromosomal DNA is not shown.)

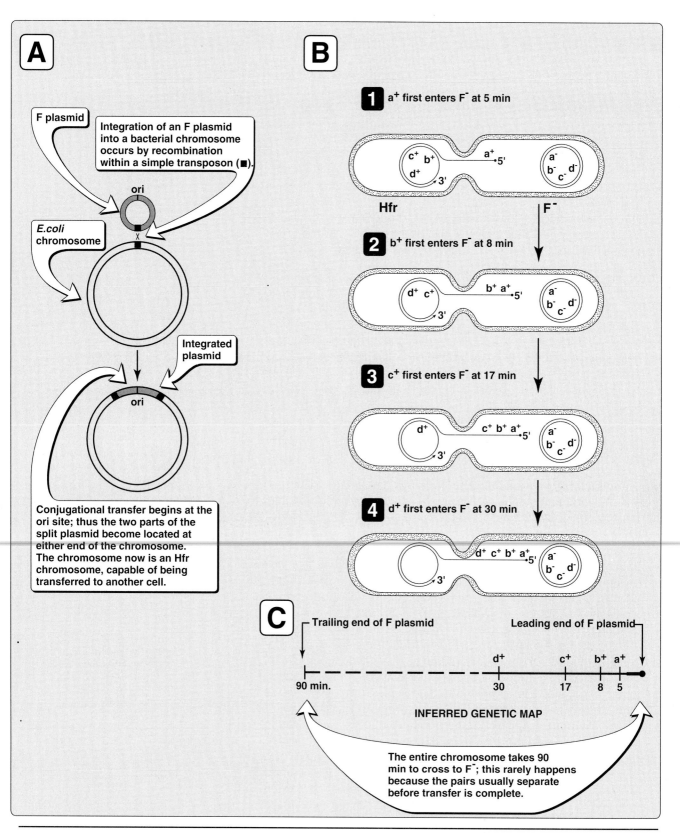

Figure 10.8
A. Integration of a conjugative plasmid into the bacterial chromosome generating an Hfr. B, C: The order of genes on the bacterial chromosome can be determined by the time of entry of the genes into a recipient cell.

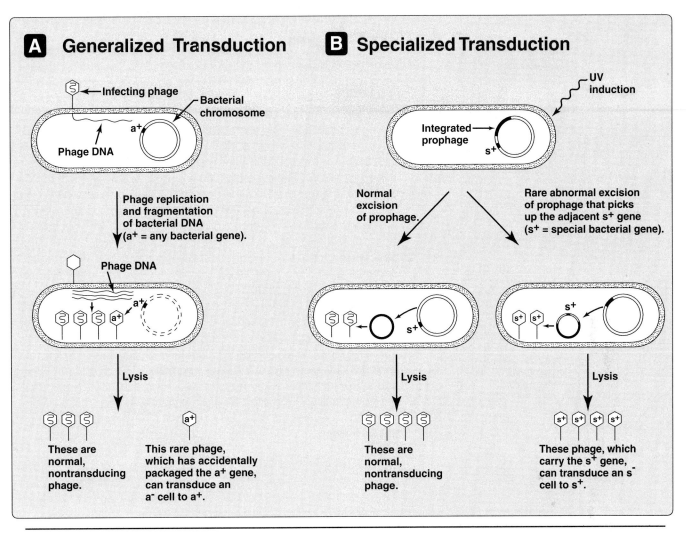

Figure 10.9
Certain phage can package bacterial genes and transfer them to other bacteria (transduction). By one mechanism (A) any bacterial gene can be transferred; by a second mechanism (B) only certain genes can be transferred, namely those in close proximity to a prophage.

B. Transduction

Transduction refers to transfer of genes from one cell to another via a phage vector without cell-to-cell contact. There are two ways in which this can occur: generalized transduction, and specialized transduction. In each case, the transducing phage is a temperate phage, so that the recipient cell survives the phage infection.

1. **Generalized transduction:** In generalized transduction, a random fragment of bacterial DNA, resulting from phage-induced cleavage of the bacterial chromosome, is accidentally encapsulated in a phage protein coat in place of the phage DNA (Figure 10.9A). When this rare phage particle infects a cell it injects the bacterial DNA fragment into the cell. If this fragment becomes integrated into the recipient chromosome by recombination, the recipient cell will be stably transduced. For example, if the recipient cell has a

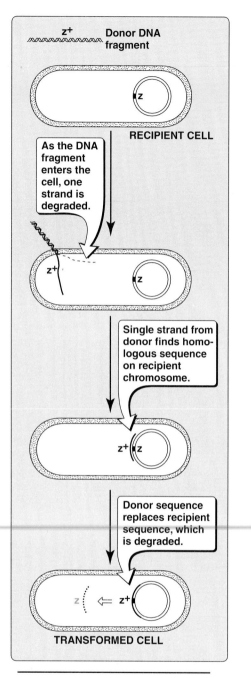

Figure 10.10
Genetic transformation of a bacterial cell by uptake of a DNA fragment.

genetic defect in leucine biosynthesis, and thus cannot grow in the absence of leucine (leu⁻), transducing phage grown on a leucine nonrequiring host (leu⁺) can cure this defect by transferring the fragment of missing DNA needed for leucine synthesis from the leu⁺ to the leu⁻ cell. Because a random fragment of bacterial DNA is packaged in a phage protein coat, any bacterial gene can be transduced in this manner. The frequency of cotransduction of two genes is a measure of their separation on the bacterial chromosome (that is, the closer two genes are located on the chromosome, the more likely they are to be transduced together). [Note: Because transducing phage package about fifty genes at a time (some one percent of the bacterial genome), generalized transduction provides a useful means for mapping bacterial genes at a finer scale than does conjugation.]

2. **Specialized transduction:** In specialized transduction, only certain bacterial genes are transduced, namely those that are located on the bacterial chromosome in close proximity to the prophage insertion site of the transducing phage (Figure 10.9B). The phage acquires the bacterial genes by a rare, abnormal excision from the bacterial chromosome. In general, a specialized transducing phage particle contains both phage and bacterial DNA joined together as a single molecule. Upon infecting another cell, this joint molecule integrates into the recipient chromosome just as the phage DNA would normally do in the process of becoming a prophage.

C. Transformation

Transformation refers to the transfer of genes from one cell to another by means of naked DNA. The discovery of transformation in 1928, one of the most important in all of biology, led eventually to the identification of DNA as the genetic material.

1. **The discovery of transformation:** Transformation was discovered in the course of studies on bacterial pneumonia caused by *Streptococcus pneumoniae* (see p. 150). Pathogenic strains of *S. pneumoniae* produce a polysaccharide that encapsulates the cells, and protects them from the host's immune system. This polysaccharide causes agar surface colonies to have a glistening, smooth (S) appearance. By contrast, mutant strains that fail to synthesize the polysaccharide are nonpathogenic, and produce rough (R) colonies. The seminal observation was that when heat-killed S cells were mixed with live R cells, some of the R cells transformed to S cells, and their progeny remained S after many generations. It was soon recognized that some substance (the "transforming principle") was released from the heat-killed S cells, and was taken up by the R cells. The transforming principle was finally identified as DNA in 1944, thus providing the first evidence that DNA is the genetic material.

2. **The transformation process:** Subsequent studies on the transformation phenomenon itself revealed that the ability of a cell to be transformed (called **competence**) depends on a transitory physio-

logic state of the cell that allows the DNA to cross the cell membrane. As the free double–stranded DNA enters the recipient cell, one of the two strands is destroyed by nucleases. The remaining single strand invades the resident chromosome, seeking a region of sequence homology. If such a sequence is found, the invading strand replaces one of the two resident strands by a complex cut-and-paste process (Figure 10.10). Transformation probably has only a minor effect on gene flow in natural bacterial populations, but it is useful experimentally for introducing a cloned gene (for example, the human gene for insulin) into bacterial cells.

VI. GENETIC VARIATION

Although all of the cells in a so-called "pure" bacterial culture are derived from a single original cell, the culture almost certainly contains rare cells that differ from the originating cell. The vast majority, if not all, of such variants (**mutants**) are due to changes (**mutations**) in their DNA.

A. Mutations

Strictly speaking, any change in the structure of the genetic material, or more specifically, any change in the base sequence of the DNA, is called a mutation. Some mutations are unstable (that is, they frequently revert back to their original state), and others do not noticeably affect the organism. Mutations that come under study are usually those that are stable, and that cause some change in the characteristics of the organism. Mutations can be classified according to the kind of chemical change that occurs in the DNA, or, when the mutation affects a protein-coding gene, by the effect the mutation has on the translation of the message. [Note: In the descriptions presented below, a knowledge of the genetic code and its mechanism of translation is assumed.[1]]

1. **Base substitutions:** A base pair in DNA, for example A=T, can be replaced with G=C, C=G, or T=A. Similarly, G=C can be replaced with A=T, T=A, or C=G. Note that in two of these substitutions, a purine (A or G) replaces a purine, and a pyrimidine (C or T) replaces a pyrimidine. These are called **transition substitutions**. In the other four substitutions, a purine replaces a pyrimidine or vice versa. These are called **transversion substitutions** (Figure 10.11A). When only a single base pair is changed, the mutation is referred to as a **"point" mutation**.

2. **Additions and deletions:** A single base pair, or a contiguous string of base pairs, can be added to or deleted from the DNA (Figure 10.11B). An **inversion** results when a string of bases is deleted followed by reinsertion of the same sequence in the opposite direction (Figure 10.11C).

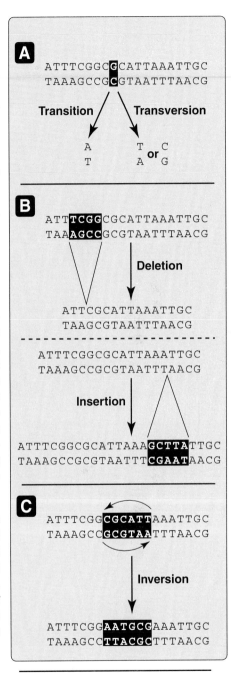

Figure 10.11
Various kinds of sequence changes (mutations) in DNA.

[1]See p. 387 in ***Lippincott's Illustrated Reviews: Biochemistry*** (2nd ed.) for a discussion of the genetic code.

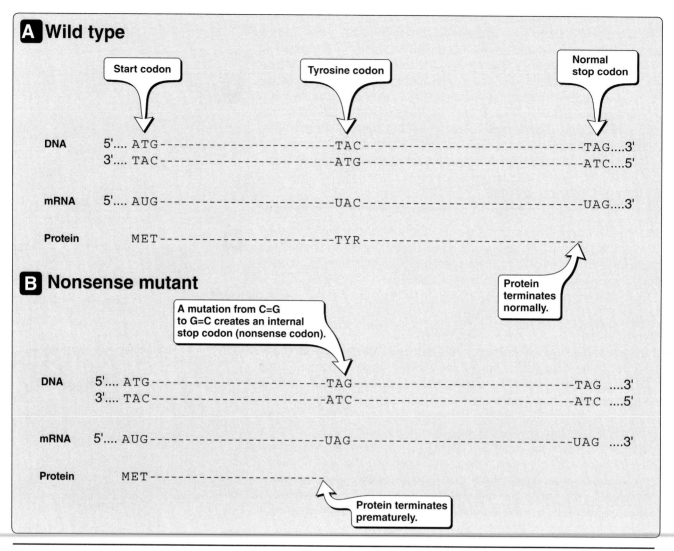

Figure 10.12
A mutation that creates an internal STOP codon (a nonsense mutation) in a gene will prematurely terminate the encoded polypeptide chain.

B. Mutants

A mutant is an organism that deviates in some recognizable characteristic (**phenotype**) from the normal, and whose progeny maintain this deviance. [Note: The term mutant should not be used interchangeably with mutation, which is the molecular change in the hereditary material responsible for the mutant phenotype.]

1. **Wild type:** To recognize a mutant bacterium, it is necessary to have an established standard for comparison. In genetic terminology, this standard is called the wild type. [Note: The term originally meant the type that is most fit to survive in the wild, but it can be any type that is chosen as a standard.] Many strains of *E. coli* can grow in a "minimal medium" whose only organic constituent is a carbon source such as glucose (a so-called minimal medium). Such organisms, which are called **prototrophs**, can obviously synthesize every organic substance they need—all amino acids, nucleotides, carbohydrates, lipids, etc. Prototrophs

are convenient wild-type strains because loss-of-function, nutritional mutants can be isolated from them.

2. **Nutritional mutants:** If a prototrophic cell suffers a mutation in any one of its hundreds of biosynthetic genes, the cell will not grow unless the missing nutrient, such as an amino acid or or some biosynthetic intermediate, is provided. Such nutritional mutants are called **auxotrophs.**

3. **Temperature-sensitive mutants:** Many kinds of mutational defects cannot be corrected simply by supplying a missing nutrient. For example, a mutation that destroys the function of DNA polymerase is lethal to the cell under all nutritional conditions, and the mutant cell could not, in general, be recovered. However, some kinds of mutations cause a mutant phenotype only in certain environments. For example, the mutation in the DNA polymerase gene might destroy the function of the polymerase at a high temperature (for example, 42°C) but not at a low temperature (for example, 30°C). Thus, the mutant appears normal and can survive when growing at low temperature, but displays the mutant phenotype at high temperature. Such a mutant is called a **temperature-sensitive mutant**, and is one example of the broader class of mutants referred to as **conditional lethal mutants**. A temperature-sensitive phenotype can often be attributed to a protein folding defect in which the protein product of the gene in question folds more or less correctly at low temperature, but is misfolded at high temperature. Temperature-sensitive mutants can, in principle, be isolated for any protein-coding gene of the organism.

4. **Missense and nonsense mutants:** If a base substitution mutation in DNA results in a replacement of one amino acid residue by another in a protein, the mutation is called **missense**. If a base substitution mutation creates an in-phase **stop codon** (UAG, UGA or UAA), and thereby prematurely terminates elongation of the polypeptide chain, the mutation is called **nonsense** (Figure 10.12). [Note: A base substitution occurring in a normal stop codon can change the stop codon to one of the 61 coding triplets, and thus prevent normal termination of the polypeptide chain.]

5. **Frame-shift mutants:** In translation, an amino acid sequence is specified by the sequence of bases in the DNA. The base sequence is translated by reading the bases three at a time. The **reading frame** is set by the first translated codon of the message. If bases are added or deleted in the interior of the message, the reading frame is shifted unless the number of bases deleted or added is an integral multiple of three. [Note: The protein produced will be missing or have gained a single amino acid, but all of the other amino acids in the chain will be correct and in proper order.] When a **frame-shift** occurs, it causes a misreading of all of the codons from the point of the deletion (or addition) to the end of the message corresponding to the C-terminus of the protein. The resulting protein appears as if its gene had suffered multiple, contiguous, missense mutations (Figure 10.13). This protein is also most likely shorter than normal, because the frame shift is likely to bring an

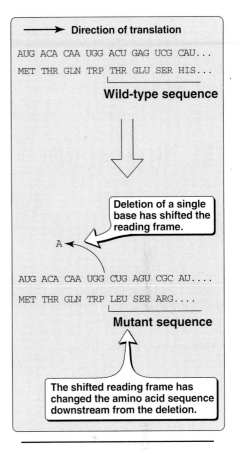

Figure 10.13
A deletion or an insertion of a single nucleotide in a gene (a frame-shift mutation) can drastically change the amino acid sequence of the encoded polypeptide chain.

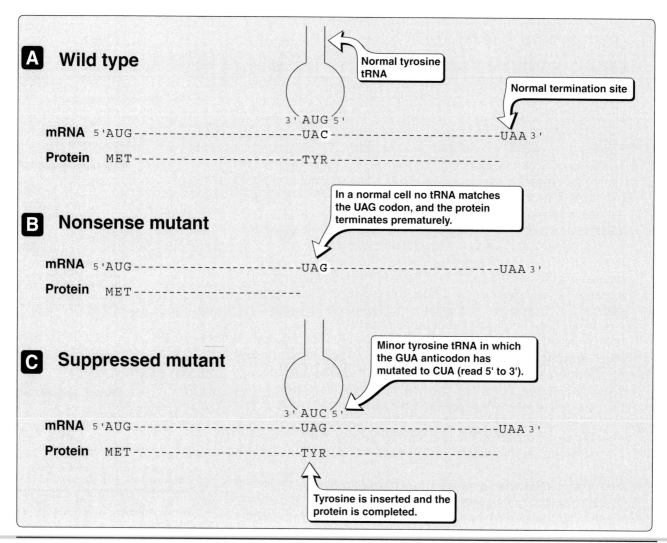

Figure 10.14
A mutation in the anticodon of certain tRNAs can nullify (suppress) the effect of a nonsense mutation.

out-of-frame stop codon into frame. More rarely, the protein may be longer than normal if translation is not terminated before the normal stop codon, which will then be out of frame.

6. **Revertants and suppressors:** A mutant can back-mutate (revert) to a form that is phenotypically indistinguishable from the standard type (wild-type). Some revertants arise by an exact restoration of the wild-type DNA sequence. Very often, however, revertants arise by a second mutation, called a **suppressor**, that nullifies the effect of the first mutation. Revertants of this type are thus, in reality, double mutants. In general, the suppressor mutation can be in the same gene as the original mutation or in a different gene. One category of suppressors frequently encountered in microbial populations is the suppressors of nonsense mutations, or simply, **nonsense suppressors**. In this case, the suppressor mutation changes the anti-codon of a transfer RNA (tRNA) so that the tRNA can recognize a nonsense (termination)

codon (UAG, UAA, or UGA), thus preventing the nonsense mutation from terminating the polypeptide chain. Instead, the amino acid carried by the mutated tRNA is inserted at the nonsense codon site. [Note: This mechanism of suppression can operate only when the tRNA is redundant (that is, when there exists a nonmutated form of this tRNA in the cell to perform the normal translating function as is true for a number of amino acids).] Figure 10.14 illustrates nonsense suppression by a mutation in the anti-codon of one of the two tyrosine tRNAs.

7. **Regulatory mutants:** All of the mutational changes described above can also occur in regions of the DNA that do not code for proteins. These may be regulatory regions that control the frequency with which a gene is transcribed (**promoter regions**), or the responsiveness of the gene to other regulatory molecules such as repressors and activators (see p. 134). Thus, in general, mutations in a regulatory region affect the strength of expression of a gene, and the conditions under which the gene is expressed.

8. **Selective methods for isolating mutants:** Mutations are rare events, and spontaneously appearing mutant cells of any one particular kind are usually present in a proportion of only one in 10^6 to 10^7 in a population. Although the use of mutagenic agents can raise the number 100- to 1000-fold, the isolation of mutants for experimental purposes requires efficient enrichment or screening techniques. One of the earliest and still useful methods of enrichment takes advantage of the fact that penicillin kills cells that are actively growing, but is harmless to cells in suspended growth. Thus, if a large population (many millions) of cells is grown in minimal medium containing penicillin, any rare auxotrophic (and therefore nongrowing) mutant cells in the population will survive, whereas the growing prototrophic wild-type cells will be killed. Removal of the penicillin, and transfer to a rich, complete medium, allows the auxotrophic mutants to be recovered. The same general method can be used to isolate temperature-sensitive, conditional lethal mutants.

C. Mutagenic agents

In nature, mutations occur "spontaneously" at a low frequency. For experimental purposes, this rate can be increased many thousandfold by various agents. The study of mutagenic agents in bacteria has been extremely useful in identifying and understanding the action of mutagenic and carcinogenic agents active in higher organisms, including humans (Figure 10.15).

1. **Base analogs:** Many natural and synthetic purines and pyrimidines can mimic the four normal bases of DNA, A, T, G, C (that is, when fed to growing cells, these analogs can be incorporated into DNA in place of the normal bases). When the DNA replicates, the base analog can sometimes mispair, thus causing a mutation. For example, 5-bromouracil (5-BU) is an analog of the normal base thymine (the large bromine atom at the 5 position mimics the normal methyl group of thymine). In fact, 5-BU is so similar to thymine that it can be made to replace almost all the thymines of

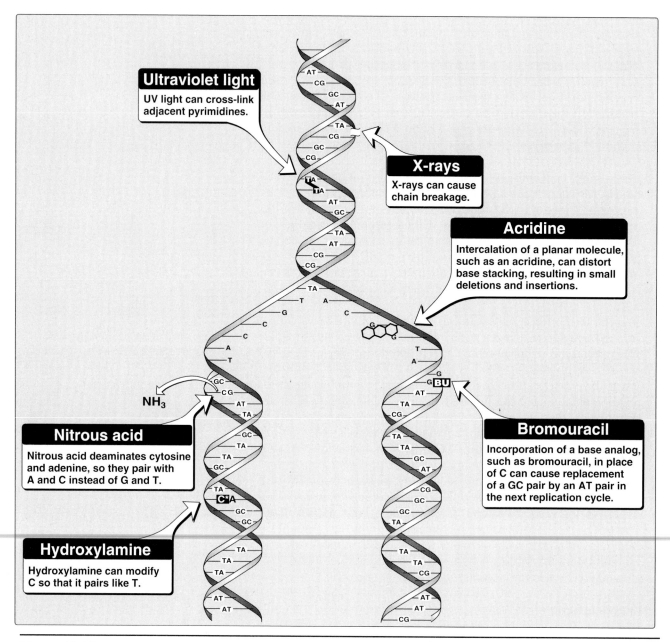

Figure 10.15
The changes in DNA caused by various mutagenic agents. [Note: C* represents the hydroxylamine-modified cyotosine.]

an organism's DNA, where it pairs with A just as T does. However, the electronegativity of the bromine atom causes 5-BU to pair with G a small fraction of the time; this mispairing causes an A=T to G=C mutation. Notice that this mutation is a transition substitution (see Figure 10.11), which is the kind of mutation that base analogs typically induce. Other analogs (for example, 2-aminopurine) are incorporated into DNA at a very low level, but once incorporated, mispair at a very high rate.

2. **Chemical modifiers:** Treatment of DNA with various chemical reagents can modify the normal bases so that they mispair with

increased frequency. For example, nitrous acid removes the amino groups from (deaminates) cytosine and adenine, converting them into uracil and guanine. In the following rounds of DNA replication, mutations will occur. Methyl (or ethyl) methane sulfonate adds alkyl groups to the bases (alkylates them). Some reagents remove the bases entirely, especially purines (depurination). All of these **mutagens** are rather nonspecific, and can induce both transitions and transversions. Hydroxylamine is a much more specific chemical mutagen that modifies cytosine so that it pairs with adenine. Thus hydroxylamine changes a G=C base pair to an A=T base pair. Treatments with chemical modifiers can be performed on isolated DNA, or on DNA contained in a living organism. When applied to bacteria, these mutagenic reagents may kill 99 percent of the cells, but the survivors include a high percentage of mutants.

3. **Frame-shift mutagens:** Mutagens that slip in between (intercalate between) the stacked bases of a DNA helix cause skipping of bases or groups of bases during replication, resulting in small insertions or deletions. Frame-shift mutagens are generally planar molecules about the size of a nucleotide, and are neither covalently incorporated into DNA, nor do they chemically modify DNA. Some examples of intercalating mutagens are acridines and ethidium bromide.

4. **Radiation:** Ultraviolet light causes mutations by creating bonds between adjacent pyrimidines in the DNA helix. These cross-linked bases (called **pyrimidine dimers**) can cause DNA replication to stop when DNA polymerase encounters the dimer on the template strand. Mutations arise during the cell's attempt to replicate the damaged DNA if, instead of ceasing DNA synthesis when the dimer is encountered, the DNA polymerase instead nonspecifically inserts any of the four nucleotides in the newly replicating strand at the site of the lesion. Not all such UV-induced dimers ultimately cause mutations, because the cell can repair UV damage by excision of the dimers, and resynthesis of the missing sequence. [Note: X-rays, which have considerably greater energy than ultraviolet rays, can cause breaks in the strands of the DNA helix.]

5. **Mobile genetic elements:** In recent years it has been recognized that the arrangement of genes in the genome of bacteria, and probably of all organisms, is not entirely static. Certain DNA segments, called transposons, have the ability to move from place to place on the chromosome and into and out of plasmids. Transposons do not exist as segments free of the genome but only as segments within the genome. There are two general kinds of transposons, replicative and nonreplicative. A **replicative transposon** leaves a copy of itself at the original location. Thus the transposition process doubles the number of copies of the transposon. A **nonreplicative transposon** does not leave a copy of itself at the original location. If transposition inserts a transposon into a functional gene, the function of the gene is generally destroyed, and this was the original basis by which transposons

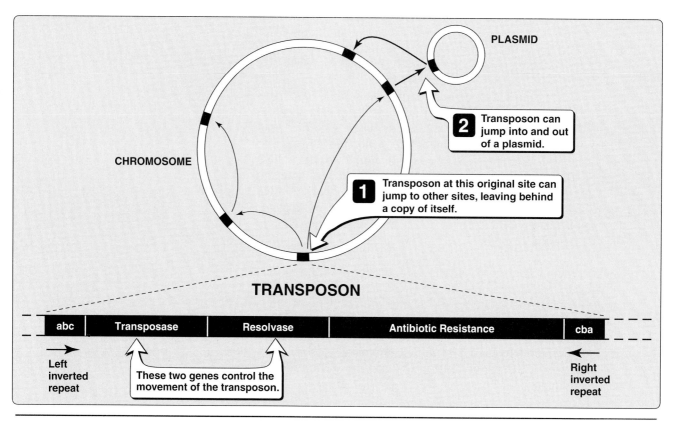

Figure 10.16
A transposon can move from place to place in the chromosome, leaving a copy of itself behind
at the previous site.

were discovered. Transposons can thus be viewed as internal mutagenic agents. The transposition process and the structure of a typical replicative transposon are shown in Figure 10.16. This transposon has three genes and a length of about five kilobases. The transposase and resolvase genes code for enzymes that are involved in the transposition process, whereas the antibiotic resistance gene is a "passenger". The transposon is bounded by short (about fifty bases) inverted repeats. These inverted repeats are the elements recognized by the transposase as it initiates the transposition. Mobile genetic elements are probably responsible for much of the genetic variability in natural bacterial populations, and for the spread of antibiotic resistance genes.

D. The Ames test for mutagenic/carcinogenic agents

A rapid laboratory test for the detection of mutagenic agents uses specially constructed mutant strains of salmonella that require histidine for growth. When such a strain is grown in the presence of a mutagenic agent, the mutagen can cause a back-mutation (reversion), resulting in a cell that grows in the absence of histidine. These revertants can be detected very sensitively (one his[+] cell among many millions of his[−] cells) by plating the treated cells on solid medium that lacks histidine. Only the revertants form colonies. The sensitivity of the test can be further enhanced by using strains with increased permeability, and decreased ability to repair DNA. Reasoning from the fact that most carcinogens are also mutagens, the Ames test is used to identify potential carcinogens.

E. Mechanisms of acquired antibiotic resistance

Acquired antibiotic resistance requires the temporary or permanent gain or alteration of bacterial genetic information. Most **resistance genes** are plasmid-mediated, but plasmid-mediated traits can interchange with chromosomal elements. Transfer of genetic material from a plasmid to the chromosome can occur by simple recombinational events, but the process is greatly facilitated by transposons (see p. 131). Many resistance genes, such as plasmid-mediated β-lactamases, tetracycline-resistance genes, and aminoglycoside-modifying enzymes are organized on transposons. Resistance to antibiotics is accomplished by three principal mechanisms (Figure 10.17).

1. **Decreased uptake (or increased efflux) of the antibiotic:** For example, gram-negative organisms can limit the penetration of certain agents, including β-lactam antibiotics, tetracyclines, and chloramphenicol, as a result of alteration in the number and structure of porins in the outer membrane.

2. **Alteration of the target site for the antibiotic:** For example, *Staphylococcus. pneumoniae* resistance to β-lactam antibiotics involves alterations in one or more of the major bacterial penicillin-binding proteins (see p. 142), which results in decreased binding of the antibiotic to its target.

3. **Acquisition of the ability to destroy or modify the antibiotic:** Examples of antibiotic inactivating enzymes include, 1) β-**lactamases** that hydrolytically inactivate the β-lactam ring of penicillins, cephalosporins, and related drugs; 2) **acetyltransferases** that transfer an acetyl group to the antibiotic, inactivating chloramphenicol or aminoglycosides; 3) **esterases** that hydrolyze the lactone ring of macrolides.

VII. GENE REGULATION

In general, bacteria can manufacture most of the organic compounds (amino acids, nucleotides, carbohydrates, lipids, etc.) that they need, and in this regard are more versatile than higher organisms. This metabolic resourcefulness is a distinct advantage to the organism when in a nutritionally poor environment, but is extremely wasteful in a nutritious environment if the bacterium had to keep all of the unneeded biosynthetic enzymes ready at hand. Bacteria thus have evolved various mechanisms for producing certain metabolic enzymes only when they are needed. Most of these mechanisms, as is the case for the following examples, involve control of transcription of the gene into messenger RNA, rather than control of translation of the messenger.

A. Negative control (repression)

Lactose is a disaccharide, composed of glucose and galactose, which is found in dairy products. The first step in the metabolism of lactose is its cleavage into monosaccharide units, a job performed by the enzyme β-galactosidase. To avoid being wasteful, bacteria synthesize β-galactosidase only when lactose is present in the growth medium. Bacteria accomplish this control by producing a **repressor protein**, which, when lactose is absent, binds to a specific

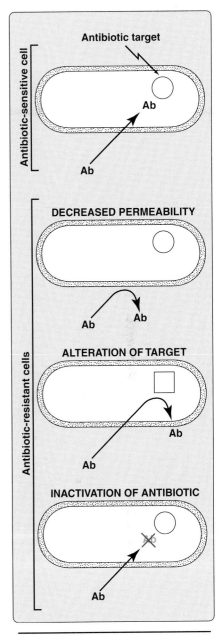

Figure 10.17
Three common mechanisms of antibiotic resistance.

site on the DNA (the **operator site**) near the start of the β-galactosidase gene. When repressor is bound, RNA polymerase—which recognizes the **promoter region** that is upstream from the operator site—is thereby blocked from initiating transcription of the genes. When lactose is present, it binds to the repressor protein, thereby preventing the repressor from binding to the DNA, and allowing transcription of the genes to occur. The β-galactosidase gene is actually one of a set of three contiguous genes, the other two being a lactose permease gene, and a β-galactoside transacetylase gene. Together, these three genes, all of which are controlled by the same repressor, comprise the **lac operon**. This mechanism is called **negative control**, because the controlling element—the repressor—acts to prevent transcription (Figure 10.18A). In this example, lactose is said to be an **inducer** of the lac operon. [Note: In other cases, the free repressor does not repress unless it is combined with another compound called a **corepressor**. For example, the repressor for the tryptophan operon is active only when it binds tryptophan.]

B. Positive control (catabolite activation)

If bacteria are grown in medium containing glucose together with some other sugar, the bacteria use the glucose exclusively as an energy source. This is due to the fact that transcription of all of the operons for utilization of sugars other than glucose fails to occur, even though the inducing sugars are present. The reason for this failure is that the sugar-utilization operons, of which the lac operon is an example, must be activated by a specific protein called **catabolite activator protein** (**CAP**), which, in turn, is only functional as an activator when complexed with cyclic AMP. [Note: CAP is also called **CRP** for **cyclic AMP receptor protein**.] Glucose, in turn, regulates CAP activity by regulating the level of cyclic AMP. When glucose is present at a high level, cyclic AMP is at a low level, and the sugar-utilization operons are not activated. When glucose is absent or at a low level, cyclic AMP is at a high level and the sugar utilization operons are activated (Figure 10.18B). Catabolite activation is thus seen to be a global regulatory mechanism by which many operons, each under individual control, are regulated by a single activator protein.

C. Modifications of RNA polymerase specificity

Microorganisms are often compelled to switch on or off large groups of genes in response to stressful environmental conditions. For example, under starvation conditions, many species sporulate, a process that requires major changes in metabolic pathways. Similarly, sudden exposure to elevated temperature (heat shock) elicits the formation of many new proteins. In both of these cases, the shift in gene expression is due to a modification of the RNA polymerase, specifically, a replacement of the normal σ (sigma) subunit with an alternative subunit that recognizes a different set of promoters.

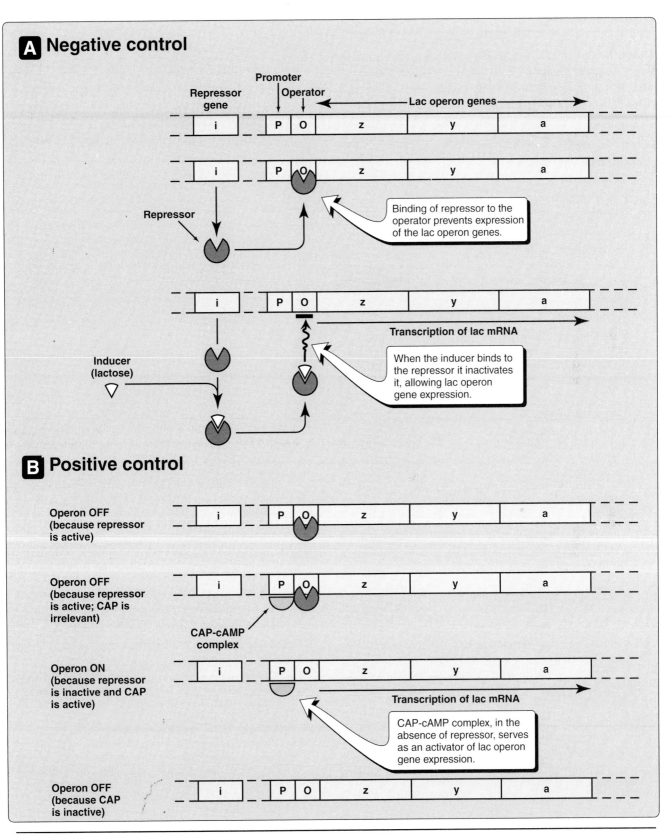

Figure 10.18
Bacterial genes can be controlled negatively by repressors or positively by activators.

Study Questions

Questions 10.1 to 10.7: For each numbered phrase, select the one lettered choice (A to R) that is most closely associated with it. Each choice (A to R) may be selected once, more than once, or not at all.

A. Temperate phage
B. Repressor
C. Suppressor mutation
D. Replicon
E. Nonsense mutation
F. Transduction
G. Transformation
H. Prototroph
I. Hfr
J. Auxotroph
K. Autotroph
L. Transposon
M. Missense mutation

10.1 Genetic transfer between bacterial cells mediated by bacteriophage

Correct answer = F.

10.2 A change in the DNA nucleotide sequence that creates a stop codon

Correct answer = E.

10.3 A strain of bacteria that requires some nutritional supplement for growth

Correct answer = J.

10.4 A contiguous segment of bacterial DNA that can move from place to place in the genome

Correct answer = L.

10.5 A protein, which when bound to DNA, blocks expression of a specific gene or group of genes

Correct answer = B.

10.6 A piece of DNA that includes an origin of replication

Correct answer = D

Choose the ONE correct answer

10.7 A lysogenic bacterium

A. carries a prophage.
B. causes the lysis of other bacteria upon contact.
C. cannot support the replication of a virulent phage.
D. is often a human pathogen.
E. is usually not capable of conjugal genetic transfer.

Correct answer = A. A lysogenic bacterium can generate phage because it carries phage genes in a latent state (the prophage). Lysogenicity does not impart any special lytic properties to the bacterium nor, in general, does it affect conjugal transfer or the ability to support the replication of other unrelated phage. The presence of a prophage can convert certain bacteria to human pathogens, but such cases are rare.

10.8 The F-plasmid of *E. coli* can fuse with the chromosome

A. at only a few specific sites.
B. at many different sites.
C. only at the origin of replication.
D. only at sites of prophage insertion.
E. at the gene that codes for the pilus protein.

Correct answer = B. The fact that fusion of the F-plasmid with the chromosome can generate many different Hfrs implies that the fusion occurs at many different, although not necessarily random, sites. The other choices are thus precluded.

10.9 Frame-shift mutations

A. are usually transversions.
B. are induced by base analogs.
C. usually affect regulatory regions.
D. cause multiple amino acid replacements.
E. usually result in a nutritional requirement.

Correct answer = D. Frame-shift mutations are either deletions or additions of a contiguous stretch of bases where the number of bases is not a multiple of three. Such mutations result in multiple contiguous amino acid replacements in the encoded protein. Transversions are a class of base-pair substitutions and do not shift the reading frame. There is no evidence or expectation that frame-shift mutations are more frequent in regulatory regions or in genes controlling nutritional pathways.

Staphylococci

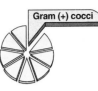

11

I. OVERVIEW

Staphylococci, with streptococci (see Chapter 12), constitute the main groups of medically important gram-positive cocci. Staphylococcal infections range from the trivial to the rapidly fatal. They can be very difficult to treat, especially those contracted in hospitals, because of the remarkable ability of staphylococci to acquire antibiotic resistance determinants. The staphylococci are ubiquitous in nature, with about a dozen species indigenous to humans occurring as part of human flora and on fomites (inanimate objects). The most virulent of the genus, *Staphylococcus aureus*, is one of the most common causes of bacterial infections, and is also an important cause of intoxications such as food poisoning and toxic shock syndrome. Among less virulent staphylococcal species, *Staphylococcus epidermidis* is an important cause of prosthetic implant infections, whereas *Staphylococcus saprophyticus* causes urinary tract infections, especially cystitis in women. Figure 11.1 summarizes the staphylococci described in this chapter.

II. GENERAL FEATURES

Staphylococci generally stain darkly gram-positive (see p. 452). They are round rather than oval, and tend to occur in bunches like grapes. Staphylococci are rather fastidious, requiring various amino acids and other growth factors, and are routinely cultured on enriched media containing broth and/or blood (see p. 25). Staphylococci are true facultatively anaerobic organisms. They produce catalase, which is one feature that distinguishes them from the catalase-negative streptococci (see p. 145). The staphylococcal cell wall, like that of other gram-positive organisms, contains a thick peptidoglycan layer, with distinctive pentaglycine bridges linking the amino acid side chains (see p. 113). Staphylococci are hardy, being relatively resistant to heat and drying, and thus can persist for long periods on fomites, which can then serve as sources of infection. The most virulent species of staphylococcus is *S. aureus*, almost all isolates of which secrete **coagulase**—an enzyme that causes citrated plasma to clot. There are other species that occasionally cause disease; these lack coagulase and are often referred to as **coagulase-negative staphylococci**.

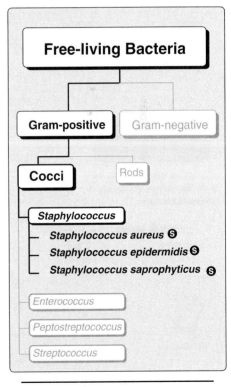

Figure 11.1
Classification of Staphylococci.
🅢 See pp. 419, 452 for summaries of these organisms.

Lippincott's Illustrated Reviews: Microbiology, by William A. Strohl, Harriet Rouse, Bruce D. Fisher. Lippincott, Williams & Wilkins, Baltimore, MD © 2001

III. STAPHYLOCOCCUS AUREUS

Although considerably more virulent than the coagulase-negative staphylococci, the degree of virulence of *S. aureus* is considered modest; generally significant host compromise is required for infection, such as a break in the skin or insertion of a foreign body (for example, wounds or surgical infections), or an obstructed hair follicle (folliculitis). *S. aureus* disease may be 1) largely or wholly the result of actual invasive infection, 2) due to toxins in the absence of infection ("pure" toxinoses), or 3) may be a combination of infection and intoxication (Figure 11.2).

A. Epidemiology

S. aureus is carried by twenty to forty percent of healthy individuals at any one time, and by almost everyone at some time. Carriage occurs most often on skin, is found abundantly on the mucous membranes of the anterior nares (a strategic site for dissemination), and on other mucous membranes such as that of the vagina. [Note: A compromised immune system significantly increases the likelihood of staphylococcal colonization leading to disease.] Carriers serve as a source of infection to themselves and others; for example, by direct contact, by contamination of fomites (objects such as a doorknob, which in turn can be a source of infection), or of food, which can then result in food poisoning. Staphylococci are hosts to a large variety of lysogenic bacteriophages (see p. 116). In the case of *S. aureus*, patterns of phage resistance and sensitivity are used in the epidemiologic tracing of strains. Phage typing separates isolates into Groups I through IV, plus "nontypeable" (by the standard phage set). [Note: Many contemporary isolates are nontypeable, thus decreasing the usefulness of this system.]

B. Pathogenesis

The virulence of *S. aureus* is dependent on a multiplicity of determinants, various combinations of which occur in different strains. The variability of the virulence factor spectrum relates to the occurrence of many of the determinants on mobile genetic elements. [Note: Coagulase is generally not considered a virulence factor because coagulase-negative mutants are as virulent as the corresponding parental strains; the association between coagulase positivity and virulence in nature is probably fortuitous.] Important virulence factors are as follows (Figure 11.3).

1. **Cell wall virulence factors:**

   a. **Protein A** is a major component of the *S. aureus* cell wall. It binds to the Fc moiety of IgG, exerting an antiopsonin (and therefore strongly antiphagocytic) effect.

   b. **Fibronectin-binding protein (FnBP)** and other staphylococcal surface proteins promote binding to mucosal cells and tissue matrices.

2. **Cytolytic exotoxins:** α, β, γ, and δ toxins attack mammalian cell (including red blood cell) membranes, and are often referred to as

Infection

S. aureus disease may be largely or wholly the result of actual invasive infection.

Colonization

S. aureus

S. aureus

Intoxication

S. aureus disease may be largely or wholly due to toxins in the absence of infection ("pure" toxicoses).

S. aureus

Toxin

Infection and intoxication

S. aureus disease may be a combination of infection and intoxication.

S. aureus

S. aureus

S. aureus

Toxin

Figure 11.2
Causes of disease due to infection with *Staphylococcus aureus*.

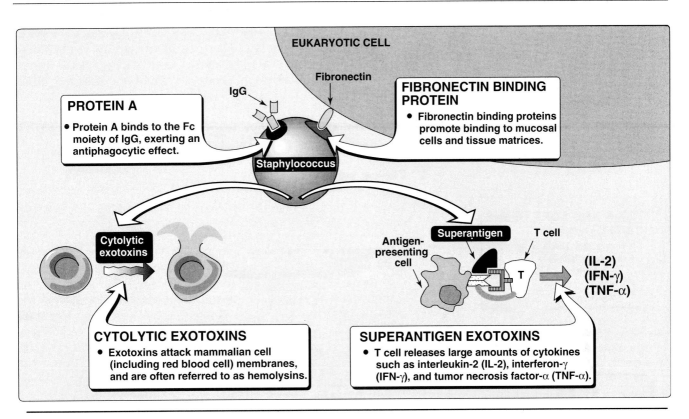

Figure 11.3
Cell wall virulence factors in *Staphylococcus aureus.*

hemolysins. α-Toxin is the best studied, and is chromosomally encoded. It polymerizes into tubes that pierce membranes, resulting in the loss of important molecules, and eventually in osmotic lysis.

3. **Superantigen exotoxins:** These toxins have an affinity for the T cell receptor–MHC Class II antigen complex (see p. 73). They thus stimulate enhanced T-lymphocyte response (as many as twenty percent of T cells respond as compared to 0.01 percent responding to the usual processed antigens) by virtue of their ability to recognize a relatively conserved region of the T cell receptor. This major T cell activation can cause toxic shock, primarily by release into the circulation of inordinately large amounts of T cell cytokines, such as interleukin-2 (IL-2), interferon-γ (IFN-γ), and tumor necrosis factor-α (TNF-α) (see p. 63).

a. **Enterotoxins:** Enterotoxins (six major antigenic types, A, B, C, D, E, and G) are produced by approximately half of all *S. aureus* isolates, most often of phage typing Group II. When these bacteria contaminate food and are allowed to grow, they secrete enterotoxin, ingestion of which can cause food poisoning. [Note: The toxin stimulates the vomiting center in the brain by binding to neural receptors in the upper GI tract.] Enterotoxins are superantigens that are even more heat-stable than *S. aureus*; therefore, organisms are not always recovered from incriminated food.

b. Toxic Shock Syndrome Toxin (TSST–1) is the classic cause of toxic shock syndrome. Because of similarities in molecular structure, it is sometimes referred to as staphylococcal enterotoxin F (SEF), although it does not cause food poisoning when ingested.

c. Exfoliatin (exfoliative toxin, ET) is also a superantigen. It causes scalded skin syndrome in children.

C. Clinical significance

S. aureus causes disease by infecting tissues—typically creating abscesses—and/or by producing toxins (Figure 11.4).

1. **Localized skin infections:** The most common *S. aureus* infections are small, superficial abscesses involving hair follicles (folliculitis) or sweat or sebaceous glands (see p. 452). For example, the common sty ("external hordeolum") is created by infection of the follicle of an eyelash. Subcutaneous abscesses called **furuncles** (boils) often form around foreign bodies, such as splinters. These generally respond to local therapy: removal of the foreign body, soaking, and drainage as indicated. **Carbuncles** are larger, deeper, multiloculated skin infections that can lead to bacteremia and require antibiotic therapy and debridement. **Impetigo** is a usually localized, superficial, spreading crusty skin lesion generally seen in children. It can be caused by *S. aureus*—although more commonly by *Streptococcus pyogenes* (see p. 146)—or both organisms together.

2. **Deep, localized infections:** These may be metastatic from superficial infections or skin carriage, or may result from trauma. [Note: An abscess in any organ or tissue should make you suspect *S. aureus*.]

   a. Osteomyelitis: *S. aureus* is the most common cause of acute and chronic infection of the bone marrow.

   b. Arthritis: *S. aureus* is the most common cause of acute infection of the joint space in children ("septic joint"). [Note: Septic joints are medical emergencies because pus can rapidly cause irreparable cartilage damage. They must be treated promptly with drainage and an antibiotic.]

3. **Acute endocarditis** is generally associated with intravenous drug abuse, and is caused by injection of contaminated preparations or by needles that are contaminated with *S. aureus*.

4. **Septicemia** is a generalized infection with sepsis or bacteremia that may be associated with a known focus (for example, a septic joint) or not ("occult" focus).

5. **Pneumonia:** *S. aureus* is a cause of severe, necrotizing pneumonia.

6. **Nosocomial infections:** *S. aureus* is one of the most common

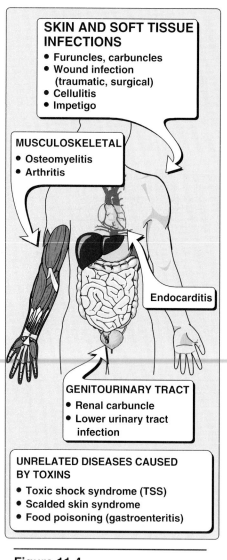

SKIN AND SOFT TISSUE INFECTIONS
- Furuncles, carbuncles
- Wound infection (traumatic, surgical)
- Cellulitis
- Impetigo

MUSCULOSKELETAL
- Osteomyelitis
- Arthritis

Endocarditis

GENITOURINARY TRACT
- Renal carbuncle
- Lower urinary tract infection

UNRELATED DISEASES CAUSED BY TOXINS
- Toxic shock syndrome (TSS)
- Scalded skin syndrome
- Food poisoning (gastroenteritis)

Figure 11.4
Some diseases caused by *Staphylococcus aureus*.

causes of hospital-acquired infections, often of wounds (surgical, decubital), or bacteremia associated with catheters. Progression to septicemia is often a terminal event.

7. **Toxinoses** are diseases caused by the action of a toxin, frequently when the organism that secreted the toxin is undetectable. Toxinoses caused by *S. aureus* include:

a. **Toxic shock syndrome**, which results in high fever, rash (resembling a sunburn, with diffuse erythema followed by desquamation), vomiting, diarrhea, hypotension, and multiorgan involvement (especially GI, renal, and/or hepatic damage). An outbreak of toxic shock syndrome occurred in the late 1970s among menstruating women. It was shown to be related to the use of hyperabsorbant tampons by women who happened to be vaginally colonized by toxic shock syndrome toxin– (TSST)–positive strains of *S. aureus*. [Note: These tampons stimulated TSST expression, resulting in entry of the toxin into the circulation in the absence of true infection.] The incidence has decreased markedly since such tampons were removed from the market. Of the few cases of toxic shock syndrome that occur currently, approximately half are associated with ordinary *S. aureus* infections, and of the latter, many are due to a circulating enterotoxin rather than to TSST.

b. **Staphylococcal gastroenteritis** is caused by ingestion of food contaminated with enterotoxin-producing *S. aureus*. Often contaminated by a food-handler, these foods tend to be protein-rich (for example, egg salad, cream pastry) and improperly refrigerated. Symptoms such as nausea, vomiting, and diarrhea are acute following a short incubation period (less than six hours), and are triggered by local actions of the toxin on the GI tract rather than from an infection. See p. 182 for a summary of food poisoning.

c. **Scalded skin syndrome** involves the appearance of superficial bullae resulting from the action of an exfoliative toxin that attacks the intercellular adhesive of the stratum granulosum, causing marked epithelial desquamation (Figure 11.5). The bullae may be infected or may result from toxin produced by organisms infecting a different site.

D. Laboratory identification

Identification of an isolate as a staphylococcus relies largely on microscopic and colony morphology, and catalase positivity. The bacteria stain strongly gram-positive, and are frequently seen in grapelikeclusters (Figure 11.6). *S. aureus* is distinguished from the coagulase-negative staphylococci primarily by coagulase positivity. In addition, *S. aureus* colonies tend to be yellow (hence the name "aureus" meaning golden) and hemolytic (Figure 11.7), rather than gray and nonhemolytic like the coagulase-negative staphylococci. *S. aureus* is also distinguished from most coagulase-negative staphylococci by being mannitol-positive.

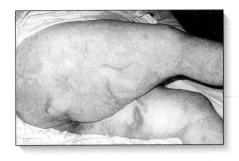

Figure 11.5
Scalded skin syndrome.

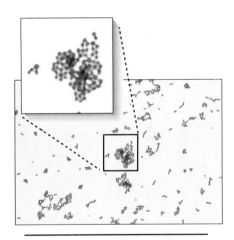

Figure 11.6
Staphylococcus aureus. Gram stain of smear from blood culture showing typical clusters.

Colonies are yellow.

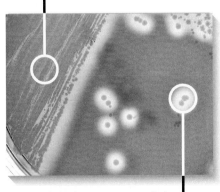

Colonies are surrounded by zone of beta hemolysis.

Figure 11.7
Staphylococcus aureus. Culture of abscess exudate on blood agar.

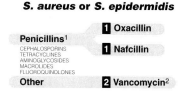

S. aureus or S. epidermidis

Penicillins[1]	**1** Oxacillin
CEPHALOSPORINS TETRACYCLINES AMINOGLYCOSIDES MACROLIDES FLUOROQUINOLONES	**1** Nafcillin
Other	**2** Vancomycin[2]

S. saprophyticus

| Penicillins | **1** Penicillin G |
| CEPHALOSPORINS TETRACYCLINES AMINOGLYCOSIDES MACROLIDES FLUOROQUINOLONES OTHER | |

[1]Most isolates resistant to penicillin G

[2]Used in methicillin-resistant isolates

Figure 11.8
Some antimicrobial agents useful in treating staphyloccal infections.

E. Immunity

S. aureus infections do not elicit strong or long-lasting immunity, as demonstrated by the continuing susceptibility of individuals to *S. aureus* infections throughout life. The reasons for this are not well understood.

F. Treatment

Serious *S. aureus* infections require aggressive treatment, including incision and drainage of localized lesions as well as systemic antibiotics. Choice of antibiotics is complicated by the frequent presence of acquired antibiotic resistance determinants (see p. 133).

1. **Acquired antibiotic resistance:** Resistance determinants are often present on mobile elements (plasmids, and transposons, see p. 131), and can be transferred among *S. aureus* strains, and between staphylococcal species.

    a. **Penicillin resistance:** Almost all *S. aureus* isolates, both community- and hospital-acquired, are now resistant to penicillin G due to penicillinase-encoding plasmids or transposons. This has required the replacement of the initial agent of choice, penicillin G, by β-lactamase-resistant penicillins such as nafcillin or oxacillin (Figure 11.8).

    b. **Methicillin-resistant S. aureus (MRSA):** In recent decades, a high percentage (often in the range of fifty percent) of hospital *S. aureus* isolates has been found to be also resistant to methicillin and/or oxacillin, due to chromosomal acquisition of the gene for a modified penicillin-binding protein ("PBP", see p. 113), PBP-2a. This protein codes for a new peptidoglycan transpeptidase with a low affinity for all currently available β-lactam antibiotics (thus contradicting its designation as a PBP), and thus renders infections with methicillin-resistant *S. aureus* unresponsive to β-lactam therapy. Unfortunately, MRSA strains are also frequently resistant to many other antibiotics, some being sensitive only to glycopeptides such as vancomycin.

    c. **Vancomycin resistance:** Vancomycin has been the agent of choice for empiric treatment of life-threatening *S. aureus* infections. Unfortunately, in 1997, several MRSAs were isolated that had also acquired low-level vancomycin resistance. The possibility that this resistance may increase in strength and spread to other species has caused considerable concern in the health care community.

G. Prevention

There is no effective vaccine against *S. aureus*. Infection control procedures such as barrier precautions, and washing of hands and fomites, are important in the control of nosocomial *S. aureus* epidemics.

IV. COAGULASE-NEGATIVE STAPHYLOCOCCI

Of twelve coagulase-negative staphylococcal species that have been recovered as normal commensals of human skin and anterior nares, the most abundant and important is *S. epidermidis*. For this reason some clinical laboratories designate all coagulase-negative staphylococci as *S. epidermidis*, a practice that is not encouraged. The second most important coagulase-negative staphylococcus is *S. saprophyticus*, which has a special medical niche. The coagulase-negative staphylococcal species are important agents of hospital-acquired infections associated with the use of implanted prosthetic devices and catheters.

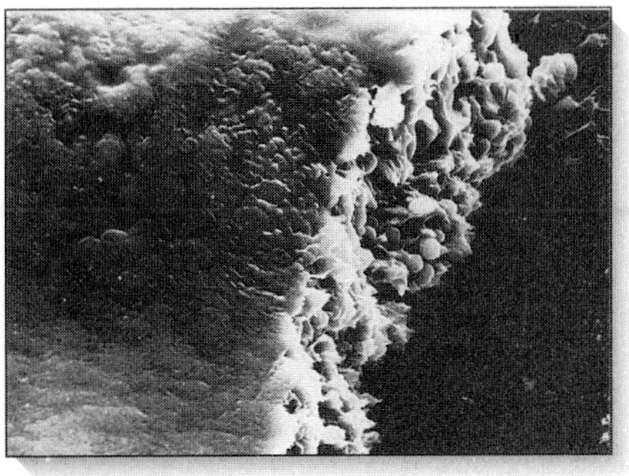

Figure 11.9
Staphylococcus epidermidis growing on extracellar slime on surface of colonized catheter.

A. Staphylococcus epidermidis

S. epidermidis is present in large numbers as part of the normal flora of the skin (see p. 7). As such it is frequently recovered from blood cultures, generally as a contaminant from skin. Despite its low virulence, it is a common cause of infection of implants such as heart valves and catheters (Figure 11.9). Cell envelope factors that facilitate attachment to plastic surfaces act as virulence factors. Acquired drug resistance by *S. epidermidis* is even more frequent than by *S. aureus*. Vancomycin sensitivity remains the rule, but vancomycin-resistant isolates have been reported.

B. Staphylococcus saprophyticus

This organism is a frequent cause of cystitis in women, probably related to its occurrence as part of normal vaginal flora (see p. 10). It tends to be sensitive to most antibiotics, even penicillin G. *S. saprophyticus* can be distinguished from *S. epidermidis* and most other coagulase-negative staphylococci by its natural resistance to novobiocin (Figure 11.10). [Note: A urinary coagulase-negative staphylococcus is often presumed to be *S. saprophyticus*; novobiocin resistance can be used for confirmation.]

Species	Frequency of disease	Coagulase	Color of colonies	Mannitol fermentation	Novobiocin resistance
S. aureus	Common	+	Golden yellow	+	−
S. epidermidis	Common	−	White	−	−
S. saprophyticus	Occasional	−	Variable	−	+

Figure 11.10
Summary of various species of staphylococci.

Study Questions

Choose the ONE correct answer

Questions 11.1 to 11.2:

A 32-year-old woman became ill four days after the onset of her menstrual period. She presented in the emergency room with fever (104°F; normal = 98.6°F), elevated white blood cell count (16,000/mm^3; normal = 4,000 to 10,000/mm^3), and a rash on her trunk and extremities. She complained of fatigue, vomiting, and diarrhea. She had recently eaten at a fast-food restaurant, but otherwise had prepared all her meals at home. The patient retained a tampon.

11.1 The patient described most likely has

    A. staphylococcal food poisoning.

    B. scalded skin syndrome.

    C. infection with a *Staphylococcus saprophyticus.*

    D. chickenpox.

    E. toxic shock syndrome.

> Correct answer = E. The patient shows the signs of toxic shock syndrome. Toxic shock syndrome as defined in the outbreak of the late '70s and early 80s included an erythematous/peeling rash (not purpuric) and was caused by overproduction of TSST-1 by colonizing *S. aureus* triggered by something in hyperabsorbant tampons. Many signs and symptoms are the results of the super-antigen activity of TSST, which activates a whole subclass of T cells, thus causing overproduction of cytokines. *Staphylococcus saprophyticus* is a frequent cause of cystitis in women, but is not associated with toxic shock syndrome.

11.2 Which one of the following laboratory criteria would establish *Staphylococcus aureus*, rather than *Streptococcus pyogenes*, as the causative organism?

    A. Growth on blood agar

    B. Production of catalase

    C. Motility

    D. Presence of gram-positive cocci

    E. Growth under anaerobic conditions

> Correct answer = B. Staphylococci produce catalase, which is one feature that distinguishes them from the catalase-negative streptococci (see p.xxx). Staphylococci and streptococci are both gram positive, nonmotile, facultatively anaerobic cocci that grows on blood agar.

11.3 *S. aureus* exfoliative toxins

    A. cause peeling of mammalian cell membranes and thus cell lysis.

    B. are important causes of toxic shock syndrome in menstruating women.

    C. cause bullous impetigo.

    D. act as virulence factors in staphylococcal pharyngitis, requiring prompt antitoxin administration.

    E. are restricted to the periplasmic space.

> Correct answer = C. These toxins attack intradermal intercellular ground substance adhesive, resulting in superficial blisters.

11.4 A 57-year-old man arrives at the emergency room complaining of weakness, fatigue and intermittent fever that has recurred for several weeks. The patient had a valvular prosthesis implanted five years previously. Physical examination reveals petechiae (pinpoint, nonraised purplish-red spots caused by intradermal hemorrhage) on the chest and stomach. Blood cultures grew catalase-positive, coagulase-negative, cocci. The gram-positive organisms failed to ferment mannitol, and their growth was inhibited by novobiocin. What is the most likely infectious agent?

    A. *Staphylococcus aureus*

    B. *Staphylococcus epidermidis*

    C. *Staphylococcus saprophyticus*

    D. *Streptococcus pneumoniae*

    E. *Staphylococcus agalactiae*

> Correct answer = B. The patient is probably suffering from bacterial endocarditis caused by *Staphylococcus epidermidis* infection of the prosthetic heart valve. *S. epidermidis* is a coagulase-negative organism that is unable to ferment mannitol, and is sensitive to novobiocin but usually resistant to penicillin. Patients with congenital heart malformations, acquired valvular defects (for example, rheumatic heart disease), prosthetic valves, and previous bacterial endocarditis show an increased incidence of bacterial endocarditis. Injection drug users also have a high risk for infection. *Streptococcus pneumoniae* and *Staphylococcus agalactiae* can be ruled out, because streptococci are catalase-negative, which is a feature that distinguishes them from the catalase-positive staphyococci.

Streptococci

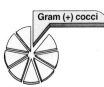

12

I. OVERVIEW

The gram-positive, nonmotile, catalase-negative cocci are a heterogeneous group of organisms, with clinically important genera that include *Streptococcus* and *Enterococcus* (Figure 12.1). They are ovoid to spherical in shape, and occur as pairs or chains. Most are facultative anaerobes, but grow fermentatively even in the presence of oxygen. Because of their complex nutritional requirements, blood-enriched medium is generally used for their isolation. The diseases caused by this group of organisms are diverse, some of the most prevalent being, for example, acute infections of the throat and skin, caused by Group A streptococci (*Streptococcus pyogenes*), genital tract colonization resulting in neonatal sepsis caused by Group B streptococci (*Streptococcus agalactiae*), endocarditis caused by the viridans group of streptococci, and pneumonia, otitis, and meningitis caused by *Streptococcus pneumoniae*.

II. CLASSIFICATION OF STREPTOCOCCI

Streptococci can be classified by several schemes, for example, by the hemolytic properties, serologic groups, and metabolic properties of streptococcal isolates.

A. Hemolytic properties on blood agar

α-Hemolytic streptococci cause a chemical change in the hemoglobin of red cells in blood agar, resulting in the appearance of a green pigment that forms a ring around the colony (see p. 453). β-Hemolytic streptococci cause gross lysis of red blood cells, resulting in a clear ring around the colony (Figure 12.2). γ-Hemolytic is a term applied to streptococci that cause no color change or lysis of red blood cells.

B. Serologic (Lancefield) groupings

Many species of streptococci have in their cell walls a polysaccharide known as the C-carbohydrate, which is antigenic and easily extractable with dilute acid. The C-carbohydrates are covalently linked to the cell wall peptidoglycan. The Lancefield scheme classifies primarily β-hemolytic streptococci into Groups A through U on the basis of their C-carbohydrate. The clinically most important groups of β-hemolytic streptococci are types A and B (Figure 12.3).

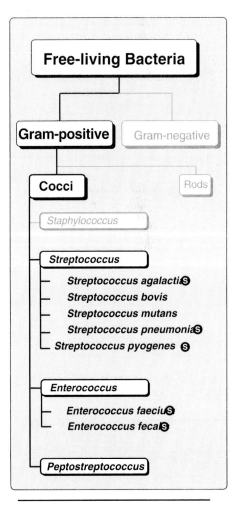

Figure 12.1
Classification of streptococci.
🅢 See pp. 420, 453 for summaries of these organisms.

Lippincott's Illustrated Reviews: Microbiology, by William A. Strohl, Harriet Rouse, Bruce D. Fisher. Lippincott, Williams & Wilkins, Baltimore, MD © 2001

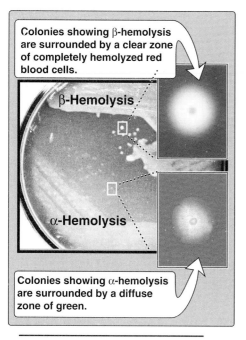

Colonies showing β-hemolysis are surrounded by a clear zone of completely hemolyzed red blood cells.

β-Hemolysis

α-Hemolysis

Colonies showing α-hemolysis are surrounded by a diffuse zone of green.

Figure 12.2
Growth on blood agar of β-hemolytic *Streptococcus* (top of culture plate); α-hemolytic *Streptococcus* (bottom of culture plate).

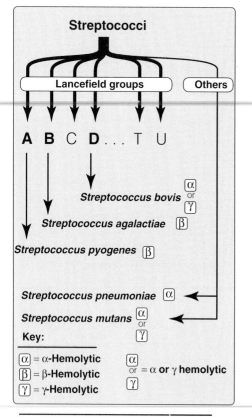

Streptococci

Lancefield groups   Others

A B C D . . . T U

Streptococcus bovis $\begin{array}{c}\alpha\\\text{or}\\\gamma\end{array}$

Streptococcus agalactiae β

Streptococcus pyogenes β

Streptococcus pneumoniae α

Streptococcus mutans $\begin{array}{c}\alpha\\\text{or}\\\gamma\end{array}$

Key:

α = α-Hemolytic
β = β-Hemolytic
γ = γ-Hemolytic

$\begin{array}{c}\alpha\\\text{or}\\\gamma\end{array}$ = α or γ hemolytic

Figure 12.3
Classification schemes for streptococci

III. GROUP A, β-HEMOLYTIC STREPTOCOCCI

Streptococcus pyogenes is the most virulent member of this group of gram-positive cocci, in that it can invade apparently intact skin or mucous membranes, causing some of the most rapidly progressive infections known. A low inoculum suffices for infection, and *S. pyogenes* must be considered a likely etiologic agent in all cases of cellulitis (diffuse spreading inflammation) anywhere in the body. Some strains of *S. pyogenes* cause postinfectious sequelae, including rheumatic fever and acute glomerulonephritis. *S. pyogenes* does not survive well in the environment. Instead it has as its habitat infected patients, and also normal human carriers in whom the organism resides on skin and mucous membranes. Nasopharyngeal carriage is common especially in colder months, and particularly among children. The most common sources of contagion are via aerosol from a nasopharyngeal carrier or someone who has streptococcal pharyngitis, or from direct contact with a skin carrier or a patient with impetigo.

A. Structure and physiology

S. pyogenes are gram-positive, nonmotile cocci. They occur as long chains when recovered from liquid culture (see p. 453), but may appear as individual cocci, pairs, or clusters of cells in Gram stains of samples from infected tissue. Structural features that are involved in the pathology or identification of the Group A streptococci include:

1. **Capsule:** Hyaluronic acid,[1] identical to that found in human connective tissue, forms the outermost layer of the cell. This capsule is not recognized as foreign by the body, and therefore is nonimmunogenic.

2. **Cell wall:** The cell wall contains a number of clinically important components. Beginning with the outer layer of the cell wall, these components include the following (Figure 12.4):

   a. **Fimbriae:** *S. pyogenes* cells are surrounded by a fringe of fimbriae (pilus-like structures). The fimbriae contain the major *S. pyogenes* virulence factor, the **M protein**. [Note: The bacterium is not infectious in the absence of M protein.] M proteins extend from an anchor in the cell membrane, through the cell wall and then the capsule, with the N-terminal end of the protein exposed on the surface of the bacterium. In the absence of specific antibodies against the M protein, this N-terminal region has antiphagocytic activity. However, it is also antigenic, and antibodies to it are opsonic. Notably, M proteins are highly variable, especially the N-terminal regions, resulting in over eighty different antigenic types. Thus, individuals may have many *S. pyogenes* infections throughout their lives, as they encounter new M protein types for which they have no antibodies. [Note: Fimbriae also contain lipoteichoic acid (LTA), which, together with M protein, plays a role in adhesion to host oral and skin epithelia.]

[1]See p. 149 in *Lippincott's Illustrated Reviews: Biochemistry* (2nd ed.) for a discussion of hyaluronic acid.

b. **The Group A–specific C-carbohydrate** is composed of rhamnose and N-acetylglucosamine. [Note: All group A streptococci, by definition, contain this antigen.]

c. **Protein F (fibronectin-binding protein)** mediates attachment to fibronectin in the pharyngeal epithelium.

3. **Extracellular products:** Like *Staphylococcus aureus* (see p. 139), *S. pyogenes* secretes a wide range of exotoxins that often vary from one strain to another, and that play roles in the pathogenesis of these organisms.

a. **Streptococcal pyrogenic exotoxins (SPEs):** Three antigenically distinct toxins, A (which corresponds to the classic erythrogenic toxin), B, and C have activity and sequence similarity to some *S. aureus* superantigen exotoxins (see p. 139). The genes for **SPE A** and **C** are carried by bacteriophage that lysogenize certain strains of *S. pyogenes* (see p. 116). **SPE B**, a cysteine protease, is encoded by a chromosomal gene that is uniformly present but variably expressed. These toxins cause a variety of effects, including the rash seen in scarlet fever, and severe streptococcal toxic shock–like disease.

b. **Cytolytic toxins and other exoenzymes: Streptolysin O** (O = "**o**xygen-labile") is a hemolysin that damages mammalian cells, including polymorphonuclear leukocytes, resulting in the release of lysosomal enzymes and degranulation. It is strongly antigenic, and antibodies formed against streptolysin O are used to document recent group A streptococcal infections (for example, the ASO test for rheumatic fever). **Streptolysin S** (S = "oxygen-**s**table") is a hemolysin that lyses erythrocytes, leukocytes, and platelets upon contact, and is responsible for lysis observed around colonies growing on the surface of blood agar. **Streptokinase** (fibrinolysin) catalyzes conversion of plasminogen to plasmin, thus causing fibrin digestion that results in lysis of clots (thrombi and emboli). It therefore facilitates the rapid spread of group A streptococci. **Streptodornases** are *S. pyogenes* DNAses that degrade the viscous DNA in necrotic tissue or exudates, thus aiding in the spread of infection. These enzymes are antigenic and can be used for diagnostic purposes. **C5a peptidase** inactivates complement component C5a, thus interfering with mobilization of white blood cells to sites of *S. pyogenes* infection. [Note: C5a has chemotactic activity that normally attracts neutrophils.] **Hyaluronidase** hydrolyzes the structural carbohydrate hyaluronic acid, which is an important component of the ground substance in connective tissue. This also aids the spread of infection. Figure 12.5 summarizes these cytolytic and other toxins.

B. Epidemiology

Respiratory droplets or skin contact spread Group A streptococcal infection from person to person, especially in crowded environments such as classrooms or children's play areas.

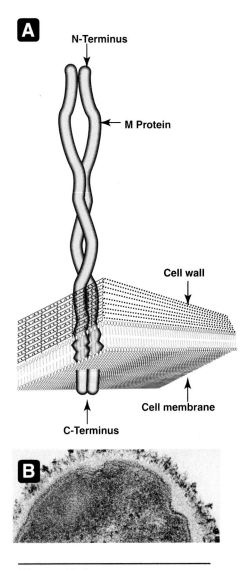

Figure 12.4
A. Schematic representation of the streptococcal M protein. B. Electron micrograph of streptococcus in which M protein appears as hairlike filament of the cell surface.

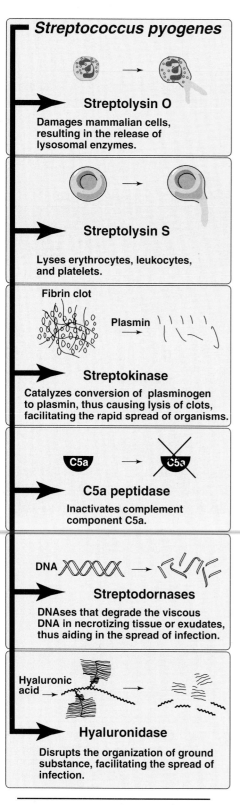

Streptococcus pyogenes

Streptolysin O

Damages mammalian cells, resulting in the release of lysosomal enzymes.

Streptolysin S

Lyses erythrocytes, leukocytes, and platelets.

Fibrin clot

Plasmin

Streptokinase

Catalyzes conversion of plasminogen to plasmin, thus causing lysis of clots, facilitating the rapid spread of organisms.

C5a → C5a

C5a peptidase

Inactivates complement component C5a.

DNA →

Streptodornases

DNAses that degrade the viscous DNA in necrotizing tissue or exudates, thus aiding in the spread of infection.

Hyaluronic acid →

Hyaluronidase

Disrupts the organization of ground substance, facilitating the spread of infection.

Figure 12.5
Cytolytic toxins and other exo-enzymes produced by *Streptococcus pyogenes*.

C. Pathology

S. pyogenes cells, perhaps in an inhaled droplet, attach to the pharyngeal mucosa via actions of protein F, lipoteichoic acid, and M protein (see Figure 12.4, p. 147). The bacteria may simply colonize (that is replicate only sufficiently to maintain themselves without causing injury); the patient is then considered **colonized**. Alternatively, the bacteria may grow and secrete toxins, causing damage to surrounding cells, invading the mucosa, and eliciting an inflammatory response with attendant influx of white cells, fluid leakage, and pus formation. The patient then has **streptococcal pharyngitis**. The bacterial hyaluronic acid capsule and M protein inhibit phagocytosis, and C5a peptidase acts to counter attraction of more white cells. Streptokinase, streptodornase, and hyaluronidase tend to decrease the viscosity of the pus, and to enhance spread through the tissues. Occasionally, there is sufficient spread that the blood stream is significantly invaded, possibly resulting in septicemia and/or seeding of distant sites, where cellulitis, fasciitis, or myonecrosis may develop rapidly or insidiously.

D. Clinical significance

S. pyogenes is a major cause of **cellulitis** (diffuse spreading skin and subcutaneous soft tissue inflammation). More specific syndromes include the following.

1. **Acute pharyngitis or pharyngotonsilitis**: *S. pyogenes* is the most common bacterial cause of sore throats, especially in patients two to twenty years old, and pharyngitis is the most common type of *S. pyogenes* infection. Florid *S. pyogenes* pharyngitis ("**strep throat**") is associated with severe, purulent inflammation of the posterior oropharynx and tonsillar areas (see p. 453). [Note: If a sunburn–like rash develops on the neck, trunk, and extremities in response to the release of pyrogenic exotoxin to which the patient does not have antibodies, the syndrome is designated **scarlet fever**.] However, many strep throats are mild, and many sore throats of other etiologies (for example, viral or mycoplasmal) are severe. Hence, laboratory confirmation is important. Antibiotic treatment (penicillin G for ten days, or a macrolide if the patient is allergic to penicillins) shortens the course of the disease, and prevents suppurative (pus-forming) complications, such as peritonsillar abscess.

2. **Impetigo:** Although *Staphylococcus aureus* is recovered from most contemporary cases of impetigo (see p. 140), *Streptococcus pyogenes* is the classic cause of this syndrome. The disease begins on any exposed surface (most commonly the legs). It usually affects children, and can cause severe and extensive lesions on the face and limbs (see p. 453). Impetigo is treated with a topical agent such as mupirocin, or systemically with penicillin or a first-generation cephalosporin, which are effective against both *Staphylococcus aureus* and *Streptococcus pyogenes*.

3. **Erysipelas:** Affecting all age groups, patients with erysipelas suffer from a fiery red, advancing erythema, especially on the face or lower limbs (see p. 453).

4. **Puerperal sepsis:** This infection is initiated during, or following soon after, the delivery of a newborn. It can occur due to exogenous transmission (for example, by nasal droplets from an infected carrier, or from contaminated instruments), or endogenously, from the patient's vaginal flora. This is a disease of the uterine endometrium in which patients suffer from a purulent vaginal discharge, and are systemically very ill.

5. **Invasive group A streptococcal (GAS) disease:** Common during the first half of the century, invasive GAS disease became rare until its resurgence during the past decade. Patients may have a deep local invasion without necrosis (cellulitis) or with it (necrotizing fasciitis/myositis, Figure 12.6). [Note: The latter disease led to the term "flesh-eating bacteria."] Invasive GAS disease often spreads rapidly, even in otherwise healthy individuals, leading to bacteremia and sepsis. Symptoms may include a toxic shock–like syndrome, fever, hypotension, multi-organ involvement, a sunburn-like rash, or a combination of these symptoms.

6. **Acute rheumatic fever:** This autoimmune disease occurs two to three weeks after the initiation of pharyngitis. It is due to cross-reactions between antigens of the heart and joint tissues, and the streptococcal antigen (especially the M protein epitopes). It is characterized by fever, rash, carditis and arthritis. Rheumatic fever is preventable if the patient is treated within the first ten days following initiation of acute pharyngitis.

7. **Acute glomerulonephritis:** This rare, postinfectious sequela occurs as soon as one week after impetigo or pharyngitis ensues, due to a few "nephritogenic" strains of group A streptococci. Antigen-antibody complexes on the basement membrane of the glomerulus initiate the disease. There is no evidence that penicillin treatment of the pyoderma or pharyngitis (to eradicate the infection) can prevent acute glomerulonephritis.

E. Laboratory identification

Depending on the form of the disease, specimens for laboratory analysis can be obtained from throat swabs, pus and lesion samples, sputum, blood, or spinal fluid. *S. pyogenes* forms characteristic small, opalescent colonies surrounded by a large zone of β hemolysis on sheep blood agar (see Figure 12.2). This organism is highly sensitive to bacitracin, and diagnostic disks with a very low concentration of the antibiotic inhibit growth in culture. Group A C-carbohydrate can be identified by the precipitin reaction. Serologic tests detect a patient's antibody titer to streptolysin-O (ASO test) after group A streptococcal infection. Anti-DNase B titers (ADB test) are particularly elevated following streptococcal infections of the skin.

F. Treatment

Drainage and debridement are very important for the treatment of necrotizing fasciitis/myositis (see Figure 12.6). Antibiotics are used for all Group A streptococcal infections. *S. pyogenes* has not acquired resistance to penicillin G, which remains the antibiotic of

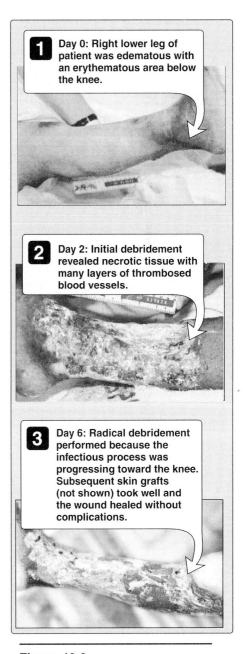

1 Day 0: Right lower leg of patient was edematous with an erythematous area below the knee.

2 Day 2: Initial debridement revealed necrotic tissue with many layers of thrombosed blood vessels.

3 Day 6: Radical debridement performed because the infectious process was progressing toward the knee. Subsequent skin grafts (not shown) took well and the wound healed without complications.

Figure 12.6
Necrotizing fasciitis in a 59-year-old woman.

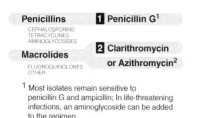

1 Most isolates remain sensitive to
penicillin G and ampicillin; In life-threatening
infections, an aminoglycoside can be added
to the regimen.

2 For penicillin-allergic patients.

Figure 12.7
Some antimicrobial agents useful
in treating infections due to
Streptococcus pyogenes.

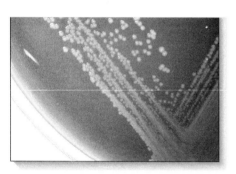

Figure 12.8
Colonies of *Streptococcus agalactiae*
grown on blood agar.

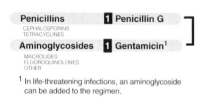

1 In life-threatening infections, an aminoglycoside
can be added to the regimen.

Figure 12.9
Some antimicrobial agents useful
in treating infections due to
Streptococcus agalactiae.

choice for acute streptococcal disease. In the case of a penicillin-allergic patient, a macrolide such as clarithromycin or azithromycin is the preferred drug (Figure 12.7).

G. Prevention

Rheumatic fever is prevented by rapid eradication of the infecting organism. Prolonged prophylactic antibiotic therapy is indicated after an episode of rheumatic fever, because having had one episode of this autoimmune disease in the past is a major risk factor for subsequent episodes if the patient is again infected with *S. pyogenes*.

IV. GROUP B, β-HEMOLYTIC STREPTOCOCCI

Group B streptococci, represented by the pathogen *Streptococcus agalactiae*, are gram-positive, catalase-negative organisms. They possess a polysaccharide capsule that is antiphagocytic, and thus allows the bacterium to infect tissue, and induce an inflammatory response. *S. agalactiae* is found in the vaginocervical tract of female carriers, and the urethral mucous membranes of male carriers, as well as in the GI tract (especially the rectum). Transmission occurs from an infected mother to her infant at birth, and venereally (propagated by sexual contact) among adults. The group B streptococci are a leading cause of meningitis and septicemia in neonates, with a high mortality rate. They are also an occasional cause of infections in post-partum women (endometritis), and individuals with impaired immune systems, in whom the organism may cause septicemia or pneumonia. Group B streptococci are also associated with lower extremity infections in diabetic patients. Samples of blood, cervical swabs, sputum, or spinal fluid can be obtained for culture on blood agar. ELISA tests (see p. 30) can also be used to demonstrate the presence of bacterial antigen in these samples. Group B streptococci are β-hemolytic, with larger colonies and less hemolysis than group A (Figure 12.8). They can also hydrolyze sodium hippurate. All isolates remain sensitive to penicillin G and ampicillin, which are still the antibiotics of choice (Figure 12.9). In life-threatening infections, an aminoglycoside can be added to the regimen. [Note: Pregnant carriers should be treated with ampicillin during labor if risk factors such as premature rupture of membranes or prolonged labor are present.]

V. STREPTOCOCCUS PNEUMONIAE (PNEUMOCOCCUS)

Streptococcus pneumoniae are gram-positive, nonmotile, encapsulated cocci (Figure 12.10). They are lancet-shaped, and their tendency to occur in pairs accounts for their earlier designation as *Diplococcus pneumoniae*. *S. pneumoniae* is the most common cause of pneumonia and otitis media, and is an important cause of meningitis and bacteremia/sepsis. The risk of disease is highest among young children, older adults, smokers, and persons with certain chronic illnesses. Like other streptococci, *S. pneumoniae* is fastidious and is routinely cultured on blood agar. It releases an α-hemolysin that damages red cell membranes, causing colonies to be α-hemolytic.

A. Epidemiology

S. pneumoniae is an obligate parasite of humans, and can be found in the nasopharynx of many healthy individuals. This organism is extremely sensitive to environmental agents. Pneumococcal infections can be either endogenous or exogenous. For example, **endogenous infection** involves the spread of *S. pneumoniae* residing in the nasopharynx of a carrier who develops impaired resistance to the organism. Susceptibility to the infection may be due, for example, to general debilitation such as that caused by malnutrition or alcoholism, to respiratory damage following a prior viral infection, or to a depressed immune system. Patients with sickle cell disease and/or those who have had their spleens removed are particularly at risk for *S. pneumoniae* infection. Infection can also be **exogenous**, for example, by droplets from the nose of a carrier. Individuals such as those described above as susceptible to endogenous infection are also the most likely to be infected by the exogenous route.

B. Pathogenesis

The bacterial capsule of *S. pneumoniae* is the most important virulence factor, and is the basis for the classification of serotypes of this organism. Cell-associated enzymes, pneumolysin, and autolysin contribute to its pathogenicity (Figure 12.11).

1. **Capsule:** The *S. pneumoniae* polysaccharide capsule is both antiphagocytic and antigenic. Antibodies to it are opsonic. The antiphagocytic properties of the capsule protect the bacteria from polymorphonuclear leukocyte attack, facilitating growth of the bacteria prior to the appearance of anti-capsular antibodies. There are approximately 85 distinct capsular serotypes, some of which endow strains with greater virulence than do others, as reflected by the fact that about twenty serotypes account for the vast majority of pneumococcal infections.

2. **Autolysin:** This peptidoglycan hydrolase is present in the bacterial cell wall, and is normally inactive. However, it is readily triggered (for example, by surface-active agents, β-lactam antibiotics, or aging), resulting in cell lysis. Autolysin is thus responsible for the release of intracellular virulence factors (notably pneumolysin).

3. **Pneumolysin:** Although retained within the cytosol of intact pneumococci, pneumolysin is thought to be an important virulence factor by virtue of its ability to attack mammalian cell membranes causing lysis once it is released by autolysin from the interior of the bacterium.

C. Clinical significance

1. **Acute bacterial pneumonia:** A leading cause of death, especially in the aged and those whose resistance is impaired, this disease is caused most frequently by *S. pneumoniae* (Figure 12.12). Pneumonia is frequently preceded by an upper or middle respiratory viral infection, which predisposes to *S. pneumoniae* infection of pulmonary parenchyma. Mechanisms by which virus infection predisposes an individual to streptococcal pneumonia include

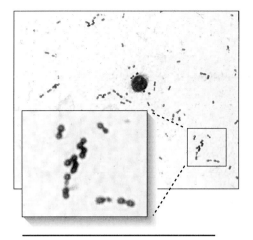

Figure 12.10
Streptoccus pneumoniae are gram-positive, nonmotile, encapsulated lancet-shaped cocci.

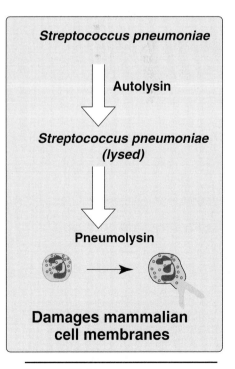

Figure 12.11
Cytolytic toxins produced by *Streptococcus pneumoniae*.

Disease Summary:"TYPICAL"PNEUMONIA[1]

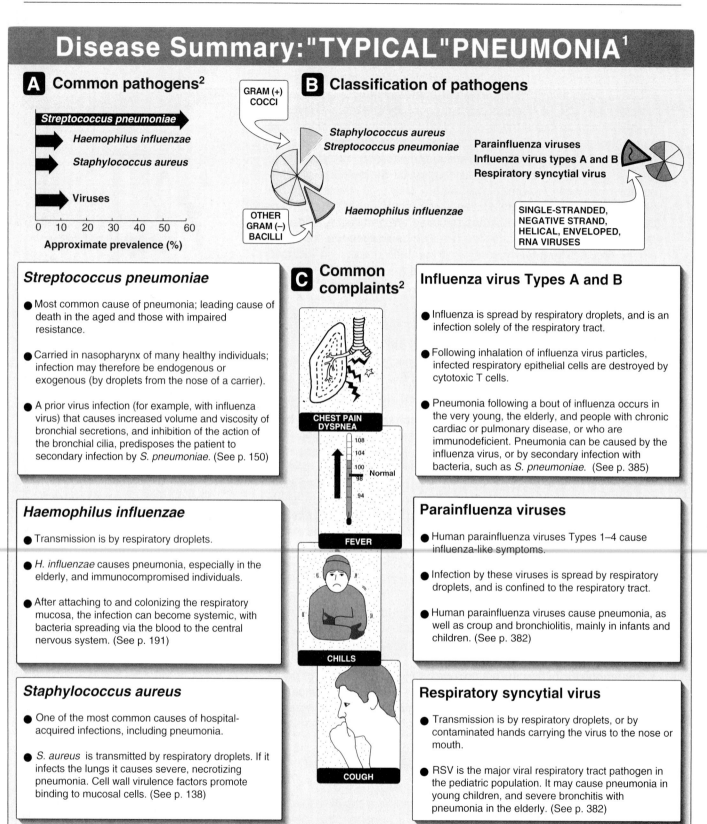

A Common pathogens[2]

Streptococcus pneumoniae
Haemophilus influenzae
Staphylococcus aureus
Viruses

0   10   20   30   40   50   60
Approximate prevalence (%)

B Classification of pathogens

GRAM (+) COCCI

Staphylococcus aureus
Streptococcus pneumoniae

Haemophilus influenzae

OTHER GRAM (–) BACILLI

Parainfluenza viruses
Influenza virus types A and B
Respiratory syncytial virus

SINGLE-STRANDED, NEGATIVE STRAND, HELICAL, ENVELOPED, RNA VIRUSES

C Common complaints[2]

CHEST PAIN DYSPNEA

108
104
100 Normal
98
94

FEVER

CHILLS

COUGH

Streptococcus pneumoniae

- Most common cause of pneumonia; leading cause of death in the aged and those with impaired resistance.

- Carried in nasopharynx of many healthy individuals; infection may therefore be endogenous or exogenous (by droplets from the nose of a carrier).

- A prior virus infection (for example, with influenza virus) that causes increased volume and viscosity of bronchial secretions, and inhibition of the action of the bronchial cilia, predisposes the patient to secondary infection by S. pneumoniae. (See p. 150)

Haemophilus influenzae

- Transmission is by respiratory droplets.

- H. influenzae causes pneumonia, especially in the elderly, and immunocompromised individuals.

- After attaching to and colonizing the respiratory mucosa, the infection can become systemic, with bacteria spreading via the blood to the central nervous system. (See p. 191)

Staphylococcus aureus

- One of the most common causes of hospital-acquired infections, including pneumonia.

- S. aureus is transmitted by respiratory droplets. If it infects the lungs it causes severe, necrotizing pneumonia. Cell wall virulence factors promote binding to mucosal cells. (See p. 138)

Influenza virus Types A and B

- Influenza is spread by respiratory droplets, and is an infection solely of the respiratory tract.

- Following inhalation of influenza virus particles, infected respiratory epithelial cells are destroyed by cytotoxic T cells.

- Pneumonia following a bout of influenza occurs in the very young, the elderly, and people with chronic cardiac or pulmonary disease, or who are immunodeficient. Pneumonia can be caused by the influenza virus, or by secondary infection with bacteria, such as S. pneumoniae. (See p. 385)

Parainfluenza viruses

- Human parainfluenza viruses Types 1–4 cause influenza-like symptoms.

- Infection by these viruses is spread by respiratory droplets, and is confined to the respiratory tract.

- Human parainfluenza viruses cause pneumonia, as well as croup and bronchiolitis, mainly in infants and children. (See p. 382)

Respiratory syncytial virus

- Transmission is by respiratory droplets, or by contaminated hands carrying the virus to the nose or mouth.

- RSV is the major viral respiratory tract pathogen in the pediatric population. It may cause pneumonia in young children, and severe bronchitis with pneumonia in the elderly. (See p. 382)

Figure 12.12
Some characteristics of community-acquired pneumonia.
[1] "Typical" penumonia is characterized by shaking chills, purulent sputum, and x-ray abnormalities that are proportional to the physical symptoms. See p. 233 for a summary of "atypical" pneumonia.
[2] Other pathogens include Legionella, Mycoplasma pneumoniae, Chlamydia pneumoniae, and gram-negative bacilli. Other complaints include anorexia, headache, nausea, diarrhea, and vomiting.

increased volume and viscosity of secretions that are more difficult to clear, and secondary inhibition of the action of bronchial cilia by viral infection.

2. **Otitis media:** The most common bacterial infection of children, this disease (which is characterized by ear ache) is most frequently caused by pneumococcus, followed by *Haemophilus influenzae* (see p. 191) and *Moraxella catarrhalis* (see p. 173). The traditional empiric treatment of pneumococcal otitis media with a β-lactam antibiotic (with or without a penicillinase-inhibitor) has been threatened by the spread of penicillin-resistant pneumococci.

3. **Bacteremia/sepsis** in the absence of a focus of infection is commonly due to pneumococcus, especially in splenectomized individuals.

4. **Meningitis:** *H. influenzae* was formerly the leading cause of bacterial meningitis in the United States. After a vaccine was developed against this organism, *S. pneumoniae* became the most common cause of bacterial meningitis (see pp. 170 to 171). This disease has a high mortality rate, even when treated appropriately.

D. Laboratory identification

Specimens for laboratory evaluation can be obtained from a nasopharyngeal swab, blood, pus, sputum, or spinal fluid. α-Hemolytic colonies appear when *S. pneumoniae* is grown on blood agar overnight under aerobic conditions at 37°C. Lancet-shaped, gram-positive diplococci are observed on a Gram stain of the sample. The growth of these bacteria is inhibited by low concentrations of the surfactant, optochin, and the cells are lysed by bile (Figure 12.13). Capsular swelling is observed when the pneumococci are treated with type-specific antisera (the Quellung reaction). [Note: This reaction was used for serotyping samples in the era of serotherapy. "Omnisera" (containing several type-specific antibodies) is useful for identifying pneumococci at the species level.]

E. Treatment

S. pneumoniae isolates were highly sensitive to penicillin G, the initial agent of choice, until the late 1980s. Since then, the incidence of penicillin resistance has been increasing worldwide. The mechanism of this resistance is due to an alteration of one or more of the bacterium's penicillin-binding proteins (PBPs, see p. 113) rather than to the production of β-lactamase. The modified PBPs have a much reduced affinity for penicillin G, and for some but not all of the other β-lactams. In 1996–7, approximately fifteen percent of *S. pneumoniae* isolates in American hospitals were classified as moderately resistant, and ten percent as highly resistant. [Note: Isolates are classified as moderately resistant if the minimal inhibitory concentration (MIC) is 0.1–1 μg/ml, or highly resistant if the MIC is greater than 2 μg/ml.] Most resistant strains remain sensitive to third generation cephalosporins (such as cefotaxime or ceftriaxone), and all are still sensitive to vancomycin; these antibiotics are therefore the agents of choice for invasive infections by penicillin-resistant strains of *S. pneumoniae* (Figure 12.14).

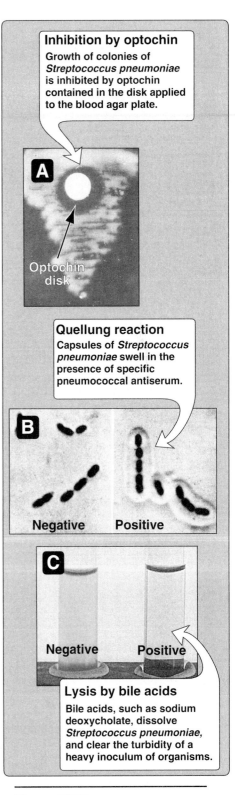

Inhibition by optochin
Growth of colonies of *Streptococcus pneumoniae* is inhibited by optochin contained in the disk applied to the blood agar plate.

Optochin disk

Quellung reaction
Capsules of *Streptococcus pneumoniae* swell in the presence of specific pneumococcal antiserum.

Negative   Positive

Negative   Positive

Lysis by bile acids
Bile acids, such as sodium deoxycholate, dissolve *Streptococcus pneumoniae*, and clear the turbidity of a heavy inoculum of organisms.

Figure 12.13
Some laboratory tests useful in the identification of *Streptococcus pneumoniae*. A. Optochin disk test. B. Quellung reaction. C. Lysis by bile salts.

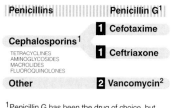

Penicillins ▓▓▓▓▓▓	**Penicillin G**[1]
	1 Cefotaxime
Cephalosporins[1]	
TETRACYCLINES AMINOGLYCOSIDES MACROLIDES FLUOROQUINOLONES	**1** Ceftriaxone
Other	**2** Vancomycin[2]

[1]Penicillin G has been the drug of choice, but resistant strains are increasingly seen.

[2]Most resistant strains remain sensitive to vancomycin; use of this antibiotic (in combination with cefotaxime or ceftriaxone) should be reserved for the critically ill patient, for example, anyone with meningitis possibly caused by *S. pneumoniae*.

Figure 12.14
Some antimicrobial agents useful in treating infections due to *Streptococcus pneumoniae*.

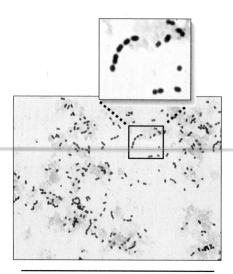

Figure 12.15
Enterococcus fecalis showing chain formation characteristic of *Streptococcus*.

F. Prevention

A "polyvalent" antipneumococcal capsular polysaccharide vaccine that immunizes against 23 serotypes of S. pneumoniae is indicated for the protection of high-risk individuals over two years of age. This vaccine protects against the pneumococcal strains responsible for 85 to 90 percent of infections, including prominent penicillin-resistant strains. The heptavalent pneumococcal conjugate vaccine (PCV7, see p. 37), effective in young children, is made up of seven pneumococcal antigens conjugated to CRM197–a mutant nontoxic diphtheria toxin. Three doses of vaccine are given at two, four, and six months of age. The PCV7 provides serotype and serogroup cross-protection for 88 percent of cases of bacteremia, 82 percent of cases of meningitis, and 71 percent of cases of pneumococcal otitis media episodes in United States children younger than six years.

VI. ENTEROCOCCI

Enterococci contain a C-carbohydrate that reacts with group D antisera. Therefore, in the past, they were considered group D streptococci. Today, DNA analysis and other properties have placed them in their own genus, *Enterococcus*. The clinically most important species are *E. faecalis* and *E. faecium*. Enterococci can be α-, β-, or nonhemolytic. As a rule, enterococci are not very virulent, but they have become prominent as a cause of nosocomial infections due to their multiple antibiotic resistance. Figure 12.15 shows the microscopic appearance of *Enterococcus faecalis*.

A. Epidemiology

Enterococci are part of the normal fecal flora. However, they can also colonize oral mucous membranes and skin, especially in hospital settings. These organisms are highly resistant to environmental and chemical agents, and can persist on fomites.

B. Diseases

Enterococci seldom cause disease in normal, healthy individuals. However, under conditions where host resistance is lowered, or where the integrity of the gastrointestinal or genitourinary tract has been disrupted, for example by instrumentation, the enterococci can spread to normally sterile sites, causing urinary tract infections, bacteremia/sepsis, subacute bacterial endocarditis, biliary tract infection, or intra-abdominal abscesses.

C. Laboratory identification

Enterococci are distinguished from the non–Group D streptococci by their ability to survive in the presence of bile, and to hydrolyze the polysaccharide esculin. Unlike nonenterococcal group D streptococci, enterococci grow in 6.5 percent NaCl, and yield a positive **pyrazin amidase** (**PYR**) test. *E. faecalis* can be distinguished from *E. faecium* by their fermentation patterns, which are commonly evaluated in clinical laboratories.

D. Treatment

Enterococci are naturally resistant to β-lactam antibiotics and amino-glycosides, but are sensitive to the synergistic action of a combination of these classes. In the past, the initial regimens of choice were penicillin + streptomycin, or ampicillin + gentamicin (Figure 12.16). However, acquired resistance determinants in many current strains negate this synergy. In addition, isolates frequently have natural or acquired resistances to many other antibiotic classes, including glycopeptide, such as vancomycin. Newer antibiotics, such as the combination of quinupristin and dalfopristin, are used to treat vancomycin-resistant infections. However, some enterococcal strains are resistant to **all** commercially available antibiotics. [Note: *E. faecium* is more likely to be vancomycin- or multiply-resistant than *E. faecalis*.]

E. Prevention

The rise of nosocomial infections by multiple drug-resistant enterococci is largely the result of selection due to high antibiotic usage in hospitals. Judicious use of antibiotics is an important factor in controlling these infections.

VII. NONENTEROCOCCAL GROUP D STREPTOCOCCI

Streptococcus bovis is the most clinically important of the nonenterococcus group D streptococci. Part of normal fecal flora, they are either α– or nonhemolytic. *S. bovis* occasionally causes urinary tract infections and subacute bacterial endocarditis, especially in association with bowel malignancy. The organism is bile- and esculin-positive, but is PYR-negative, and does not grow in 6.5 percent salt (unlike the enterococci). It tends to be sensitive to penicillin and other antibiotics.

VIII. VIRIDANS STREPTOCOCCI

The viridans group of streptococci includes many gram-positive, catalase-negative, α– or γ–hemolytic species that constitute the main facultative **oral flora**. The viridans streptococci are relatively avirulent, but *Streptococcus mutans* and other members of the viridans group cause dental caries. In patients with abnormal or damaged heart valves, they can also infect these valves during a bacteremia, causing subacute bacterial endocarditis (Figure 12.17). Therefore, at-risk patients with rheumatic, congenital, or arteriosclerotic valvular disease should receive prophylactic penicillin before undergoing dental procedures.

IX. PEPTOSTREPTOCOCCI

Anaerobic streptococci are more properly designated as members of the genus *Peptostreptococcus*. They are present on mucous membranes of the genitourinary and GI tracts, and are particularly abundant among the normal oral, especially periodontal, flora. Relatively avirulent, they contribute to mixed anaerobic infections of soft tissues, where they are involved in wound infections, abscesses, pneumonia, and genital tract disease.

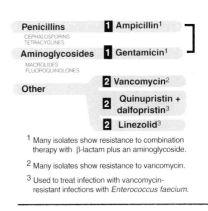

Penicillins	[1] Ampicillin[1]
CEPHALOSPORINS TETRACYCLINES	
Aminoglycosides	[1] Gentamicin[1]
MACROLIDES FLUOROQUINOLONES	
Other	[2] Vancomycin[2]
	[2] Quinupristin + dalfopristin[3]
	[2] Linezolid[3]

[1] Many isolates show resistance to combination therapy with β-lactam plus an aminoglycoside.

[2] Many isolates show resistance to vancomycin.

[3] Used to treat infection with vancomycin-resistant infections with *Enterococcus faecium*.

Figure 12.16
Some antimicrobial agents useful in treating infections due to Enterococci.

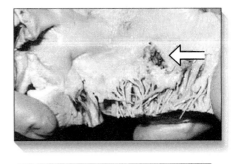

Figure 12.17
Streptoccal endocarditis showing vegetation of the mitral valve leaflet [Note: Vegetation is a tissue outgrowth composed of fibrin and aggregated blood platelets adherent to a diseased heart valve.]

Study Questions

Questions 12.1 to 12.6: For each numbered phrase, select the one statement (A to I) that is most closely associated with it. Each statement (A to I) may be selected once, more than once, or not at all.

A. Mediates infection of vascular implants
B. Forms tubules that pierce mammalian cell membranes
C. Corresponds to Lancefield Group B antigen
D. Induced by sex pheromones
E. Released only after autolysis
F. Combines with Fc portion of IgG classes
G. Polysaccharide virulence factor
H. Correlated with necrotizing fasciitis

12.1 *Staphylococcus aureus* protein A

Correct answer = F. This activity is antiopsonic and contributes to the virulence of *S. aureus*.

12.2 *Streptococcus pyogenes* pyrogenic toxin B (SPE B)

Correct answer = H. Processing of this exoprotein yields a protease that may play a role in pathogenesis of the necrotizing lesion.

12.3 *Streptococcus pneumoniae* capsule

Correct answer = G. The pneumococcal polysaccharide capsule is its most important virulence factor.

12.4 *Staphylococcus aureus* α-toxin

Correct answer = B The α-toxin is an important *S. aureus* virulence factor and a prototype of bacterial toxins that attack mammalian cell membranes.

12.5 *Staphylococcus epidermidis* cell envelope

Correct answer = A. Capsular polysaccharide and protein adhesins mediate adherence to the surface of various plastics.

Choose the ONE correct answer

12.6 A 52-year-old homosexual man, generally in good health, is diagnosed as having colon carcinoma and is scheduled for surgery. While waiting for his HMO to arrange for a bed, he develops persistent low-grade fever and constitutional symptoms. Physical examination is unremarkable save for a heart murmur not previously present. Outpatient blood cultures yield gram-positive, α-hemolytic cocci. The most likely cause for the clinical picture is:

A. spread of his carcinoma.
B. anxiety, with skin flora contamination of the blood cultures.
C. subacute endocarditis due to *Streptococcus bovis*.
D. subacute endocarditis due to Group B streptococci.
E. AIDS.

Correct answer = C. *S. bovis*, a member of normal fecal flora, is a hemolytic and not uncommon cause of subacute endocarditis seen in association with bowel neoplasms.

12.7 A 55-year-old male was admitted to a local hospital with fever and chills. The patient was HIV positive and had received multiple courses of antibiotics. Blood cultures grew a gram-positive cocci, which tested positive with Group D streptococcal antisera. The isolate was resistant to penicillin and vancomycin. Which one of the following is the most likely pathogen?

A. *Streptococcus pneumoniae*
B. *Enterococcus faecium*
C. *Streptococcus pyogenes*
D. *Streptococcus agalactiae*
E. *Enterococcus faecalis*

Correct answer = B. *Enterococcus faecium* is most likely to be vancomycin- or multiply drug-resistant.

Facultative and Aerobic Gram-positive Rods

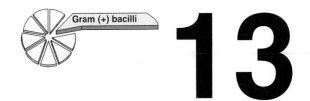

13

I. OVERVIEW

The organisms discussed in this chapter are grouped on morphologic grounds (that is, they are gram-positive rods). They are not closely related, nor do they cause similar clinical conditions. The genus *Corynebacterium* includes *Corynebacterium diphtheriae*, the cause of the prototypic toxin-mediated disease, diphtheria, as well as several usually harmless human commensals. The genus *Bacillus* is a large genus of spore-forming bacteria, principally of soil origin; however anthrax (a zoonotic septicemia) and a type of food poisoning are caused by species in this group. *Listeria monocytogenes* is a cause of infections including meningitis in populations such as newborns, pregnant women, and the immunocompromised. Organisms discussed in this chapter are summarized in Figure 13.1.

II. CORYNEBACTERIA

Corynebacteria are small, slender, pleomorphic, gram-positive rods of distinctive morphology that tend to stain unevenly but do not form spores. They are nonmotile and unencapsulated. They occur in characteristic clumps that look like Chinese characters or picket fence patterns (Figure 13.2), presumably created by the snapping motion with which the cells complete their division. *Corynebacterium* is a large genus of diverse habitat. Most species are facultative anaerobes, and those found associated with humans, including the pathogen *Corynebacterium diphtheriae*, grow aerobically on standard laboratory media such as blood agar.

A. Corynebacterium diphtheriae

Diphtheria, caused by *Corynebacterium diphtheriae*, is a life-threatening illness that is among the best studied of bacterial diseases. An early consequence of this interest was the development of effective vaccination protocols, and widespread immunization beginning in early childhood has made the disease rare in developed countries. Early presumptive diagnosis is critical, but few present-day clinicians have seen a case of the disease.

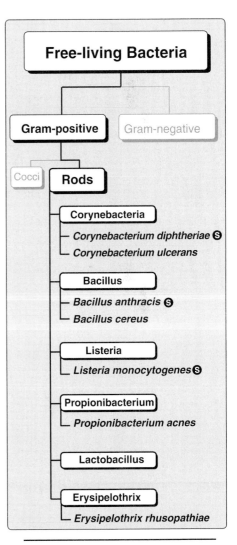

Figure 13.1
Classification of facultative and aerobic gram-positive rods.
Ⓢ See pp. 408, 443 (*C.diphtheriae*), pp. 402, 438 (*B. anthracis*), pp. 413, 447 (*L. monocytogenes*) for summaries of these organisms.

Lippincott's Illustrated Reviews: Microbiology,
by William A. Strohl, Harriet Rouse, Bruce D. Fisher.
Lippincott, Williams & Wilkins, Baltimore, MD © 2001

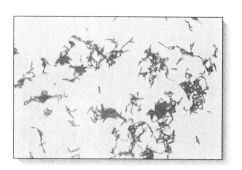

Figure 13.2
Corynebacterium diphtheriae.

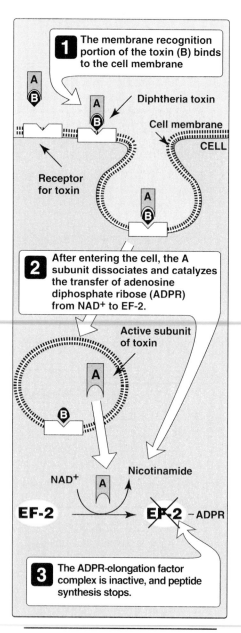

1 The membrane recognition portion of the toxin (B) binds to the cell membrane

A
B

A
B   Diphtheria toxin

Cell membrane

CELL

Receptor for toxin

A
B

2 After entering the cell, the A subunit dissociates and catalyzes the transfer of adenosine diphosphate ribose (ADPR) from NAD+ to EF-2.

Active subunit of toxin

A

B

NAD+   Nicotinamide

A

EF-2 ⟶ EF-2 –ADPR

3 The ADPR-elongation factor complex is inactive, and peptide synthesis stops.

Figure 13.3
Action of diphtheria toxin.

1. **Epidemiology:** *C. diphtheriae* is found in the throat and nasopharynx of carriers and patients with diphtheria. This disease is a local infection, usually of the throat. Therefore the organism is primarily spread by respiratory droplets, usually by convalescent or asymptomatic carriers. It is less frequently spread by direct contact with an infected carrier or a contaminated fomite.

2. **Pathogenesis:** Diphtheria is caused by the local and systemic effects of a single exotoxin that inhibits eukaryotic protein synthesis. The toxin molecule is a heat labile polypeptide that is composed of two fragments, A and B. Fragment B binds to susceptible cell membranes and mediates the delivery of fragment A to its target. Inside the cell, fragment A separates from fragment B, and catalyzes a reaction between nicotine adenine dinucleotide (NAD+) and the eukaryotic polypeptide chain elongation factor, EF-2[1] (Figure 13.3). The resulting ADP-ribosylation of EF-2 inactivates it and blocks the translocation of a polypeptidyl-tRNA from the acceptor site (A site) to the donor site (P site) on the ribosome. [Note: A single molecule of diphtheria toxin can inhibit all protein synthesis in a eukaryotic cell within hours of its introduction.] Recent genetic studies have identified the cell receptor for diphtheria toxin as being identical to the receptor for a heparin-binding epidermal growth factor, a member of a common family of receptors found in many eukaryotic cell membranes. The structural gene for diphtheria toxin (*tox*) is encoded in the genome of a corynebacterial bacteriophage, β phage. Only those strains of *C. diphtheriae* that are lysogenic (see p. 116) for a β phage can produce toxin and are therefore virulent. The phage's *tox* gene is regulated by a host bacterium-encoded repressor, DtxR, which itself is repressed under conditions of limited iron (in other words, low intracellular concentrations of iron allow maximum expression of the *tox* gene).

3. **Clinical significance**

   a. **Upper respiratory tract infection:** Diphtheria consists of a strictly local infection, usually of the throat. The infection produces a distinctive thick, grayish, adherent exudate (called a pseudomembrane) that is composed of cell debris from the mucosa, and inflammatory products. It coats the throat and may extend into the nasal passages or downward in the respiratory tract, where the exudate sometimes obstructs the airways, even leading to suffocation. As the disease progresses, generalized symptoms occur due to production and absorption of toxin. Although all human cells are sensitive to diphtheria toxin, the major clinical effects involve the heart and peripheral nerves. Cardiac conduction defects and myocarditis may lead to congestive heart failure and permanent heart damage. Neuritis of cranial nerves and paralysis of muscle groups, such as those that control movement of the palate or the eye, are seen late in the disease.

[1]See pp. 397 and 398 in *Lippincott's Illustrated Reviews: Biochemistry* (2nd ed.) for a discussion of polypeptide chain elongation.

b. Cutaneous diphtheria: A puncture wound or cut in the skin can result in the introduction of *C. diphtheriae* into the subcutaneous tissue. Rarely, colonization and exotoxin production lead to tissue degeneration and death.

4. Immunity: Diphtheria toxin is antigenic, and stimulates the production of antibodies that neutralize the toxin's activity. [Note: Formalin treatment of the toxin produces a **toxoid** that retains the antigenicity but not the toxicity of the molecule. This is the material that is used for immunization against the disease (see p. 38).]

5. Laboratory identification: The initial diagnosis and decision to treat for diphtheria must be made based on clinical observation, because no reliable, rapid laboratory test is available. However, a definitive diagnosis requires isolation of the organism, which must then be tested for virulence, using either animal inoculation or, more commonly, an immunologic precipitin reaction to demonstrate toxin production. *C. diphtheriae* can be isolated most easily from a selective medium, such as Tinsdale's agar, which contains potassium tellurite, an inhibitor of other respiratory flora, and on which the organism produces several distinctive colony types (Figure 13.4). *C. diphtheriae* from clinical material or culture has a distinctive morphology when stained, for example, with methylene blue. This morphology includes characteristic bands and reddish (polychromatic) granules that are often seen in thin, sometimes club-shaped rods that appear in clumps, suggestive of Chinese characters or picket fences (see Figure 13.2). This method of visual identification is not very useful, however, for a diagnostic microbiologist who has never before seen a specimen of *C. diphtheriae*—a situation that is becoming increasingly common due to the low incidence of diphtheria cases in the United States today.

6. Treatment: Treatment of diphtheria requires prompt neutralization of toxin, followed by eradication of the organism. A single dose of horse serum antitoxin inactivates any circulating toxin, although it does not affect toxin that is already bound to a cell-surface receptor. [Note: Serum sickness caused by a reaction to the horse protein may cause complications (see p. 36).] *C. diphtheriae* is sensitive to several antibiotics, such as erythromycin, or penicillin (Figure 13.5).

7. Prevention: The cornerstone of prevention of diphtheria is immunization with toxoid, usually administered in the DPT triple vaccine together with tetanus toxoid and pertussis antigens (see p. 40). The initial series of injections should be started in infancy. Booster injections of diphtheria toxoid (with tetanus toxoid) should be given at approximately ten-year intervals throughout life. It might be noted that control of an epidemic outbreak of diphtheria involves rigorous immunization, and also a search for healthy carriers among patient contacts.

B. Diphtheroids

A number of other corynebacterium species that morphologically resemble the type species, *C. diphtheriae*, are common commensals

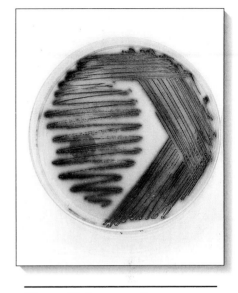

Figure 13.4
Corynebacterium diphtheriae grown on Tinsdale's agar.

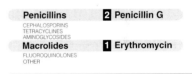

Figure 13.5
Summary of antibiotic therapy for *Corynebacterium diphtheriae* infection.

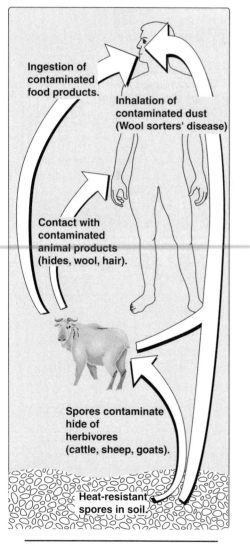

PENICILLINS
CEPHALOSPORINS
TETRACYCLINES
AMINOGLYCOSIDES
MACROLIDES
FLUOROQUINOLONES
Other   **1** Vancomycin

Figure 13.6
Antimicrobial agent useful in treating
infections due to diphtheroids.

Ingestion of
contaminated
food products.

Inhalation of
contaminated dust
(Wool sorters' disease)

Contact with
contaminated
animal products
(hides, wool, hair).

Spores contaminate
hide of
herbivores
(cattle, sheep, goats).

Heat-resistant
spores in soil.

Figure 13.7
Anthrax in animal and human hosts.

of the nose, throat, nasopharynx, skin, urinary tract, and conjunctiva. They are therefore called diphtheroids, and are generally unable to produce exotoxin, but a few cause disease in rare circumstances such as in immunosuppressed individuals. For example, *C. ulcerans* is sensitive to the β phage, and produces small amounts of diphtheria toxin if lysogenized; it has been implicated in a mild, diphtheria-like illness. Several species of corynebacteria have been recovered in infections such as endocarditis of prosthetic valves, lung abscesses, and urinary tract infections. Most strains have been shown to be multiple drug-resistant; the only common antimicrobial agent to which they are susceptible is vancomycin (Figure 13.6).

III. BACILLUS

Species of the genus *Bacillus* are gram-positive, form endospores, and are either strictly or facultatively aerobic. Most of the seventy or so species of *Bacillus* are found in soil and water, and are usually encountered in the medical laboratory as airborne contaminants. *Bacillus anthracis*, the cause of the disease **anthrax**, is an exception.

A. Bacillus anthracis

B. anthracis has an illustrious place in medical history. It was the first bacterium shown to be the causative agent of an infectious disease by Koch in 1877. In 1881, Pasteur produced the first vaccine by using attenuated live *B. anthracis* to protect sheep against anthrax.

1. **Epidemiology:** Anthrax is an enzootic disease of worldwide occurrence. [Note: An **enzootic** disease is endemic to a population of animals (that is, its occurrence changes little over time). This is as compared to an **epizootic** disease, which attacks a large number of animals at the same time (similar to a human epidemic).] Anthrax affects principally domestic herbivores—sheep, goats, and horses—and is transmitted to humans by contact with infected animal products or contaminated dust (Figure 13.7). Infection is usually initiated by the subcutaneous inoculation of spores through incidental skin abrasions. Less frequently, the inhalation of spore-laden dust causes a pulmonary form of anthrax. [Note: Sometimes an occupational hazard, this form of pneumonia is known as "wool-sorter's disease."] *B. anthracis* spores may remain viable for many years in contaminated pastures, or in bones, wool, hair, hides, or other animal materials. These spores, like those of clostridia (see p. 209), are highly resistant to physical and chemical agents. In the United States, a veterinary vaccine in widespread use makes domestic animal sources of the disease quite rare. Contaminated agricultural imports may account for the few cases seen, and lead occasionally to the quarantine of goods from endemic areas.

2. **Pathogenesis:** *B. anthracis* possesses a capsule that is antiphagocytic, and is essential for full virulence. It is composed

of polymers of D-glutamic acid, and is not immunogenic by itself. The organism also produces two plasmid-coded exotoxins. The first, **edema factor**, is a calmodulin-dependent adenylate cyclase that causes the elevation of intracellular cAMP, and is responsible for the severe edema usually seen in *B. anthracis* infections. A second toxin, called **lethal toxin**, is responsible for additional adverse effects. The exotoxins elicit protective antibodies.

3. Clinical significance

a. **Cutaneous anthrax:** About 95 percent of human cases of anthrax are of the cutaneous form. Upon introduction of organisms, or spores that germinate, a papule develops. It rapidly evolves into a painless, black, severely swollen "malignant pustule", which eventually crusts over. The organisms may invade regional lymph nodes, and then the general circulation, leading to a fatal septicemia. Although some cases remain localized and heal, the overall mortality in untreated cutaneous anthrax is about twenty percent.

b. **Pulmonary anthrax** ("**woolsorter's disease**") is caused by inhalation of spores. It is characterized by progressive hemorrhagic lymphadenitis (inflammation of the lymph nodes), and has a mortality rate approaching 100 percent if left untreated.

c. **Gastrointestinal form:** This unusual form of anthrax is caused by the ingestion of spores, for example, by eating raw or inadequately cooked meat containing *B. anthracis* spores. This is the portal of entry commonly seen in animals.

4. **Laboratory identification:** *B. anthracis* is easily recovered from clinical materials, where it is often present in massive numbers. Microscopically, the organisms appear as blunt-ended bacilli, and occur singly, in pairs, or frequently in long chains. They do not sporulate often in clinical samples, but do so in culture (Figure 13.8). The spores are oval and centrally located. On blood agar, the colonies are large, grayish, non-hemolytic, and have an irregular border. Unlike many bacillus species, *B. anthracis* is non-motile, and is encapsulated *in vivo*. A direct immunofluorescence assay aids in the identification of the organism. In the laboratory, suspected anthrax should be handled with extreme caution, particularly to prevent transmission via aerosols.

5. **Treatment:** *B. anthracis* is sensitive to penicillin, doxycycline, and ciprofloxacin. However, these antibiotics are effective in cutaneous anthrax only when administered early in the course of the infection (Figure 13.9).

6. **Prevention:** It is important to note that because of the resistance of endospores to chemical disinfectants, autoclaving is the most reliable means of decontamination. A cell-free vaccine is available for workers in highrisk occupations (see p. 39).

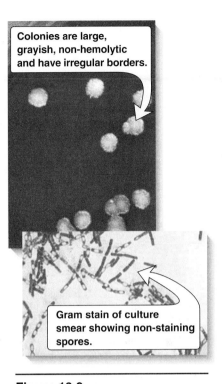

Colonies are large, grayish, non-hemolytic and have irregular borders.

Gram stain of culture smear showing non-staining spores.

Figure 13.8
Bacillus anthracis. A. Culture; B. Microscopy of culture smear. Spores appear as clear areas within the individual bacilli.

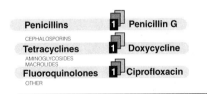

Penicillins — Penicillin G
CEPHALOSPORINS
Tetracyclines — Doxycycline
AMINOGLYCOSIDES
MACROLIDES
Fluoroquinolones — Ciprofloxacin
OTHER

Figure 13.9
Some antimicrobial agents useful in treating infections due to *Bacillus anthracis*.

B. Other species of bacillus

Uncommonly, other species of bacillus are implicated in opportunistic lesions, particularly following trauma or the placement of artificial devices and catheters. A commonly identified species is *B. cereus*. Strains of this species produce a tissue-destructive exotoxin. *B. cereus* also causes food poisoning by means of enterotoxins with either emetic or diarrheal effects. The latter of these has a cAMP-stimulatory mechanism like that of cholera toxin (see p. 185) or the coliform LT toxin (see p. 176). [Note: Food poisoning by *B. cereus* is most likely far more frequent than is diagnosed.]

IV. LISTERIA

Listeria species are slender, short, gram-positive rods (Figure 13.10). They do not form spores. Sometimes they occur as diplobacilli or in short chains, and are avid intracellular parasites that may be seen within host cells in tissue samples. *Listeria* species are catalase-positive, and displays a distinctive tumbling motility in liquid medium, which is most active after growth at 25°C; these characteristics distinguish it from streptococcus (catalase-negative) or corynebacterium (nonmotile) species, both of which may be confused morphologically with listeria. *Listeria* species grow facultatively on a variety of enriched media.

A. Epidemiology

Listeria species, including the pathogenic *L. monocytogenes*, are widespread among animals in nature. Listeria infections, which may occur as sporadic cases or in small epidemics, are usually food-borne. For example, studies have shown that two to three percent of processed dairy products (including ice cream and cheese), twenty to thirty percent of ground meats, and a majority of retail poultry samples are contaminated with *L. monocytogenes*. [Note: *L. monocytogenes* is capable of growth at 4°C, thus refrigeration does not reliably suppress its growth in food.] One to fifteen percent of healthy humans are asymptomatic intestinal carriers of the organism. Listeria infections are most common in pregnant women, their fetuses or newborns, and in immunocompromised individuals such as the elderly or AIDS patients. In the United States, some 2000 cases are reported each year.

B. Pathogenesis

L. monocytogenes is a facultative, intracellular parasite, and has been used extensively to study phagocytosis and immune activation of macrophages. The organism attaches to and enters a variety of mammalian cells, apparently by normal phagocytosis, and once internalized, escapes from the phagocytic vacuole by elaborating a membrane-damaging toxin called **listeriolysin O**. This is a sulfhydryl-activated, pore-forming cytolysin with amino acid sequence similarities to streptolysin O (see p. 147) and pneumococcal pneumolysin (see p. 151). [Note: Mutants lacking a functional listeriolysin O are avirulent.] *L. monocytogenes* grows in the cytosol, and stimulates changes in cell function that facilitate its direct passage from cell to cell. The organisms induce a reorganization of cel-

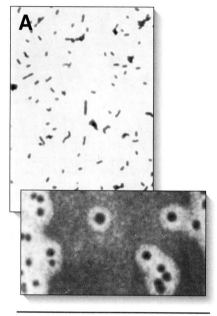

Figure 13.10
Listeria monocytogenes. A. Gram stain of spinal-fluid culture. B. Sheep blood agar culture showing β-hemolysis.

lular actin such that short filaments and actin-binding proteins cohere to the bacteria, creating a comet-like "tail". This complex appears to propel the organisms through the cell to pseudopods in contact with adjacent cells. Bacterium-produced membrane-degrading phospholipases then mediate the passage of the organism directly to a neighboring cell, allowing avoidance of the intercellular milieu, including cells of the immune system (Figure 13.11).

C. Clinical significance

Septicemia and meningitis are the most commonly reported forms of *L. monocytogenes* infection (**listeriosis**). A variety of focal lesions are less frequently seen, such as granulomatous skin lesions. Lymphadenitis and endocarditis may also occur. Pregnant women, usually in the third trimester, may have a milder "flu-like" illness. In this as well as in asymptomatic vaginal colonization, the organism can be transmitted to a newborn (*L. monocytogenes* is a relatively common cause of newborn meningitis) or to the fetus and initiate abortion. Immunocompromised individuals, especially those with defects in cellular immunity, are susceptible to serious generalized infections.

D. Laboratory identification

The organism can be isolated from blood, cerebrospinal fluid, and other clinical specimens by standard bacteriologic procedures. On blood agar, *L. monocytogenes* produces a small colony surrounded by a narrow zone of β hemolysis (see Figure 13.10). *Listeria* species can be distinguished from various streptococci by morphology, positive motility, and the production of catalase.

E. Treatment and prevention

A variety of antibiotics have been successfully used to treat *L. monocytogenes* infections, including ampicillin and trimethoprim-sulfamethoxazole (Figure 13.12). Prevention of *L. monocytogenes* infections can be accomplished by proper food preparation and handling.

V. OTHER NON-SPORE-FORMING, GRAM-POSITIVE RODS

Propionibacterium is a genus of anaerobic or microaerophilic rods of diphtheroid-like morphology. They are common inhabitants of normal skin, and, in rare instances, have been reported as causes of endocarditis or infections of plastic implants. *P. acnes*, often a strict anaerobe, has been implicated as a contributing cause of acne. Various species of *Lactobacillus* are part of the commensal flora of human mucous membranes. These organisms are usually long and slender with squared ends, and frequently occur in chains. They produce quantities of lactic acid during fermentation, and have been thought to assist in maintaining the acid pH of normal mucous epithelia. On the other hand, acid production by oral lactobacilli may play a role in the production of dental caries. *Erysipelothrix rhusopathiae* is a filamentous, gram-positive rod that causes disease in animals and, rarely, a skin infection called **erysipeloid** in people who commonly handle animal products, for example, butchers, veterinarians, and fishermen. The organism is sensitive to penicillin, erythromycin, and tetracycline.

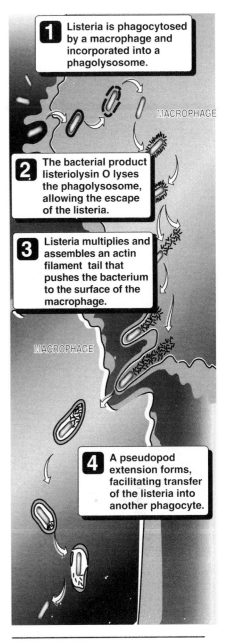

Figure 13.11
Life cycle of *Listeria monocytogenes* in host macrophages.

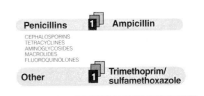

Figure 13.12
Some antimicrobial agents useful in treating infections caused by *Listeria monocytogenes*.

Study questions

Choose the ONE correct answer

13.1 All of the following are important to the epidemiology or pathogenesis of anthrax except:

 A. production of endospores.

 B. a reservoir of healthy human carriers.

 C. infection being possible by the respiratory route.

 D. production of a highly lethal exotoxin.

 E. possession of an antiphagocytic capsule.

> Correct answer = B. As far as is known, *B. anthracis* does not grow in any healthy mammalian tissue. *B. anthracis* spores can contaminate soil from products of infected animals, and be introduced to humans in dirt via skin abrasions, inhalation, etc. It then causes severe local or generalized infection both by resisting phagocytosis and by the elaboration of a toxin that causes hemolysis, massive edema, and other effects.

13.2 A diagnosis of diphtheria is confirmed by:

 A. microscopic appearance of organisms stained with methylene blue.

 B. isolation of a typical colony on Tinsdale's agar.

 C. isolation of typical organisms from materials such as blood, showing invasiveness.

 D. detection of β phage plaques in cultures of suspicious isolates.

 E. demonstration of toxin production by a suspicious isolate.

> Correct answer = E. Observation of diphtheria toxin production (E) is required to prove the diagnosis. Items (A) and (B) are presumptive indicators. β phage (D) is a temperate phage, and lytic activity is not observed. *C. diphtheriae* is noninvasive, and the organism (but not the toxin) is recovered only from surface infections such as those of the oropharynx, skin lesions, etc.

13.3 *Listeria monocytogenes* shows which of the following characteristics?

 A. It can grow at refrigerator temperatures (4°C).

 B. It is an extracellular pathogen.

 C. It is catalase-negative.

 D. It is a gram-negative coccus.

 E. It is strictly a human pathogen.

> Correct choice = A. *Listeria monocytogenes* grows optimally at 30 to 37°C, but is capable of growth at 4°C. Thus refrigeration does not reliably suppress its growth in food. *Listeria monocytogenes* is a catalase-positive, gram-positive, obligate intracellular pathogen. These organisms are found in cattle, other warmblooded animals, and fish, where they can cause disease.

Questions 13.4 and 13.5

13.4 A 26-year-old woman, eight months pregnant, visits her obstetrician complaining of fever, myalagia and backache of recent onset. Three weeks earlier the patient had been a weekend guest at a rural farmhouse, where all the food was reported to be "unprocessed" and "natural". A culture of the patient's blood shows gram-positive rods that are catalase-positive, and display a distinctive tumbling motility in liquid medium. What is the most likely source of the woman's infection?

 A. Well-done roast beef

 B. Fresh, raw cow's milk

 C. Home baked bread

 D. Home-made apple sauce

 E. Baked apple pie

> Correct answer = B. The woman is most likely suffering from listerosis. *Listeriae* are common in the GI tract and milk of cattle, but are normally killed by pasteurization. Unpasteurized milk was presumably consumed at the farm.

Questions 13.5 – 13.6

Match the appropriate bacterium from the following list with the statement to which it most closely corresponds. Each bacterium can match one, more than one, or none of the statements.

 A. *Bacillus cereus*

 B. *Bacillus subtilis*

 C. *Corynebacteria* other than *diphtheriae*

 D. *Lactobacillus* species

 E. *Listeria monocytogenes*

 F. *Propionibacter* species

13.5 Several guests at a birthday picnic experience sudden onset of vomiting and/or diarrhea some eight to eighteen hours after leaving the party.

> Correct answer = A.

13.6 Organisms commonly recovered on blood agar (routine culture procedure) from nasopharyngeal cultures of normal people.

> Correct answer = C.

Neisseriae

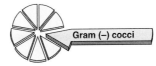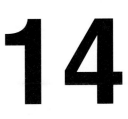

I. OVERVIEW

The genus *Neisseria* consists of gram-negative, aerobic cocci. Two *Neisseria* species are pathogenic for humans—*Neisseria gonorrhoeae* (commonly called **gonococcus**), the causal agent of **gonorrhea**; and *Neisseria meningitidis* (commonly called **meningococcus**), a frequent cause of **meningitis**. Gonococci and meningococci are nonmotile diplococci, and cannot be distinguished from each other under the microscope. However they can be differentiated in the laboratory by their sugar utilization patterns, and by the sites of their primary infections. Both bacteria are classified as pyogenic cocci, because infections by these organisms are also characterized by the production of purulent (pus-like) material made up largely of white blood cells. The neisseriae, and organisms that are easily confused with neisseriae and which are also discussed in this chapter, are listed in Figure 14.1.

II. NEISSERIA GONORRHOEAE

Gonorrhea is one of the most frequently reported infectious diseases in the United States. The causal agent, *N. gonorrhoeae*, a gram-negative diplococcus, is frequently observed inside polymorphonuclear leukocytes of clinical samples obtained from infected patients (Figure 14.2). *N. gonorrhoeae* is usually transmitted during sexual contact, or more rarely, during the passage of a baby through an infected birth canal. It does not survive long outside the human body because it is highly sensitive to dehydration.

A. Structure

Gonococci are unencapsulated (unlike the meningococci, see p. 168), piliated and nonmotile, and resemble a pair of kidney beans.

1. **Pili:** These hairlike surface appendages are made of helical aggregates of repeating peptide subunits, called pilin. Pili enhance attachment of the organism to host epithelial and mucosal cell surfaces, and confer resistance to phagocytosis; they are therefore among the most important virulence factors. Pili are also antigenic. At least twenty gonococcal genes code for pilin, most of which are not expressed at any given time because they lack promoters[1] (that is, they are "silent"). By shuffling and

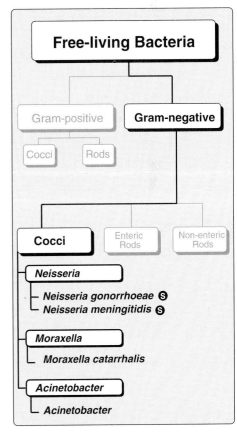

Figure 14.1
Classification of neisseria and related organisms. ⑤ See pp. 415, 449 for summaries of these organisms.

Lippincott's Illustrated Reviews: Microbiology, by William A. Strohl, Harriet Rouse, Bruce D. Fisher. Lippincott, Williams & Wilkins, Baltimore, MD © 2001

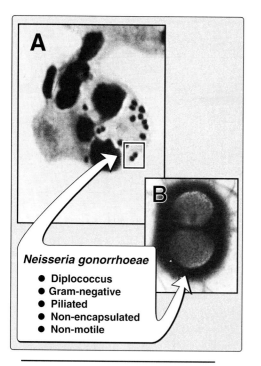

Neisseria gonorrhoeae

- **Diplococcus**
- **Gram-negative**
- **Piliated**
- **Non-encapsulated**
- **Non-motile**

Figure 14.2
A. Presence of *Neisseria gonorrhoeae* in polymorphonuclear leukocytes in urethral discharge.
B. Gonococcus (electron microscope) showing pili.

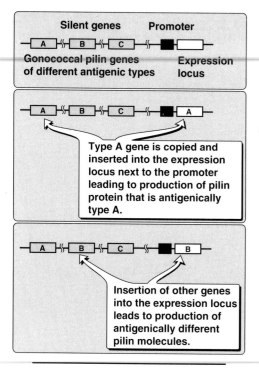

Type A gene is copied and inserted into the expression locus next to the promoter leading to production of pilin protein that is antigenically type A.

Insertion of other genes into the expression locus leads to production of antigenically different pilin molecules.

Figure 14.3
Antigenic variation in the gonococcus.

recombining chromosomal regions of these genes, a single strain of *N. gonorrhoeae* can at different times synthesize ("express") multiple pilins that have different amino acid sequences. This process, known as **gene conversion**, allows the organism to produce antigenically different pilin molecules over time (Figure 14.3). In addition, if a gene is moved into an expression locus so that the reading frame is shifted,[2] then no pilin is made (that is, the organism is nonpiliated). This is called **phase variation**. Gene conversion and phase variation are two mechanisms by which the gonococcus can avoid the host's immune response, and thereby cause repeated infections in the same individual.

2. **Lipooligosaccharide:** Gonococcal lipooligosaccharides (LOS) have shorter, more highly branched, nonrepeat O-antigenic side chains than do lipopolysaccharides found in other gram-negative bacteria (LPS, see p. 13). The bactericidal antibodies in normal human serum are IgM molecules directed against the LOS antigens.

3. **Outer membrane proteins (OMPs):** OMP I functions as a porin in complex with OMP III, and is antigenically diverse in different strains of gonococci. OMP II is referred to as the "opacity protein" because its presence renders gonococcal colonies less translucent. OMP II, along with the pili, mediates attachment of the organism to a host cell. Because of OMP II's ability to undergo extensive antigenic variation, it also contributes significantly to the ability of the organism to evade the immune response and cause repeated infections.

B. Pathogenesis

Pili and OMP II facilitate the adhesion of the gonococcus to epithelial cells of the urethra, rectum, cervix, pharynx, or conjunctiva, and thus make possible colonization. Pili also enable the bacterium to resist phagocytosis. [Note: Only piliated gonococci are virulent.] In addition, both gonococci and meningococci produce an IgA protease that cleaves IgA_1 (see p. 84), thus helping the pathogen to evade immunoglobulins of this subclass.

C. Clinical significance

Gonococci most often colonize the mucous membrane of the genitourinary tract or rectum. For example, Figure 14.4 shows gonococci growing in the fallopian tube. There the organisms may cause a localized infection with the production of pus, or may lead to tissue invasion, chronic inflammation, and fibrosis. A higher proportion of females than males are generally asymptomatic; these individuals act as the reservoir for maintaining and transmitting gonococcal infections. [Note: More than one sexually transmitted disease may be acquired at the same time, for example gonorrhea in combination with syphilis (*Treponema pallidum* infection), chlamydia, human immunodeficiency virus, or hepatitis B virus. Patients with gonorrhea may therefore have to be treated for more than one pathogen.]

[1]See p. 384 in *Lippincott's Illustrated Reviews: Biochemistry* (2nd ed.) for a discussion of promoters.
[2]See p. 391 in *Lippincott's Illustrated Reviews: Biochemistry* (2nd ed.) for a discussion of reading frame.

1. **Genitourinary tract infections:** Symptoms of gonococcal infection are more acute and easier to diagnose in males. The patient typically presents with a yellow, purulent exudate and painful urination. In females, infection occurs in the endocervix and extends to the urethra and vagina. A greenish-yellow cervical discharge is most common, often accompanied by intermenstrual bleeding. The disease may progress to the uterus, causing **salpingitis** (inflammation of the fallopian tubes), **pelvic inflammatory disease** (**PID**), and **fibrosis**. *N. gonorrhoeae* is the most common cause of PID in females. Infertility occurs in approximately twenty percent of women with gonococcal salpingitis, due to tubal scarring.

2. **Rectal infections,** prevalent in male homosexuals, are characterized by constipation, painful defecation, and purulent discharge.

3. **Pharyngitis** is contracted by oral-genital contact. Infected individuals may show a purulent exudate, and the condition may mimic a mild viral or a streptococcal sore throat (see p. 148).

4. **Ophthalmia neonatorum** is an infection of the conjunctival sac that is acquired by a newborn during passage through the birth canal of a mother infected with gonococcus (Figure 14.5). If untreated, acute conjunctivitis may lead to blindness. For many years, routine prevention was performed immediately after birth by the instillation of a dilute solution of silver nitrate into the eye. Today, clinicians prefer the use of erythromycin in place of silver nitrate, because the antibiotic also eradicates *Chlamydia trachomatis*, if present. [Note: Gonococcal conjunctivitis can also occur in adults.]

5. **Disseminated infection:** Most strains of gonococci have a limited ability to multiply in the bloodstream. Therefore, bacteremia with gonococci is rare. [Note: In contrast, meningococci multiply rapidly in blood (see p. 169).] However, some strains do invade the bloodstream, and may result in a disseminated infection in which the organism can cause fever, erythematous or maculopapular lesions on the skin, and a painful, purulent arthritis. [Note: Gonococcal infection is the most common cause of **septic arthritis** in sexually active adults.] Disseminated infections are seen in both men and women, but are more common in women, particularly during pregnancy and menses. Figure 14.6 compares the incidence of the common sexually transmitted diseases (STDs) with the incidence of other infectious diseases. (A summary of organisms causing the most common STDs is presented in Figure 20.6 on p. 238.)

D. Laboratory identification

In the male, the finding of numerous neutrophils containing gram-negative diplococci in a smear of urethral exudate permits a provisional diagnosis of gonococcal infection, and indicates that the individual should be treated. In contrast, to diagnose gonococcal infection in the female, or at other sites in the male, a positive culture is needed. If disseminated gonococcal infection is suspected, appropriate cultures should be set up as indicated, for example, of skin lesions, joint fluid, and blood.

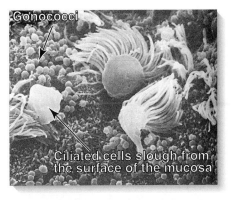

Figure 14.4
Human fallopian tube tissue twenty hours after infection with *Neisseria gonorrhoeae*.

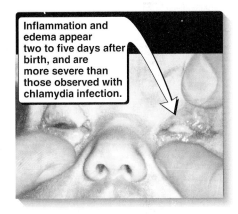

Figure 14.5
Gonococcal ophthalmia neonatorum.

**Disease cases
(cases reported)**

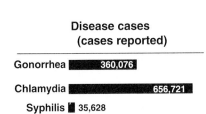

Figure 14.6
Incidence of some sexually transmitted diseases in the United States (1999).

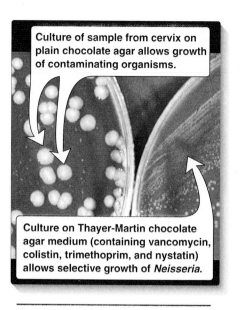

Culture of sample from cervix on plain chocolate agar allows growth of contaminating organisms.

Culture on Thayer-Martin chocolate agar medium (containing vancomycin, colistin, trimethoprim, and nystatin) allows selective growth of *Neisseria*.

Figure 14.7
Left: Mixed growth on plain chocolate agar. Right: Pure culture on Thayer-Martin chocolate agar medium.

PENICILLINS
Cephalosporins   **1**-Ceftriaxone
TETRACYCLINES
AMINOGLYCOSIDES
MACROLIDES
FLUOROQUINOLONES
OTHER

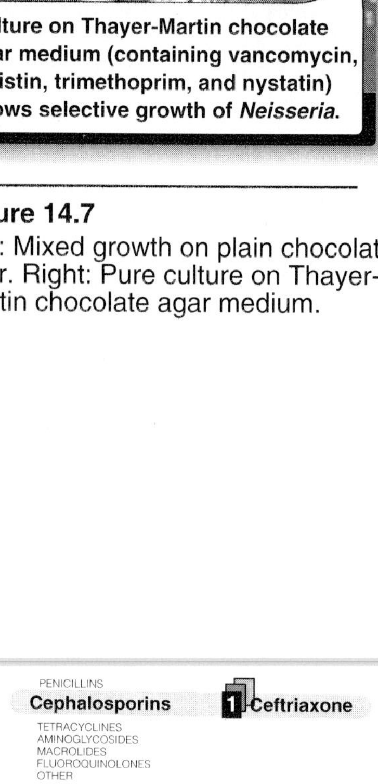

Figure 14.8
Summary of antibiotic therapy for *Neisseria gonorhoeae* infections.

1. **Growth conditions for cell culture:** *N. gonorrhoeae* grows best under aerobic conditions, and most strains require enhanced CO_2. *N. gonorrhoeae* ferments glucose, but not maltose, lactose, or sucrose. [Note: *N. meningitidis* does ferment maltose (see p. 172).] All members of the genus are oxidase-positive as shown by a test in which the colonies turn pink and then black when flooded with one percent dimethyl- or tetramethyl-*p*-phenylenediamine solution. [Note: The oxidase test (see p. 27) is used to identify neisseriae, but does not distinguish between gonococci, meningococci, and nonpathogenic neisseriae.]

2. **Selective media:** Gonococci, like pneumococci, are very sensitive to heating or drying. Cultures must be plated promptly, or if this is not possible, transport media must be used to extend the viability of the organism to be cultured. **Thayer-Martin medium** (chocolate agar supplemented with several antibiotics that suppress the growth of nonpathogenic neisseriae and other normal and abnormal flora) is normally used to isolate gonococci (Figure 14.7). The use of this medium is important for cultures that are typically obtained from sites such as the genitourinary tract or rectum, where there is normally an abundance of flora. In nonselective medium, the normal flora overgrows the gonococci.

E. Treatment and prevention

Over twenty percent of current isolates of *N. gonorrhoeae* are resistant to penicillin, tetracycline, cefoxitin, and/or spectinomycin. Penicillin-resistant organisms are called PPNG—penicillinase-producing *N. gonorrhoeae*. These strains contain plasmids that carry the gene for β-lactamase of the TEM (encoded in a transposable element) type, such as is seen in *E. coli* and *H. influenzae*. The frequency of PPNG in the United States is now sufficiently high that penicillin is no longer recommended for the treatment of gonorrhea. However, most organisms still respond to treatment with third-generation cephalosporins; for example, a single intramuscular dose of ceftriaxone is recommended therapy for uncomplicated gonococcal infections of the urethra, endocervix, or rectum (Figure 14.8). Intramuscular spectinomycin is indicated in patients who are allergic to cephalosporins. [Note: Many patients with gonorrhea—ten to twenty percent of males, and thirty to fifty percent of females—have coexisting chlamydial infections. Therefore, doxycycline, a tetracycline effective against chlamydia, is often included as part of the treatment regimen for gonorrhea.]

III. NEISSERIA MENINGITIDIS

Neisseria meningitidis is one of the most frequent causes of **meningitis.** Infection with *N. meningitidis* can also take the form of a fulminant **meningococcemia**, with intravascular coagulation, circulatory collapse, and potentially fatal shock, but without meningitis. In each case, symptoms can occur with extremely rapid onset and great intensity. Outbreaks of meningitis are most common in winter and early spring, and are favored by close contact between individuals, for example, in schools, institutions, and military barracks. Severe epidemics also occur periodically in developing nations, for example, in sub-Saharan Africa and in Latin America.

A. Structure

Like *N. gonorrhoeae*, *N. meningitidis* is a nonmotile, gram-negative diplococcus, shaped like a kidney bean, which always appears in pairs (see Figure 14.9). It is also piliated; the pili allow attachment of the organism to the nasopharyngeal mucosa where it is harbored both in carriers and in those with meningococcal disease. When meningococcus is isolated from blood or spinal fluid it is invariably encapsulated. The meningococcal polysaccharide capsule is antiphagocytic, and is therefore the most important virulence factor. [Note: Antibodies to the capsule carbohydrate are bactericidal.]

1. **Serogroups:** The lipooligosaccharide capsule (LOS) is antigenically diverse, which has allowed the identification of at least 14 capsular polysaccharide types, called serogroups (Figure 14.10). Most infections are due to serogroups A, B, C, W, and Y, although approximately ninety percent of cases of meningococcal disease are caused by serogroups A, B, and C. Serogroup A is usually responsible for massive epidemics in developing countries. In the United States, *N. meningitidis* serogroup B is the predominant cause of disease and mortality, followed by group C. Organisms that do not have a capsule are called "ungrouped."

2. **Serotypes:** A second classification system called serotyping (1, 2, ...20) is also a serologic classification (see Figure 14.10), but is based on the properties of the outer membrane proteins (OMPs, see p. 166) and LOS. There is no predicable relationship between the serogroups and the serotypes.

B. Epidemology

Transmission occurs through inhalation of respiratory droplets from a carrier or a patient in the early stages of the disease. In addition to contact with a carrier, risk factors include recent viral or mycoplasma upper respiratory tract infection, active or passive smoking, and complement deficiency. The transmission rate among family members of an infected individual is 1000–fold higher than in the general population. In susceptible persons, pathogenic strains may invade the bloodstream and cause systemic illness after an incubation period of two to ten days. The incidence of meningococcal disease in the United States is highest among infants less than one year of age (Figure 14.11). Humans are the only natural host.

C. Pathogenesis

The antiphagocytic properties of the meningococcal capsule aid in the maintenance of infection. LOS also is released during autolysis and bacterial cell division, and is responsible for many of the toxic effects found in disseminated meningococcal disease. As noted on p. 166, gonococci and meningococci make an IgA protease that cleaves IgA$_1$, and thus helps the pathogens to evade immunoglobulins of this subclass. [Note: The nonpathogenic neisseriae do not make this protease.]

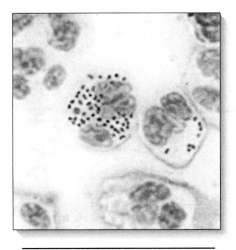

Figure 14.9
Smear of purulent cerebrospinal fluid showing *Neisseria meningitidis*.

EPIDEMIOLOGIC CLASSIFICATION	ANTIGENIC DETERMINANT
Serogroups (>13)	Polysaccharide capsule
Serotypes (>20)	Outer membrane proteins and lipo-oligosaccharides

Figure 14.10
Antigenic determinants of *Neisseria meningitidis*.

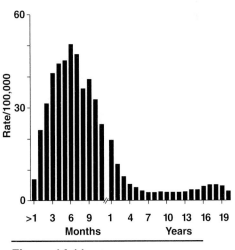

Figure 14.11
Incidence of meningococcal infection according to the age.

D. Clinical significance

N. meningitidis initially colonizes the nasopharynx, resulting in a largely asymptomatic meningococcal pharyngitis. In young children and other susceptible individuals, the organism can cause disseminated disease by spreading through the blood, leading to meningitis and/or fulminating septicemia. [Note: *Haemophilus influenzae* was previously a common cause of meningitis in children, but with the introduction of a vaccine, the incidence of meningitis due to *H. influenzae* infection has decreased 90 to 95 percent. Therefore, *N. meningitidis* is currently a leading cause of meningitis]

1. **Meningitis:** The epithelial lining of the nasopharynx normally serves as a barrier to bacteria. Thus, most persons colonized by *N. meningitides* remain well. As a rare event, the meningococci penetrate this barrier, and enter the bloodstream where they rapidly multiply (**meningococcemia**). In patients with fulminating septicemia, meningococci can be detected in blood smears—an unusual occurrence. If not severe, the patient may have only a fever and other nonspecific symptoms. However, the organism can seed from the blood to other sites, for example, crossing the blood-brain barrier and infecting the meninges. There they multiply and induce an acute inflammatory response, accompanied by an influx of polymorphonuclear leukocytes, resulting in a purulent meningitis. Joint symptoms are also commonly seen in meningococcal infections, and a petechial rash is commonly observed (Figure 14.12). Within several hours the initial fever and malaise can evolve into severe headache, a rigid neck, vomiting, and sensitivity to bright lights—symptoms characteristic of meningitis. Coma can occur within a few hours. A summary of the major organisms causing meningitis is shown in Figure 14.13.

2. **Septicemia:** Meningococci can cause a life-threatening septicemia in an apparently healthy individual in less than twelve hours. Up to thirty percent of patients with meningitis go on to **fulminant septicemia**. In this condition, the clinical presentation is one of severe septicemia and shock, for which the bacterial endotoxin (LOS, see p. 169) is largely responsible. An acute fulminating meningococcal septicemia seen mainly in very young children is referred to as the **Waterhouse-Friderichsen syndrome**. It is characterized by large, purple, blotchy skin hemorrhages, vomiting and diarrhea, circulatory collapse, necrosis of the adrenals, and death within ten to twelve hours.

E. Laboratory identification

Under the light microscope, *N. meningitidis* obtained from cerebrospinal fluid (CSF) and skin lesion aspirates appear as gram-negative diplococci, often in association with polymorphonuclear leukocytes. [Note: In performing a Gram stain on CSF, the clinical sample is centrifuged to concentrate the organisms, because 10^5 to 10^6 bacteria per ml are required for this test.] Carriers can be detected by culturing swabs from the nasopharyngeal region.

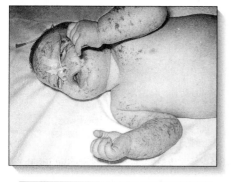

Figure 14.12
Petechial rash and neck extension characteristic of meningococcal meningitis.

Disease Summary: BACTERIAL MENINGITIS

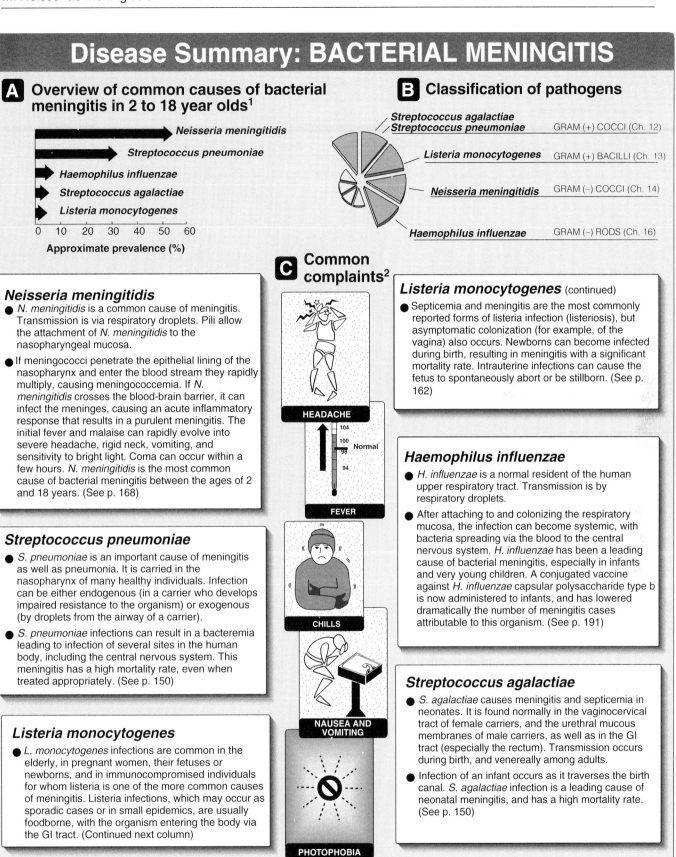

A Overview of common causes of bacterial meningitis in 2 to 18 year olds[1]

Neisseria meningitidis
Streptococcus pneumoniae
Haemophilus influenzae
Streptococcus agalactiae
Listeria monocytogenes

0   10   20   30   40   50   60
Approximate prevalence (%)

B Classification of pathogens

Streptococcus agalactiae
Streptococcus pneumoniae   GRAM (+) COCCI (Ch. 12)

Listeria monocytogenes   GRAM (+) BACILLI (Ch. 13)

Neisseria meningitidis   GRAM (–) COCCI (Ch. 14)

Haemophilus influenzae   GRAM (–) RODS (Ch. 16)

C Common complaints[2]

HEADACHE

FEVER

CHILLS

NAUSEA AND VOMITING

PHOTOPHOBIA

Neisseria meningitidis

● N. meningitidis is a common cause of meningitis. Transmission is via respiratory droplets. Pili allow the attachment of N. meningitidis to the nasopharyngeal mucosa.

● If meningococci penetrate the epithelial lining of the nasopharynx and enter the blood stream they rapidly multiply, causing meningococcemia. If N. meningitidis crosses the blood-brain barrier, it can infect the meninges, causing an acute inflammatory response that results in a purulent meningitis. The initial fever and malaise can rapidly evolve into severe headache, rigid neck, vomiting, and sensitivity to bright light. Coma can occur within a few hours. N. meningitidis is the most common cause of bacterial meningitis between the ages of 2 and 18 years. (See p. 168)

Streptococcus pneumoniae

● S. pneumoniae is an important cause of meningitis as well as pneumonia. It is carried in the nasopharynx of many healthy individuals. Infection can be either endogenous (in a carrier who develops impaired resistance to the organism) or exogenous (by droplets from the airway of a carrier).

● S. pneumoniae infections can result in a bacteremia leading to infection of several sites in the human body, including the central nervous system. This meningitis has a high mortality rate, even when treated appropriately. (See p. 150)

Listeria monocytogenes

● L. monocytogenes infections are common in the elderly, in pregnant women, their fetuses or newborns, and in immunocompromised individuals for whom listeria is one of the more common causes of meningitis. Listeria infections, which may occur as sporadic cases or in small epidemics, are usually foodborne, with the organism entering the body via the GI tract. (Continued next column)

Listeria monocytogenes (continued)

● Septicemia and meningitis are the most commonly reported forms of listeria infection (listeriosis), but asymptomatic colonization (for example, of the vagina) also occurs. Newborns can become infected during birth, resulting in meningitis with a significant mortality rate. Intrauterine infections can cause the fetus to spontaneously abort or be stillborn. (See p. 162)

Haemophilus influenzae

● H. influenzae is a normal resident of the human upper respiratory tract. Transmission is by respiratory droplets.

● After attaching to and colonizing the respiratory mucosa, the infection can become systemic, with bacteria spreading via the blood to the central nervous system. H. influenzae has been a leading cause of bacterial meningitis, especially in infants and very young children. A conjugated vaccine against H. influenzae capsular polysaccharide type b is now administered to infants, and has lowered dramatically the number of meningitis cases attributable to this organism. (See p. 191)

Streptococcus agalactiae

● S. agalactiae causes meningitis and septicemia in neonates. It is found normally in the vaginocervical tract of female carriers, and the urethral mucous membranes of male carriers, as well as in the GI tract (especially the rectum). Transmission occurs during birth, and venereally among adults.

● Infection of an infant occurs as it traverses the birth canal. S. agalactiae infection is a leading cause of neonatal meningitis, and has a high mortality rate. (See p. 150)

Figure 14.13
Some characteristics of organisms causing bacterial meningitis.

[1]Escherichia coli is a major cause of meningitis in the newborn. Viral meningitis is often due to enteroviruses and sometimes herpes simplex virus.
[2]Other complaints include nuchal rigidity (profound stiffness of the neck that prevents flexion), and cardiac arrhythmias.

	GLUCOSE FERMENTATION	MALTOSE FERMENTATION	PLASMIDS	VACCINE AVAILABLE	POLY-SACCHARIDE CAPSULE	β-LACTAMASE PRODUCTION	OXIDASE
Neisseria gonorrhoeae	+	–	Common	–	–	Common	+
Neisseria meningitidis	+	+	Rare	Serogroups A, C, W, Y	+	None	+

Figure 14.14
Differential bacteriologic features of *Neisseria gonorrhoeae* and *Neisseria meningitidis*.

1. **Culture conditions:** Meningococci are cultured on chocolate agar with increased CO_2. The sample must be plated promptly, or if this is not possible, transport medium must be used to extend the viability of the organism to be cultured. Unlike gonococci, meningococci are usually cultured from cerebrospinal fluid or blood, which are normally sterile, so a selective medium is not required and plain chocolate agar is sufficient. Thayer-Martin medium (see p. 168) is required for samples obtained from a skin lesion or nasopharyngeal swab, in order to eliminate contaminating organisms.

2. **Additional tests:** All *Neisseria* species are oxidase-positive. To differentiate between species, sugar fermentation tests are used (Figure 14.14). *N. meningitidis* ferments both glucose and maltose, whereas *N. gonorrhoeae* ferments only glucose. In bacterial meningitis, the CSF shows increased pressure, elevated protein, decreased glucose (due in part to its consumption as a bacterial nutrient), and many neutrophils. The presence of an infecting organism or of antigenic capsular substance confirms the diagnosis.

F. Treatment and prevention

Bacterial meningitis is a medical emergency. Accordingly, antibiotic treatment cannot await a definitive bacteriologic diagnosis. High fever, headache, and a rash typical of meningococcal infection are treated immediately in an effort to prevent fulminant septicemia where the mortality rate is high. In the past, meningitis was treated with penicillin G or ampicillin (both of which can pass the inflamed blood-brain barrier) in large intravenous doses pending the result of cultures. Most infectious disease specialists now prefer to use cefotaxime or ceftriaxone (Figure 14.15). Prompt treatment reduces mortality to about ten percent.

1. **Diagnosis:** Prompt action is important. Gram stains on cerebrospinal fluid can be performed immediately, and latex agglutination tests with serogroup-specific anticapsular antibody can be used to obtain rapid presumptive identification of serogroup-specific meningococci in CSF.

2. **Vaccines:** A capsular vaccine for serogroups A, C, W, and Y is very effective, and is used routinely by the military or during an

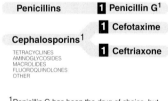

Penicillins   **1** Penicillin G[1]
                   1 Cefotaxime
Cephalosporins[1]
TETRACYCLINES   **1** Ceftriaxone
AMINOGLYCOSIDES
MACROLIDES
FLUOROQUINOLONES
OTHER

[1]Penicillin G has been the drug of choice, but resistant strains are increasingly common. Sensitivity testing should be performed.

Figure 14.15
Summary of antibiotic therapy of *Neisseria meningitidis* infections.

outbreak of meningococcal meningitis due to serogroup A or C in the civilian population. Unfortunately, the polysaccharide of serogroup B does not elicit an effective immune response. Protection generated by vaccines to polysaccharide capsules is short-lived in young children, the target group in which most meningococcal infections occur. Figure 14.16 summarizes vaccines and serogroups.

3. **Prophylaxis:** Rifampin is usually used to treat family members of an infected individual; the drug is effective in eliminating the carrier state.

IV. MORAXELLA

Members of the genus *Moraxella* are nonmotile, gram-negative coccobacilli that are generally found in pairs (Figure 14.17). They are related to the neisseriae, and the two organisms can be confused on Gram stain. *Moraxella* are aerobic, oxidase-positive, fastidious organisms that do not ferment carbohydrates. The genus *Moraxella* includes a variety of organisms that are part of the normal human flora (particularly the respiratory and genital tracts), some of which were formerly classified in the genus *Branhamella*. Disease most commonly occurs in immunologically-compromised hosts. The most important pathogen in the genus is *Moraxella* (formerly *Branhamella*) *catarrhalis*. This organism can cause infections of the respiratory system, middle ear, eye, CNS, and joints. Other moraxellae cause a comparably broad spectrum of infections. These organisms can be cultured on blood or chocolate agar, and identified by a battery of biochemical tests. Treatment depends on clinical presentation and results of sensitivity testing, because β-lactamase production in *M. catarrhalis* is increasing.

V. ACINETOBACTER

Members of the genus *Acinetobacter* are nonmotile coccobacilli that are frequently confused with neisseriae in gram-stained samples. They are generally encapsulated, oxidase-negative, obligately aerobic, and they do not ferment carbohydrates. *Acinetobacter* are widely distributed in nature, and are commonly found in soil, water, and foodstuff, on inanimate objects (fomites), and as part of the normal flora of humans and other animals. These organisms commonly colonize the skin, and may transiently colonize the pharynx. Although *Acinetobacter* are well-adapted to survival in diverse environments, a relative lack of virulence factors (for example, they have no known cytotoxins) limits their pathogenic potential to patients whose immunologic defenses are compromised. In such individuals, *Acinetobacter* are capable of infecting virtually any body site, organ system, or tissue. The organisms may be cultured on a variety of relatively simple laboratory media. However, as is the case for other organisms that are widely distributed in nature and/or are part of the normal flora, isolation of *Acinetobacter* in a clinical specimen does not, alone, signify etiology. Because *Acinetobacter* strains are frequently resistant to a variety of antibiotics, the treatment of choice depends on clinical presentation and the results of sensitivity testing.

SEROGROUP CLASSIFICATION	COMMENT
A	Usually responsible for massive epidemics in developing countries.
B	Does not elicit an effective immune response.
B, C	Responsible for most of endemic meningitis in the United States.
A, C	Effective capsular vaccine is available.

Figure 14.16
Characteristics of the common serogroups of *Neisseria meningitidis*.

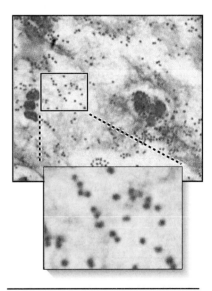

Figure 14.17
Moraxella catarrhalis. Gram stain of sputum showing large gram-negative cocci.

Study Questions

Choose the ONE correct answer

14.1 A 14-month-old boy boy presented to his family physician with fever, vomiting, and lethargy of 24 hours duration. There was no neck stiffness or photophobia, but a nonblanching rash was found on the boy's chest. The boys tonsils were inflamed. The child was diagnosed with upper respiratory viral infection, and was transported to the hospital. That evening the child became increasingly irritable and drowsy. He was started on parenteral fluids and ceftriaxone. Several hours later the patient developed seizures. The boy was transfered to the pediatric intensive care unit, where he developed unreactiive pupils and central nonresponsive hypothermia. Later that next day, he showed no recordable brainstem activity. The child died two days after admission. Group B meningococcal infection was diagnosed by rapid antigen screen, and was confirmed on blood culture. The most likely source of the meningococcal infection was:

A. activation of endogenous *Neisseria meningitidis*.

B. close contact with a carrier.

C. contaminated fomites.

D. close contact with an infected pet.

E. contaminated food

> Correct answer = B. Transmission occurs through inhalation of respiratory droplets from close contact with a carrier, or a patient in the early stages of the disease.

14.2 A gram-negative diplococcus was isolated from a chocolate agar culture of a cerebrospinal fluid sample. Which one of the following tests or observations would be most informative in identifying the organism as *Neisseria meningitidis*?

A. Appearance of colonies

B. Growth on Thayer-Martin medium

C. Direct oxidase test on spinal fluid

D. Growth in air

E. Positive oxidase test and ability of culture isolate to ferment glucose and maltose

> Correct answer = E. A gram-negative diplococcus may be identified definitively on the basis of positive oxidase test and ability to ferment both glucose and maltose. Growth on Thayer-Martin medium is a nonspecific result because this medium allows growth of neisseriae and several other species. Biochemical determinations are rarely conducted directly on spinal fluid specimens because of the presence of interfering substances which affect the accuracy of the tests. Growth in air only eliminates obligate anaerobes.

14.3 Which one of the following is characteristic of *Neisseria meningitidis*, but not *Neisseria gonorrhoeae*?

A. Ferments glucose

B. Contains a polysaccharide capsule

C. Is oxidase-positive

D. Most isolates show resistance to penicillin

E. No effective vaccines are available

> Correct answer = B. *Neisseria meningitidis* contains a polysaccharide capsule, whereas *Neisseria gonorrhoeae* does not. *Neisseria meningitidis* ferments both glucose and maltose, but *Neisseria gonorrhoeae* metabolizes only glucose. Most isolates of *Neisseria meningitidis* remain sensitive to penicillin, although resistance is increasing. Effective vaccines exist for *Neisseria meningitidis* serogroups A and C, but not for *Neisseria gonorrhoeae*.

14.4 Meningococcal vaccine

A. is effective in infants less than two years of age.

B. provides protection against disease due to serogroup B

C. is prepared from capsular polysaccharide of *N. meningitidis*.

D. does not prevent disseminated meningococcal disease.

E. contains heat-inactivated *N. meningitidis*.

> Correct answer = C. A capsular vaccine for serogroups A, C, W, and Y is available. It is prepared from capsular polysaccharide of *N. meningitidis*. The polysaccharide of serogroup B does not elicit an effective immune response. Protection generated by vaccines to polysaccharide capsules is weak and short-lived in young children, the target group in which most meningococcal infections occur.

Enteric Gram-negative Rods

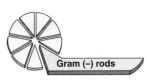

Gram (–) rods

15

I. OVERVIEW

All of the organisms covered in this chapter are routinely found in the gastrointestinal tract of humans or other animals. Many also have alternative habitats in soil or water. All are relatively hardy, but are sensitive to drying, and all grow well in the presence of oxygen, being true facultative anaerobes. They contain lipopolysaccharide (LPS), which is both antigenic and a potential virulence factor (endotoxin). These gram-negative rods belong to diverse taxonomic groups. They constitute only a minor fraction of the total microbial flora of the GI tract (most of the bowel organisms are either gram-positive or gram-negative anaerobes). Different enteric gram-negative rods cause diseases in the gastrointestinal (GI) tract, outside of the GI tract, or in both locations. For example, diseases caused by members of the genera *Escherichia, Salmonella, Yersinia, and Campylobacter* can be both gastrointestinal and extraintestinal, those caused by members of the genera *Shigella, Helicobacter,* and *Vibrio* are primarily gastrointestinal, and those caused by members of the genera *Enterobacter, Klebsiella, Serratia,* and *Proteus* are primarily extraintestinal. Fecal contamination is frequently important in the transmission of those organisms that cause gastrointestinal diseases. The gram-negative rods discussed in this chapter are listed in Figure 15.1.

II. ESCHERICHIA COLI

Escherichia is a genus of the family Enterobacteriaceae, which also includes the genera *Salmonella, Shigella, Enterobacter, Klebsiella, Serratia,* and *Proteus,* among others. Members of this family are classified into genera and species on the basis of DNA relatedness and biochemical characteristics, such as substrate utilization and fermentation end products. *E. coli* is part of the normal flora of the colon in humans and other animals, but can be pathogenic both within and outside of the gastrointestinal tract. [Note: The differences in the degree of virulence of different *E. coli* strains are caused by the individual plasmid and integrated prophage repertoire associated with each strain.] *E. coli* has fimbriae or pili that are frequently important for adherence to host mucosal surfaces, and different strains of the organism may be motile or non-motile. Most strains can ferment lactose (that

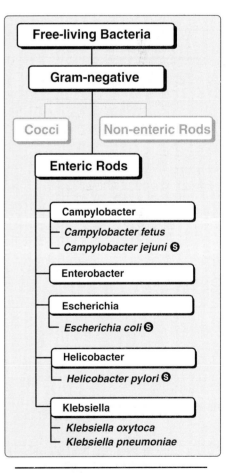

Figure 15.1
Classification of enteric gram-negative rods (figure continues on the next page). **ⓈⒶ** See pp. 401, 437 for summaries of these organisms.

Lippincott's Illustrated Reviews: Microbiology,
by William A. Strohl, Harriet Rouse, Bruce D. Fisher.
Lippincott, Williams & Wilkins, Baltimore, MD © 2001

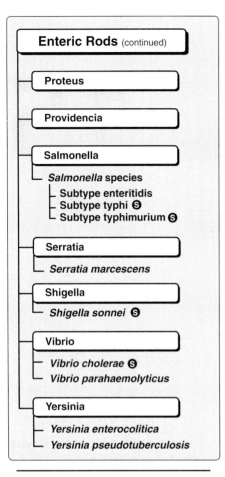

Figure 15.1 (continued)
Classification of enteric gram-
negative rods. ❺ See pp. 401, 437
for summaries of these organisms.

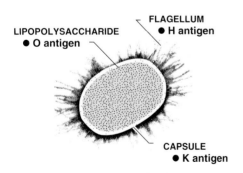

Figure 15.2
Structure of *Escherichia coli* showing
virulence factors.

is, they are Lac⁺), in contrast to the major intestinal pathogens, *Salmonella* (see p. 179) and *Shigella* (see p. 183), which cannot ferment lactose (that is, they are Lac⁻). *E. coli* produces both acid and gas during fermentation of carbohydrates.

A. Structure and physiology

E. coli shares many properties with the other Enterobacteriaceae. They are all true **facultative anaerobes** (see p. 110). They all **ferment glucose**, and can **generate energy by reducing nitrates to nitrites**. They all lack cytochrome oxidase (that is, they are **oxidase-negative**). Typing of strains is based on differences in three structural antigens: O, H, and K (Figure 15.2). The **O antigens** (**somatic** or **cell wall antigens**) are found on the polysaccharide portion of the LPS. These antigens are heat-stable, and may be shared among different Enterobacteriaceae genera. O antigens are commonly used to serologically type many of the enteric gram-negative rods. The **H antigens** are associated with **flagella**; therefore, only flagellated (motile) Enterobacteriaceae such as *E. coli* have them. The **K antigens** are most often associated with the **capsule** or less commonly, with the **fimbriae**. Among *E. coli* species, there are many serologically distinct O, H, and K antigens, and specific serotypes are associated with particular diseases. For example, a serotype of *E. coli* possessing O157 and H7 (designated O157:H7) causes a severe form of hemorrhagic colitis (see p. 177).

B. Clinical significance: intestinal disease

Transmission of intestinal disease is commonly by the fecal/oral route, with contaminated food and water serving as vehicles for transmission. At least five types of intestinal infections that differ in their pathogenic mechanisms have been identified.

1. **Enterotoxigenic *E. coli* (ETEC):** ETEC are a common cause of **traveler's diarrhea**. Transmission occurs through food and water contaminated with human waste, or by person-to-person contact. ETEC colonize the small intestine (pili facilitate the binding of the organism to the intestinal mucosa). In a process mediated by **enterotoxins** (see p. 13), ETEC cause prolonged hypersecretion of chloride ions and water by the intestinal mucosal cells, while inhibiting the reabsorption of sodium. The gut becomes full of fluid, resulting in significant watery diarrhea that continues over a period of several days. Enterotoxins include a heat-stable toxin (ST) that works by causing an elevation in cellular cGMP levels, whereas a heat-labile toxin (LT) causes elevated cAMP (Figure 15.3). [Note: LT is essentially identical to cholera toxin (see p. 185).]

2. **Enteropathogenic *E. coli* (EPEC):** EPEC are an important cause of diarrhea in infants, especially in locations with poor sanitation. The newborn becomes infected during birth, or *in utero*. The EPEC attach to mucosal cells in the small intestine, causing destruction of microvilli and development of characteristic lesions. Watery diarrhea results, which on rare occasions may become chronic. Shiga-like toxins are responsible for this destruction (see p. 184).

3. **Enterohemorrhagic _E. coli_ (EHEC):** EHEC bind to cells in the large intestine, where they produce an exotoxin (**verotoxin**, or **Shiga-like toxin**), causing a severe form of copious, bloody diarrhea (**hemorrhagic colitis**) in the absence of mucosal invasion or inflammation. Serotype O157:H7 is the most common strain of _E. coli_ that produces verotoxin (Figure 15.4). [Note: This strain is also associated with outbreaks of a potentially life-threatening, acute renal failure (**hemolytic uremic syndrome**).] The primary reservoir of EHEC is cattle. Therefore the possibility of infection can be greatly decreased by thoroughly cooking ground beef, and pasteurizing milk.

4. **Other _E. coli_ infections: Enteroinvasive _E. coli_ (EIEC)** cause a dysentery-like syndrome with fever and bloody stools. **Enteroadherent _E. coli_ (EAEC)** also cause traveler's diarrhea, and persistent diarrhea of young children.

C. Clinical significance: extraintestinal disease

The source of infection for extraintestinal disease is frequently the patient's own flora, where the individual's own _E. coli_ is non-pathogenic in the intestine, but causes disease in that individual when the organism is found, for example, in the bladder or blood stream (normally sterile sites).

1. **Urinary tract infections (UTI):** _E. coli_ is the most common cause of UTI, including cystitis and pyelonephritis (Figure 15.5). Women are particularly at risk for infection. **Uncomplicated cystitis** (the most commonly encountered UTI) is caused by uropathogenic strains of _E. coli_, characterized by P fimbriae (an adherence factor) and, frequently, hemolysin, colicin V, and resistance to the bactericidal activity of serum complement. **Complicated UTI (pyelonephritis)** typically occur in settings of obstructed urinary flow, and may be caused by nonuropathogenic strains.

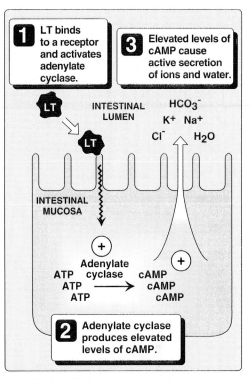

Figure 15.3
The action of _Escherichia coli_ LT (heat-labile toxin). [Note: ST (heat-stable toxin) activates guanylate cyclase, causing production of cGMP that also causes secretion.]

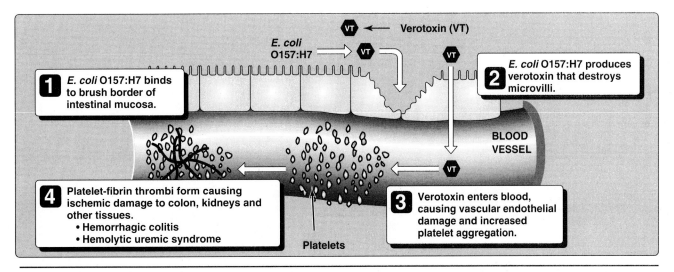

Figure 15.4
Pathogenesis of _E. coli_ O157:H7 infection.

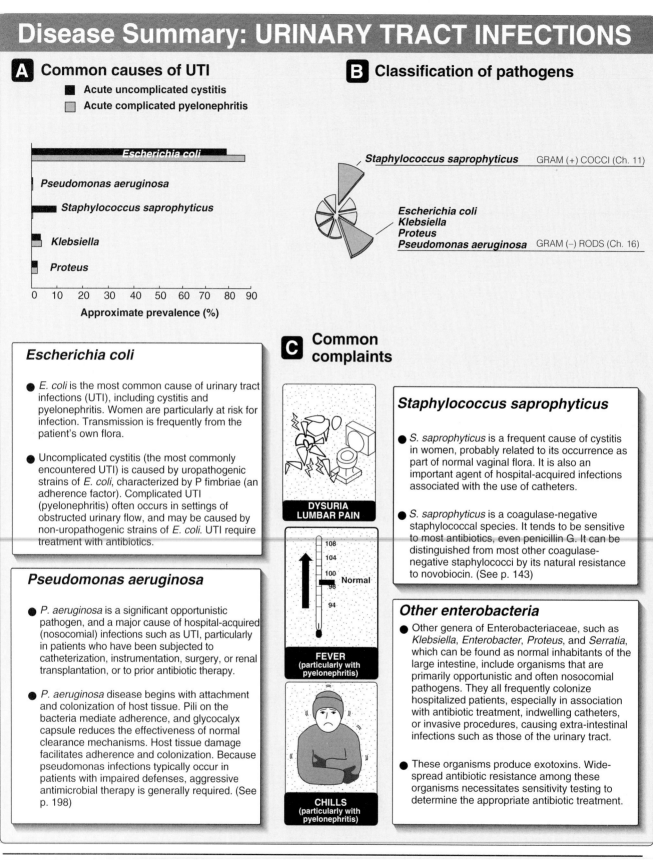

Figure 15.5
Disease summary of urinary tract infections.

2. **Neonatal meningitis:** *E. coli* is a major cause of this disease occurring within the first month of life. The K1 (capsular) antigen is particularly associated with such infections.

3. **Nosocomial (hospital-acquired) infections:** These include **sepsis/bacteremia**, **endotoxic shock**, and **pneumonia**.

D. Laboratory identification

Intestinal disease: Because *E. coli* is normally part of the intestinal flora, detection in stool cultures of disease-causing strains is generally difficult. EIEC strains often do not ferment lactose, and may be detected on media such as MacConkey agar (see p. 25). EHEC, unlike most other strains of *E. coli*, ferment sorbitol slowly if at all, and may be detected on MacConkey sorbitol agar. **Extraintestinal disease:** Isolation of *E. coli* from normally sterile body sites (for example, the bladder or CSF) is diagnostically significant. Specimens may be cultured on MacConkey agar. Strains of *E. coli* can be further characterized on the basis of serologic tests.

E. Treatment and prevention

Intestinal disease can best be prevented by care in selection, preparation, and consumption of food and water. Maintenance of fluid and electrolyte balance is of primary importance in treatment. Antibiotics may shorten duration of symptoms; however, resistance is widespread. Extraintestinal diseases require antibiotic treatment (Figure 15.6). Antibiotic sensitivity testing of isolates is necessary to determine the appropriate choice of drugs.

III. SALMONELLA

Members of the genus *Salmonella* can cause a variety of diseases, including **gastroenteritis** and **enteric (typhoid) fever**. *Salmonella* classification has undergone numerous revisions; currently, all strains are grouped in a single species, *S. enterica*. This species is further divided into over 1500 serotypes based on the cell wall (O), flagellar (H), and capsular (Vi, analogous to K) antigens (Figure 15.7). Originally thought to be different species, serotypes typhimurium and typhi are of particular clinical significance. Lipopolysaccharide (both lipid A and O antigen) and the Vi antigen are virulence factors. Most strains of *Salmonella* are Lac⁻, and produce acid and gas during fermentation of glucose. They also produce H₂S from sulfur-containing amino acids.

A. Epidemiology

Salmonella are widely distributed in nature. Serotype typhi is the exclusively human pathogen, whereas other strains are associated with animals and foods (for example, eggs and poultry). Fecal/oral transmission occurs, and may involve chronic carriers. Pet turtles have also been implicated as sources of infection. Young children and the elderly are particularly susceptible to *Salmonella* infection. Individuals in crowded institutions may also sustain *Salmonella* epidemics.

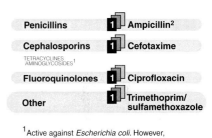

Penicillins	**1** Ampicillin[2]
Cephalosporins	**1** Cefotaxime
TETRACYCLINES AMINOGLYCOSIDES[1]	
Fluoroquinolones	**1** Ciprofloxacin
Other	**1** Trimethoprim/ sulfamethoxazole

[1] Active against *Escherichia coli*. However, less toxic drugs may be effective.

[2] *Escherichia coli* often shows significant resistance to antimicrobial agents, particularly to ampicillin. Ampicillin/clavulanate or ampicillin/sulbactam are alternates. Sensitivity testing is an essential part of therapy.

Figure 15.6
Some antimicrobial agents useful in therapy of infections caused by *Escherichia coli*.

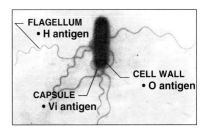

Figure 15.7
Salmonella species with peritrichous flagella (flagella over the entire surface of cell).

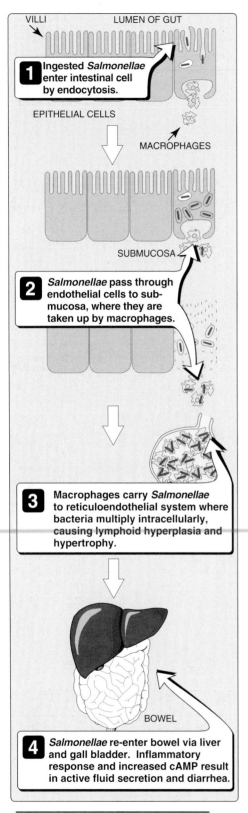

VILLI   **LUMEN OF GUT**

1 Ingested *Salmonellae* enter intestinal cell by endocytosis.

EPITHELIAL CELLS

MACROPHAGES

SUBMUCOSA

2 *Salmonellae* pass through endothelial cells to submucosa, where they are taken up by macrophages.

3 Macrophages carry *Salmonellae* to reticuloendothelial system where bacteria multiply intracellularly, causing lymphoid hyperplasia and hypertrophy.

BOWEL

4 *Salmonellae* re-enter bowel via liver and gall bladder. Inflammatory response and increased cAMP result in active fluid secretion and diarrhea.

Figure 15.8
Mechanism of salmonella infection causing diarrhea.

B. Pathogenesis

Salmonella invade epithelial cells of the small intestine. Disease may remain localized or become systemic, sometimes with disseminated foci. The organisms are facultative, intracellular parasites that survive in phagocytic cells (Figure 15.8). Development of clinical symptoms depends on: 1) the **infectious dose** (this is strain-dependent), 2) **bacterial factors** including proteins that induce the intestinal epithelial cells to endocytose the organisms and promote survival within phagocytic cells, and 3) **host factors** including achlorhydria (absence of HCl from the gastric juice), sickle cell disease, and reduced cell-mediated immunity.

C. Clinical significance

Salmonella infection can cause both intestinal and extraintestinal diseases.

1. **Gastroenteritis:** This is a localized disease, caused primarily by serotypes enteriditis and typhimurium. It is characterized by nausea, vomiting, and diarrhea (usually nonbloody), which develop generally within 48 hours of ingesting contaminated food or water. Fever and abdominal cramping are common. In uncompromised patients, disease is generally self-limiting (48 to 72 hours), although convalescent carriage of organisms may persist for a month or more.

2. **Enteric (typhoid) fever:** This is a severe, life-threatening systemic illness, characterized by fever and, frequently, abdominal symptoms. It is caused primarily by serotype typhi, but other serotypes can also cause this disease. Nonspecific symptoms may include chills, sweats, headache, anorexia, weakness, sore throat, cough, and myalgias. About thirty percent of patients have a faint maculopapular rash on the trunk (**rose spots**). The incubation period varies from 5 to 21 days. Untreated, mortality is approximately fifteen percent; among survivors, the symptoms generally resolve in three to four weeks. Timely and appropriate antibiotic therapy reduces mortality to less than one percent, and speeds resolution of the fever. Complications can include intestinal hemorrhage and, rarely, focal infections and endocarditis. A small percentage of patients become chronic carriers. [Note: Infected gallbladders are the main source of fecal contamination.]

3. **Other sites of Salmonella infection: Sustained bacteremia** is often associated with vascular *Salmonella* infections that occur when bacteria seed atherosclerotic plaque. *Salmonella* can also cause abdominal infections (often of the hepatobiliary tract and spleen), osteomyelitis, septic arthritis, and, rarely, infections of other tissues or organs. Chronic carriage may, rarely, develop.

D. Laboratory identification

In patients with diarrhea, *Salmonella* can typically be isolated from stools on MacConkey agar or moderately selective media (Figure 15.9). For patients with enteric fever, appropriate specimens include blood, bone marrow, urine, and tissue from typical rose spots.

E. Treatment and prevention

For gastroenteritis in uncompromised hosts, antibiotic therapy is often not needed, and may prolong the convalescent carrier state. For enteric fever, appropriate antibiotics include β-lactams and fluoroquinolones (Figure 15.10). Prevention of salmonella infection is accomplished by proper sewage disposal, correct handling of food, and good personal hygeine.

IV. CAMPYLOBACTER

Members of the genus *Campylobacter* are curved, spiral, or S-shaped organisms that microscopically resemble vibrios (Figure 15.11). A single, polar flagellum provides the organism with its characteristic darting motility. Somatic, flagellar, and capsular antigens all contribute to the numerous serotypes. Most *Campylobacter* are microaerophilic (that is, they require oxygen, but at lower concentrations than that found in air). Members of this genus utilize a respiratory pathway, and do not ferment carbohydrates. *Campylobacter* infect the intestine, and can cause ulcerative, inflammatory lesions in the jejunum, ileum, or colon. Bacteremia may occur.

A. Epidemiology

Campylobacter are widely distributed in nature as commensals of many different vertebrate species, including mammals and fowl, both wild and domestic. These serve as reservoirs of infection. *Campylobacter* can be transmitted to humans primarily via the fecal/oral route—through direct contact, exposure to contaminated meat (especially poultry), or contaminated water supplies.

B. Pathogenesis and clinical significance

Campylobacter may cause both intestinal and extraintestinal disease. They are currently the leading cause of food-borne disease in the United States (Figure 15.12). [Note: Characteristics of some common forms of bacterial food poisoning are shown in Figure 15.13.] *C. jejuni* typically causes an **acute enteritis** in otherwise healthy individuals following a one-to-seven day incubation. The disease lasts days to several weeks, and generally is self-limiting. Symptoms may be both systemic (fever, headache, myalgia) and intestinal (abdominal cramping and diarrhea, which may or may not be bloody). *C. jejuni* is a cause of both **traveler's diarrhea** and **pseudoappendicitis**. Bacteremia (often transient) may occur, most often in infants and the elderly. Sustained bacteremia usually reflects host compromise. Complications include septic abortion, reactive arthritis, and Guillain-Barre syndrome. Less common than *C. jejuni*, other enteric *Campylobacter* may cause a similar clinical presentation. *C. fetus* may also cause intestinal infections, but has a greater propensity than *C. jejuni* to cause bacteremia and infections of other sites (perhaps because *C. fetus* is resistant to the bactericidal activity of serum complement, whereas most *C. jejuni* strains are sensitive). *C. fetus* particularly causes infection of vascular sites, but may also infect the CNS and other local sites. In compromised hosts, **campylobacteriosis** is more likely to result from infection with *C. fetus* than with *C. jejuni*.

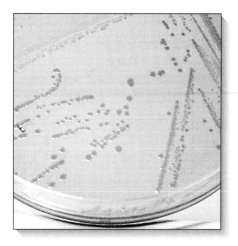

Figure 15.9
Salmonella species on MacConkey agar.

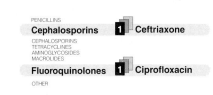

Figure 15.10
Some antimicrobial agents useful in empiric therapy of infections due to *Salmonella* serotype typhi.

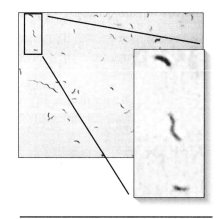

Figure 15.11
Micrograph showing the S-shaped cells of *Campylobacter jejuni*.

Disease Summary: FOOD POISONING (bacterial)

A Some common causes of food poisoning

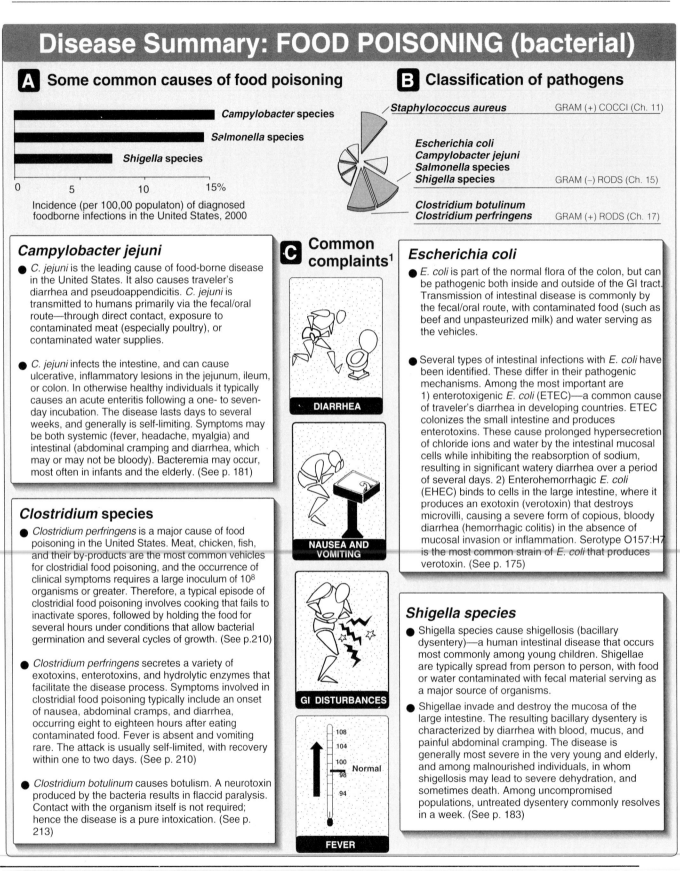

Campylobacter species
Salmonella species
Shigella species

0   5   10   15%

Incidence (per 100,00 populaton) of diagnosed
foodborne infections in the United States, 2000

B Classification of pathogens

Staphylococcus aureus   GRAM (+) COCCI (Ch. 11)

Escherichia coli
Campylobacter jejuni
Salmonella species
Shigella species   GRAM (−) RODS (Ch. 15)

Clostridium botulinum
Clostridium perfringens   GRAM (+) RODS (Ch. 17)

C Common complaints[1]

DIARRHEA

NAUSEA AND VOMITING

GI DISTURBANCES

108
104
100
98   Normal
94

FEVER

Campylobacter jejuni

- C. jejuni is the leading cause of food-borne disease in the United States. It also causes traveler's diarrhea and pseudoappendicitis. C. jejuni is transmitted to humans primarily via the fecal/oral route—through direct contact, exposure to contaminated meat (especially poultry), or contaminated water supplies.

- C. jejuni infects the intestine, and can cause ulcerative, inflammatory lesions in the jejunum, ileum, or colon. In otherwise healthy individuals it typically causes an acute enteritis following a one- to seven-day incubation. The disease lasts days to several weeks, and generally is self-limiting. Symptoms may be both systemic (fever, headache, myalgia) and intestinal (abdominal cramping and diarrhea, which may or may not be bloody). Bacteremia may occur, most often in infants and the elderly. (See p. 181)

Clostridium species

- Clostridium perfringens is a major cause of food poisoning in the United States. Meat, chicken, fish, and their by-products are the most common vehicles for clostridial food poisoning, and the occurrence of clinical symptoms requires a large inoculum of 10^8 organisms or greater. Therefore, a typical episode of clostridial food poisoning involves cooking that fails to inactivate spores, followed by holding the food for several hours under conditions that allow bacterial germination and several cycles of growth. (See p.210)

- Clostridium perfringens secretes a variety of exotoxins, enterotoxins, and hydrolytic enzymes that facilitate the disease process. Symptoms involved in clostridial food poisoning typically include an onset of nausea, abdominal cramps, and diarrhea, occurring eight to eighteen hours after eating contaminated food. Fever is absent and vomiting rare. The attack is usually self-limited, with recovery within one to two days. (See p. 210)

- Clostridium botulinum causes botulism. A neurotoxin produced by the bacteria results in flaccid paralysis. Contact with the organism itself is not required; hence the disease is a pure intoxication. (See p. 213)

Escherichia coli

- E. coli is part of the normal flora of the colon, but can be pathogenic both inside and outside of the GI tract. Transmission of intestinal disease is commonly by the fecal/oral route, with contaminated food (such as beef and unpasteurized milk) and water serving as the vehicles.

- Several types of intestinal infections with E. coli have been identified. These differ in their pathogenic mechanisms. Among the most important are 1) enterotoxigenic E. coli (ETEC)—a common cause of traveler's diarrhea in developing countries. ETEC colonizes the small intestine and produces enterotoxins. These cause prolonged hypersecretion of chloride ions and water by the intestinal mucosal cells while inhibiting the reabsorption of sodium, resulting in significant watery diarrhea over a period of several days. 2) Enterohemorrhagic E. coli (EHEC) binds to cells in the large intestine, where it produces an exotoxin (verotoxin) that destroys microvilli, causing a severe form of copious, bloody diarrhea (hemorrhagic colitis) in the absence of mucosal invasion or inflammation. Serotype O157:H7 is the most common strain of E. coli that produces verotoxin. (See p. 175)

Shigella species

- Shigella species cause shigellosis (bacillary dysentery)—a human intestinal disease that occurs most commonly among young children. Shigellae are typically spread from person to person, with food or water contaminated with fecal material serving as a major source of organisms.

- Shigellae invade and destroy the mucosa of the large intestine. The resulting bacillary dysentery is characterized by diarrhea with blood, mucus, and painful abdominal cramping. The disease is generally most severe in the very young and elderly, and among malnourished individuals, in whom shigellosis may lead to severe dehydration, and sometimes death. Among uncompromised populations, untreated dysentery commonly resolves in a week. (See p. 183)

Figure 15.12 (continued on next page)
Disease summary of some major organisms causing bacterial food poisoning.
[1]Other complaints may include headache and myalgias.

Disease Summary: FOOD POISONING (bacterial)

Staphylococcus aureus

- *S. aureus* gastroenteritis is caused by ingestion of food containing the bacterial enterotoxin. Often contaminated by a food-handler, these foods tend to be protein-rich (for example, egg salad, cream pastry) and improperly refrigerated.
- The toxin stimulates the vomiting center in the brain by binding to neural receptors in the upper GI tract. Symptoms such as nausea, vomiting, and diarrhea are acute following a short incubation period (less than six hours). The attack is usually self-limiting. (See p.xxx)

Salmonella species

- Non-typhoidal Salmonella serotypes, particularly *S. typhimurium* and *S. enteritidis*, cause a localized gastroenteritis where the symptoms result from the causative bacteria proliferating in the intestine of affected individuals. Transmission is usually via food, especially chickens, eggs, and egg products.
- These organisms all produce exotoxins. Widespread antibiotic resistance among these organisms requires sensitivity testing to determine the appropriate antibiotic treatment, if any is given.

Figure 15.12 (continued)
Disease summary of major organisms causing bacterial food poisoning.

C. Laboratory identification

Campylobacter can be isolated from feces using special selective media and microaerophilic conditions. Because of their small size, these organisms are not retained by bacteriologic filters that hold back most other bacteria. Thus, filtration of the fecal suspension may enhance recovery rate. Presumptive diagnosis can be made on the basis of finding curved organisms with rapid, darting motility in a wet mount of feces.

D. Treatment and prevention

Diarrhea should be treated symptomatically with fluid and electrolyte replacement. For patients with more severe symptoms (for example, high fever, bloody diarrhea, worsening illness, or illness of more than a week's duration), or for patients with systemic illness, antibiotics should be administered. For *C. jejuni*, ciprofloxacin is the drug of choice; other antibiotics are also effective (Figure 15.14). For *C. fetus*, ampicillin or third-generation cephalosporins are effective. Thorough cooking of potentially contaminated foods (for example, poultry) and pasteurization of milk and milk products is essential to prevention of campylobacteriosis.

ONSET: 1 TO 6 HOURS

Bacillus cereus
Staphylococcus aureus

ONSET: 8 TO 16 HOURS

Clostridium perfringens
Bacillus cereus[1]

ONSET: > 16 HOURS

Campylobacter jejuni
Clostridium botulinium
Escherichia coli
Salmonella species
Shigella species

[1]Illness due to diarrheal enterotoxin, rather than preformed enterotoxin)

Reverse type = Illness commonly caused by toxin in food; viable bacteria may or may not be present in the food.

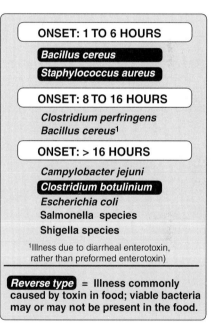

Figure 15.13
Characteristics of some common forms of bacterial food poisoning.

PENICILLINS
CEPHALOSPORINS
TETRACYCLINES
AMINOGLYCOSIDES
Macrolides — 1 Erythromycin
Fluoroquinolones — 2 Ciprofloxacin
OTHER

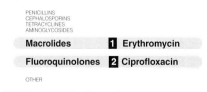

Figure 15.14
Some antimicrobial agents useful in empiric therapy of infections due to *Campylobacter jejuni*.

V. SHIGELLA

Shigella species cause **shigellosis** (**bacillary dysentery**)—a human intestinal disease that occurs most commonly among young children. Shigellae are nonmotile, unencapsulated, and Lac^{-}. Most strains do not produce gas in a mixed acid fermentation of glucose.

A. Epidemiology

Shigellae are typically spread from person to person, with contaminated stools serving as a major source of organisms. Flies and contaminated food or water can also transmit the disease. Shigellosis has a low infectious dose (fewer than 200 viable organisms are suf-

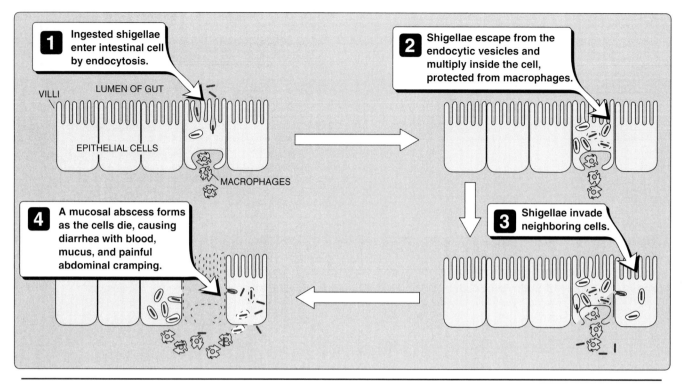

Figure 15.15
Mechanism of shigella infection causing diarrhea.

ficient to cause disease). Hence secondary cases within a household are common, particularly under conditions of crowding and/or poor sanitation. The forty serotypes of shigella are organized into four groups (A, B, C, and D) based on the serologic relatedness of their polysaccharide O antigens. Group D (*S. sonnei*) is the serogroup that is found most commonly in the United States.

B. Pathogenesis and clinical significance

Shigellae invade and destroy the mucosa of the large intestine. Infection rarely penetrates to deeper layers of the intestine, and does not lead to shigella bacteremia (Figure 15.15). An exotoxin (**Shiga toxin**) with enterotoxic and cytotoxic properties has been isolated from these organisms, and its toxigenicity may play a secondary role in development of intestinal lesions. Shigellae cause classic **bacillary dysentery**, characterized by diarrhea with blood, mucus, and painful abdominal cramping. The disease is generally most severe in the very young and elderly, and among malnourished individuals, in whom shigellosis may lead to severe dehydration, and sometimes death. Among uncompromised populations, untreated dysentery commonly resolves in a week, but may persist longer.

C. Laboratory identification

During acute illness, organisms can be cultured from stools using differential, selective Hektoen agar or other media specific for intestinal pathogens.

D. Treatment and prevention

Antibiotics (for example, ciprofloxacin or azithromycin) can reduce the duration of illness and the period of shedding organisms, but usage is controversial because of widespread antibiotic resistance (Figure 15.16). Protection of the water and food supply, and personal hygiene are crucial for preventing *Shigella* infections. Vaccine development is currently experimental.

VI. VIBRIOS

Members of the genus *Vibrio* are short, curved, rod-shaped organisms. *Vibrios* are closely related to the family Enterobacteriaceae. They are rapidly motile by means of a single polar flagellum (Figure 15.17). [Note: This contrasts with the peritrichous flagella (distributed all over the surface) of the motile Enterobacteriaceae.] O and H antigens are both present, but only O antigens are useful in distinguishing strains of vibrios that cause epidemics. Vibrios are facultative anaerobes. The growth of many *Vibrio* strains either requires or is stimulated by NaCl. Pathogenic vibrios include: 1) *V. cholerae*, serogroup O1 strains that are associated with epidemic cholera; 2) non-O1 *V. cholerae* and related strains that cause sporadic cases of cholera-like and other illnesses; and 3) *V. parahaemolyticus* and other halophilic vibrios, which cause gastroenteritis and extraintestinal infections.

A. Epidemiology

V. cholerae is transmitted by contaminated water and food. There are no known animal reservoirs, nor animal or arthropod vectors. Among humans, long-term carriage is considered uncommon. There are two biotypes (subdivisions) of the species, *V. cholerae*: classic and El Tor. In contrast to the classic strain, the El Tor strain is distinguished by the production of hemolysins, higher carriage rates, and the ability to survive in water for longer periods. Outbreaks of both strains have been associated with raw or undercooked seafood harvested from contaminated waters.

B. Pathogenesis

Following ingestion, *V. cholerae* infects the small intestine. Adhesion factor(s) are important for colonization and virulence. Achlorhydria, or treatments that lessen gastric acidity, greatly reduce the infectious dose. The organism is noninvasive, and causes disease through the action of an enterotoxin that initiates an outpouring of fluid (Figure 15.18). **Cholera toxin** is a multimeric protein composed of an A and a B subunit. The B subunit (consisting of five identical monomers) binds to the GM_1 ganglioside receptor of cells lining the intestine. The A subunit has two components: A2, which facilitates penetration of the cell membrane, and A1, an ADP-ribosyl transferase that ADP-ribosylates the membrane-bound G_s protein.[1] G_s protein activates adenylate cyclase, which produces elevated levels of intracellular cAMP. This in turn causes an outflowing of ions and water to the lumen of the intestine.

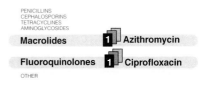

Figure 15.16
Some antimicrobial agents useful in therapy of infections caused by shigella species.

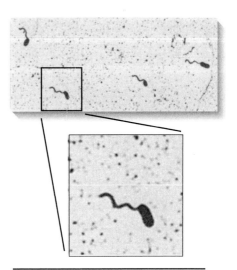

Figure 15.17
Light micrograph showing the curved, rod-shaped cells characteristic of vibrio species.

 [1]See p. 82 in *Lippincott's Illustrated Reviews: Biochemistry* (2nd ed.) for a discussion of the mechanism of action of G_s proteins.

C. Clinical significance

Full-blown **cholera** is characterized by massive loss of fluid and electrolytes from the body. After an incubation period ranging from hours to a few days, profuse **watery diarrhea** (**rice-water stools**) begins. Untreated, the death from severe dehydration causing hypovolemic shock may occur in hours to days, and the death rate may exceed fifty percent. Appropriate treatment reduces the death rate to under one percent. [Note: Non-O1 *Vibrio cholerae* and other non-halophilic vibrios cause sporadic cases of cholera indistinguishable from that caused by *V. cholerae*, serotype O1. They also cause milder illness, comparable to that caused by enterotoxigenic *E. coli*.]

D. Laboratory identification

V. cholerae grows on standard media such as blood and MacConkey agars. Thiosulfate–citrate–bile salts–sucrose (TCBS) medium can enhance isolation. The organism is oxidase-positive, but further biochemical testing is necessary for specific identification of *V. cholerae*.

E. Treatment and prevention

Replacement of fluids and electrolytes is crucial in preventing shock, and does not require bacteriologic diagnosis. Antibiotics (tetracycline is the drug of choice) can shorten the duration of diarrhea and excretion of the organism (Figure 15.19). Prevention relies primarily on public health measures that reduce fecal contamination of water supplies and food. Adequate cooking of foods can minimize transmission.

F. Vibrio parahaemolyticus and other halophilic, noncholera vibrios

These organisms are characterized by a requirement for higher-than-usual concentrations of NaCl, and their ability to grow in ten percent NaCl. They are common in coastal sea waters. *V. parahaemolyticus* is associated with outbreaks of **gastrointestinal illness** that result from ingestion of contaminated and inadequately cooked seafood, especially shellfish and crustaceans. The disease is self-limiting, and antibiotics do not alter the course of infection. Neither human carriers nor other mammalian reservoirs have been identified. Other halophilic, noncholera vibrios are associated with **soft tissue infections**, septicemia (resulting either from contact of wounds with contaminated sea water or from ingestion of contaminated seafood), **otitis media** and **otitis externa** (**swimmer's ear**). For soft tissue infections, prompt administration of antibiotics such as tetracycline or cefotaxime is important, and surgical drainage/debridement may be required. Bacteremia is associated with high mortality.

VII. YERSINIA

The genus *Yersinia* includes three species of medical importance: *Y. enterocolitica* and *Y. pseudotuberculosis*, both potential pathogens of the GI tract that are discussed in this chapter, and *Y. pestis*, the etiologic agent of bubonic plague, which is discussed in Chapter 16 (see p. 205). *Y. enterocolitica* and *Y. pseudotuberculosis* are both motile when

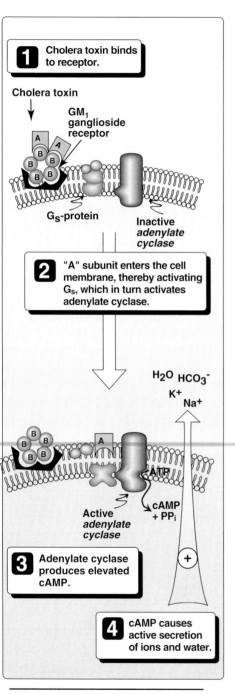

1 Cholera toxin binds to receptor.

Cholera toxin

GM$_1$ ganglioside receptor

G$_s$-protein

Inactive adenylate cyclase

2 "A" subunit enters the cell membrane, thereby activating G$_s$, which in turn activates adenylate cyclase.

H$_2$O HCO$_3^-$
K$^+$
Na$^+$

Active adenylate cyclase

ATP

cAMP + PP$_i$

3 Adenylate cyclase produces elevated cAMP.

4 cAMP causes active secretion of ions and water.

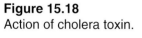

Figure 15.18
Action of cholera toxin.

grown at 25°C but not at 37°C. Multiple serotypes of both strains exist, and the V and W antigens are virulence factors. In contrast to most pathogenic Enterobacteriaceae, these strains of *Yersinia* grow well at room temperature as well as at 37°C. Most strains are Lac⁻.

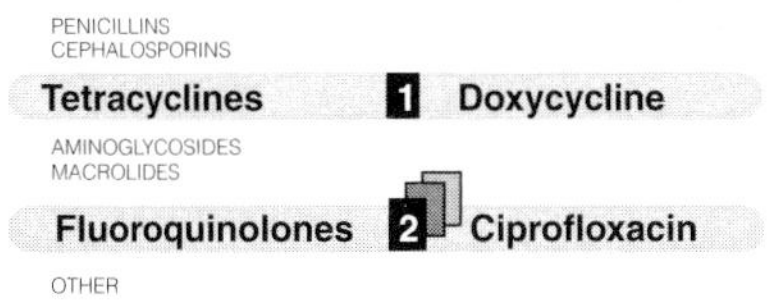

A. Pathogenesis and clinical significance

Infection occurs via ingestion of food that has become contaminated through contact with colonized domestic animals, abattoirs, or raw meat (especially pork). *Y. enterocolitica* is a relatively uncommon cause of enterocolitis in the United States, and *Y. pseudotuberculosis* is even rarer. Infection results in ulcerative lesions in the terminal ileum, necrotic lesions in Peyer's patches, and enlargement of mesenteric lymph nodes. **Enterocolitis** caused by *Yersinia* is characterized by fever, abdominal pain, and diarrhea. When accompanied by right lower quadrant tenderness and leukocytosis, the symptoms are clinically indistinguishable from appendicitis. Symptoms commonly resolve in one to three weeks. Sequelae may include **reactive polyarthritis** and **erythema nodosum**. Other, less common clinical presentations include **exudative pharyngitis** and, in compromised patients, **septicemia**.

B. Laboratory identification

Yersinia can be cultured from appropriate specimens on MacConkey or CIN (a medium selective for *Yersinia*) agars. Identification is based on biochemical screening. In the absence of a positive culture, serologic tests for anti-*Yersinia* antibodies may assist in diagnosis.

C. Treatment and prevention

Reducing infections and outbreaks rests on measures to limit potential contamination of meat, and to ensure its proper handling and preparation. Antibiotic therapy, for example, with ciprofloxacin or trimethoprim-sulfamethoxazole, is essential for systemic disease (sepsis), but is of questionable value for self-limited disease such as enterocolitis (Figure 15.20).

VIII. HELICOBACTER

Members of the genus *Helicobacter* are curved or spiral organisms. They have a rapid, corkscrew motility due to multiple polar flagella (Figure 15.21). *H. pylori*, the species of human significance, is microaerophilic, and produces urease. It causes acute gastritis, and duodenal and gastric ulcers. *H. pylori* (and several other *Helicobacter* species) are unusual in their ability to colonize the stomach, whose low pH normally protects against bacterial infection. *H. pylori* infections are relatively common, and world-wide in distribution.

A. Pathogenesis

Transmission of *H. pylori* is thought to be from person to person; the organism has not been isolated from food or water. Untreated, infec-

PENICILLINS
CEPHALOSPORINS
Tetracyclines   **1** **Doxycycline**
AMINOGLYCOSIDES
MACROLIDES
Fluoroquinolones **2** Ciprofloxacin
OTHER

Figure 15.19
Some antimicrobial agents useful in therapy of infections caused by *Vibrio cholerae*.

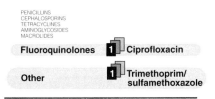

PENICILLINS
CEPHALOSPORINS
TETRACYCLINES
AMINOGLYCOSIDES
MACROLIDES
Fluoroquinolones **1** Ciprofloxacin

Other **1** Trimethoprim/ sulfamethoxazole

Figure 15.20
Some antimicrobial agents useful in therapy of infections caused by *Yersina entercolitica*.

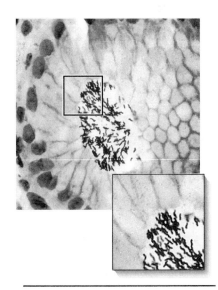

Figure 15.21
Helicobacter pylori in association with gastric mucosa.

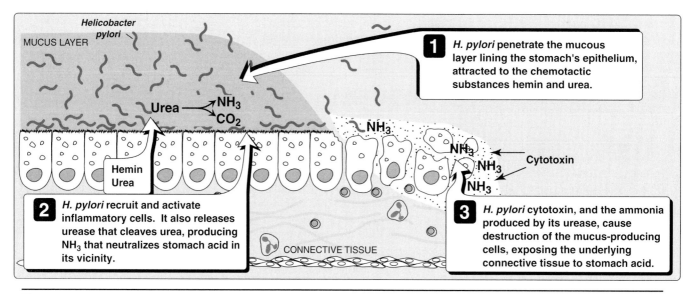

Figure 15.22
Helicobacter pylori infection resulting in ulceration of the stomach.

tions tend to be chronic and life-long. *H. pylori* colonizes gastric mucosal (epithelial) cells in the stomach, and metaplastic gastric epithelium in the duodenum or esophagus, but does not colonize the rest of the intestinal epithelium. The organism survives in the mucus layer that coats the epithelium, and causes a chronic inflammation of the mucosa (Figure 15.22). Although the organism is noninvasive, it recruits and activates inflammatory cells. Urease released by *H. pylori* produces ammonia ions that neutralize stomach acid in the vicinity of the organism, thus favoring bacterial multiplication. Ammonia may also both cause injury and potentiate the effects of a cytotoxin produced by *H. pylori*.

B. Clinical significance

Initial infection with *H. pylori* causes **acute gastritis**, sometimes with **diarrhea** that lasts about one week. The infection usually becomes chronic, with diffuse, superficial gastritis that may be associated with epigastric discomfort. Both **duodenal ulcers** and **gastric ulcers** are closely correlated with infection by *H. pylori*. [Note: *H. pylori* infection is found in over 95 percent of duodenal ulcer patients, and in nearly all patients with gastric ulcers who do not use aspirin or other nonsteroidal antiinflammatory drugs, both risk factors for gastric ulcers.] *H. pylori* infection appears to be a risk factor for development of **gastric carcinoma** and **gastric B-cell lymphoma**.

C. Laboratory identification

Noninvasive diagnostic tests include serologic tests (ELISA for serum antibodies to *H. pylori*, see p. 29) and breath tests for urease. [Note: Breath tests involve administering radioactively labeled urea by mouth. If *H. pylori* are present in the patient's stomach, the urease produced by the organism will split the urea to CO_2 (radioactively labeled and exhaled) and NH_3.] Invasive tests involve gastric biopsy specimens obtained by endoscopy. *H. pylori* can be detected in such specimens histologically, by culture, or by a test for urease.

D. Treatment and prevention

Elimination of *H. pylori* requires combination therapy with two or more antibiotics. Although *H. pylori* is innately sensitive to many antibiotics, resistance readily develops. A typical regimen includes metronidazole, tetracycline, and bismuth (Figure 15.23).

IX. OTHER ENTEROBACTERIACEAE

Other genera of *Enterobacteriaceae*, such as *Klebsiella*, *Enterobacter*, *Proteus*, and *Serratia*, which can be found as normal inhabitants of the large intestine, include organisms that are primarily opportunistic, and often nosocomial pathogens. Wide-spread antibiotic resistance among these organisms necessitates sensitivity testing to determine the appropriate antibiotic treatment.

A. Enterobacter

Enterobacter species are motile and Lac⁺. They rarely cause primary disease in humans, but frequently colonize hospitalized patients, especially in association with antibiotic treatment, indwelling catheters, or invasive procedures. These organisms may infect burns, wounds, the respiratory tract (causing pneumonia), or the urinary tract.

B. Klebsiella

Klebsiellae are large, nonmotile bacilli that possess a luxurious capsule (Figure 15.24). They are Lac⁺. *K. pneumoniae* and *K. oxytoca* cause a **necrotizing lobar pneumonia** in individuals compromised by alcoholism, diabetes, or chronic obstructive pulmonary disease. *K. pneumoniae* also causes **urinary tract infections** and **bacteremia**, particularly in hospitalized patients.

C. Serratia

Serratia are motile, and ferment lactose slowly, if at all. The species of *Serratia* that most frequently causes human infection is *S. marcescens*. *Serratia* can cause extraintestinal infections such as those of the lower respiratory and urinary tracts, especially among hospitalized patients.

D. Proteus, Providencia, and Morganella

Members of these genera are agents of urinary tract and other extraintestinal infections. *Proteus* species are relatively common causes of uncomplicated as well as nosocomial UTIs. Other extraintestinal infections, such as wound infections, pneumonias, and septicemias, are associated with compromised patients.

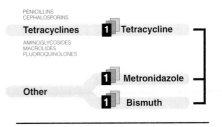

Figure 15.23
One of a number of combinations of drugs useful in treating gastric ulcer caused by *Helicobacter pylori*.

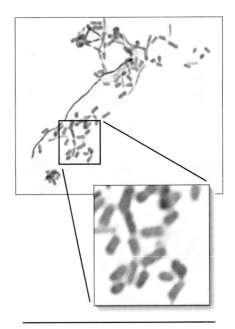

Figure 15.24
Micrograph showing the rod-shaped cells of *Klebsiella pneumonia*.

Study Questions

Choose the ONE correct answer

15.1 A Lac$^+$, glucose-fermenting gram-negative rod isolated from a previously healthy child with bloody diarrhea is most likely to be:

    A. *Shigella sonnei.*

    B. *Pseudomonas aeruginosa.*

    C. *Escherichia coli.*

    D. *Salmonella cholerae.*

    E. *Helicobacter pylori.*

> Correct answer = C. Shigella characteristically causes bloody diarrhea (dysentery) but is Lac$^-$. Pseudomonas characteristically causes infections in compromised hosts, and is Lac$^-$. Salmonella is also Lac$^-$. *Helicobacter pylori* causes gastritis. *Escherichia coli* is Lac$^+$, and enteroinvasive strains characteristically cause a dysentery-like syndrome.

15.2 An elderly man, hospitalized and recovering from cardiac bypass surgery, develops pneumonia. Sputum culture reveals a gram-negative rod that produces a green pigment, but does not ferment carbohydrates. The most likely organism is:

    A. *Klebsiella pneumoniae.*

    B. *Serratia* species.

    C. *Proteus* species.

    D. *Enterobacter* species.

    E. *Pseudomonas aeruginosa.*

> Correct answer = E. All five organisms are opportunists capable of causing pneumonia in compromised patients. However, the first four are members of the family *Enterobacteriaceae* and, by definition, can ferment carbohydrates. In addition, none of the organisms is known to produce a green pigment, although serratia may produce a red pigment. *Pseudomonas aeruginosa* is an obligate aerobe that utilizes respiratory pathways exclusively. Production of green pyocyanin pigment regularly occurs.

15.3 An elderly alcoholic male develops a severe, necrotizing lobar pneumonia. The organism is Lac$^+$ and produces a luxuriant capsule. The most likely agent is:

    A. *Klebsiella pneumoniae.*

    B. *Serratia* species.

    C. *Yersinia pseudotuberculosis.*

    D. *Pseudomonas aeruginosa.*

    E. *Campylobacter fetus.*

> Correct answer = A. The combination of necrotizing pneumonia and an alcoholic patient suggests *Klebsiella pneumoniae*, and the laboratory data (Lac$^+$ and a luxuriant capsule) are consistent. Serratia can cause pneumonia in compromised patients; necrosis is not a characteristic feature; the organism ferments lactose slowly if at all, and does not have a luxuriant capsule. *Yersinia pseudotuberculosis* is lac$^-$, and rarely causes pneumonia. *Pseudomonas aeruginosa* can cause pneumonia in compromised patients, but does not ferment lactose. *Campylobacter fetus* typically causes bacteremia and disseminated infections.

15.4 Which of the following organisms produces toxins that ADP-ribosylate host cell proteins?

    A. *Escherichia coli*, *Salmonella* species, and *Shigella* species.

    B. *Escherichia coli*, *Vibrio cholerae*, and *Pseudomonas aeruginosa.*

    C. *Campylobacter fetus*, *Proteus* species, and *Shigella* species.

    D. *Campylobacter jejuni*, *Pseudomonas aeruginosa*, and *Salmonella* species.

    E. *Vibrio cholerae*, *Campylobacter jejuni*, and *Proteus* species.

> Correct answer = B. Cholera toxin and *E. coli* LT are ADP-ribosyl transferases that cause elevated levels of cAMP. *Pseudomonas aeruginosa* exotoxin A ADP-ribosylates elongation factor-2 required for eukaryotic protein synthesis.

Other Gram-negative Rods

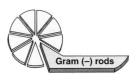
Gram (–) rods

16

I. OVERVIEW

Although not part of a closely related family, the organisms covered in this chapter do share two significant features of structure and physiology. First, they all have a gram-negative cell envelope, and thus contain lipopolysaccharide (LPS), which is a virulence factor. Second, they all are able to grow in the presence of oxygen, and therefore cause infections at sites where oxygen tension is high (for example, in the lungs, and other vital tissues). It is helpful to consider these organisms as follows: 1) those that are primarily or exclusively pathogens of the human respiratory tract (*Haemophilus*, *Bordetella*, and *Legionella*), 2) one genus that includes an extremely successful opportunistic pathogen (*Pseudomonas*), and 3) those that are primarily pathogens of animals (that is, zoonotic organisms such as *Brucella, Francisella,* and *Pasteurella,* for which humans are accidental hosts). Although *Yersinia pestis* is a member of the family Enterobacteriaceae (covered in Chapter 15), it is included in this chapter because it is a nonenteric, gram-negative rod. *Bartonella*, another unusual gram-negative rod that is responsible for trench fever and cat-scratch disease, is also described here. The organisms covered in this chapter are listed in Figure 16.1.

II. HAEMOPHILUS

Cells of *Haemophilus influenzae*—the major human pathogen of this genus—are pleomorphic, ranging from coccobacilli to long, slender filaments. *H. influenzae* may produce a capsule (six capsular types have been distinguished), or may be unencapsulated (Figure 16.2). The capsule is an important virulence factor. Serious, invasive *H. influenzae* disease is associated particularly with capsular type b (Hib), which is composed of polyribose phosphate. Hib is especially important as a pathogen of young children, although it can cause disease in individuals of all age groups. Nontypeable (unencapsulated) strains may also cause serious disease, and are a significant cause of pneumonia among the elderly and individuals with chronic lung disease.

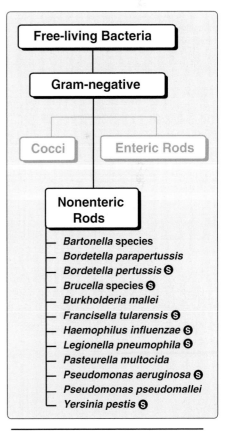

Free-living Bacteria

Gram-negative

Cocci | Enteric Rods

Nonenteric Rods

- *Bartonella* species
- *Bordetella parapertussis*
- *Bordetella pertussis* Ⓢ
- *Brucella* species Ⓢ
- *Burkholderia mallei*
- *Francisella tularensis* Ⓢ
- *Haemophilus influenzae* Ⓢ
- *Legionella pneumophila* Ⓢ
- *Pasteurella multocida*
- *Pseudomonas aeruginosa* Ⓢ
- *Pseudomonas pseudomallei*
- *Yersinia pestis* Ⓢ

Figure 16.1
Classification of other gram-negative rods. Ⓢ See pp. 401, 437 for summaries of these organisms.

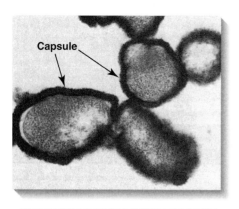

Figure 16.2
Haemphilus influenzae (electron micrograph) showing thick capsule.

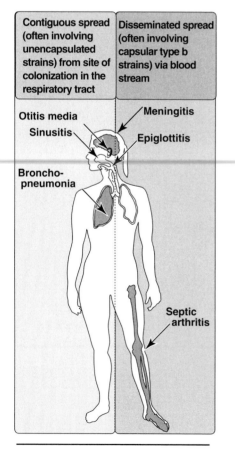

Figure 16.3
Infections caused by *Haemophilus influenzae.*

A. Epidemiology

H. influenzae is a normal component of the upper respiratory tract flora in humans, and may also colonize the conjunctiva and genital tract. Humans are the only natural hosts, and colonization begins shortly after birth, with unencapsulated strains and capsular type b being carried most frequently. *H. influenzae* illnesses are usually sporadic in occurrence.

B. Pathogenesis

H. influenzae is transmitted by respiratory droplets. IgA protease produced by the organism degrades secretory IgA, thus facilitating colonization of the upper respiratory tract mucosa. From this site, *H. influenzae* can enter the bloodstream and disseminate to distant sites. Diseases caused by *H. influenzae* therefore fall into two categories (Figure 16.3). First, disorders such as otitis media, sinusitis, epiglottitis, and bronchopneumonia result from contiguous spread of the organism from its site of colonization in the respiratory tract. Second, disorders such as meningitis, septic arthritis, and cellulitis result from invasion of the bloodstream, followed by localization of *H. influenzae* in other areas of the body. Contiguous spread is more commonly associated with unencapsulated strains in a setting where there has been a breakdown in natural host defenses, whereas severe, invasive disease is more commonly associated with encapsulated type b strains.

C. Clinical significance

H. influenzae has been a leading cause of **bacterial meningitis**, primarily in infants and very young children, frequently in conjunction with an episode of otitis media. A vaccine against *H. influenzae* type B, administered to infants, has dramatically decreased the frequency of such infections (see p. 37). Clinically, *H. influenzae* meningitis is indistinguishable from other purulent meningitides, and may be gradual in onset or fulminant (sudden onset with great severity). Mortality is high in untreated patients, but appropriate therapy reduces mortality to about five percent. Survivors may be left with permanent neurologic sequelae. **Epiglottitis** (cellulitis of the epiglottis and surrounding tissues) is a rare but life-threatening condition, primarily of younger children, for whom death may result from either airway obstruction or sepsis. Other presentations include **bacteremia** (which may result in **cellulitis** or **septic arthritis**, or may occur without localized disease), **otitis media**, and **pneumonia**. *H. aegyptius* (sometimes referred to as an *H. influenzae* biotype, or the Koch-Weeks bacillus) infection can cause outbreaks of a **purulent conjunctivitis**, and may also cause a life-threatening bacteremia, **Brazilian purpuric fever**.

D. Laboratory identification

The diagnosis of *H. influenzae* infection must be considered in each of the conditions listed above. However, a definitive diagnosis generally requires identification of the organism, for example, by culture on chocolate agar. [Note: Laboratory culture of *H. influenzae* requires enriched medium containing X factor (hemin) and V factor (NAD$^+$).]

Isolation from normally sterile sites and fluids (for example, blood, CSF, or synovial fluid) is significant, whereas isolation from pharyngeal cultures is inconclusive. Rapid diagnosis is crucial because of the potentially fulminant course of type b infections. In cases of meningitis, Gram staining of CSF commonly reveals pleomorphic gram-negative coccobacilli (Figure 16.4). Type b capsule may be demonstrated directly in CSF, either by the capsular swelling (quellung) reaction (see p. 28), or by immunofluorescent staining (see p. 31). Capsular antigen may be detected in CSF or other body fluids using immunologic tests, such as latex agglutination, countercurrent immunoelectrophoresis, and radioimmune assay.

E. Treatment

When invasive *H. influenzae* is suspected, a suitable antibiotic (for example, a third-generation cephalosporin such as ceftriaxone or cefotaxime) should be started as soon as appropriate specimens have been taken for culture (Figure 16.5). Antibiotic sensitivity testing is necessary because of emergence of strains resistant to antibiotics commonly used to treat *H. influenzae* (for example, strains with β-lactamase-mediated ampicillin resistance). Sinusitis, otitis media, and other upper respiratory tract infections are treated with trimethoprim-sulfamethoxazole or ampicillin plus sulbactam.

F. Prevention

Active immunization against Hib is effective in preventing invasive disease, and also reduces respiratory carriage of Hib (Figure 16.6). The current vaccine, generally given to children under the age of two, consists of Hib polyribose phosphate (PRP) capsular carbohydrate conjugated to a carrier protein (see p. 37). Rifampin is given prophylactically to individuals in close contact with a patient infected with *H. influenzae*—particularly those patients with invasive disease (for example, *H. influenzae* meningitis).

G. Other *Haemophilus* species

H. ducreyi causes **chancroid** (**soft chancre**), a sexually transmitted ulcerative disease (see p. 239). In addition to the painful genital lesions, inguinal lymphadenopathy may occur. Untreated, this progresses to formation of a bubo (a swollen lymph node), which then suppurates (forms pus). Azithromycin is effective against *H. ducreyi* infections.

III. BORDETELLA

Bordetella pertussis and *B. parapertussis* are the human pathogens of this genus. The former causes the disease **pertussis** (also known as **whooping cough**), and the latter causes a clinically similar illness. Whooping cough is a highly contagious disease and a significant cause of morbidity and mortality worldwide (51 million cases and 600,000 deaths each year). Members of the genus *Bordetella* are aerobic. They are small, encapsulated coccobacilli that grow singly or in pairs. They can be serotyped on the basis of cell-surface molecules termed "**agglutinogens.**"

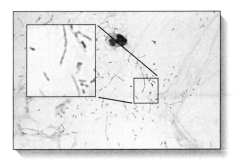

Figure 16.4
Haemophilus influenzae from spinal fluid. Gram-negative, pleomorphic bacilli and coccobacilli.

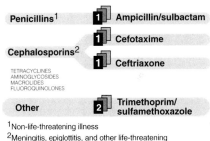

Penicillins[1]   Ampicillin/sulbactam

Cephalosporins[2]   Cefotaxime

Ceftriaxone

TETRACYCLINES
AMINOGLYCOSIDES
MACROLIDES
FLUOROQUINOLONES

Other   Trimethoprim/ sulfamethoxazole

[1]Non-life-threatening illness
[2]Meningitis, epiglottitis, and other life-threatening illness.

Figure 16.5
Some antimicrobial agents useful in treating infections caused by *Haemophilus influenzae*.

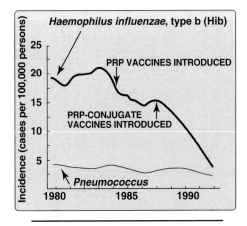

Figure 16.6
Incidence of *Haemophilus influenzae* type b meningitis in a pediatric population in the United States (compared to the nearly constant number of pneumococcal infections).

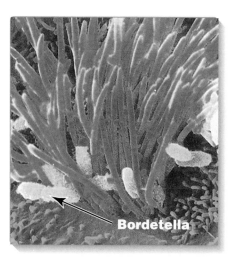

Figure 16.7
Ciliated cells of the respiratory system infected with *Bordetella pertussis* (scanning electron micrograph).

A. Epidemiology

The major mode of transmission of *Bordetella* is via droplets spread by coughing, but the organism survives only briefly outside of the human respiratory tract. The incidence of whooping cough among different age groups can vary substantially, depending on whether or not active immunization of young children is widespread in the community. In the absence of an immunization program, disease is most common among young children (ages one to five). Very young infants are at somewhat lower risk because of passive transfer of maternal antibodies. In such populations, the immunity generated in childhood is maintained in adults because of repeated exposure to the organism through cases in children. Widespread immunization markedly reduces the incidence of disease overall, but shifts the age distribution to adults who have lost the protection conferred by childhood immunization, and to young infants who have not yet been vaccinated.

B. Pathogenesis

B. pertussis binds to ciliated epithelium in the upper respiratory tract (Figure 16.7). There, the bacteria produce a variety of toxins and other virulence factors that interfere with ciliary activity, eventually causing death of these cells (Figure 16.8). These factors include: 1) **pertussis toxin**, a major virulence factor whose effects include lymphocytosis, sensitization to histamine, and activation of the insulin-secreting islet cells, leading to hypoglycemia. The toxin is comprised

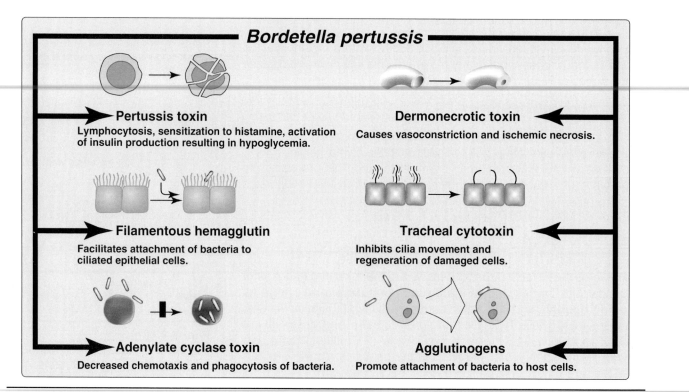

Figure 16.8
Toxins produced by *Bordetella pertussis*.

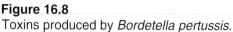

of a binding subunit, and an active subunit that catalyzes the ADP ribosylation of several host cell G regulatory proteins; 2) **filamentous hemagglutinin**, a protein that facilitates attachment of the bacteria to ciliated epithelial cells in the respiratory tract; 3) **adenylate cyclase toxin**, which is, in fact, adenylate cyclase secreted by *B. pertussis* that is taken up by leukocytes, resulting in the accumulation of large amounts of intracellular cAMP that interferes with leukocyte functions such as killing and chemotaxis; 4) **dermonecrotic toxin**, which causes ischemic necrosis when injected intradermally into suckling mice; 5) **tracheal cytotoxin**, which inhibits cilia movement and prevents regeneration of damaged cells, thus causing an accumulation in the lungs of mucus, bacteria, and inflammatory debris, leading at least in part to the severity of the whooping cough; and 6) **agglutinogens**, which contribute to attachment of the bacteria to host cells.

C. Clinical significance

The incubation period for **pertussis** generally ranges from one to three weeks (Figure 16.9). The disease can be divided into two phases: catarrhal and paroxysmal.

1. **Catarrhal phase:** This phase begins with relatively nonspecific symptoms such as rhinorrhea, mild conjunctival injection (hyperemia, or "blood shot"), malaise, and/or mild fever, and then progresses to include a dry, nonproductive cough.

2. **Paroxysmal phase:** With worsening of the cough, the paroxysmal phase begins. The name **whooping cough** derives from the paroxysms of coughing followed by a "whoop" as the patient inspires rapidly. Large amounts of mucus may be produced. Paroxysms may cause cyanosis and/or end with vomiting. [Note: Whooping may not occur in all patients.] Pertussis typically causes an elevated white blood count, sometimes in excess of 50,000 cells/μL (normal range = 4500–11,000 white blood cells/μL) during the latter part of the catarrhal or early paroxysmal phase. This reflects an increase in lymphocytes (both T and B cells), and a smaller increase in neutrophils. Following the paroxysmal phase, convalescence requires at least an additional three to four weeks. During this period, secondary complications such

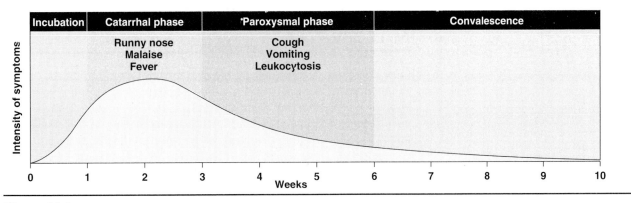

Figure 16.9
Clinical presentation of *Bordetella pertussis* disease.

as infections (for example, otitis media and pneumonia) and CNS dysfunction (for example, encephalopathy or seizures). Disease is generally most severe in infants.

D. Laboratory identification

Presumptive diagnosis may be made on clinical grounds once the paroxysmal phase of classic pertussis begins. Pertussis may be suspected in an individual who has onset of catarrhal symptoms within one to three weeks of exposure to a diagnosed case of pertussis. Culture of *B. pertussis* from the nasopharynx of a symptomatic patient supports the diagnosis. The organism produces pinpoint colonies in three to six days on selective agar medium, for example, one that contains blood and charcoal (which serves to absorb and/or neutralize inhibitory substances), and is supplemented with antibiotics to inhibit growth of normal flora.] More rapid diagnosis may be accomplished using a direct fluorescent antibody (DFA) test to detect *B. pertussis* in smears of nasopharyngeal specimens. In combination, culture and DFA offer fifty to eighty percent diagnostic sensitivity. Serologic tests for antibodies to *B. pertussis* are primarily useful for epidemiologic surveys.

E. Treatment

Erythromycin is the drug of choice for infections with *B. pertussis*, both as chemotherapy (where it reduces both the duration and severity of disease), and as chemoprophylaxis for household contacts (Figure 16.11). [Note: Supportive therapy is also very important during the paroxysmal phase.] For erythromycin treatment failures, trimethoprim-sulfamethoxazole is an alternative choice.

F. Prevention

Two forms of vaccine are currently available that have had a significant effect on lowering the incidence of whooping cough. One form consists of killed whole cells, and a second form is acellular, containing proteins purified from *B. pertussis*. Both are formulated in combination with diphtheria and tetanus toxoids (see p. 41). To protect infants who are at greatest risk of life-threatening *B. pertussis* disease, immunization is generally initiated when the infant is two months old.

IV. LEGIONELLA

Legionellaceae are facultative intracellular parasites that cause primarily respiratory tract infections. In nature, *Legionella* cells are unencapsulated, relatively slender rods; however, in clinical material, they appear coccobacillary in shape (Figure 16.12). Members of the Legionellaceae family are aerobic and fastidious, and have a particular requirement for L-cysteine.

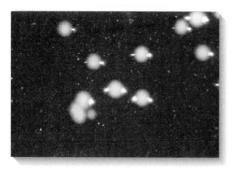

Figure 16.10
Pure culture of *Bordetella pertussis* on Regan-Lowe medium after 72 hours of incubation.

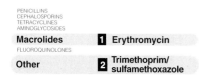

Figure 16.11
Some antimicrobial agents useful in therapy of infections caused by *Bordetella pertussis*.

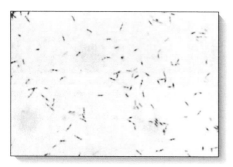

Figure 16.12
Gram stain of *Legionella pneumophila* obtained from pure culture.

A. Epidemiology

The Legionellaceae family includes 34 species whose normal habitat is water and soil, and which can colonize cooling towers and water distribution systems. About 85 to 90 percent of human disease is caused by a single species, *Legionella pneumophila*. Most infections result from inhalation of aerosolized organisms, but occasionally may follow other exposures (for example, swimming in contaminated water). Both sporadic cases and localized outbreaks may occur. One famous outbreak occurred in 1976 during a convention of American Legion members (hence the name, *Legionella*). The organism is chlorine tolerant, and thus survives water treatment procedures.

B. Pathogenesis

The organism gains entry to the upper respiratory tract by aspiration of water containing the organism, or by inhalation of a contaminated aerosol. Failure to clear the organisms permits them to reach the lungs. [Note: Such failure is more common in hosts that are already ill, for example, those with diabetes or pulmonary compromise.] Alveolar macrophages in the lung bed normally constitute an important line of defense for clearing invading organisms. Although the macrophages do phagocytose *L. pneumophila*, the resulting phagosome fails to fuse with a lysosome. Instead, the organisms multiply within the protected environment of the phagosome until the cell ruptures, releasing a new crop of bacteria.

C. Clinical significance

Legionellaceae primarily cause respiratory tract infections. There are two distinctly different presentations: Legionnaires' disease and Pontiac fever. The factors that determine which presentation will occur are not understood, although the condition of the host likely plays a role.

1. **Legionnaires' disease (LD):** This is an atypical, acute lobar pneumonia with multisystem symptoms. It may occur sporadically or in outbreaks (for example, nosocomial outbreaks have occurred). Predisposing factors include immunocompromise (for example, immunosuppressive therapy), pulmonary compromise (for example, heavy smoking or chronic lung disease), consumption of large amounts of alcohol, and debilitation brought on by age or surgery. LD typically develops in only one to five percent of individuals exposed to a common source. Legionellae are estimated to cause one to five percent of the cases of community-acquired pneumonias in adults (Figure 16.13). The case fatality rate for LD ranges from five to thirty percent, a high rate that may reflect the fact that many LD patients have additional contributing factors as listed above. Symptoms develop after an incubation period ranging from two to ten days. Early symptoms may be relatively nonspecific: fever, malaise, myalgia, anorexia, and/or headache. The severity and range of symptoms associated with LD vary substantially. A cough that is only slightly productive then appears, sometimes with respiratory compromise. Diarrhea (watery rather than bloody stools) occurs in 25 to 50 percent of cases. Nausea, vomiting, and neurologic symptoms may also occur.

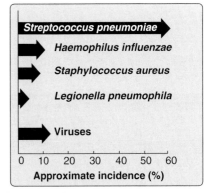

Figure 16.13
Some common pathogens causing community-acquired pneumonia.

2. Pontiac fever: This is an influenza-like illness that characteristically infects otherwise healthy individuals. The attack rate among those exposed to a common source is typically ninety percent or more. Recovery is usually complete within one week. No specific therapy is required.

3. Nonrespiratory infections: Legionellaceae occasionally cause a small number of nonrespiratory infections. These include wound infections following immersion of a wound in contaminated water, and infection of extrapulmonary sites as a result of hematogenous spread in a patient with Legionnaires' disease.

D. Laboratory identification

LD cannot be diagnosed unambiguously on the basis of clinical presentation or radiologic appearance of lungs. Although the organism can be Gram stained, the Gimenez stain is more useful for visualization. The definitive method of diagnosis involves the culturing of *Legionella* from respiratory secretions, using buffered (pH 6.9) charcoal yeast extract (BCYE, see p. 446) enriched with L-cysteine, iron, and α-ketoglutarate. Visible colonies form in three to five days. Other tests include: 1) direct fluorescent antibody test; 2) radioimmunoassay for bacterial antigen in the urine; 3) DNA probe for hybridization with legionella ribosomal RNA; and 4) detection of antibodies to legionella (this test is useful only for epidemiologic purposes because antibodies to legionella develop slowly).

E. Treatment

Macrolides, such as erythromycin or azithromycin, are the drugs of choice for Legionnaires' disease. Fluoroquinolones are also effective (Figure 16.14). Pontiac fever is usually treated symptomatically, without antibiotics.

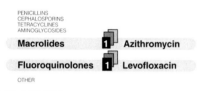

PENICILLINS
CEPHALOSPORINS
TETRACYCLINES
AMINOGLYCOSIDES

| Macrolides | **1** | Azithromycin |
| Fluoroquinolones | **1** | Levofloxacin |

OTHER

Figure 16.14
Some antimicrobial agents useful in therapy of infections caused by *Legionella pneumophila*.

V. PSEUDOMONAS

Pseudomonas aeruginosa, the primary human pathogen in the genus *Pseudomonas*, is widely distributed in nature (it is found in soil, water, plants, and animals). It may colonize healthy humans without causing disease, but is also a significant opportunistic pathogen, and a major cause of nosocomial (hospital-acquired) infections. *P. aeruginosa* is regularly a cause of nosocomial pneumonia, nosocomial urinary tract infections, surgical site infections, infections of severe burns, and infections of patients undergoing either chemotherapy for neoplastic diseases or antibiotic therapy. *P. aeruginosa* is motile (it has polar flagella), encapsulated, and obligately aerobic (it oxidizes but does not ferment carbohydrates). Nutritional requirements are minimal, and the organism can grow on a wide variety of organic substrates. In fact, *P. aeruginosa* can even grow in laboratory water baths, hot tubs, wet IV tubing, and other water-containing vessels. This explains why the organism is responsible for so many nosocomial infections. *P. aeruginosa* produces diffusible green and blue pigments (pyoverdin and pyocyanin, respectively), and may also produce red and black pigments. Figure 16.15 shows the rod-shaped cells of *P. aeruginosa*.

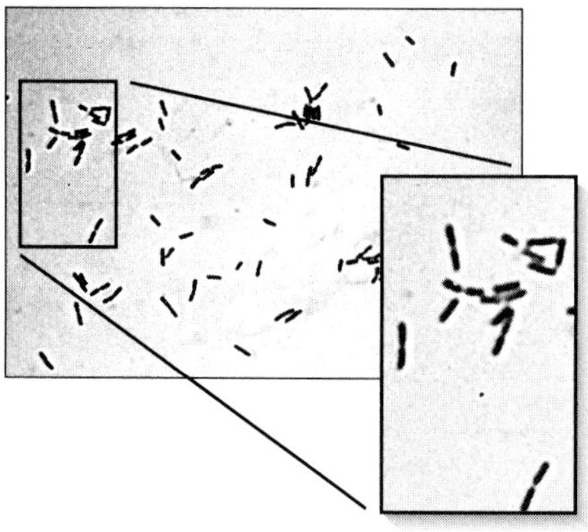

Figure 16.15
Micrograph showing the rod-shaped cells of *Pseudomonas aeruginosa*.

A. Pathogenesis

P. aeruginosa disease begins with attachment to and colonization of host tissue. Pili on the bacteria mediate adherence, and a glycocalyx capsule reduces the effectiveness of normal clearance mechanisms. Host tissue damage facilitates adherence and colonization. *P. aeruginosa* produces numerous toxins and extracellular products that promote local invasion and dissemination of the organism. These include extracellular proteases (for example elastase, alkaline protease), cytotoxin (formerly called leukocidin), hemolysins (phospholipase C and rhamnolipid), and pyocyanin. Systemic disease is promoted by an antiphagocytic capsule, endotoxin (particularly the lipid A moiety), exotoxin A (an inhibitor of mammalian protein synthesis that ADP-ribosylates elongation factor), and exotoxin S (that ADP-ribosylates specific GTP-binding proteins).

B. Clinical significance

P. aeruginosa causes both localized and systemic illness. Virtually any tissue or organ system may be affected. Individuals most at risk include those with impaired immune defenses. A prior treatment with antibiotics that eliminate normal flora can also provide *P. aeruginosa* with increased access for colonizing tissue.

1. **Localized infections:** These may occur in the eye (keratitis and endophthalmitis, following trauma), ear (external otitis or swimmer's ear; invasive and necrotizing otitis externa, particularly in elderly diabetic patients or trauma patients), skin (wound sepsis, Figure 16.16, purulent rashes occurring in epidemics associated with use of contaminated whirlpools, hot tubs, and swimming pools), urinary tract (particularly in hospitalized patients who have been subjected to catheterization, instrumentation, surgery, or renal transplantation), respiratory tract (pneumonia in individuals with chronic lung disease, congestive heart failure, or cystic fibrosis, and particularly in patients who have been intubated or are on ventilators), gastrointestinal tract (infections range from relatively mild diarrheal illness in children to severe, necrotizing enterocolitis in infants and neutropenic cancer patients), and the central nervous system (meningitis and brain abscesses, particularly in association with trauma, surgery, or tumors of the head or neck). Localized infections have the potential to lead to disseminated infection.

2. **Systemic infections:** Infections reflecting systemic spread of the organism include bacteremia (most common in patients whose immune system has been compromised by hematologic malignancies, congenital or acquired immunodeficiencies, neutropenia, severe burns, or diabetes mellitus), secondary pneumonia (particularly in patients with hematologic malignancies), bone and joint infections (in IV drug users and patients with urinary tract or pelvic infections), endocarditis (in IV drug users and patients with prosthetic heart valves), central nervous system (in already-compromised patients), and skin/soft tissue infections (erythematous necrotic lesions known as ecthyma gangrenosum, abscesses, cellulitis, bullae, and necrotizing fasciitis).

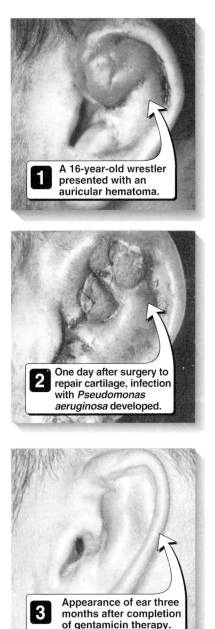

1 A 16-year-old wrestler presented with an auricular hematoma.

2 One day after surgery to repair cartilage, infection with *Pseudomonas aeruginosa* developed.

3 Appearance of ear three months after completion of gentamicin therapy.

Figure 16.16
Pseudomonas infection of the pinna of the ear.

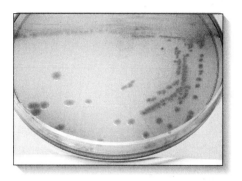

Figure 16.17
Pseudomonas aeruginosa cultured on MacConkey agar. Organisms grow as flat, blue-green colonies with distinct feathered edges.

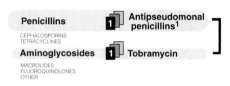

[1] Piperacillin, ticarcillin, ticarcillin + clavulanic acid, or piperacillin + taxobactam

Figure 16.18
Some antimicrobial agents useful in therapy of infections caused by *Pseudomonas aeruginosa*.

C. Laboratory identification

P. aeruginosa can be isolated by plating on a variety of media, both nonselective (for example blood agar) and moderately selective (for example, MacConkey agar, Figure 16.17). Identification is based on the results of a battery of biochemical and other diagnostic tests. Serologic typing is used in the investigation of clusters of cases, which may stem from exposure to a common source.

D. Treatment and Prevention

Specific therapy varies with the clinical presentation and the antibiotic sensitivity pattern of the isolate. It is difficult to find antibiotics that are effective against *P. aeruginosa*, due to its rapid development of resistance mutations and its own innate mechanisms of antibiotic resistance. *Pseudomonas* infections typically occur in patients with impaired defenses. Therefore aggressive antimicrobial therapy (often a combination of two bactericidal antibiotics such as an aminoglycoside, an antipseudomonal β-lactam, or a quinolone) is generally required (Figure 16.18).

E. Other pseudomonads

1. Burkholderia mallei

Burkholderia mallei (formerly called *P. mallei*) differs from *P. aeruginosa* and most other members of the genus *Pseudomonas* in being nonmotile. It is the etiologic agent of **glanders**, a serious infection that affects primarily horses, donkeys, and mules, but occasionally infects other animals and, rarely, humans. Human-to-human transmission can occur. In humans, the clinical presentation depends on the route of infection. For example, it may be 1) an acute, localized, suppurative infection (such as those of the mucous membranes leading to mucopurulent discharge and ulcerating granulomatous lesions, typically of the eye, nose, or lips), 2) an acute pulmonary infection (characterized by lung abscesses, or lobar or bronchopneumonia); 3) an acute septicemic infection, which is nearly always fatal; or 4) a chronic suppurative infection (characterized by multiple subcutaneous or intramuscular abscesses, often of the arms and legs). Culture and serologic tests are useful diagnostically. Treatment depends on presentation and the results of sensitivity testing.

2. Pseudomonas pseudomallei

P. pseudomallei is a normal inhabitant of soil and water. It is endemic to southeast Asia, as well as parts of Africa and the Middle East. Transmission occurs when the organism is introduced into wounds or abrasions of the skin, and may also occur through inhalation or ingestion. Rare instances of human-to-human transmission have been described. Although exposure to the organism in endemic areas may be common (based on seroconversion rates), the disease caused by the organism, **melioidosis**, is much less common. Melioidosis has varied presentations similar to those described for *B. mallei*. Culture and serologic tests are useful diagnostically, although negative serology does not rule out infection. Treatment depends on presentation and the results of sensitivity testing.

VI. BRUCELLA

Members of the genus *Brucella* are primarily pathogens of animals (domestic and feral). Thus, **brucellosis (undulant fever)** is a **zoonosis** (a disease of animals that may be transmitted to humans under natural conditions). Different species of *Brucella* are each associated with particular animal species, for example, *B. abortus* (cattle), *B. melitensis* (goats and sheep), *B. suis* (swine), *B. canis* (dogs), *B. ovis* (sheep), etc. All but *B. ovis* are known to cause disease in humans. The brucellae are aerobic, facultative, intracellular parasites that can survive and multiply within host phagocytes. Cells of the genus *Brucella* are unencapsulated, small coccobacilli arranged singly or in pairs (Figure 16.19). Lipopolysaccharide is the major virulence factor as well as the major cell wall antigen.

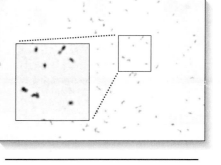

Figure 16.19
Gram stain of *Brucella melitensis.*

A. Epidemiology

Brucellosis is a chronic, life-long infection in animals. Organisms localize in reproductive organs (male and female), and are shed in large numbers in milk, urine, and the placenta and other tissues discharged during delivery or spontaneous abortion. The primary manifestations of infection in animals are sterility and abortion. Transmission to humans characteristically occurs as a result of either direct contact with infected animal tissues or ingestion of unpasteurized milk or milk products (Figure 16.20). [Note: Although *Brucella* occurs throughout the world, it is rare in the United States due to pasteurization of milk—a process that kills the organism.] Brucellosis is also an occupational risk for laboratory personnel working with these organisms. Because few organisms are found in muscle, meat products are rarely sources of infection. Human-to-human transmission is rare; outbreaks within families generally reflect common food source exposure.

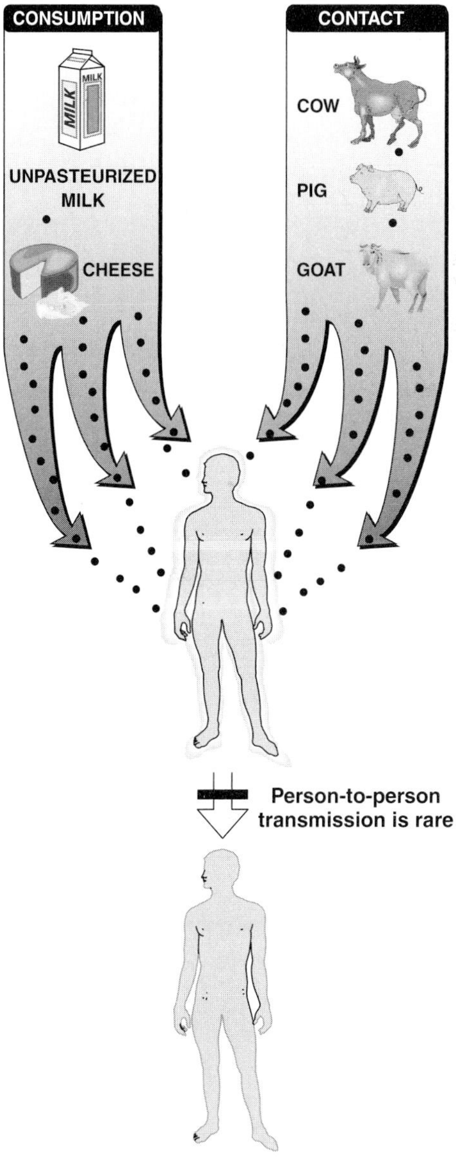

B. Pathogenesis

Brucellae typically enter the body through cuts and abrasions in the skin, or through the GI tract. [Note: Drugs that decrease gastric acidity may increase the likelihood of transmission via the GI route.] Inhalation of infected aerosols can also lead to disease among abattoir workers. Once the organisms gain entry, they are transported via the lymphatic system to the regional lymph nodes, where they multiply. The organisms are then carried by the blood to organs that are involved in the reticuloendothelial system, including the liver, spleen, kidneys, bone marrow, and other lymph nodes.

C. Clinical significance

The incubation period for *Brucella* infections can range from five days to several months, but typically lasts several weeks. Symptoms are nonspecific and flu-like (malaise, fever, sweats, anorexia and GI symptoms, headache, and back pains), and may also include depression. Their onset may be abrupt or insidious. Objective clinical findings are often few and mild, in contrast to the patient's subjective evaluation. Untreated, patients may develop an undulating pattern of fever (their temperatures repeatedly rise then fall, hence the name "**undulant fever**" as the traditional name for brucellosis).

Figure 16.20
Transmission of *Brucella.*

Subclinical infections occur. Manifestations of brucellosis may involve any of a variety of organ systems including the GI tract, and the skeletal, neurologic, cardiovascular, and pulmonary systems.

D. Laboratory identification

Although the nonspecific symptoms may not point to a diagnosis of brucellosis, a detailed history is often crucial, including the patient's occupation, exposure to animals, travel to countries where brucella infection is prevalent, or ingestion of potentially contaminated foods. The organism can be cultured from blood and other body fluids, or from tissue specimens. Multiple blood specimens should be cultured. For plated materials, colonies may appear in four to five days; however, longer times are required for blood cultures, and these are routinely examined for up to one month before being declared negative. Because isolation of organisms is difficult and time consuming, and there are no rapid diagnostic methods available, brucellosis is a disease for which serologic tests for agglutinating antibodies are diagnostically useful. Titers greater than 1:160 and rising are considered indicative of brucella infection.

E. Treatment

Combination therapy involving doxycycline and gentamicin (or streptomycin) is generally recommended for brucellosis (Figure 16.21). Prolonged treatment (for example, six weeks) is generally necessary to prevent relapse, and to reduce the incidence of complications.

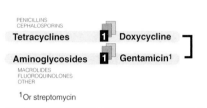

PENICILLINS
CEPHALOSPORINS

Tetracyclines 🔳 **Doxycycline**

Aminoglycosides 🔳 **Gentamicin**[1]

MACROLIDES
FLUOROQUINOLONES
OTHER

[1]Or streptomycin

Figure 16.21
Some combinations of antimicrobial agents useful in treating infections caused by Brucella.

VII. FRANCISELLA TULARENSIS

Francisella tularensis is primarily a pathogen of animals. Thus **tularemia** (also known as **rabbit fever** and **deerfly fever**) is a **zoonosis**. The cells are small, pleomorphic coccobacilli that possess a lipid-rich capsule, which, although nontoxic, may be a virulence factor (Figure 16.22). Members of the genus *Francisella* are facultative intracellular parasites that can survive and multiply within host macrophages as well as in other types of cells. The organisms are strict aerobes.

A. Epidemiology

The host range of *F. tularensis* is broad, and includes wild and domestic mammals, birds, and house pets. A number of biting or blood-sucking arthropods (for example, ticks, lice, and mites) can serve as vectors. [Note: Ticks can also serve as reservoirs of the organism, passing the bacteria to progeny via their eggs (**transovarian transmission**).] Infection of humans occurs as a result of contact with infected animal tissues (Figure 16.23), or the bite of an infected arthropod. Within particular geographic regions, specific vertebrates and invertebrate vectors are associated with transmission. For example, in the United States, the major (but not exclusive) endemic tularemic area encompasses Arkansas, Missouri, and Oklahoma. Incidence is most common in the summer months, a fact that reflects the arthropod transmission of the disease. During the

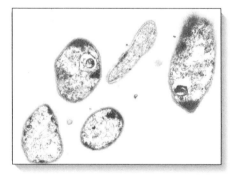

Figure 16.22
Electron micrograph showing the pleomorphic cells of *Francisella tularenis*.

winter months, a smaller peak incidence occurs, which reflects exposure of hunters to infected animal carcasses. Infection is also more common in males (they have a greater exposure risk). Tularemia is an occupational risk for veterinarians, hunters and trappers, domestic livestock workers, and meat handlers. Recreational activities that increase exposure to ticks and biting flies also increase the risk of acquiring tularemia.

B. Pathogenesis

In cases involving cutaneous inoculation, the organism multiplies locally for three to five days. It typically produces a papule that ulcerates after several days, and may persist for weeks or longer. Organisms spread from the local lesion to the regional lymph nodes, where they cause enlarged, tender nodes that may suppurate. From the lymph nodes, the organisms spread via the lymphatic system to various organs and tissues, including lungs, liver, spleen, kidneys, and the CNS.

C. Clinical significance

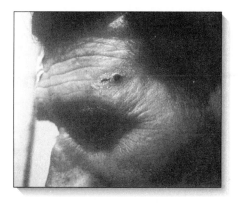

Figure 16.23
Tularemia in muskrat trapper. The healing ulcer above the patient's left eyebrow is the site of entry of *Francisella tularensis.*

Tularemia varies in severity from mild to fulminant and fatal. Clinical presentation, infectious dose, and length of the incubation period depend on the virulence of the organism, the portal of entry, and host immunity. Onset of symptoms is usually abrupt. The most common symptoms are flu-like (chills, fever, headache, malaise, anorexia, and fatigue), although respiratory and gastrointestinal symptoms may also occur.

1. **Ulceroglandular tularemia:** The most common presentation of tularemia is ulceroglandular. Ulcers may result from contact with contaminated animal products (typically on the hands and/or forearms), or from insect bites (commonly on the trunk and/or lower extremities). Multiple lesions may occur. The location of affected lymph nodes also reflects the type of exposure. Lymphadenopathy is characteristic.

2. **Other forms of tularemia:** Tularemia characterized by lymphadenopathy without evidence of ulceration is known as **glandular tularemia**. In these cases, the ulcer may have been minimal or have healed prior to the patient's having sought medical attention. In **oculoglandular tularemia,** the organism gains entry through the conjunctiva, which becomes inflamed. In **pharyngeal tularemia**, the organism gains entry through the pharynx, and causes a severe sore throat. In **pneumonic tularemia**, the prominent feature of initial presentation is pulmonary. The pneumonia may be primary, a result of inhalation of infectious aerosols, or secondary, a result of hematogenous dissemination of the organisms from a primary site elsewhere in the body to the lungs.

D. Laboratory identification

Clinical presentation and history consistent with possible exposure is of primary importance in diagnosis. Results of routine laboratory tests are not specific to tularemia. The organism may be cultured from ulcer scrapings, lymph node biopsies, gastric washings, and

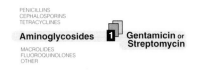

Figure 16.24
Some antimicrobial agents useful in treating infections caused by *Francisella tularensis*.

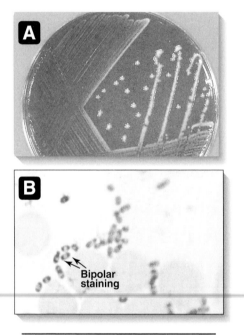

Figure 16.25
Pasteurella multocida. A. Culture on blood agar showing small, translucent, non-hemolytic colonies. B. Blood smear, Wright stain. (Note bipolar staining.)

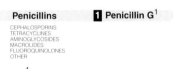

Figure 16.26
Some antimicrobial agents useful in empiric therapy of infections caused by *Pasteurella multocida*.

sputum, but rarely from blood. *F. tularensis* is nutritionally fastidious, and requires a sulfhydryl source such as cysteine. The organism is highly infectious, and laboratories must take special precautions when culturing specimens to avoid laboratory transmission. For this reason, the lab should be notified when there is a suspicion of tularemia. Confirmation of the clinical diagnosis is most commonly made serologically. Antibodies to *Francisella* can be readily detected by agglutination or ELISA tests (see pp. 30 to 31).

E. Treatment

The drug of choice for treatment of the forms of tularemia discussed above is streptomycin or, as an alternate, gentamicin (Figure 16.24).

VIII. PASTEURELLA

Members of the genus *Pasteurella* primarily colonize mammals and birds, both domestic and feral. Thus, pasteurellae infections are considered zoonoses. The major human pathogen in this genus is *Pasteurella multocida*, which can cause either disease or asymptomatic infections. Pasteurellae are coccobacilli or rods that often exhibit bipolar staining, and some strains are encapsulated (Figure 16.25). Virulence factors include the organism's capsule and endotoxin. Pasteurellae are aerobes/facultative anaerobes.

A. Epidemiology

The majority of pasteurellae infections in humans are soft tissue infections that follow an animal bite or a cat scratch. A smaller fraction of human pasteurellae infections occur either following a non-bite animal exposure, or in the absence of any known animal exposure. The source of pasteurellae in the latter infections is suspected to be nasopharyngeal colonization of the patient.

B. Clinical significance

P. multocida infection should be suspected in cases of acute, painful cellulitis that develop within 24 hours of an animal bite or cat scratch, or an infected animal licking an open wound. Soft tissue infections are characterized by the rapid onset of acute local inflammation within hours of the bite or scratch. Lesions often begin to drain within one to two days. Manifestations of *P. multocida* infection can include lymphangitis, lymphadenitis, fever, and local complications such as osteomyelitis or arthritis, which can result in extended disability.

C. Laboratory identification

Laboratory diagnosis (essential in non–bite/scratch-associated cases) can be accomplished by culturing the organism on blood agar, and performing appropriate biochemical tests.

D. Treatment

For soft tissue infections, wounds should be cleansed, irrigated, and debrided. Deep-seated infections require surgical drainage and prolonged antibiotic treatment. Penicillin is the drug of choice (Figure 16.26). Fatal infections are uncommon, and usually reflect underlying compromise.

IX. YERSINIA PESTIS

The genus *Yersinia* is a member of the family Enterobacteriaceae, which is presented in Chapter 15. The most clinically notorious member of this genus is *Yersinia pestis*, which causes **plague** rather than enteric disease, and therefore is being discussed separately from the rest of the family. In common with other yersiniae, *Y. pestis* is a small rod that stains bipolarly (Figure 16.27). It produces V and W antigens, which are virulence factors, as are its endotoxin and antiphagocytic capsule.

A. Epidemiology

Plague is predominantly a zoonosis with worldwide distribution. In the United States, the Southwest has been a primary focus of *Y. pestis* infection, although the distribution of human cases has been expanding into the Northwest and South-central states. The organism can infect a variety of mammals. For example, rats are common reservoirs in urban areas of some countries (**urban plague**). However, in the United States, plague is predominantly found in the wild, where prairie dogs and ground squirrels are the most important reservoirs (**sylvatic plague**). Household pets, particularly cats allowed to roam in plague-endemic areas, may also become infected. Plague is characteristically transmitted by fleas, which serve to maintain the infection within the animal reservoir. Humans are generally accidental and dead-end hosts. Plague can also be transmitted by ingestion of contaminated animal tissues, or via the respiratory route (**pneumonic plague**). [Note: The latter occurs either when organisms reach the lung and establish a secondary pneumonia, or following exposure to respiratory secretions from a patient or animal with plague pneumonia (Figure 16.28).]

B. Pathogenesis

Organisms are carried by the lymphatic system from the site of inoculation to regional lymph nodes, where they are ingested by phagocytes. However, the organisms are resistant to intracellular killing by phagocytes, and instead may multiply within these cells. Furthermore, the bacteria released from lysed phagocytes have synthesized a new envelope antigen that confers increased resistance to phagocytosis. The affected lymph nodes display hemorrhagic necrosis accompanied by high concentrations of both polymorphonuclear leukocytes and extracellular bacteria. Hematogenous spread of bacteria to other organs or tissues may occur, resulting in additional hemorrhagic lesions at these sites.

C. Clinical significance

Plague may present several clinically different pictures. Most common is the bubonic/septicemic form. Pneumonic plague may develop during epidemics. Less common presentations include

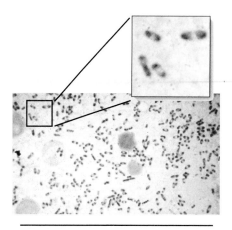

Figure 16.27
Gram stain of *Yersinia pestis*. This organism is typically seen as straight rods or cocobacilli. (Note bipolar staining.)

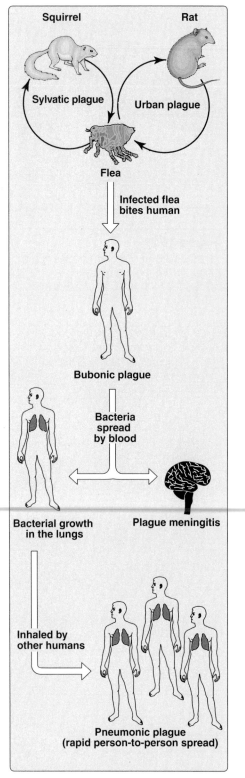

Figure 16.28
Epidemiology and pathology of plague.

plague meningitis (typically a secondary focus resulting from hematogenous spread of the organisms), cutaneous plague, and pharyngitis (the latter two generally acquired by handling or ingesting contaminated animal tissues).

1. **Bubonic (septicemic) plague:** The infectious cycle begins when a flea ingests a blood meal from an animal that is infected and bacteremic. *Y. pestis* produces a coagulase that causes the blood to clot in the flea's foregut. The organism multiplies in this environment. When the flea next attempts to feed, it regurgitates these bacteria from its foregut into the new animal's skin. The incubation period (from flea bite to development of symptoms) is generally two to eight days. Onset of nonspecific symptoms, such as high fever, chills, headache, myalgia, and weakness that proceeds to prostration, is characteristically sudden. Within a short time, a characteristic, painful **bubo** develops (Figure 16.29). Buboes (pronounced swellings comprised of one or more infected nodes and surrounding edema that led to the name "bubonic plague") are typically located in the groin, but may also occur in axillae or on the neck. As the disease proceeds, blood pressure generally drops, potentially leading to septic shock and death. Mortality of untreated bubonic plague generally exceeds fifty percent, with untreated and highly contagious pneumonic plague being invariably fatal unless rapidly treated. Other manifestations associated with bubonic plague include pustules or vesicles containing leukocytes and *Y. pestis*. Purpura and necrosis of extremities may occur during systemic disease. [Note: Ingestion of contaminated meat or exposure to airborne bacilli can result in primary lesions in the pharynx. These produce a severe tonsillitis and cervical buboes.] **Septicemic plague** is a variation in which the patient is overwhelmed by massive bacteremia before the characteristic buboes develop.

2. **Pneumonic plague:** If plague bacilli reach the lungs they cause a purulent pneumonia that, if untreated, is rapidly fatal. It is also highly contagious, and the organisms cause pneumonic plague directly when inhaled.

3. **Plague meningitis:** This results from hematogenous dissemination of organisms to the meninges. It may occur following inadequately treated bubonic plague or, like septicemic plague, may occur without or prior to development of a bubo. Organisms can be demonstrated in the CSF.

D. **Laboratory identification**

Diagnosis of *Y. pestis* infection may be made on the basis of clinical presentation. Laboratory identification can be initiated by a gram-stained smear, and culture of an aspirate from a bubo (or from CSF or sputum in the case of meningitis or pneumonic presentations). The organism grows on both MacConkey and blood agars, although colonies grow somewhat more slowly than do those of other Enterobacteriaceae.

E. Treatment and prevention

Streptomycin is the drug of choice; gentamicin and tetracycline are acceptable alternatives (Figure 16.30). For plague meningitis, chloramphenicol offers good penetration into the CSF. Because of the potential for overwhelming septicemia, rapid institution of antibiotic therapy is crucial. Supportive therapy is essential for patients with signs of shock. A formalin-killed vaccine is available for those at high risk of acquiring plague. For individuals in enzootic areas, efforts to minimize exposure to rodents and fleas is important.

X. BARTONELLA

Members of the genus *Bartonella* (formerly *Rochalimaea*) are facultative, intracellular parasites, and can be cultivated on special media in the laboratory. Three species have been implicated in human diseases.

A. Bartonella quintana

Bartonella quintana causes **trench fever**, an often mild, relapsing fever with maculopapular rash. The organism has a reservoir in humans, and its vector is the human body louse. The disease is therefore associated with humans living in poor sanitary conditions. Specific diagnosis can be aided by culture of clinical materials and by serologic tests. Broad-spectrum antibiotics are effective in the treatment of the disease (Figure 16.31).

B. Bartonella henselae

B. henselae was recently shown to be associated with most cases of **cat-scratch disease**, a syndrome that has been familiar to physicians for decades, but whose etiology had been elusive. The illness is characterized by small abscesses at the site of a cat (less commonly other pets) scratch or bite. This is followed by fever and localized lymphadenopathy. *B. henselae* is also responsible for several other types of infections, such as **bacillary angiomatosis**—a disease of small blood vessels of the skin and visceral organs—seen primarily in immunocompromised patients, such as those with AIDS. *B. henselae* infections are successfully treated with rifampin in combination with doxycycline (see Figure 16.31).

C. Bartonella bacilliformis

B. bacilliformis causes **Oroya fever**—a serious, infectious anemia in which the organism destroys red blood cells while causing damage to the liver and spleen. This disease is transmitted through the bite of a sandfly, and occurs primarily in regions of South America. Diagnosis can be made based on the appearance of blood smears. Treatment includes blood transfusion and administration of antibiotics (see Figure 16.31). Prevention involves controlling the sandfly population.

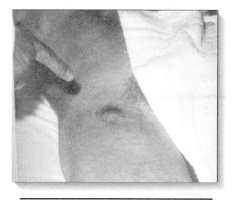

Figure 16.29
Bubo characteristic of infections due to *Yersinia pestis*.

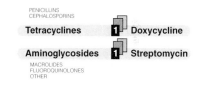

Figure 16.30
Antimicrobial agent useful in treating infections caused by *Yersinia pestis*.

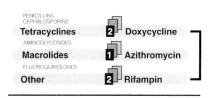

Figure 16.31
Some antimicrobial agents useful in empiric therapy of infections caused by *Bartonella* species.

Study Questions

Choose the ONE correct answer

16.1 Which of the following is true of *Haemophilus influenzae*?

A. Invasive infections are most commonly associated with encapsulated strains.

B. Most invasive infections occur in infants during the neonatal period.

C. Most human infections are acquired from domestic pets.

D. The organism can be readily cultured on sheep blood agar in an environment of elevated CO_2.

E. Older adults are rarely at risk for infection with this organism because they typically have a high level of immunity.

Correct answer = A. The capsule is antiphagocytic, and facilitates hematogenous dissemination of *H. influenzae*. Although *H. influenzae* is an important pathogen of infants and young children, passive transfer of maternal IgG may afford neonates protection. Immunity begins to wane in the elderly, increasing the risk of infection for this population. Humans are the only natural host for *H. influenzae*. *H. influenzae* requires both hemin (X factor) and NAD (V factor), which are not available in sheep blood agar. Heating the blood lyses the erythrocytes, releasing both X and V factors, and simultaneously inactivates an NAD-inactivating enzyme present in blood. Media made with such heated blood is termed chocolate agar. The organism does prefer elevated CO_2.

16.2 Which of the following organisms is typically transmitted sexually?

A. *Brucella suis*

B. *Legionella pneumophila*

C. *Yersinia pestis*

D. *Haemophilus ducreyi*

E. *Pasteurella multocida*

Correct answer = D. Brucella species are characteristically transmitted by contaminated dairy products or animal tissues. *Legionella pneumophila* is most commonly transmitted by inhalation of aerosolized organisms. *Yersinia pestis* is typically transmitted by the bite of an infected flea; less commonly by inhalation of aerosolized organisms. *Pasteurella multocida* is transmitted by an animal bite or cat scratch.

16.3 For which of the following organisms is there no known animal reservoir?

A. *Francisella tularensis*

B. *Pasteurella multocida*

C. *Bordetella pertussis*

D. *Brucella melitensis*

E. *Yersinia pestis*

Correct answer = C. *Francisella tularensis* has a broad host range, including wild and domestic mammals, birds, and house pets. *Pasteurella multocida* primarily colonizes mammals and birds, both domestic and feral. *Brucella melitensis* primarily infects sheep and goats. *Yersinia pestis* infects a variety of mammals.

16.4 Which of the following statements about *Bordetella pertussis* infection is true?

A. Infection causes a leukocytosis characterized primarily by a marked elevation in polymorphonuclear leukocytes.

B. Isolation of the organism from clinical specimens is greatest during the early stages of illness.

C. Clinical diagnosis of whooping cough can usually be made within a few days of onset of initial symptoms.

D. Children who receive a full series of immunizations with the pertussis vaccine generally develop solid, lifelong immunity to pertussis.

E. The organism can be cultured on standard laboratory media such as sheep blood agar.

Correct answer = B. *Bordetella pertussis* typically causes a lymphocytic leukocytosis. Initial symptoms of *Bordetella* infection are relatively nonspecific (rhinorrhea, etc.). The characteristic paroxysmal coughing begins somewhat later. Maintenance of solid immunity depends on repeated exposure to the organism, either through natural causes or by administration of booster shots. Growth of *Bordetella* requires a medium containing a substance such as charcoal to absorb or neutralize inhibitory substances, and also antibiotics that inhibit the growth of normal flora.

16.5 For which of the following organisms is human disease typically acquired by drinking contaminated, unpasteurized cow's milk?

A. *Brucella abortus*

B. *Francisella tularensis*

C. *Legionella pneumophila*

D. *Bordetella pertussis*

E. *Haemophilus influenzae*

Correct answer = A. *Francisella* is typically acquired either by the bite of a blood-sucking arthropod or by exposure to infected animal tissues. *Legionella pneumophila* is most commonly acquired by inhalation of aerosolized organisms. *Bordetella pertussis* is acquired by inhalation of aerosolized organisms. *Haemophilus influenzae* is a normal component of the upper respiratory tract of humans.

Clostridia and Other Anaerobic Rods

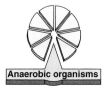

Anaerobic organisms

17

I. OVERVIEW

The organisms discussed in this chapter are all **obligate anaerobes** [that is, they are microorganisms that obtain energy exclusively by fermentation because they cannot utilize molecular oxygen (aerobic metabolism) for the production of energy]. They are also, in varying degrees, damaged by free oxygen, which limits the conditions under which these organisms can colonize the human body or cause disease. The obligate anaerobic genus, *Clostridium*, consists of gram-positive, spore-forming rods that are associated with soft tissue and skin infections (for example, cellulitis and fasciitis), and antibiotic-associated colitis and diarrhea. These organisms also synthesize some of the most potent exotoxins known. For example, the toxins of specific clostridial species cause botulism, tetanus, gas gangrene, and pseudomembranous colitis. A number of anaerobic, gram-negative rods and cocci such as *Bacteroides* and related genera are frequently involved in visceral and other abscesses, although these are generally polymicrobic (mixed) infections where some facultative bacteria are also involved. The organisms discussed in this chapter are listed in Figure 17.1. [Note: Other important anaerobic bacteria are discussed elsewhere in this book, for example, the anaerobic *Actinomyces* are discussed in Chapter 21.]

II. CLOSTRIDIA

Clostridia are the anaerobic gram-positive rods of greatest clinical importance. [Note: Other clinically important gram-positive rods are aerobic.] Clinically significant species of *Clostridium* include *C. perfringens*, which causes histotoxic (tissue destructive) infections (**myonecrosis**) and **food poisoning**; *C. difficile*, which causes **pseudomembranous colitis** associated with antibiotic use; *C. tetani*, which causes **tetanus** ("lockjaw"); and *C. botulinum*, which causes **botulism**.

A. General features of clostridia

Clostridia are large, gram-positive, blunt-ended rods. They form endospores, and the position of the developing spore within the vegetative cell is useful in identifying the species (Figure 17.2). Most species are motile.

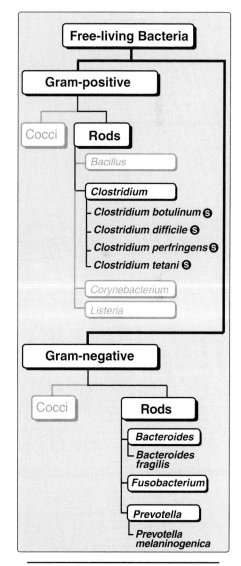

Figure 17.1
Classification of organisms in this chapter. ❺ See pp. 406, 442 for summaries of these organisms.

Lippincott's Illustrated Reviews: Microbiology,
by William A. Strohl, Harriet Rouse, Bruce D. Fisher.
Lippincott, Williams & Wilkins, Baltimore, MD © 2001

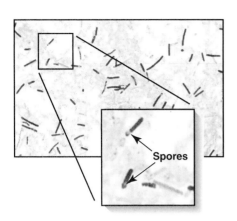

Figure 17.2
Clostridium difficile Gram stain. [Note subterminal non-staining spores.]

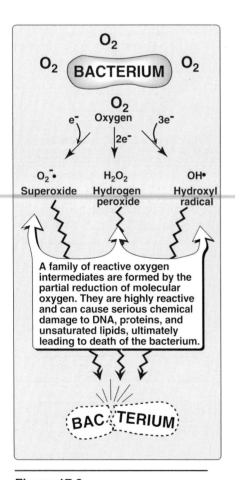

A family of reactive oxygen intermediates are formed by the partial reduction of molecular oxygen. They are highly reactive and can cause serious chemical damage to DNA, proteins, and unsaturated lipids, ultimately leading to death of the bacterium.

Figure 17.3
Toxic effects of reactive oxygen intermediates on anaerobic bacteria.

1. Physiology: Clostridia cannot use free oxygen as the terminal electron acceptor in energy production as do aerobic organisms (see p. 110). Instead, they use a variety of small organic molecules such as pyruvate as the final electron acceptors in the generation of energy.[1] In the vegetative state, clostridia are also variably inhibited or damaged by O_2 (Figure 17.3). [Note: The reasons for this damage are not entirely clear. One explanation is that these organisms produce oxygen radicals and peroxides, and some of them cannot detoxify these reactive molecules because they lack enzymes such as peroxidases, catalase, or superoxide dismutase[2].] Clostridia grow on enriched media in the presence of a reducing agent such as cysteine or thioglycollate (to maintain a low oxidation-reduction potential), or in an O_2-free, gaseous atmosphere provided by an air-evacuated glove box, sealed jar, or other device.

2. Epidemiology: Clostridia, including the potential pathogens, are common in the human environment. They are part of the intestinal flora in humans and other mammals, and are found in soil, sewage, and aquatic settings, particularly those with high organic content. However, a number of clostridial species can produce destructive and invasive infections when introduced into tissues, for example, by a break in the skin due to surgery or trauma. Their presence in infectious processes is opportunistic and often derives from the patient's own normal flora. Endospore formation facilitates their persistent survival in the environment because spores are resistant to chemical disinfectants, and may withstand ultraviolet irradiation or boiling temperature for some time, although not standard autoclaving conditions (121°C for fifteen minutes). In addition to causing infections and intoxications, clostridia also frequently occur as commensals or contaminants in clinical materials; they thus can complicate the interpretation of cultured samples from such sources.

B Clostridium perfringens

C. perfringens is a large, rod-shaped, nonmotile, gram-positive, encapsulated bacillus. It is ubiquitous in nature, with its vegetative form as part of the normal flora of the vagina and gastrointestinal tract. Its spores are found in soil. [Note: Spores are rarely seen in the body or following *in vitro* cultivation.] When introduced into tissues, however, *C. perfringens* can cause **anaerobic cellulitis**, and **myonecrosis (gas gangrene)**. Some strains of *C. perfringens* also cause a common form of **food poisoning**.

1. Pathogenesis: *C. perfringens* secretes a variety of exotoxins, enterotoxins, and hydrolytic enzymes that facilitate the disease process (Figure 17.4).

[1]See p. 95 in *Lippincott's Illustrated Reviews: Biochemistry* (2nd ed.) for a discussion of anaerobic glycolysis.
[2]See p. 114 in *Lippincott's Illustrated Reviews: Biochemistry* (2nd ed.) for a discussion of reactive oxygen intermediates.
[3]See pp.192 and 197 in *Lippincott's Illustrated Reviews: Biochemistry* (2nd ed.) for a discussion of phopholipases and lecithin.

a. **Exotoxins:** *C. perfringens* elaborates at least twelve exotoxins, designated by Greek letters. The most important of these, and the one that seems to be required for virulence in tissues, is **alpha toxin**. Alpha toxin is a lecithinase (phospholipase C[3]) that degrades lecithin in mammalian cell membranes, causing lysis of endothelial cells as well as erythrocytes, leukocytes, and platelets. Other *C. perfringens* exotoxins have hemolytic or other cytotoxic and necrotic effects, either locally or when dispersed in the bloodstream. *C. perfringens* strains can be grouped, A through E, on the basis of their spectrum of exotoxins. Type A strains, which produce both alpha toxin and enterotoxin, are responsible for most human clostridial infections.

b. **Enterotoxin:** *C. perfringens* enterotoxin, a small, heat-labile protein, acts in the lower portion of the small intestine. The molecule binds to receptors on the epithelial cell surface and alters the cell membrane, disrupting ion transport (primarily in the ileum), and leading to loss of fluid and intracellular proteins. Interestingly, enterotoxin-producing strains are unusually heat resistant, the spores remaining viable for over an hour at 100°C, thus enhancing their threat as enteropathogens.

c. **Degradative enzymes:** *C. perfringens* is a metabolically vigorous organism that produces a variety of hydrolytic enzymes including proteases, DNases, hyaluronidase, and collagenases, which liquefy tissue and promote the spread of infection.

2. Clinical significance

The disease processes initiated by *C. perfringens* result from a combination of infection with the production of exo- and/or enterotoxins and degradative enzymes.

a. **Myonecrosis (gas gangrene):** Clostridial spores are introduced into tissue, for example, by contamination with dirt, or by endogenous transfer from the intestinal tract. Severe and open wounds, such as compound fractures and other necrotizing injury (for example, in car accidents) are a prime predisposing condition. If the normal tissue oxidation-reduction potential is lowered, as occurs when there is considerable cell injury or compromise of circulation, the spores germinate and grow rapidly. These lesions almost always involve coinfection with several species of organisms, including clostridia and other anaerobes, and facultative species that use up available O_2, thus protecting the anaerobes from oxygen's toxic effects. Alpha toxin and other exotoxins are secreted and extensive cell killing ensues. The production of enzymes that break down ground substance facilitates the spread of infection. Fermentation of tissue carbohydrates yields gas, and an accumulation of gas bubbles in the subcutaneous spaces produces a crinkling sensation on palpation (**crepitation**), hence the name gas gangrene, although this finding is not unique to clostridial infections (Figure 17.5). The exudates are copious and foul smelling. As the disease progresses, increased capil-

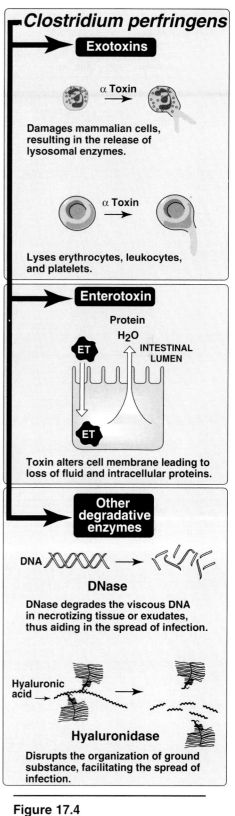

Figure 17.4
Toxins and degradative enzymes produced by *Clostridium perfringens*. [ET = enterotoxin.]

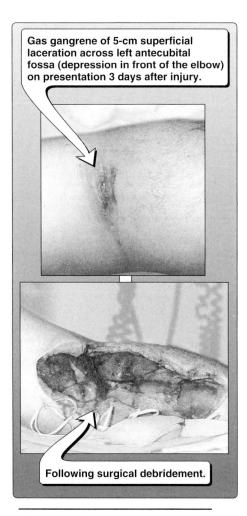

Gas gangrene of 5-cm superficial laceration across left antecubital fossa (depression in front of the elbow) on presentation 3 days after injury.

Following surgical debridement.

Figure 17.5
Gas gangrene of arm.

lary permeability leads to the exotoxins being carried by the circulation from damaged tissue to other organs, resulting in systemic effects such as shock, renal failure, and intravascular hemolysis. Untreated clostridial myonecrosis is uniformly fatal within days of the initiation of gangrene.

b. **Anaerobic cellulitis:** This is a clostridial infection of connective tissue in which the spread of bacterial growth along fascial planes (fasciitis) does not involve invasion of muscle substance. Necrotic processes play a more limited role, but surgical intervention is generally unsuccessful because of the rapidity of spread of the infection.

c. **Food poisoning:** *C. perfringens* is a common cause of food poisoning in the United States. Typically, the onset of nausea, abdominal cramps, and diarrhea occurs eight to eighteen hours after eating contaminated food. Fever is absent and vomiting rare. The attack is usually self-limited, with recovery within one to two days. Meat, chicken, fish, and their by-products are the most common vehicles for clostridial food poisoning, and the occurrence of clinical symptoms requires a large inoculum of 10^8 organisms or greater. Therefore a typical episode of clostridial enterotoxin food poisoning involves cooking that fails to inactivate spores, followed by holding the food for several hours under conditions that allow bacterial germination and several cycles of growth.

d. **Enteritis necroticans:** Outbreaks of a necrotizing bowel disease with high mortality (greater than fifty percent) caused by *C. perfringens* have been sporadically reported. The disease is known as pigbel in New Guinea and darmbrand in Germany, and a clinically similar illness is known, but unusual, in the United States.

e. **Clostridial endometritis:** This condition is a grave complication of incomplete abortion, or the use of inadequately sterilized instruments. Gangrenous infection of uterine tissue is followed by toxemia and bacteremia.

3. **Laboratory identification:** Diagnosis of clostridial myonecrosis or cellulitis rests largely on clinical impression. The presence of clostridia in clinical materials may be adventitious (that is, an accidental contamination). However, specimens from diseased tissue, when gram-stained, usually show vegetative clostridial forms (large, gram-positive rods), accompanied by other bacteria and cellular debris. Because of the extensive necrosis, intact host cells, including inflammatory cells, are rare in exudates. When cultured anaerobically on blood agar, *C. perfringens* grows rapidly, producing colonies with a unique double zone of hemolysis (Figure 17.6). Diagnostic tests are available for identifying characteristic clostridial biochemical reactions (for example, sugar fermentation, organic acid production, and the production of enterotoxin). In food poisoning, the organism can be sought in suspected food and patient's feces. Quantitative cultures are

required to show heavy growth (greater than 10^5 organisms/gram of food or feces), which suggests causal significance.

4. **Treatment and prevention:** The key to both prevention and treatment of gas gangrene is immediate and thorough removal of foreign material and devitalized tissue, and exposure of the wound to O_2. Hyperbaric oxygen chambers increase the tissue O_2 tension in the affected part, and probably inhibit the pathologic process. If debridement is unable to control the progression of the gangrene, amputation, when anatomically possible, is still mandatory in gangrene. Supplementary to this is the administration of antibiotics in high dose. *C. perfringens* is sensitive to penicillin and several of the common inhibitors of prokaryotic protein synthesis (Figure 17.7). [Note: It should be borne in mind that clostridial infections usually involve a mixture of species; therefore, a broad-spectrum approach is important.] The administration of antitoxin has not proven to be clinically useful, and such antisera are not presently available. Clostridial food poisoning is almost always self-limited, and requires only supportive care. Prevention is a matter of appropriate food handling practice.

C Clostridium botulinum

C. botulinum causes botulism, which occurs in several clinical forms. Botulism is caused by the action of a neurotoxin that is one of the most potent poisons known. It causes a flaccid paralysis. Contact with the organism itself is not required; hence the disease can be a pure intoxication.

1. **Epidemiology:** *C. botulinum* is found worldwide in soil and aquatic sediments, and the spores frequently contaminate vegetables, and meat or fish. Under appropriate conditions, including a strictly anaerobic environment at neutral or alkaline pH, the organism germinates, and toxin is produced during vegetative growth. Because the toxin is often elaborated in food, outbreaks frequently occur in families or other eating groups.

2. **Pathogenesis:** There are a number of types of botulinum toxin, designated A through G, but human disease is almost always caused by types A, B, or E. The botulinum serotypes and tetanus toxin constitute a homologous set of proteins whose neurotoxicity arises from proteolytic cleavage of specific synaptic vesicle peptides, causing subsequent failure of neurotransmission. In contrast to tetanus toxin, which causes constant contraction (spasms, see p. 214), botulinum toxins affect peripheral cholinergic synapses by blocking the neuromuscular junction and inhibiting release of the neurotransmitter, acetylcholine, thus preventing contraction and causing flaccid paralysis (Figure 17.8). [Note: In minute doses, botulinum toxin preparations have been used therapeutically to relieve spastic conditions such as post-stroke spasticity and strabismus.]

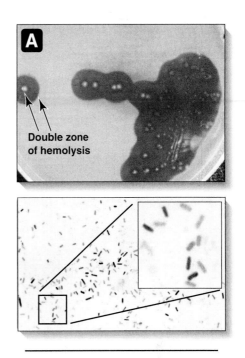

Double zone of hemolysis

Figure 17.6
Clostridium perfringens. A. Colonies on blood agar showing double zone of hemolysis. B. Photomicrograph of Gram stain.

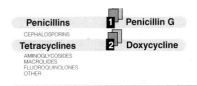

Penicillins	1	Penicillin G
CEPHALOSPORINS		
Tetracyclines	2	Doxycycline
AMINOGLYCOSIDES MACROLIDES FLUOROQUINOLONES OTHER		

Figure 17.7
Some antimicrobial agents useful in empiric therapy of infections due to *Clostridium perfringens*.

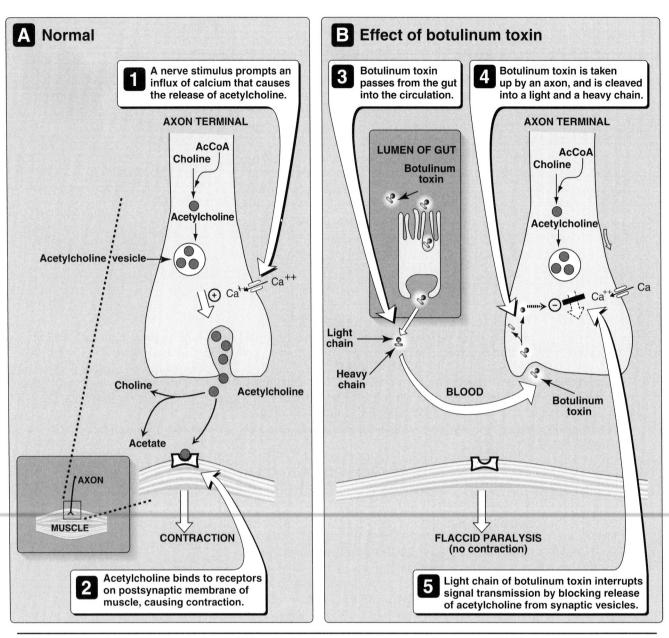

Figure 17.8
Mechanism of botulinum toxin. [AcCoA = acetyl-CoA.]

3. Clinical significance:

a. **Classic botulism** is a food poisoning in which a patient first begins to experience difficulties in focusing vision, in swallowing, and in other cranial nerve functions, 12 to 36 hours after ingesting toxin-containing food but not necessarily viable organisms. There is no fever or sign of sepsis. A progressive paralysis of striated muscle groups develops, and mortality is about fifteen percent, the patient usually succumbing to respiratory paralysis. Recovery is protracted, lasting several weeks.

b. Infant botulism: The most common form of botulism in the United States today is infant botulism or a cause of **floppy baby syndrome** (Figure 17.9). *C. botulinum* colonizes the large bowel of infants, 3 to 24 weeks of age, and the toxin produced is slowly absorbed. Constipation, feeding problems, lethargy, and poor muscle tone are common early signs. Certain formula supplements, such as honey contaminated with *C. botulinum* spores, may transmit the organism. The condition is possibly a cause of sudden infant death syndrome, but recovery is the usual outcome, following symptomatic treatment that may be prolonged.

c. Wound botulism: A rare form of botulism occurs when a wound becomes contaminated with the organism, and toxin is absorbed from that site.

4. Laboratory identification: The organism can be cultured and identified by standard anaerobic methods (see p. 25).

5. Treatment and prevention: Antitoxin, which neutralizes unbound botulinum toxin, should be administered as soon as possible in suspected botulinal intoxication. A trivalent (A, B, E) horse antiserum is available from the CDC. [Note: The risk of adverse reactions to horse serum must be kept in mind.] A variety of supportive measures, including mechanical ventilation, may be required. In wound botulism, the infection can be treated with penicillin or other antibiotics to which the organism is sensitive. This treatment has had ambiguous success in infant botulism. Non-acid, canned foods are the best known sources of botulinal food poisoning, with most cases associated with home processing. Other methods of food preservation, such as smoking, have also been implicated. The toxin is inactivated by boiling temperature, although killing of botulinal spores requires moist heat under pressure (autoclaving).

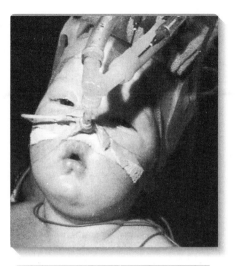

Figure 17.9
Infant botulism. Patient has ptosis (droop of upper eyelids) and dilated pupils. Nasograstic feeding tube is in place, and patient is on respirator.

D Clostridium tetani

The introduction of *C. tetani* spores into even small wounds via contaminated dirt is probably a common occurrence. But a combination of the extreme O_2 sensitivity of vegetative *C. tetani* and widespread immunization against its exotoxin, make the resulting disease, **tetanus**, rare in developed countries. In the United States, the disease is seen most often in older individuals who have not received their immunization boosters regularly, and whose immunity has therefore waned. Growth of the organism is completely local, but it produces a very powerful neurotoxin that is transported to the central nervous system, where it causes a spastic paralysis.

1. Epidemiology: *C. tetani* spores are common in barnyard, garden, and other soils. The most typical focus of infection in tetanus is a puncture wound caused, for example, by a splinter. Introduced foreign bodies or small areas of cell killing create a nidus of devitalized material in which tetanus spores can germinate and grow. Special circumstances may also lead to infection, for example, after severe burns or surgery. Illicit drugs often contain spores that

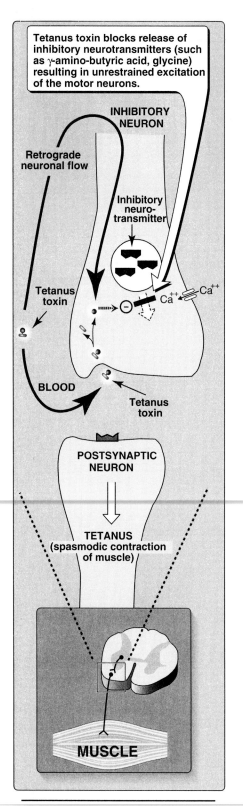

Figure 17.10
Mechanism of tetanus toxin.

are introduced by injection. In less developed countries, tetanus is a common complication of birth, where the umbilical wound becomes infected from unclean cutting instruments or dressings.

2. **Pathogenesis:** Tetanus toxin, called **tetanospasmin**, is an extremely potent toxin. It is transported from an infected locus by retrograde neuronal flow or by blood. It is a plasmid-coded exotoxin of a single antigenic type, and is produced as a single polypeptide that is cleaved to generate the mature toxin of two chains held together by a disulfide bond. The heavy fragment (B) mediates binding to neurons and cell penetration of the light fragment (A). The A fragment blocks neurotransmitter release at inhibitory synapses, and thus causes severe, prolonged muscle spasms (Figure 17.10). The A fragment has been shown to be a protease; it cleaves a small synaptic vesicle protein, synaptobrevin, and abolishes the flow of inhibitory neurotransmitters. [Note: Patients who recover from tetanus do not have an antibody response, presumably because the dose of toxin was too small to be immunogenic.]

3. **Clinical significance:** Tetanus has an incubation period varying from four days to several weeks. A shorter period is usually associated with more severe disease and wounds closer to the brain. Tetanus presents as a spastic paralysis, in which muscle spasms often first involve the site of infection. In the early stages of the disease, the jaw muscles are affected, so that the mouth cannot open (**trismus** or "**lockjaw**"). Gradually other voluntary muscles become involved (Figure 17.11), and any external stimulus (for example, noise or bright light) precipitates a painful spasm, and sometimes convulsions. Death, which occurs in fifteen to sixty percent of cases, is usually the result of paralysis of chest muscles leading to respiratory failure.

4. **Laboratory identification:** Because treatment must be initiated immediately, the diagnosis of tetanus is based largely on clinical findings. The focus of infection is often a trivial wound that may be difficult to locate. *C. tetani* has a characteristic morphology, with a long, slender rod and round, terminal spore (the "racquet-shaped" bacillus, Figure 17.12), and characteristic swarming growth on anaerobic blood agar. However, a smear or culture of clinical material does not always reveal the organism because the disease can be caused by relatively few organisms, and the bacteria are killed by oxygen if not properly transported and cultured.

5. **Treatment:** Prompt administration of antitoxin to neutralize any toxin not yet bound to neurons is the first order of treatment. Treatment with human hyperimmune globulin (tetanus immune globulin) is preferred, but in countries where it is not available, horse antitoxin is used. Vigorous treatment with sedatives and muscle relaxants to minimize spasms, and attention to maintenance of ventilation, are important. The organism is sensitive to penicillin, and this drug can be used to eradicate the infection. Prophylactic management of tetanus-prone wounds requires debridement and immunologic treatment appropriate to the patient's vaccination history as discussed below.

6. **Prevention:** Active immunization with tetanus toxoid (formalin-inactivated toxin) prevents tetanus. It is usually administered to children as a triple vaccine with diphtheria toxoid and pertussis antigens, called DPT. The currently recommended regimen calls for injections of infants at two, four, six, and eighteen months of age, followed by a booster upon entering school, at about age five years. Recent studies have confirmed that circulating antibody levels gradually decline, and that many older individuals lose protection. Therefore booster immunizations with a preparation of diphtheria and tetanus toxoids given every ten years throughout life are recommended. Tetanus immune globulin can be used to give immediate passive immunity to injury victims with no history of immunization. Active immunization should also be started. Antitoxin and toxoid, administered in different areas of the body, can be given simultaneously.

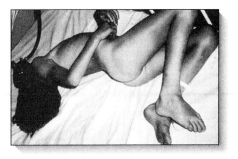

Figure 17.11
Tetanus with opisthotonos (muscle spasms causing rigidity of the neck and back, and arching of the back).

E. Clostridium difficile

Diarrhea is a common complication of antimicrobial and antineoplastic drug treatment, and it can range from loose stools to life-threatening **pseudomembranous colitis** (PMC, Figure 17.13). *C. difficile* is estimated to be responsible for about a quarter of **antibiotic-associated diarrheas** (AAD) in hospitalized patients, and almost all cases of PMC. Small numbers of *C. difficile* are part of the normal fecal flora in two to three percent of healthy adults. In hospitalized or nursing home patients, however, the organism is much more common. After its introduction to a site, the environment—dust, bedding, toilets—becomes persistently contaminated with spores, and new residents are easily colonized. They are then at higher risk for developing intestinal side effects of antibiotic treatments.

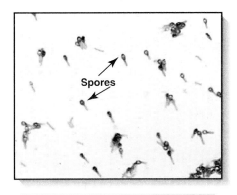

Figure 17.12
Photomicrograph of *Clostridium tetani* showing terminal spores.

1. **Pathogenesis:** *C. difficile* is a minor component of the normal flora of the large intestine. When antimicrobial treatment suppresses more predominant species in this community, *C. difficile* proliferates. Pathogenic strains produce two toxic polypeptides, designated A and B. Toxin A is an enterotoxin that causes excessive fluid secretion, but also stimulates an inflammatory response, and has some cytopathic effect in tissue culture. Toxin B is a cytotoxin; in tissue culture it disrupts protein synthesis and causes disorganization of the cytoskeleton. [Note: Both toxins are encoded by linked chromosomal genes.]

2. **Clinical significance:** Virtually all antimicrobial drugs have been reported as predisposing to clostridial AAD and colitis. The three drugs most commonly implicated are clindamycin, ampicillin and the cephalosporins. The severity of disease varies widely from mild diarrhea through varying degrees of inflammation of the large intestine to a fulminant PMC. The pseudomembranous exudate, composed of mucus, fibrin, inflammatory cells and cell debris overlying an ulcerated epithelium, is best demonstrated by endoscopy. Milder disease often lasts some time after cessation of drug treatment, or may reoccur. Infants born in a hospital are rapidly colonized by *C. difficile*, yet very rarely suffer diarrhea caused by this organism. It is postulated that in the immature large intestine, exotoxin receptors may not yet be present or accessible.

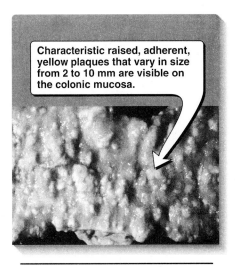

Characteristic raised, adherent, yellow plaques that vary in size from 2 to 10 mm are visible on the colonic mucosa.

Figure 17.13
Pseudomembranous colitis in a colon specimen obtained during a colectomy.

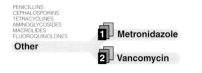

Figure 17.14
Some antimicrobial agents useful in treating infections due to *Clostridium difficile*.

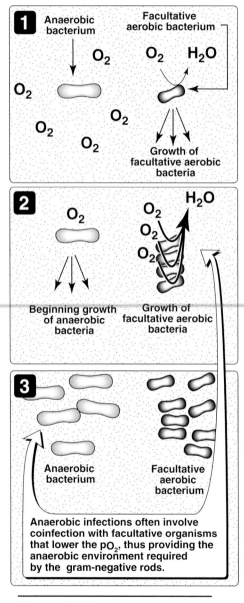

Figure 17.15
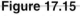
Anaerobic organisms' growth is facilitated by facultative aerobic bacteria.

3. **Laboratory identification:** *C. difficile* can be cultured from stools and identified by routine anaerobic procedures; however, the more rapid and useful tests are directed at demonstrating toxin production in stool extracts. Recently developed enzyme immunoassays (ELISA, see p. 30) for exotoxins A and B have largely replaced earlier immunologic or tissue culture cytotoxicity assays.

4. **Treatment:** Discontinuance of the predisposing drug, and fluid replacement, usually lead to resolution of the symptoms. Relapses, however, are common. Oral administration of metronidazole or vancomycin may be added in severe cases, or those with lack of response Figure 17.14).

III. ANAEROBIC GRAM-NEGATIVE RODS

Anaerobic gram-negative rods are normally the most common organisms in the oral cavity (particularly the gingiva), the female genital tract, and the lower gastrointestinal tract, where they outnumber *E. coli* 1000:1. They are therefore frequently recovered from infections in various parts of the body, for example, gram-negative anaerobic rods are recovered in about ten percent of bacteremias. Gram-negative rods generally constitute the majority of organisms associated with anaerobic abscesses. Organisms in this group may breach the host epithelial barrier and establish infection in any body tissue. This usually occurs because of trauma, an incident such as a ruptured appendix, or because of compromised immune status. A localized abscess is the most common lesion, and the infectious process often involves two or more species of organisms. For example, various facultative organisms help to lower the pO$_2$, thus providing the anaerobic environment required by the coinfecting gram-negative rods (Figure 17.15).

A Bacteroides

Members of the genus *Bacteroides* are the predominant anaerobes found in the human colon. They are part of the normal flora, and only cause disease when they gain access to the blood during bowel penetration, for example, during surgery or trauma. They are, however, the most common cause of serious infections by anaerobic organisms. Bacteroides are slender rods or coccobacilli. Their polysaccharide capsule is an important virulence factor, conveying resistance to phagocytosis.

1. **Epidemiology:** *Bacteroides* are transmitted from the colon to the blood or peritoneum following abdominal trauma. Thus the source of infection is endogenous (it is not transmitted from person to person).

2. **Pathology and clinical significance:** The major disease-causing bacteroides species is *B. fragilis*. [Note: *B. fragilis* has been divided into five subspecies, which are referred to more properly as the *B. fragilis* group.] The bacterial cell wall lipopolysaccharide has little or no endotoxic activity, but several enzymes (for example, heparinase, collagenase, etc.) probably contribute to tissue destruction.

When released from the colon into the blood, *B. fragilis* multiplies rapidly, causing bacteremia. If it is introduced into the abdominal cavity, *B. fragilis* causes peritonitis, and/or abdominal abscesses.

3. **Laboratory identification:** Exudates from mixed anaerobic lesions are often copious and noticeably foul smelling. Such material should be collected with the possibility of anaerobes in mind. Special anaerobic transport tubes are available to protect O_2-sensitive bacteria during transit to the laboratory, although many bacteroides strains are considerably O_2 tolerant. A Gram stain of such exudates shows numerous faint, slender gram-negative rods, usually in mixed flora. The organisms are easily obscured by debris and polymorphonuclear leukocytes. *B. fragilis* can be cultured on blood agar under anaerobic conditions. Gas chromatography can be used to identify the characteristic short-chain fatty acids produced by the organism, and biochemical tests can determine its sugar fermentation pattern.

4. **Treatment and prevention:** Drug resistance is common among the *Bacteroides*. Metronidazole is the antibiotic of choice for *B. fragilis* infections. Alternative choices include ampicillin-sulbactam, imipenem-cilastin, ticarcillin-clavulanate, chloramphenicol, cefoxitin, or clindamycin (Figure 17.16). Aminoglycosides are, of course, ineffective against anaerobes (see p. 45). Surgical drainage of any abscesses is essential to assure penetration of drugs. To prevent *Bacteroides* contamination of a surgical wound, a preoperative antibiotic such as cefoxitin can be administered.

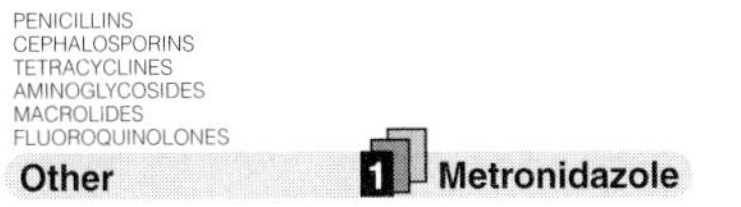

PENICILLINS
CEPHALOSPORINS
TETRACYCLINES
AMINOGLYCOSIDES
MACROLIDES
FLUOROQUINOLONES
Other　　　　　　**1 Metronidazole**

Figure 17.16
Some antimicrobial agents useful in treating infections due to *Bacteroides fragilis*.

B Prevotella

Prevotella melaninogenica is part of the normal flora of the mouth and upper alimentary and respiratory tracts. Its cell wall contains a strong endotoxin. *Prevotella* infections are usually associated with the upper respiratory tract, causing, for example, dental and sinus infections, pulmonary infections and abscesses, brain abscesses, and infections caused by a human bite. The source of these infections is generally the oral flora. Laboratory identification is similar to that of *B. fragilis*. In addition, *P. melaninogenica* forms black colonies on blood agar—a characteristic from which its name was derived. *P. melaninogenica* exhibits less drug resistance than do the bacteroides, and are usually susceptible to penicillin.

C Fusobacterium

Fusobacteria are spindle-shaped bacilli with pointed ends (Figure 17.17). They are found as part of the normal flora of the mouth, female genital tract, and colon. They grow slowly *in vivo*, and are therefore of limited virulence. These organisms are involved in a great variety of clinical presentations, for example, in peritonitis and abdominal abscesses, and can cause pelvic inflammatory disease, empyema (accumulation of pus in a cavity such as the thoracic cavity), bronchiectasis, a necrotizing aspiration pneumonia, brain abscesses, osteomyelitis, peridontal disease, and an inflammation of the tonsils known as **Vincent's angina** or "**trench mouth**".

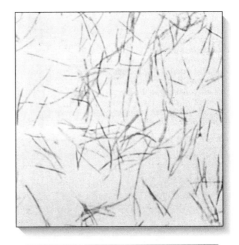

Figure 17.17
Fusobacterium nucleatum showing spindle-shaped bacilli with pointed ends.

Study Questions

Choose the ONE correct answer

17.1 The most common form of infection caused by *Clostridium botulinum* in this country is:

A. infant botulism.

B. wound infection.

C. food poisoning.

D. primary septicemia.

E. anaerobic cellulitis.

> Correct answer = A. Presently the most common form of botulism in the United States occurs in infants (A). Malignant food poisoning (C) was the first described form of infection, and is probably the best known; a wound focus is rare. *Clostridium botulinum* is noninvasive, and causes neither septicemia (D) nor cellulitis (E).

17.2 *Clostridium perfringens* infections are commonly associated with:

A. contamination of wounds.

B. antibiotic treatment.

C. consumption of water contaminated with sewage.

D. immunosuppression.

E. pre-existing lung disease.

> Correct answer = A. Contamination of wounds is the most common route of infection by this organism. However, the symptoms of gastroenteritis associated with some strains of *C. perfringens* are usually caused by the contamination of food.

17.3 Specific antitoxin is an important part of treatment in:

A. gas gangrene.

B. tetanus.

C. enteritis necroticans.

D. pseudomembranous colitis.

E. Bacteroides and Prevotella infections.

> Correct answer = B. Tetanus antitoxin (B) is an essential reagent in wound prophylaxis and the treatment of clinical disease. It neutralizes only that toxin that has not bound the neuronal receptors. In the case of gas gangrene (A), numerous clinical studies have shown no advantage in the use of antitoxin preparations; presumably the same would be true for enteritis necroticans and pseudomembranous colitis (C and D). Possible toxins among the gram-negative anaerobes are poorly described, and no therapeutic antisera are available (E).

17.4 A predisposing factor in pseudomembranous colitis (PMC) is:

A. clindamycin treatment.

B. neonatal age.

C. diet high in dairy products.

D. cholecystitis.

E. old age (more than sixty years of age).

> Correct answer = A. Antibiotic or antineoplastic treatment is often complicated by gastrointestinal disturbance, including PMC. Certain drugs, including clindamycin, are more likely to cause this complication.

17.5 The normal habitat of *Bacteroides fragilis* is:

A. soil.

B. birds.

C. cattle and dairy products.

D. human colon.

E. human upper respiratory tract.

> Correct answer = D. Other gram-negative anaerobes are common in the upper respiratory tract and mouth.

17.6 Which one of the following statements best describes *Bacteroides fragilis*?

A. These organisms are not found in the colon.

B. Infections by these organism are treated with aminoglycosides.

C. Infections by these organisms often produce a foul-smelling discharge.

D. These organisms are routinely culture on blood agar in room air.

E. Infections by these organisms produce severe neurologic symptoms.

> Correct answer = C. Exudates from mixed anaerobic lesions are often copious and noticeably foul smelling. Aminoglycosides inhibit bacterial protein synthesis. Susceptible organisms have an oxygen-dependent system that transports the antibiotic across the cell membrane. They are effective only against aerobic organisms because anaerobes, such as *Bacteroides* species lack the oxygen-requiring transport system. *B. fragilis* can be cultured on blood agar under anaerobic conditions. The bacterial cell wall lipopolysaccharide has little or no endotoxic activity, but several enzymes (for example, heparinase, collagenase, etc.) probably contribute to tissue destruction. Neurotoxicity is not a characteristic finding in infection by this organism.

Spirochetes

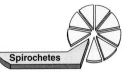

18

I. OVERVIEW

The spirochetes are long, slender, motile, flexible, undulating, gram-negative bacilli that have a characteristic corkscrew or helical shape. Depending on the species, they can be aerobic, anaerobic, or facultatively anaerobic. Some species can be grown in laboratory culture (either cell-free culture or tissue culture), whereas others cannot. Some species are free-living, and some are part of the normal flora of humans and animals. Spirochetes that are important human pathogens are confined to three genera (Figure 18.1): *Treponema* (*T. pallidum* is the cause of **syphilis**), *Borrelia* (*B. burgdorferi* causes **Lyme disease**, *B. recurrentis* causes **relapsing fever**), and *Leptospira* (*L. interrogans* causes **leptospirosis**).

II. STRUCTURAL FEATURES OF SPIROCHETES

Spirochetes have a unique structure that is responsible for their motility. As illustrated in Figure 18.2, the spirochete cell has a central **protoplasmic cylinder** bounded by a plasma membrane and a typical gram-negative cell wall. Unlike other bacilli, this cylinder is enveloped by an outer sheath composed of glycosaminoglycans.[1] Between the cell wall and the outer sheath are located multiple **periplasmic flagella** that do not protrude from the cell but are oriented axially. Bundles of these endoflagella, called **axial filaments**, span the entire length of the cell and are anchored at both ends. Although the mechanics are not totally clear, it is likely that these axial periplasmic flagella rotate like the external flagella of other motile bacteria, thereby propelling the cell in a cork-screw-like manner. Spirochetes can move through highly viscous solutions with little impediment, and it is theorized that this kind of motion is responsible for the ability of spirochete pathogens to penetrate and invade host tissue, just as a corkscrew penetrates cork.

III. TREPONEMA PALLIDUM

Syphilis is primarily a sexually transmitted disease caused by the spirochete *Treponema pallidum*. Starting with a small lesion (chancre), the several progressive stages of the disease can span a period of thirty

[1]See p.147 in *Lippincott's Illustrated Reviews: Biochemistry* (2nd ed.) for a discussion of glycosaminoglycans.

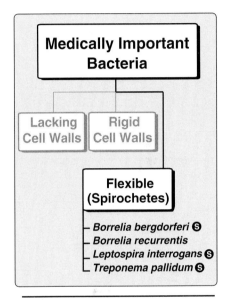

Figure 18.1
Classification of Spirochetes.
Ⓢ See pp. 404, 439 (*B. bergdorferi*), pp. 412, 447 (*L. interrogans*), pp. 422, 454 (*T. pallidium*) for summaries of these organisms.

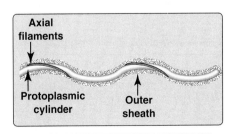

Figure 18.2
Spirochete morphology.

Lippincott's Illustrated Reviews: Microbiology,
by William A. Strohl, Harriet Rouse, Bruce D. Fisher.
Lippincott, Williams & Wilkins, Baltimore, MD © 2001

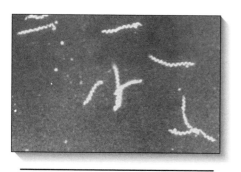

Figure 18.3
Dark-ground microscopy of *Treponema pallidum.*

years or more, often ending in syphilitic dementia (paresis) or cardiovascular damage. The causative organism of syphilis is extremely fastidious and fragile. It cannot be cultured routinely in the laboratory, and is very sensitive to disinfectants, heat, and drying. *T. pallidum* is so thin that it cannot be observed by conventional light microscopy, but requires immunofluorescent or dark-field techniques (Figure 18.3). The outer surface of the spirochete is very sparse in proteins, and the organism is only weakly antigenic. *T. pallidum* appears to produce neither endotoxins nor exotoxins, although it does secrete hyaluronidase, an enzyme that disrupts the ground substance, and probably facilitates dissemination of the organism.

A. Pathogenesis

Transmission of *T. pallidum* is almost always by sexual contact or transplacentally (**congenital syphilis**). This is understandable from the fact that the organism is so sensitive to environmental factors that survival outside of the host for more than a few minutes is highly unlikely. The organism enters the body through a break in the skin, or by penetrating mucous membranes, such as those of the genitalia.

B. Clinical significance

1. **Syphilis:** The disease syphilis occurs in three stages (Figure 18.4). The first symptom of **primary stage** syphilis is a hard genital or oral ulcer (**chancre**) that develops at the site of inoculation. The average period between infection and the appearance of the chancre is about three weeks, but varies with the number of infecting organisms. This primary lesion heals spontaneously, but the organism continues to spread throughout the body via the lymph and blood. An asymptomatic period ensues, lasting as long

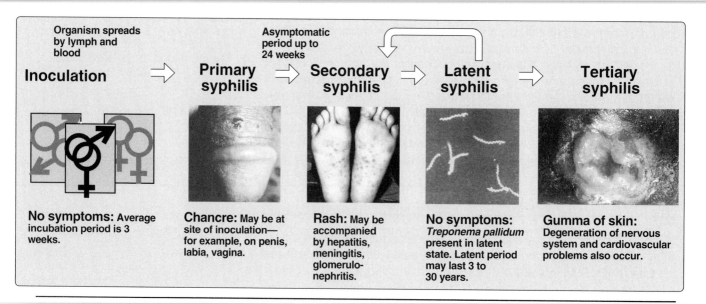

Figure 18.4
Clinical stages of untreated syphilis.

as 24 weeks, and is followed by the **secondary stage**. This stage is characterized by the appearance of a red, maculopapular rash on almost any part of the body, including on the palms of the hands and soles of the feet. Also present are pale, moist papules seen primarily in the anogenital region (where they are called **condylomas**), the armpits, and the mouth. Both primary and secondary lesions teem with *T. pallidum*, and are extremely infectious. The secondary stage may be accompanied by systemic involvement, causing hepatitis, meningitis, nephritis, or chorioretinitis. Upon healing of the secondary lesions, the disease enters a latent period that can last for many years. In approximately forty percent of infected individuals, the disease progresses to a **tertiary stage**, characterized by degeneration of the nervous system, cardiovascular lesions such as aneurysms, and granulomatous lesions (**gummas**) in the liver, skin, and bones. [Note: Some individuals remain asymptomatic through the primary and/or secondary stages, and yet develop tertiary syphilis.] Immunity to reinfection is quickly established in the early stages of syphilis, but is lost if the disease is treated successfully. In later stages, immunity is more long-lasting. Both antibody and cell-mediated immunity play a role in the acquisition of immunity, but in most cases are not sufficient to eradicate the disease.

2. **Congenital syphilis:** *T. pallidum* can be transmitted through the placenta to a fetus after the first ten to fifteen weeks of pregnancy. Infection can cause death and spontaneous abortion of the fetus, or cause it to be stillborn. Infected infants that live develop a condition similar to secondary syphilis, including a variety of central nervous system and structural abnormalities. Treatment of the pregnant mother with appropriate antibiotics prevents congenital syphilis.

3. **Other treponemal infections:** Three geographically localized treponemal diseases closely mimic syphilis. They include **bejel** (found in hot, arid areas of Africa, Southeast Asia, and the Middle East), **yaws** (found in humid, tropical countries, Figure 18.5), and **pinta** (found in South and Central America, Mexico, and the Phillipines). The causative organisms are *Treponema* species or subspecies that are morphologically and antigenically indistinguishable from *T. pallidum*, and the diseases exhibit primary, secondary, and tertiary stages similar to those of syphilis. However, unlike syphilis, direct skin contact, crowded living conditions, and poor hygiene contribute to the spread of these diseases. Sexual contact is usually not the mode of transmission, and congenital infections occur rarely if at all. All three diseases are curable with penicillin.

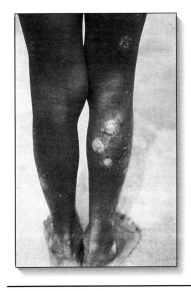

Figure 18.5
Yaws: early stage.

C. Laboratory identification

Although treponemal spirochetes from primary and secondary lesions can be detected microscopically using immunofluorescent stain or dark-field illumination (see Figure 18.3), syphilis is usually diagnosed serologically. Infection with *T. pallidum* elicits two kinds of antibodies: 1) antitreponemal antibodies that are specific to the treponemal surface proteins, and 2) nontreponemal antibodies, called **reagin**, that are directed against normal phospholipid compo-

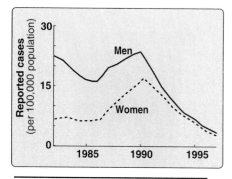

Penicillins   **1** Penicillin G[1]

CEPHALOSPORINS
TETRACYCLINES
AMINOGLYCOSIDES
MACROLIDES
FLUOROQUINOLONES
OTHER

[1]In cases of patient sensitivity to penicillin, alternate therapy with erythromycin or tetracyclines may also effective for some stages of syphilis.

Figure 18.6
Antimicrobial agents useful in therapy of infections due to *Treponema pallidum*.

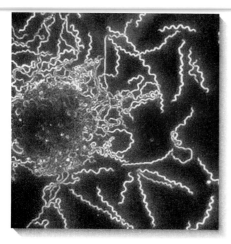

Figure 18.7
Incidence of primary and secondary syphilis.

nents—such as cardiolipin[2]—of mammalian membranes. Serologic tests utilizing both kinds of antibodies are available. Antitreponemal antibody tests are more specific than reagin-based tests, but remain positive during successful treatment, and are thus not useful for monitoring therapy. Cardiolipin-based tests are less specific, and are liable to give more false positives. They are nevertheless useful in screening and for monitoring therapy, because tests for reagin become negative about a year after successful treatment.

D. Treatment and prevention

A single treatment with penicillin is curative for primary and secondary syphilis, and no antibiotic resistance has been reported. In cases of patient sensitivity to penicillin, alternate therapy with erythromycin or tetracyclines may also be effective (Figure 18.6). In spite of an inexpensive and highly effective cure, there are still over 8000 new cases of syphilis in the United States each year (Figure 18.7). There is no vaccine against *T. pallidum*, and prevention depends on safe sexual practices. [Note: More than one sexually transmitted disease (STD) can be passed on at the same time. Therefore, when any STD has been diagnosed, the possibility of the infected individual also having syphilis should be considered.]

IV. BORRELIA BURGDORFERI

Members of the genus *Borrelia* are relatively large spirochetes, which, like the *Treponema*, have endoflagella that make them highly motile (Figure 18.8). *Borrelia* species are unusual among bacteria in that they have linear rather than circular plasmid and chromosomal DNA. Like *T. pallidum*, *Borrelia* do not appear to produce endotoxins or exotoxins.

A. Pathogenesis

Lyme disease is caused by the spirochete *Borrelia burgdorferi*, which is transmitted by the bite of a small tick of the genus *Ixodes* (Figure 18.9). [Note: The tick must be attached for at least 24 hours before there is transmission of the bacterium.] Mice and other small rodents serve as primary reservoirs for the spirochete, but deer and other mammals serve as hosts for the ticks. Lyme disease is currently the most common arthropod-transmitted disease in the United States, averaging at least 10,000 cases per year.

B. Clinical significance

The **first stage** of Lyme disease begins 3 to 32 days after a tick bite, when a characteristic red, circular lesion with a clear center (**erythema chronicum migrans**) appears at the site of the bite (Figure 18.10). Flu-like symptoms often accompany the erythema. The organism spreads via the lymph or blood to musculoskeletal sites,

[2]See p.192 in *Lippincott's Illustrated Reviews: Biochemistry* (2nd ed.) for a discussion of the structure of cardiolipin.

Figure 18.8
Dark-field microscopic image of *Borrelia burgdorferi* taken from a culture of the organism in the laboratory.

skin, central nervous system, heart, and other tissues and organs. Weeks to months after the onset, the **second stage** of the disease begins, with symptoms such as arthritis, arthralgia, cardiac complications, and neurologic complications such as meningitis. Months to years later, the **third stage** begins with the appearance of chronic arthritis, and progressive central nervous system disease. Lyme disease is rarely fatal, but can result in a poor quality of life if untreated. IgM antibodies, which are directed against flagellar antigens, appear early after the onset of the disease, whereas IgG antibodies appear later. These antibodies offer protective immunity to reinfection, but the immunity is lost if the disease is treated early and successfully. Although caused by different spirochetes, the general similarities in the progression of Lyme disease and syphilis are striking.

C. Laboratory identification

Unlike *T. pallidum*, *B. burgdorferi* can be cultured, but the procedure is difficult, and takes six to eight weeks. Serologic tests have been used to diagnose Lyme disease, but the number of false positives can outnumber the true positives. Such tests thus should be used only as confirmatory of a strong clinical suspicion. The most definitive test today is the polymerase chain reaction assay, which is rapid, sensitive, and specific (see p. 32).

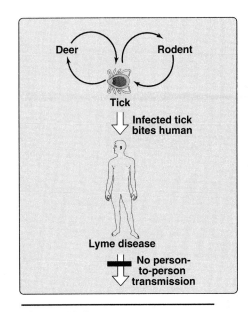

Figure 18.9
Transmission of Lyme disease.

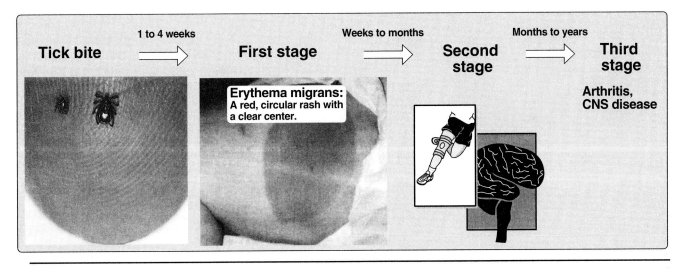

Figure 18.10
Clinical stages of untreated Lyme disease.

D. Treatment and prevention

Amoxicillin and doxycycline are useful treatments in the early stages of the disease (Figure 18.11). If arthritic symptoms have already appeared, longer courses of antibiotics are used. In 1998, a ninety percent–effective vaccine became available. Prevention of infection also includes use of insect repellents, and wearing clothing that sufficiently protects the body from tick bites.

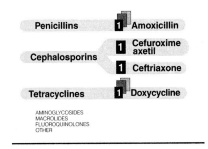

Figure 18.11
Summary of antibiotic therapy of Lyme disease.

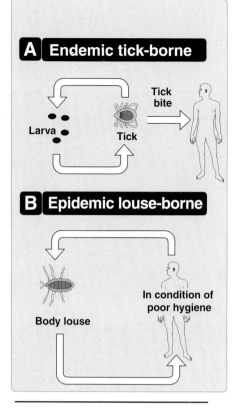

Figure 18.12
Endemic versus epidemic
relapsing fever.

V. BORRELIA RECURRENTIS

The spirochete *Borrelia recurrentis* is a large, culturable spirochete. The organism is responsible for the disease known as **relapsing fever**, which is characterized by several cycles of apparent recovery, each followed by a relapse. A most striking property of *B. recurrentis* is its ability to change its surface protein antigens. This ability accounts for the relapsing nature of the disease, because with each relapse a new antigenic variant arises.

A. Pathogenesis

A distinction is often made between **endemic** and **epidemic relapsing fever**. The endemic disease, which occurs in most areas of the world, is tick-borne (*B. recurrentis* is passed from the mother tick to her progeny), whereas the epidemic disease is transmitted from human to human by body lice (Figure 18.12). Fatalities from the endemic disease are rare, but during epidemics in crowded, unsanitary, louse-infested environments, fatalities can be as high as thirty percent if untreated.

B. Clinical significance

The first symptoms of relapsing fever appear three to ten days after exposure to an infected arthropod (Figure 18.13). These symptoms include an abrupt onset of high fever accompanied by severe headache, muscle pain, and general malaise. During this febrile period, which lasts three to five days, abundant spirochetes are present in the blood. The fever abates along with the number of spirochetes, and apparent recovery is experienced for a period of four to ten days, but is followed by a recurrence of the initial symptoms. There may be as many as ten such recurrences, generally with decreasing severity. In fatal cases, the spirochete invades many organs of the body (heart, spleen, liver, kidney), with death generally due to myocarditis.

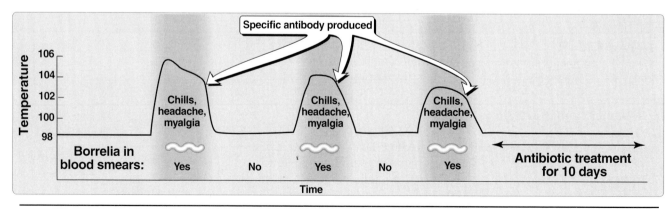

Figure 18.13
Clinical stages of relapsing fever.

C. Diagnosis and treatment

Diagnosis is usually based on the appearance of Giemsa- or Wright-stainable, loosely coiled spirochetes in the blood during the febrile stage of the disease. Tetracyclines, erythromycin, and penicillin have proven effective treatments (Figure 18.14). However, the relapsing nature of the disease makes it difficult to distinguish spontaneous remissions from response to therapy. No vaccines are available, and prevention is best accomplished by protecting against ticks and lice.

VI. LEPTOSPIRA INTERROGANS

Leptospira interrogans infection causes the disease **leptospirosis**. The organism is a very slender (lepto = slender), tightly coiled, culturable spirochete with a single, thin, axial filament, and hooked ends (Figure 18.15). Many serogroups and serotypes (serovars) are recognized, and are specific to distinct geographic locales. *L. interrogans* is sensitive to drying and to a broad range of disinfectants; it can, however, survive for weeks in slightly alkaline water.

A. Epidemiology and Pathogenesis

Leptospirosis is essentially an animal disease that is coincidentally transmitted to humans—primarily by water or food contaminated with animal urine or feces. Entrance to the body can also occur via small skin abrasions or via the conjunctiva. Although leptospirosis occurs worldwide (under various local names, such as **infectious jaundice**, **marsh fever**, **Weil's disease**, and **swineherd's disease**), the incidence of the disease today in developed countries is very low; less than 100 cases of clinically significant *L. interrogans* infections are reported annually in the United States.

B. Clinical significance

Fever occurs one to two weeks after infection, at which time spirochetes appear in the blood. These symptoms decrease after about one week. However, in cases of biphasic disease (that is, the disease having two stages), spirochetes reappear, accompanied by invasion of the liver, kidneys, and central nervous system. This results in jaundice, hemorrhage, tissue necrosis, and/or aseptic meningitis. This second stage of the disease, which lasts three or more weeks, involves a rise in circulating IgM antibodies. In severe cases of the disease, mortality can be as high as ten percent.

C. Diagnosis and treatment

Although *L. interrogans* can be cultured, diagnosis is usually based on serologic agglutination tests (see p. 30) and visual demonstration of the spirochetes in urine, blood, or cerebrospinal fluid. Penicillin or doxycycline is useful if administered during the first stage of the disease, but both are ineffective later (Figure 18.16). No vaccine is currently available. Prevention of exposure to potentially contaminated water and food helps control the transmission of *L. interrogans*.

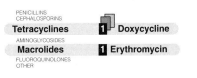

Figure 18.14
Some antimicrobial agents useful in empiric therapy of infections due to *Borrelia recurrentis*.

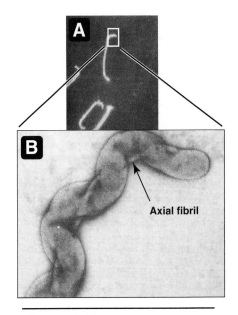

Figure 18.15
A. Dark-field micrograph of *Leptospira interrogans*. B. Electron micrograph of one end of a negatively stained leptospira showing the axial fibril.

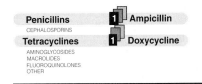

Figure 18.16
Some antimicrobial agents useful in treating *Leptospira interrogans* infections.

Study Questions

Choose the ONE correct answer

18.1 The probable cause for the relapsing nature of relapsing fever caused by *Borrelia recurrentis* is:

   A. the sequential appearance of new antibiotic resistant variants.

   B. periodic spore dormancy and activation.

   C. successive appearance of antigenic variants.

   D. periodic hormonal fluctuations in the host.

   E. organisms that survive and propagate after spirochete-induced fever.

Correct answer = C. Any of these mechanisms are conceivable with various degrees of plausibility. The weight of evidence, however, favors the mechanism whereby new antigenic variants arise that can elude, for a period, the host's immune defenses and then be replaced by another variant.

18.2 Which of the following spirochete-caused diseases is transmitted by an arthropod?

   A. Leptospirosis

   B. Pinta

   C. Relapsing fever

   D. Yaws

   E. Syphilis

Correct answer = C. *Borrelia recurrentis*, the cause of relapsing fever, is borne by ticks or lice. Pinta, yaws and syphilis are transmitted by direct human-to-human contact, whereas leptospirosis is transmitted via water contaminated with animal urine.

18.3 A distinctive feature of spirochetes is the presence of:

   A. fimbriae.

   B. endoflagella.

   C. helically arranged pili.

   D. nucleosomes.

   E. variable surface antigens.

Correct answer = B. The endoflagella are thought to be responsible for the corkscrew motion of spirochetes. The other structural features are not specific to spirochetes.

18.4 Syphilis and Lyme disease are strikingly similar in which of the following aspects?

   A. Their modes of transmission are similar.

   B. Both diseases display three similar, distinct phases.

   C. Both causative agents share many antigenic markers.

   D. The diseases show cross-immunity.

   E. Both causative agents can be cultured.

Correct answer = B. Syphilis, like Lyme disease, has three distinct phases including the initial primary-stage lesion (chancre) at the site of entry of the pathogen. The other listed properties are either irrelevant or false. Unlike *T. pallidum*, *B. burgdorferi* can be cultured, but the procedure is difficult, and takes six to eight weeks.

18.5 A 22-year-old male presents to his physician, complaining of a two week history of a sore on his penis. Physical examination shows a firm, raised, red, non-tender chancre midway between the base and glans of the penis. Which of the following is the most appropriate course of action for the physician?

   A. Test a serum sample for antibodies to Herpes simplex virus.

   B. Swab the chancre and culture on Thayer-Martin agar.

   C. Swab the chancre and perform a Gram stain.

   D. Perform a dark-field examination on a swab of the active lesion.

   E. Swab the chancre and culture on blood agar.

Correct answer = D. The patient most likely has primary syphilis rather than herpes simplex virus because the penile chancre is not tender. Herpes lesions are typically very painful. *Treponema pallidum*, the etiologic agent of syphilis, cannot be readily cultured in the routine clinical microbiology laboratory. Treponemal spirochetes from primary and secondary lesions can be detected microscopically using immunofluorescent stain or dark-field illumination. However, syphilis is usually diagnosed serologically by detection of 1) antitreponemal antibodies that are specific to the treponemal surface proteins, and 2) nontreponemal antibodies, called reagin, that are directed against normal phospholipid components.

Mycoplasma 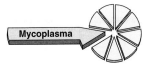 19

I. OVERVIEW

Mycoplasmas are small, prokaryotic organisms with no peptidoglycan cell walls. Instead, they are enclosed in a single, trilaminar plasma membrane. Because of their extremely small size, mycoplasmas frequently pass through bacteriologic filters. The many *Mycoplasma* species are widely distributed in nature, and include several commensals commonly found in the mouth and genitourinary tract of humans and other mammals. For these reasons, mycoplasmas are often recovered as contaminants or adventitious flora from biologic materials including clinical samples. Three *Mycoplasma* species are definitively associated with human disease, namely *Mycoplasma pneumoniae*, which is the cause of a primary atypical pneumonia, and *Mycoplasma hominis* and *Ureaplasma urealyticum*, which are associated with a variety of genitourinary diseases such as urethritis, pelvic inflammatory disease, and intrapartum infections (Figure 19.1). Lacking cell walls, mycoplasmas are insensitive to antibiotics that inhibit cell division by preventing cell wall synthesis (such as penicillin, see p. 44). However, they are susceptible to other inhibitors of prokaryotic metabolism.

II. GENERAL FEATURES OF MYCOPLASMAS

Lacking cell walls, mycoplasmas are enclosed instead by a membrane composed of a lipid bilayer (Figure 19.2). They are therefore plastic and very pleomorphic, and thus cannot be classified as either cocci or rods. Mycoplasmas are also the smallest of known free-living, self-replicating prokaryotic cells. Their double-stranded DNA genomes often measure less than 10^9 daltons. [Note: This may approach the minimum DNA coding capacity required for the free-living state.]

A. Physiology

Mycoplasmas have limited biosynthetic capabilities, and require a variety of small organic molecules for growth. Unlike other prokary-

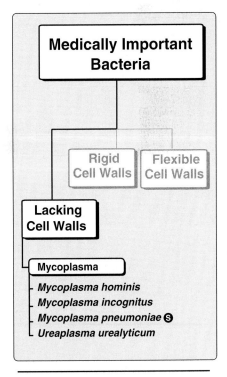

Figure 19.1
Classification of Mycoplasma.
🅢 See pp. 414, 448 for a summary of this organism.

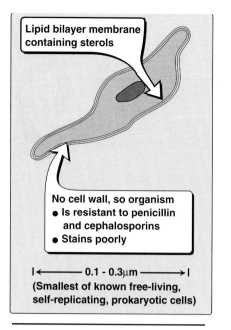

Figure 19.2
Structural features of mycoplasma.

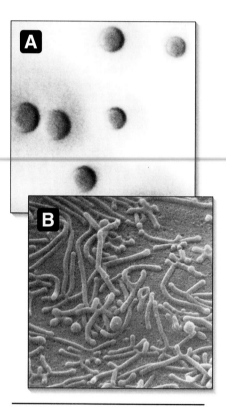

Figure 19.3
A. Colonies of *Mycoplasma pneumoniae* showing "fried egg" appearance. B. Scanning electron micrograph of *Mycoplasma pneumoniae.*

otes, mycoplasmas contain sterols in their cell membranes. Because most mycoplasma species cannot synthesize the sterol ring, they require an external source of cholesterol from serum or a similar medium supplement. Given appropriate supplementation, they can be grown in cell-free media. The medically important species of mycoplasmas are facultative anaerobes (see p. 110), although some genus members are strict anaerobes.

B. Colony production

Mycoplasmas produce minute colonies on specialized agar after several days of incubation. These are best visualized under 30 to 100x magnification. The central portion of the colony penetrates the agar while the periphery spreads over the adjacent surface, in some cases giving the colony a characteristic "fried egg" appearance (Figure 19.3).

III. MYCOPLASMA PNEUMONIAE

Mycoplasma pneumoniae is transmitted by respiratory droplets, and causes a lower respiratory tract infection called **primary atypical pneumonia** (so named because the signs and symptoms are unlike typical lobar pneumonia). The organism accounts for approximately twenty percent of pneumonia cases as well as causing milder infections such as bronchitis, pharyngitis, and nonpurulent otitis media. Infections occur worldwide and year around, with increased incidence in late fall and winter. Cases are usually sporadic, although occasional epidemics among individuals in close contact are reported in both civilian settings (for example, schools and prisons) and among military populations. The highest incidence of clinical disease is seen in older children and young adults (six to twenty years of age).

A. Pathogenesis

Mycoplasma pneumoniae possesses a membrane-associated protein, P1, which functions as a cytoadhesin. It is concentrated in a specialized organelle, visible under electron microscopy, which binds sialic acid-rich glycolipids found on certain host cell membranes. Among susceptible cell types are ciliated bronchial epithelial cells. The organisms grow closely attached to the host cell luminal surface and inhibit ciliary action. Eventually patches of affected mucosa desquamate, and an inflammatory response develops in bronchial and adjacent tissues involving lymphocytes and other mononuclear cells. The clinical disease is thus largely an expression of host-specific immune response rather than of damage created by the organism itself. In infected individuals, organisms are shed in saliva for several days before onset of clinical illness. Reinfection is common, and symptoms are more severe in older children and young adults who have previously encountered the organism.

B. Clinical significance

Primary atypical pneumonia (lower respiratory tract disease) is the best known form of *M. pneumoniae* infection. However, this disease accounts for a minority of the infectious episodes with this organism, upper respiratory tract and ear infection being much more frequent. Primary atypical pneumonia clinically resembles pneumonias caused by a number of viruses and bacteria such as *Chlamydia* species. Onset is usually gradual, beginning with nonspecific symptoms such as unrelenting headache, accompanied by fever, chills, and malaise. After two to four days, a dry or scantily productive cough develops. Earache is sometimes an accompanying complaint. Chest X-rays reveal a patchy, diffuse bronchopneumonia involving one or more lobes (Figure 19.4). The infiltration is usually more extensive than physical examination might suggest. Patients often remain ambulatory throughout the illness, hence the name "**walking pneumonia**." In the absence of pre-existing compromise (immunodeficiency, emphysema, etc.), the disease remits after three to ten days without specific treatment. X-ray abnormalities resolve more slowly in two weeks to two months. Complications are rare, but include central nervous system disturbances, a rash known as erythema multiforme, and a mild hemolytic anemia (the latter associated with the production of cold agglutinins, see below).

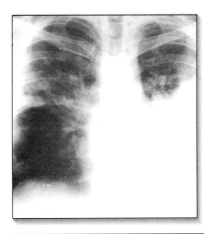

Figure 19.4
X-ray of lung of an individual with *M. pneumoniae*–induced primary atypical pneumonia.

C. Immunity

Infection with *M. pneumoniae* elicits both local and systemic immune responses. Only one *M. pneumoniae* serotype has been described. Serum antibody to outer membrane glycolipids and to the P1 adhesin can be demonstrated, with antibody peaking two to four weeks after infection, and gradually disappearing over the following year. An IgM antibody, the **cold agglutinin**, is produced by approximately sixty percent of infected patients. [Note: The name of this antibody is derived from the fact that it reacts with the human erythrocyte antigen I, reversibly agglutinating I^+ red blood cells at temperatures of $0°$ to $4°C$ but not at $37°C$.]

D. Laboratory identification

Direct microscopic examination of clinical material for *M. pneumoniae* is of limited value. Sputum is scanty and nonpurulent, and the pathogen stains poorly or not at all using standard bacteriologic stains. Nucleic acid hybridization of such material, probing for mycoplasmal 16S ribosomal RNA, has been commercially developed. It is quite sensitive but not widely used because of technical demands and expense. Sputum samples or throat swabs can be cultured on special media, but isolation of the organism usually requires eight to fifteen days, and thus cannot aid in early treatment decisions. Serologic tests are therefore the most widely used procedures for establishing a diagnosis of primary atypical pneumonia. Specific antibody is commonly detected by complement fixation using an extract of mycoplasmal glycolipids. A diagnosis is established by a four-fold rise in titer between acute and convalescent samples. Because symptoms of illness develop slowly, the initial serum sample may be positive. [Note: Nonspecific cold agglutinins also develop in more than sixty percent of patients, but similar serologic responses (false positives) are occasionally seen in diseases such as infectious mononucleosis, rubella, influenza, adenovirus

M. pneumoniae

PENICILLINS
CEPHALOSPORINS

Tetracyclines   **1** Tetracycline

AMINOGLYCOSIDES

Macrolides   **1** Erythromycin

FLUOROQUINOLONES
OTHER

Figure 19.5

Summary of antibiotic therapy of *Mycoplasma pneumoniae*.

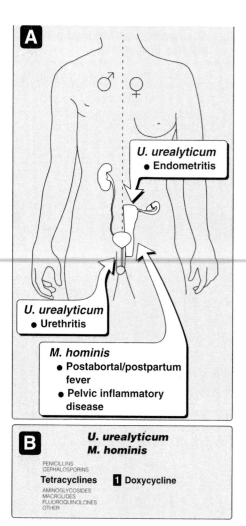

A

U. urealyticum
● Endometritis

U. urealyticum
● Urethritis

M. hominis
● Postabortal/postpartum fever
● Pelvic inflammatory disease

B   *U. urealyticum*
          M. hominis

PENICILLINS
CEPHALOSPORINS

Tetracyclines   **1** Doxycycline

AMINOGLYCOSIDES
MACROLIDES
FLUOROQUINOLONES
OTHER

Figure 19.6

A. Diseases caused by *M. hominis* and *U. urealyticum*. B. The antibiotic used to treat these infections.

and listeria infections. Therefore, either positive or negative results must be interpreted with caution.]

E. Treatment

M. pneumoniae is sensitive to doxycycline or erythromycin (Figure 19.5). When given early, either antibiotic shortens the course of disease, although symptoms may only be eliminated gradually with such treatment. The organisms, however, may persist in the convalescent upper respiratory tract for a number of weeks. A summary of organisms causing atypical pneumonia is presented in Figure 19.7.

IV. GENITAL MYCOPLASMAS

Mycoplasma hominis and *Ureaplasma urealyticum* are common inhabitants of the genitourinary tract, particularly in sexually active adults. Because colonization rates in some populations are in excess of fifty percent, it is difficult to establish an unequivocal causal role in various disease states with which the organisms are associated. Both agents can be cultured. They grow more rapidly than *M. pneumoniae*, and can be distinguished by their carbon utilization patterns; *M. hominis* degrades arginine, *U. urealyticum* hydrolyses urea. [Note: *Ureaplasma* is sometimes referred to as a "T-strain" of mycoplasma because it produces **t**iny colonies, not visible to the naked eye.] The major clinical condition associated with *M. hominis* is **postpartum** or **postabortal fever** (Figure 19.6). The organism has been isolated from blood cultures in up to ten percent of women so affected. It is also recovered locally in cases of **pelvic inflammatory disease**, although sometimes in mixed culture. A number of serotypes of *M. hominis* have been described. It is important to note that *M. hominis* isolates, in contrast to other mycoplasmas, are uniformly resistant to erythromycin. Tetracycline is effective for specific treatment. *U. urealyticum* is a common cause of **urethritis** when neither gonococcus nor chlamydia can be demonstrated, particularly in men. In women, the organism has been isolated from cases of endometritis and from vaginal secretions of women who undergo premature labor or deliver low-birth-weight babies. The infants are often colonized, and *U. urealyticum* has been isolated from the infant's lower respiratory tract, and the central nervous system both with and without evidence of inflammatory response.

V. OTHER MYCOPLASMAS

Several other species of mycoplasma can be recovered from human sources, for which, to date, no pathogenic role is established. One such organism, the AIDS-associated mycoplasma, or *M. incognitus*, has been isolated in high frequency from patients with that disease, where the organism may play a role, possibly as a secondary invader.

Disease Summary: "ATYPICAL" PNEUMONIA[1]

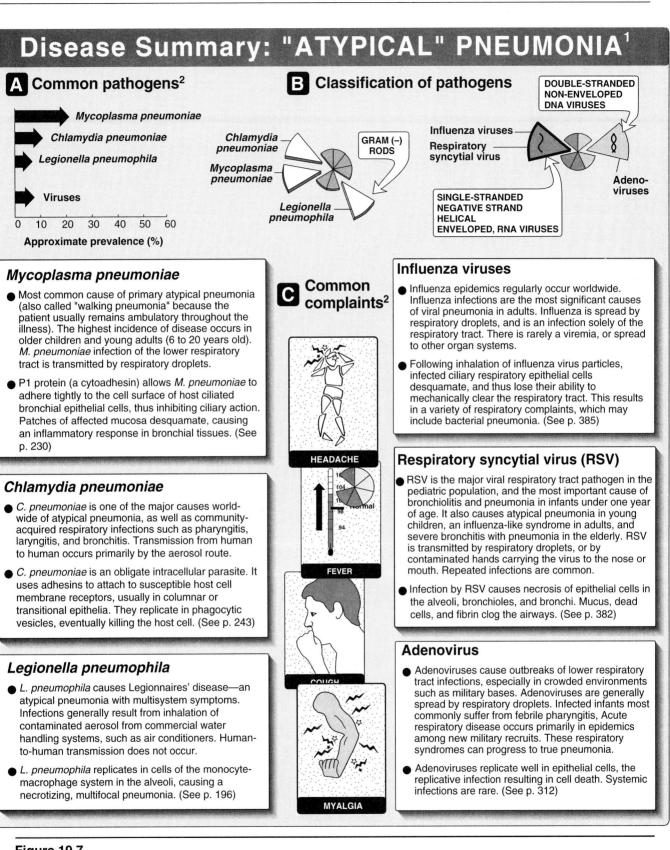

A Common pathogens[2]

Mycoplasma pneumoniae

Chlamydia pneumoniae

Legionella pneumophila

Viruses

0   10   20   30   40   50   60
Approximate prevalence (%)

B Classification of pathogens

Chlamydia pneumoniae

Mycoplasma pneumoniae

GRAM (−) RODS

Legionella pneumophila

DOUBLE-STRANDED NON-ENVELOPED DNA VIRUSES

Influenza viruses

Respiratory syncytial virus

Adeno-viruses

SINGLE-STRANDED NEGATIVE STRAND HELICAL ENVELOPED, RNA VIRUSES

C Common complaints[2]

HEADACHE

FEVER

COUGH

MYALGIA

Mycoplasma pneumoniae

● Most common cause of primary atypical pneumonia (also called "walking pneumonia" because the patient usually remains ambulatory throughout the illness). The highest incidence of disease occurs in older children and young adults (6 to 20 years old). M. pneumoniae infection of the lower respiratory tract is transmitted by respiratory droplets.

● P1 protein (a cytoadhesin) allows M. pneumoniae to adhere tightly to the cell surface of host ciliated bronchial epithelial cells, thus inhibiting ciliary action. Patches of affected mucosa desquamate, causing an inflammatory response in bronchial tissues. (See p. 230)

Chlamydia pneumoniae

● C. pneumoniae is one of the major causes worldwide of atypical pneumonia, as well as community-acquired respiratory infections such as pharyngitis, laryngitis, and bronchitis. Transmission from human to human occurs primarily by the aerosol route.

● C. pneumoniae is an obligate intracellular parasite. It uses adhesins to attach to susceptible host cell membrane receptors, usually in columnar or transitional epithelia. They replicate in phagocytic vesicles, eventually killing the host cell. (See p. 243)

Legionella pneumophila

● L. pneumophila causes Legionnaires' disease—an atypical pneumonia with multisystem symptoms. Infections generally result from inhalation of contaminated aerosol from commercial water handling systems, such as air conditioners. Human-to-human transmission does not occur.

● L. pneumophila replicates in cells of the monocyte-macrophage system in the alveoli, causing a necrotizing, multifocal pneumonia. (See p. 196)

Influenza viruses

● Influenza epidemics regularly occur worldwide. Influenza infections are the most significant causes of viral pneumonia in adults. Influenza is spread by respiratory droplets, and is an infection solely of the respiratory tract. There is rarely a viremia, or spread to other organ systems.

● Following inhalation of influenza virus particles, infected ciliary respiratory epithelial cells desquamate, and thus lose their ability to mechanically clear the respiratory tract. This results in a variety of respiratory complaints, which may include bacterial pneumonia. (See p. 385)

Respiratory syncytial virus (RSV)

● RSV is the major viral respiratory tract pathogen in the pediatric population, and the most important cause of bronchiolitis and pneumonia in infants under one year of age. It also causes atypical pneumonia in young children, an influenza-like syndrome in adults, and severe bronchitis with pneumonia in the elderly. RSV is transmitted by respiratory droplets, or by contaminated hands carrying the virus to the nose or mouth. Repeated infections are common.

● Infection by RSV causes necrosis of epithelial cells in the alveoli, bronchioles, and bronchi. Mucus, dead cells, and fibrin clog the airways. (See p. 382)

Adenovirus

● Adenoviruses cause outbreaks of lower respiratory tract infections, especially in crowded environments such as military bases. Adenoviruses are generally spread by respiratory droplets. Infected infants most commonly suffer from febrile pharyngitis, Acute respiratory disease occurs primarily in epidemics among new military recruits. These respiratory syndromes can progress to true pneumonia.

● Adenoviruses replicate well in epithelial cells, the replicative infection resulting in cell death. Systemic infections are rare. (See p. 312)

Figure 19.7
Some characteristics of atypical pneumonia.

[1]"Atypical" pneumonia is characterized by insidious onset, scant sputum and x-ray abornalities greater than predicted by physical symptoms. See p. 152 for summary of "typical" pneumonia.

[2]Other pathogens include Chlamydia psittaci, Pneumocystis carinii, varicella-zoster virus and parainfluenza viruses.

Study Questions

Choose the ONE correct answer

19.1 A distinguishing feature of human mycoplasma species is that they:

A stain well with Giemsa, but not by Gram stain.

B. contain no bacterial peptidoglycan.

C. are not immunogenic because they mimic host cell membrane components.

D. cannot be cultivated *in vitro*.

E. are dependent on host sources of ATP.

Correct answer = B. The distinguishing feature of mycoplasmas is their complete lack of a cell wall.

19.2 Which of the following is most characteristic of *Mycoplasma pneumoniae* infection?

A. Infection results in a fever of sudden onset accompanied by a productive cough.

B. Infection most commonly occurs in the upper respiratory tract.

C. Infection is definitively diagnosed by direct microscopic examination of sputum.

D. Reinfection is rare and less severe than primary infection.

E. Infection causes extensive scarring and calcification of affected lung tissue.

Correct answer = B. Primary atypical pneumonia is the best known form of *M. pneumoniae* infection. However, upper respiratory tract and ear infection are much more frequent. Atypical pneumonia is characterized by a gradual onset and a scantily productive cough. Direct microscopic examination of clinical material for *M. pneumoniae* is of limited value. Sputum is scanty and nonpurulent, and the pathogen stains poorly or not at all using standard bacteriologic stains. Reinfection causes more severe lesions and a more extensive chronic inflammatory response. Recovery is slow, but without residual damage.

19.3 Postpartum fever due to *Mycoplasma hominis* is treated with:

A. tetracycline.

B. erythromycin.

C. penicillin G.

D. a second-generation cephalosporin.

E. vancomycin.

Correct answer = A. Mycoplasmas are small, prokaryotic organisms with no peptidoglycan cell walls. Thus inhibitors of cell wall synthesis, such as penicillins, cephalosporins, and vancomycin are not effective. *M. hominis* isolates, in contrast to other mycoplasmas, are uniformly resistant to erythromycin. Tetracycline is effective for specific treatment.

19.4 A 30-year-old woman complained of unrelenting headache, accompanied by fever, chills, and malaise. After two to four days, a dry cough developed. Chest X-rays reveal a patchy, diffuse bronchopneumonia involving both lobes. Her white cell count was not elevated. Which of the following is the most likely diagnosis?

A. Legionellosis

B. Infection with parainfluenza virus

C. Infection with *Streptococcus pneumoniae*

D. Infection with *Haemophilus influenzae*

E. Infection with *Mycoplasma pneumoniae*

Correct answer = E. The description suggests primary atypical pneumonia caused by *Myoplasma pneumoniae*. Patients often remain ambulatory throughout the illness, hence the name "walking pneumonia." In the absence of preexisting compromise (immunodeficiency, emphysema, etc.), the disease remits after three to ten days without specific treatment. X-ray abnormalities resolve more slowly in two weeks to two months.

19.5 Which of the following laboratory tests for *Mycoplasma pneumoniae* is the most specific and sensitive.

A. Cold agglutinin

B. Complement fixation test

C. Gram stain.

D. A DNA probe to the *Mycoplasma pneumoniae* 16S ribosomal RNA

E. Culture of sputum

Correct answer = D: Direct microscopic examination of clinical material for *M. pneumoniae* is of limited value. Sputum is scanty and non-purulent, and the pathogen stains poorly or not at all using standard bacteriologic stains. Nucleic acid hybridization of such material, probing for mycoplasmal 16S ribosomal RNA, is sensitive and shows high specificity. Sputum samples or throat swabs can be cultured on special media, but isolation of the organism usually requires eight to fifteen days, and thus cannot aid in early treatment decisions.

Chlamydiae

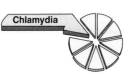

20

I. OVERVIEW

Chlamydia is a genus of very small bacteria that are obligate intracellular parasites, depending on the host cell for energy in the forms of ATP and NAD^+. They grow in cytoplasmic vacuoles in a limited number of host cell types. The genus is divided into three species: *Chlamydia trachomatis*, *Chlamydia psittaci* and *Chlamydia pneumoniae*. *C. trachomatis* infections cause diseases of the genitourinary tract and of the eye, including many cases of non-gonococcal urethritis and ocular infections such as trachoma. *C. psittaci* and *C. pneumoniae* infect various levels of the respiratory tract. For example, *C. psittaci* causes psittacosis and *C. pneumoniae* causes atypical pneumonia. Figure 20.1 summarizes the clinically significant chlamydiae.

II. GENERAL FEATURES OF CHLAMYDIAE

Chlamydiae are small, round to ovoid organisms that vary in size during the different stages of their replicative cycle (Figure 20.2). The chlamydial cell envelope consists of two lipid bilayers with associated cell wall material that resembles a gram-negative envelope. However, it contains no peptidoglycan, and muramic acid is not present. The chlamydial DNA genome is less than 10^9 daltons in size, making it among the smallest found in prokaryotic cells. Chlamydiae possess ribosomes and synthesize their own proteins, and therefore are sensitive to antibiotics that inhibit this process, such as tetracyclines and macrolides (see pp. 45 to 46).

A. Physiology

Chlamydiae are energy parasites, hence their requirement for growth in living cells. They are unable to synthesize their own pools of ATP, or regenerate NAD^+ by oxidation. With these high energy molecules exogenously supplied, chlamydia produce CO_2 from compounds such as glucose, pyruvate or glutamate, and carry out the usual bacterial metabolic activities.

B. Pathogenesis

Chlamydiae have a unique life cycle, with morphologically distinct infectious and reproductive forms (Figure 20.3). The extracellular infectious form, called the **elementary body**, is a tiny, condensed,

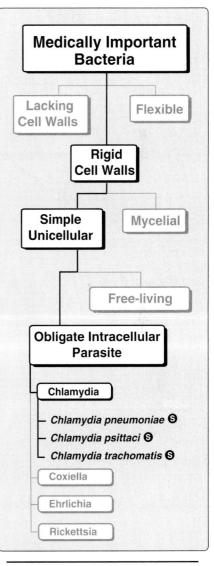

Figure 20 .1
Classification of *Chlamydia*.
Ⓢ See pp. 405, 441 for summaries of these organisms.

Lippincott's Illustrated Reviews: Microbiology,
by William A. Strohl, Harriet Rouse, Bruce D. Fisher.
Lippincott, Williams & Wilkins, Baltimore, MD © 2001

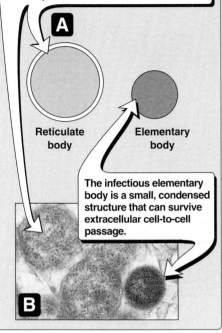

The noninfectious reticulate body is metabolically active, and divides repeatedly by binary fission, forming inclusion bodies. The cell envelope has two lipid bilayers with an associated cell wall material (similar to gram-negative cells), but no peptidoglycan or muramic acid is present.

A

Reticulate body

Elementary body

The infectious elementary body is a small, condensed structure that can survive extracellular cell-to-cell passage.

B

Figure 20.2
Structural features of *Chlamydia*.
A. Schematic drawing. B. Electron micrograph.

apparently inert structure that can survive extracellular cell-to-cell passage, and initiates an infection. The elementary body is taken up by phagocytosis into susceptible host cells, a process facilitated by proteins in the chlamydial cell envelope that function as adhesins, directing attachment to glycolipid or glycopolysaccharide receptors on the host cell membrane. Once inside the cell, the elementary body prevents fusion of the phagosome and lysosome, protecting itself from enzymatic destruction. The particle reorganizes over the next eight hours into a larger, noninfectious **reticulate body**, which becomes metabolically active, and divides repeatedly by binary fission within the cytoplasm of the host cell. As the reticulate body divides, it fills the endosome with its progeny, forming an **inclusion body**. After 48 hours, multiplication ceases and reticulate bodies condense to become new infectious elementary bodies. The elementary bodies are then released from the cell by cytolysis, ending in host cell death.

C. Laboratory identification

1. **Useful stains:** Chlamydiae are not stained using the Gram stain, but can be visualized under light microscopy by stains that preserve the host cell architecture. Direct immunofluorescence is also a common and useful procedure. In *C. trachomatis* only, a matrix of glycogen-like material accumulates in the inclusions, which can be shown by staining with iodine. Other species do not give this reaction.

2. **Chlamydial antigens:** Although DNA homology among chlamydial species is less than thirty percent, they share lipopolysaccharide antigens that delineate the genus. In addition, there is a class of abundant outer membrane proteins that have species or subspecies specificity, and elicit protective antibody. Antigenic classification in this genus is usually done by immunofluorescence, using monoclonal antibodies.

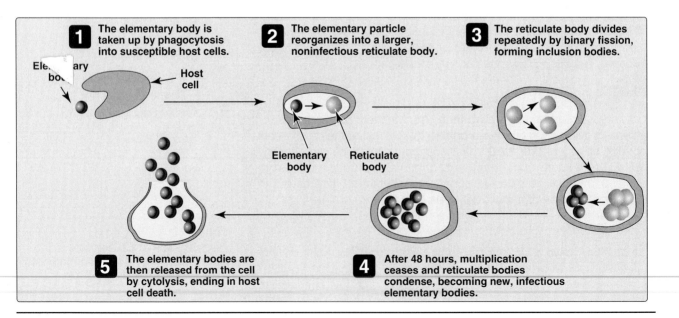

1 The elementary body is taken up by phagocytosis into susceptible host cells.

Elementary body

Host cell

2 The elementary particle reorganizes into a larger, noninfectious reticulate body.

Elementary body   Reticulate body

3 The reticulate body divides repeatedly by binary fission, forming inclusion bodies.

5 The elementary bodies are then released from the cell by cytolysis, ending in host cell death.

4 After 48 hours, multiplication ceases and reticulate bodies condense, becoming new, infectious elementary bodies.

Figure 20.3
Reproduction cycle of *Chlamydia*.

III. CHLAMYDIA TRACHOMATIS

Chlamydia trachomatis is divided into a number of serotypes, which correlate with the clinical syndrome they cause (Figure 20.4). For example, *C. trachomatis* is the major causal agent of the syndrome, **non-gonococcal urethritis** (**NGU**), and is currently the most common sexually transmitted bacterial disease in the United States (Figure 20.5). *C. trachomatis* can also cause eye infections, with symptoms ranging from irritation to blindness. **Trachoma**, which is a very ancient disease, was well described in Egyptian writings around 3800 B.C. It remains widely prevalent in developing areas of the world.

A. Clinical significance

C. trachomatis causes a range of genitourinary and eye infections.

1. **Nongonococcal urethritis (NGU):** Annually, more than four million urogenital *Chlamydia trachomatis* infections occur in the United States, in young, sexually active individuals of all socioeconomic groups. In males, the urethra is the principal locus of infection. Females may present with cervicitis and/or urethritis (see p. 441). Infections are often asymptomatic, although communicable. [Note: Among women, the asymptomatic rate is higher than fifty percent.] Whether locally symptomatic or not, contiguous spread of infection may involve the epididymis in men, and fallopian tubes and adjacent tissues in women (**pelvic inflammatory disease**). Infection with *C. trachomatis* confers little protection against reinfection, which commonly occurs. Repeated or chronic episodes may lead to sterility in both sexes, and to ectopic pregnancies. Chlamydial NGU is symptomatically similar to infections caused by *Neisseria gonorrhoeae* (see p. 167), although the average incubation time is longer (two to three weeks), and the discharge tends to be more mucoid and contains fewer pus cells. In addition, the two infections often occur simultaneously or sequentially. Therefore, patients suspected of chlamydial infection should be treated for neisserial infection as well. NGU is caused by serotypes D–K of *C. trachomatis* (see Figure 20.4). These serotypes also cause eye infections, for example, in infants born to genitally infected women (Figure 20.5, see p. 242).

2. **Lymphogranuloma venereum (LGV):** *C. trachomatis* serotypes L_1, L_2, and L_3 cause LGV, a more invasive sexually transmitted disease (see p. 441). It is uncommon in the United States, but is endemic in Asia, Africa, and South America. LGV is characterized by transient papules on the external genitalia followed in one to two months by painful swelling of inguinal and perirectal lymph nodes. Adenopathy (swelling of the lymph nodes) is often accompanied by mild constitutional symptoms. The affected lymph nodes suppurate, and chronic inflammation and fibrosis lead to extensive ulceration and blockage of regional lymphatic drainage. (See Figure 20.6 for a summary of sexually transmitted diseases.)

Species and serotype	Disease
C. trachomatis A, B, C	● Trachoma
D – K	● Cervicitis ● Endometritis ● Epididymitis ● Inclusion conjunctivitis of the newborn (ICN) or adult ● Infant pneumonia syndrome ● Nongonococcal urethritis ● Proctitis ● Salpingitis
L_1, L_2, L_3	● Lymphogranuloma venereum (LGV)
C. psittaci Many	● Pneumonia (psittacosis)
C. pneumoniae One	Acute respiratory diseases including: ● Bronchitis ● Pharyngitis ● Pneumonia ● Sinusitis

Figure 20.4
Correlation between chlamydial species/serotypes and disease.

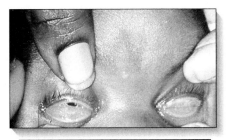

Figure 20.5
Neonatal conjunctivitis due to chlamydial infection.

Disease Summary: Sexually Transmitted Diseases

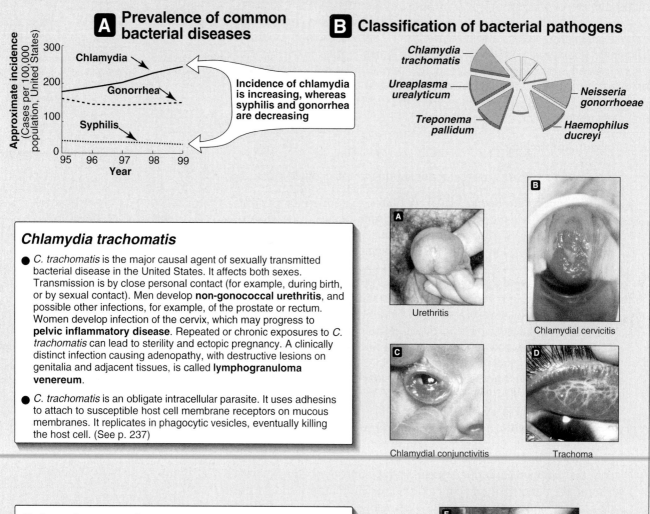

A Prevalence of common bacterial diseases

Incidence of chlamydia is increasing, whereas syphilis and gonorrhea are decreasing

B Classification of bacterial pathogens

Chlamydia trachomatis
Ureaplasma urealyticum
Treponema pallidum
Neisseria gonorrhoeae
Haemophilus ducreyi

Chlamydia trachomatis

- *C. trachomatis* is the major causal agent of sexually transmitted bacterial disease in the United States. It affects both sexes. Transmission is by close personal contact (for example, during birth, or by sexual contact). Men develop **non-gonococcal urethritis**, and possible other infections, for example, of the prostate or rectum. Women develop infection of the cervix, which may progress to **pelvic inflammatory disease**. Repeated or chronic exposures to *C. trachomatis* can lead to sterility and ectopic pregnancy. A clinically distinct infection causing adenopathy, with destructive lesions on genitalia and adjacent tissues, is called **lymphogranuloma venereum**.

- *C. trachomatis* is an obligate intracellular parasite. It uses adhesins to attach to susceptible host cell membrane receptors on mucous membranes. It replicates in phagocytic vesicles, eventually killing the host cell. (See p. 237)

Urethritis

Chlamydial cervicitis

Chlamydial conjunctivitis

Trachoma

Neisseria gonorrhoeae

- *N. gonorrhoeae* causes **gonorrhea**. It is transmitted by sexual contact. In males, symptoms include infection of the urethra (**gonococcal urethritis**), purulent discharge, and pain during urination. In females, infection is usually localized to the endocervix, often causing a purulent vaginal discharge. If the woman's disease progresses to the uterus, **gonococcal salpingitis** (which may lead to tubal scarring and infertility), **pelvic inflammatory disease**, and fibrosis can occur. Alternatively, the infection may be asymptomatic in women.

- *N. gonorrhoeae* is highly sensitive to cool temperatures and dehydration. Bacterial proteins (pili and outer membrane proteins) enhance the attachment of the bacterium to host epithelial and mucosal cell surfaces, such as those of the urethra, rectum, cervix, pharynx, or conjunctiva, causing colonization and infections. (See p. 165)

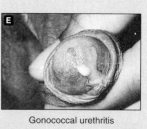

Gonococcal urethritis

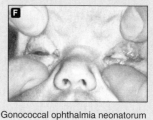

Gonococcal ophthalmia neonatorum

BACTERIA

Figure 20.6

Some characteristics of sexually transmitted diseases: bacterial pathogens (continued on next page).

Disease Summary: Sexually Transmitted Diseases

Treponema pallidum

- *T. pallidum* infection causes **syphilis**. It is transmitted primarily by sexual contact, where the infectious lesion is generally on the skin or mucous membrane of the genitalia. Within two to ten weeks after infection, a painless, hard ulcer (**chancre**) forms. Up to ten weeks later, a secondary rash occurs that may be accompanied by systemic involvement, such as syphilitic hepatitis, meningitis, nephritis, or chorioretinitis. In about 40 percent of infected individuals, a tertiary stage occurs after a latent (asymptomatic period). Tertiary syphilis is characterized by degenerative changes in the nervous system, cardiovascular lesions, and granulomatous lesions (gummas) in the liver, skin, and bones.

- *T. pallidum* can be transmitted across the placenta of an infected woman to her fetus, causing death and spontaneous abortion of the fetus, or causing it to be stillborn. Those infants that live have the symptoms of congenital syphilis, which include a variety of central nervous system and structural abnormalities. (See p. 221)

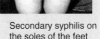
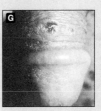

Primary syphilis chancres of the penis

Secondary syphilis on the soles of the feet

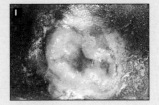

A gumma of tertiary syphilis

Ureaplasma urealyticum

- *U. urealyticum* causes **non-gonococcal urethritis**, particularly in men. The organism has a high colonization rate among sexually active men and women.

- In women, *U. urealyticum* causes **postpartum fever** and **chorioamnionitis**. The organism has been isolated from cases of endometritis, and from vaginal secretions of women who undergo premature labor or deliver low-birth-weight babies. These infants are often colonized, and *U. urealyticum* has been isolated from the infant's lower respiratory tract and the central nervous system of infants, both with and without evidence of inflammatory response. (See p. 232)

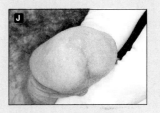

Non-gonococcal urethritis

Haemophilus ducreyi

- *H. ducreyi* causes **chancroid (soft chancre)**, a sexually-transmitted, ulcerative disease. Chancroid is a major health problem in developing countries, and its incidence is increasing in the United States. *H. ducreyi* infection causes painful, ragged ulcers on the genitalia, and lymphadenopathy may occur. Untreated, this progresses to formation of a bubo (a swollen, painful lymph node), which then suppurates.

- Open genital sores facilitate the transmission of HIV, and *H. ducreyi* infection is frequently associated with AIDS. (See p. 193)

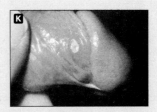

Chancroid

BACTERIA

Figure 20.6 (continued)
Some characteristics of sexually transmitted diseases: bacterial pathogens.

Disease Summary: Sexually Transmitted Diseases

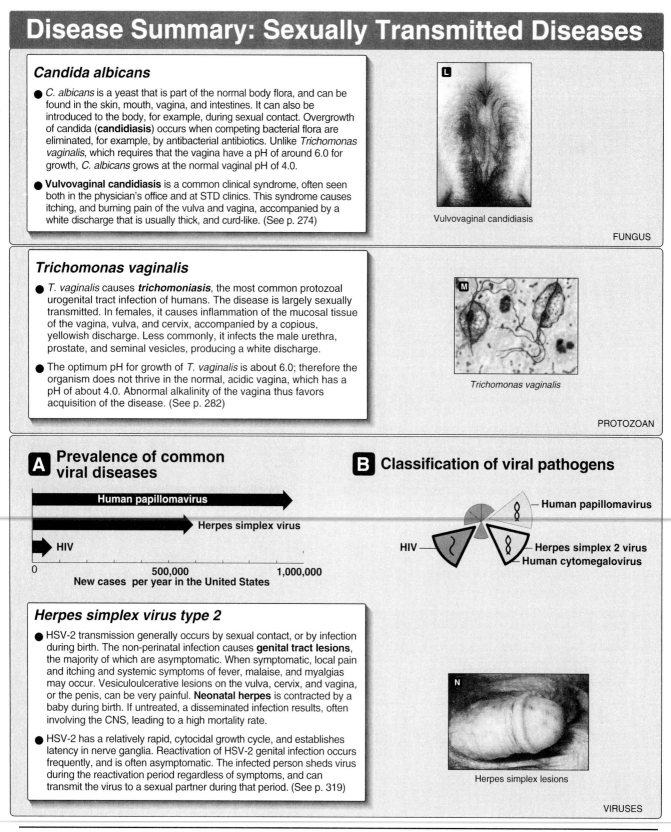

Candida albicans

- *C. albicans* is a yeast that is part of the normal body flora, and can be found in the skin, mouth, vagina, and intestines. It can also be introduced to the body, for example, during sexual contact. Overgrowth of candida (**candidiasis**) occurs when competing bacterial flora are eliminated, for example, by antibacterial antibiotics. Unlike *Trichomonas vaginalis*, which requires that the vagina have a pH of around 6.0 for growth, *C. albicans* grows at the normal vaginal pH of 4.0.

- **Vulvovaginal candidiasis** is a common clinical syndrome, often seen both in the physician's office and at STD clinics. This syndrome causes itching, and burning pain of the vulva and vagina, accompanied by a white discharge that is usually thick, and curd-like. (See p. 274)

Vulvovaginal candidiasis

FUNGUS

Trichomonas vaginalis

- *T. vaginalis* causes **trichomoniasis**, the most common protozoal urogenital tract infection of humans. The disease is largely sexually transmitted. In females, it causes inflammation of the mucosal tissue of the vagina, vulva, and cervix, accompanied by a copious, yellowish discharge. Less commonly, it infects the male urethra, prostate, and seminal vesicles, producing a white discharge.

- The optimum pH for growth of *T. vaginalis* is about 6.0; therefore the organism does not thrive in the normal, acidic vagina, which has a pH of about 4.0. Abnormal alkalinity of the vagina thus favors acquisition of the disease. (See p. 282)

Trichomonas vaginalis

PROTOZOAN

A Prevalence of common viral diseases

Human papillomavirus

Herpes simplex virus

HIV

0   500,000   1,000,000
New cases per year in the United States

B Classification of viral pathogens

Human papillomavirus

HIV ———

Herpes simplex 2 virus
Human cytomegalovirus

Herpes simplex virus type 2

- HSV-2 transmission generally occurs by sexual contact, or by infection during birth. The non-perinatal infection causes **genital tract lesions**, the majority of which are asymptomatic. When symptomatic, local pain and itching and systemic symptoms of fever, malaise, and myalgias may occur. Vesiculoulcerative lesions on the vulva, cervix, and vagina, or the penis, can be very painful. **Neonatal herpes** is contracted by a baby during birth. If untreated, a disseminated infection results, often involving the CNS, leading to a high mortality rate.

- HSV-2 has a relatively rapid, cytocidal growth cycle, and establishes latency in nerve ganglia. Reactivation of HSV-2 genital infection occurs frequently, and is often asymptomatic. The infected person sheds virus during the reactivation period regardless of symptoms, and can transmit the virus to a sexual partner during that period. (See p. 319)

Herpes simplex lesions

VIRUSES

Figure 20.6 (continued)
Some characteristics of sexually transmitted diseases: fungi, protozoa, and viruses (continued on next page).

Disease Summary: Sexually Transmitted Diseases

VIRUSES

Human papillomavirus

● Infection by some types of human papillomavirus causes **anogenital warts (condylomata acuminata)** and **periungual verruca vulgaris**. Transmission is through sexual contact, or from a mother to her baby during its birth.

● Lesions appear around the external genitalia, on the cervix, and/or inside the urethra or vagina, four to six weeks after infection. Some HPV infections are benign, but several types of HPV have been implicated as causes of cervical cancer. (See p. 307)

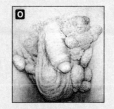
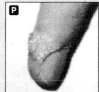

Condyloma acuminatum   Periungual verruca vulgaris (on a finger)

Human cytomegalovirus

● HCMV is the most common intrauterine viral infection. It is also the most common viral infection of neonates. HCMV is transmitted by infected individuals through their tears, urine, saliva, semen or vaginal secretions, and breast milk. Of infants born to women experiencing their first HCMV infection during pregnancy, 35 percent to 50 percent will become infected, of which 10 percent will be symptomatic (**cytomegalic inclusion disease**). Manifestations of the latter can include various degrees of damage to liver, spleen, blood-forming organs, and components of the nervous system (a common cause of hearing loss and mental retardation) or fetal death. Invasive opportunistic HCMV infections are common in AIDS patients. Such infections are also a danger to transplant recipients and other immunocompromised individuals.

● HCMV replicates initially in epithelial cells, usually of the respiratory and GI tracts. This is followed by viremia and infection of all organs of the body. Latency is established in non-neural tissues, primarily lymphoreticular cells and glandular tissues. (See p. 326)

A single renal tube contains large intranuclear virus inclusion bodies that have a typical "owl-eye" appearance.

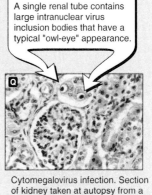

Cytomegalovirus infection. Section of kidney taken at autopsy from a three-month-old boy.

Opportunistic Infections of AIDS

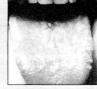
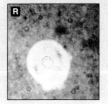

Cryptococcus present in the cerebrospinal fluid.   Oral thrush or candidiasis

Human immunodeficiency virus

● HIV infects CD4+ T cells, T cell precursors, and cells of the monocyte/macrophage lineage, resulting in a state of immunodeficiency. Transmission of HIV occurs by three routes: 1) sexually (the virus is present in both semen and vaginal secretions); 2) via blood or blood products; and 3) perinatally. Several weeks after the initial infection, some individuals experience symptoms similar to those of infectious mononucleosis. The acute-phase viremia resolves into a clinically asymptomatic latent period lasting from months to many years. The progression from asymptomatic infection to **acquired immunodeficiency syndrome** occurs as a continuum of progressive clinical states. Infected cells of the monocyte/macrophage system transport the virus into other organs including the brain. Death usually occurs from opportunistic infections, such as those shown to the right.

● HIV is a nononcogenic retrovirus. It binds to a surface CD4 molecule, located primarily on helper T cells. HIV enters the cell by fusion of the virus envelope with the plasma membrane, following which, reverse transcription occurs. This results in formation of a molecule of double-stranded DNA that is integrated into a host cell chromosome. Progeny virus are produced continuously, and the process eventually kills the host cell. (See p. 359)

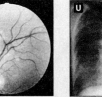
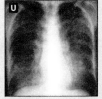

Cytomegalovirus retinitis   Pneumocystis pneumonia

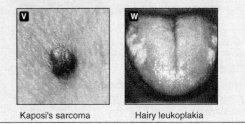

Kaposi's sarcoma   Hairy leukoplakia

Figure 20.6 (continued)
Some characteristics of sexually transmitted diseases: viruses.

3. **Trachoma:** *C. trachomatis*, serotypes A, B, B$_a$, and C cause a chronic keratoconjunctivitis that often results in blindness (see p. 441). Trachoma is transmitted by personal contact, for example, by eye to eye via droplets, by contaminated surfaces touched by hands and conveyed to the eye, or by flies. Because of persistent or repeated infection over several years, the inflammatory response with attendant scarring leads to permanent opacities of the cornea, and distortion of eyelids (Figure 20.6; also see Figure 28.6, p. 321).

4. **Neonatal conjunctivitis and other infections:** Over fifty percent of infants born to women infected with *C. trachomatis*, serotypes D–K (see Figure 20.4) will contract symptomatic infection on passage through the birth canal. The most common presentation is **inclusion conjunctivitis of the newborn** (**ICN**, see Figure 20.5). This acute, purulent conjunctivitis [named for the inclusion bodies (see p. 236) seen in infected conjunctival epithelial cells] usually heals without permanent damage to the eye. Approximately one in ten infected infants will present with or develop an **interstitial pneumonitis**, which is usually mild and self-limiting.

5. **Inclusion conjunctivitis in adults:** Individuals of any age may develop a transient purulent conjunctivitis due to *C. trachomatis* serotypes D–K (see Figure 20.4). Such individuals are often found to be genitally infected as well.

B. Laboratory identification

C. trachomatis can be demonstrated in clinical material by several direct procedures, and by culturing in human cell lines. Samples, particularly from urethra and cervix in genitourinary infection, and conjunctivae in ocular disease, should be obtained by cleaning away overlying exudate, and gently scraping to exfoliate infected epithelial cells.

1. **Direct tests:** Microscopic examination using direct fluorescent antibody staining reveals the characteristic cellular cytoplasmic inclusions. *C. trachomatis* infections can now be detected with high sensitivity and specificity using DNA-amplification performed on urine specimens. This permits cost-effective screening of large numbers of individuals without the need for access to a medical clinic and a pelvic examination. For example, Figure 20.7 shows the high prevalence of infection among young female military recruits detected by polymerase chain reaction assay performed on patient-collected urine samples.

2. **Culturing methods:** *C. trachomatis* can be cultivated by tissue culture in a number of human cell lines. In the standard procedure, using McCoy cells, addition to the culture medium of a eukaryotic metabolic inhibitor such as cycloheximide enhances growth of the parasite. The presence of chlamydial inclusions can be demonstrated after two to seven days of incubation.

3. **Detection of serotypes:** Serotypes of *C. trachomatis* can be determined by immunofluorescence staining with monoclonal antibodies. However, the procedure is not widely used because it adds little to clinical impressions. Serologic testing for specific antibodies

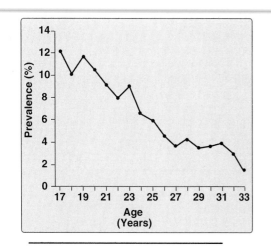

Figure 20.7
Prevalence of chlamydial infection among 13,204 female military recruits, according to age.

is similarly not very helpful except in suspected lymphogranuloma venereum, where a single high-titer response is diagnostic.

C. Treatment and prevention

Chlamydiae are sensitive to a number of broad-spectrum antibacterials. Azithromycin and tetracyclines are currently the drugs of choice. Resistant strains have not been reported in the clinical setting. Erythromycin should be used in small children and in pregnant women because of the effects of tetracyclines on calcification (Figure 20.8). [Note: These drugs are also effective in the simultaneous treatment of gonococcal infections that may accompany chlamydial infections.] A topical ocular preparation containing erythromycin provides moderately effective prophylaxis in newborns. Detection—a particular problem in asymptomatic individuals—followed by specific treatment are the key means of control.

IV. CHLAMYDIA PSITTACI

Psittacosis or, more broadly, **ornithosis**, denotes a zoonotic disease that is transmitted to humans by inhalation of dust contaminated with respiratory secretions or feces of infected birds. The human disease usually targets the lower respiratory tract (Figure 20.9). There is an acute onset of fever, hacking dry cough, and flu-like symptoms. Bilateral patchy pulmonary infiltrates are observed. Enlargement of liver and spleen is a frequent accompanying feature. Frank hepatitis, encephalitis, or myocarditis sometimes ensues. The severity of illness ranges from essentially asymptomatic infection to, rarely, a fatal outcome, usually for older patients. A wide variety of bird species including psittacines (the parrot family) carry *Chlamydia psittaci*, often latently, and contact with either diseased or healthy birds is an important item in differential diagnosis. A specific diagnosis can be made by showing a four-fold rise in antibody titer with either complement fixation (see p. 29) or indirect immunofluorescence tests (see p. 31). The organism can be grown in tissue culture from sputum and other clinical materials; however, this is not routinely attempted. Some strains are highly contagious and impose a considerable laboratory risk. If given early in the disease, doxycycline or erythromycin is effective in eradicating symptoms, but the organisms sometimes persist well into convalescence, because the drugs are bacteriostatic, not bacteriocidal (see p. 45).

V. CHLAMYDIA PNEUMONIAE

Chlamydia pneumoniae is a respiratory pathogen causing pharyngitis, sometimes followed by laryngitis, bronchitis, or interstitial pneumonia. It is a significant cause of **community-acquired respiratory infection**, occurring worldwide and without seasonal incidence. Epidemic outbreaks have been reported. About fifty percent of adults in the United States have antibodies to *C. pneumoniae*. Nevertheless, reinfection is known to occur. Several recent studies have linked *C. pneumoniae* antigens (or higher antibody titers to the organism) with atherosclerotic processes and asthma. However, a role for the organism in these diseases has not been established. Neither serologic tests nor recovery by culturing is routinely available. The organism is sensitive to doxycycline and erythromycin.

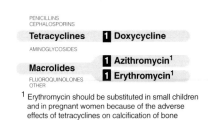

PENICILLINS
CEPHALOSPORINS
Tetracyclines   ▊ Doxycycline
AMINOGLYCOSIDES
Macrolides   ▊ Azithromycin[1]
FLUOROQUINOLONES   ▊ Erythromycin[1]
OTHER

[1] Erythromycin should be substituted in small children and in pregnant women because of the adverse effects of tetracyclines on calcification of bone and teeth formation.

Figure 20.8
Some antimicrobial agents useful in treating infections due to *Chlamydia trachomatis.*

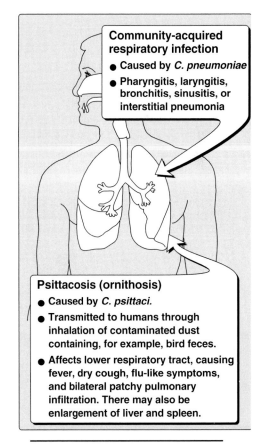

Community-acquired respiratory infection
● Caused by *C. pneumoniae*
● Pharyngitis, laryngitis, bronchitis, sinusitis, or interstitial pneumonia

Psittacosis (ornithosis)
● Caused by *C. psittaci.*
● Transmitted to humans through inhalation of contaminated dust containing, for example, bird feces.
● Affects lower respiratory tract, causing fever, dry cough, flu-like symptoms, and bilateral patchy pulmonary infiltration. There may also be enlargement of liver and spleen.

Figure 20.9
Diseases caused by *C. psittaci* and *C. pneumoniae.*

Study Questions

Choose the ONE correct answer

20.1 Which one of the following is characteristic of chlamydiae?

A. Reticulate bodies are infectious, extracellular form
of the organism.

B. Most genital tract infections are asymptomatic and
are undiagnosed and untreated.

C. Sensitive to β-lactam antibiotics.

D. Stain gram positive.

E. Inclusion bodies are formed from division of elementary bodies.

> Correct answer = B. The extracellular infectious
> form is called the elementary body, not the reticu-
> late body. Once inside the cell, the elementary
> body reorganizes into a larger, noninfectious
> reticulate body, which becomes metabolically
> active, and divides repeatedly by binary fission
> within the cytoplasm of the host cell forming an
> inclusion body. Chlamydiae are not stained using
> the Gram stain. The chlamydial cell envelope con-
> tains no peptidoglycan, thus β-lactam antibiotics
> have no effect on cell growth.

20.2 A feature of *Chlamydia* that is unique to this genus is:

A. the requirement of an obligate intracellular habitat.

B. its replicative cycle is distinguished by two morphologic forms that develop in cytoplasmic vacuoles.

C. the lack of muramic acid in its cell envelope.

D. its use of host coenzymes of energy metabolism.

E. all of the above.

> Correct answer = B. Extracellularly, chlamydiae
> exist as small, dense elementary bodies that are
> highly infective, but metabolically inert. In host cell
> cytoplasmic vacuoles, they develop into larger,
> metabolically active reticulate bodies that divide,
> and the progeny finally mature into elementary
> bodies that are released. Rickettsiae are also
> obligately intracellular (A), and use certain host
> energy coenzymes (D). Certain other unrelated
> species appear to require living host cells for
> growth. Mycoplasmas, having no peptidoglycan,
> lack muramic acid (C).

20.3 All of the following are true statements about
Chlamydia trachomatis EXCEPT which one?

A. It infects several types of epithelial cells.

B. It has a reservoir in domestic fowl.

C. It has a number of serotypes (about fifteen) that
correlate with the syndrome produced on infection.

D. It presently causes the most common sexually
transmitted disease in the United States.

E. It can be detected by direct immunofluorescence
on clinical material.

> Correct answer = B. All other items are correct.
> Whereas other chlamydia species are principally
> parasites of birds, *C. trachomatis* is a strictly
> human pathogen.

Questions 20.4 to 20.7:

Match the appropriate bacterium from the following list with
the statement to which it most closely corresponds. Each
bacterium can match one, more than one, or none of the
statements.

A. *Chlamydia pneumoniae*

B. *Chlamydia psittaci*

C. *Haemophilus influenzae*

D. *Legionella pneumophila*

E. *Mycoplasma pneumoniae*

G. *Streptococcus pneumoniae*

20.4. A college student visits the outpatient clinic, complaining of headache, malaise developing over several
days, and a hacking, nonproductive cough. He is
mildly febrile. A chest x-ray shows a greater degree
of bronchopulmonary infiltration than suggested by
the physical findings.

> Correct answer = E.

20.5 What is the next most probable alternative etiology in
item 20.3?

> Correct answer = A.

20.6 A 55-year-old man experiences the abrupt onset of
high fever, general myalgia, pleurisy, and a dry
cough. He also complains of diarrhea. He is a building superintendent, and has been servicing air condi-
tioning equipment.

> Correct answer = D.

20.7 A 35-year-old small animal veterinarian presents with
severe headache, myalgia, and splenomegaly in
addition to pulmonary findings. A scanty sputum was
obtained, containing a few mixed bacteria and scattered mononuclear cells on routine Gram staining.

> Correct answer = B.

Mycobacteria and Actinomycetes

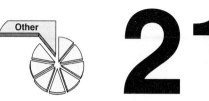

21

I. OVERVIEW

Mycobacteria are slender rods with lipid-rich cell walls that are resistant to penetration by chemical dyes, such as those used in the Gram stain. They therefore stain poorly, but once stained, cannot be easily decolorized by treatment with acidified organic solvents. Hence they are termed "**acid-fast**" (see p. 24). Mycobacterial infections are **intracellular**, and generally result in the formation of slow-growing granulomatous lesions that are responsible for major tissue destruction. For example, *Mycobacterium tuberculosis* causes tuberculosis, the principal chronic bacterial disease in humans, and a leading cause worldwide of death from infection. This organism has increasingly become a cause for special concern in immunocompromised patients. Members of the genus *Mycobacterium* also cause **leprosy**, as well as several tuberculosis-like human infections. This genus belongs to the order of organisms (Actinomycetales) that also includes the genera *Actinomyces* and *Nocardia*. These organisms all cause granulomatous lesions with various clinical presentations. Mycobacteria and other clinically significant Actinomycetales discussed in this chapter are listed in Figure 21.1.

II. MYCOBACTERIA

Mycobacteria are long, slender rods that are nonmotile and do not form spores (Figure 21.2). Mycobacterial cell walls are unusual in that they are approximately sixty percent lipid, including a unique class of very long-chain (75 to 90 carbons), β-hydroxylated fatty acids called **mycolic acids**. These complex with a variety of polysaccharides and peptides, creating a waxy cell surface that makes mycobacteria strongly hydrophobic, and accounts for their acid-fast staining characteristic. Their unusual cell walls make mycobacteria impervious to many chemical disinfectants, and convey resistance to the corrosive action of strong acids or alkalis as well. Use is made of this fact in decontaminating clinical specimens such as sputum, where nonmycobacterial organisms are digested by such treatments. Mycobacteria are also very resistant to drying, but not to heat or ultraviolet irradiation. Mycobacteria are strictly aerobic. Most species grow slowly with generation times of 8 to 24 hours, in part because their hydrophobic surface promotes clumped growth and slow uptake of nutri-

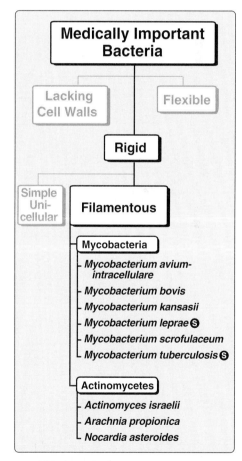

Figure 21.1
Classification of mycobacteria and Actinomycetes.
Ⓢ See pp. 414, 448 for summaries of these organisms.

Lippincott's Illustrated Reviews: Microbiology,
by William A. Strohl, Harriet Rouse, Bruce D. Fisher.
Lippincott, Williams & Wilkins, Baltimore, MD © 2001

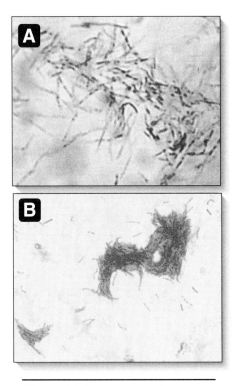

Figure 21.2
Mycobacterium tuberculosis.
A. Acid-fast stain of sputum from a patient with tuberculosis. B. Typical growth pattern showing "cording", (that is, growing in strings).

ents. Most mycobacteria grow on fairly simple artificial media (see p. 448). Species are differentiated by rate and optimal temperature of growth, production of pigments, and other biochemical tests. Animal inoculation is rarely used nowadays, except in the case of *Mycobacterium leprae*, which has never been successfully maintained except in animals.

A. Mycobacterium tuberculosis

It is currently estimated that about one third of the world's population is infected with *M. tuberculosis* (the **tubercle bacillus**), with thirty million people having active disease. Eight million new cases occur, and two million people die of the disease, each year. Figure 21.3 shows the estimated number of tuberculosis cases by country in 1997.

1. **History of the disease:** Tuberculosis is a disease of great antiquity in both the western and eastern hemispheres. It achieved epidemic proportions, however, in the late 18th and 19th centuries as populations increased and urbanization developed. Because of a rise in the standard of living, and the success of public health strategies in the United States and western Europe, the incidence of infection began to decline steadily before the turn of the century, and this raised hopes that tuberculosis might be eradicated early in the 21st century. It is disappointing that the yearly decline ended in I984, and after several years of stationary incidence, annual numbers in the West actually increased from 1988 to 1994. Also, once a disease mainly of the elderly, clinical tuberculosis has become more prevalent among younger individuals (25 to 44 years old) and among children (Figure 21.4). The increased incidence and the shift in age distribution in the United States was attributed to the large numbers of infected immigrants (particularly from southeast Asia), homeless persons, intravenous drug users,

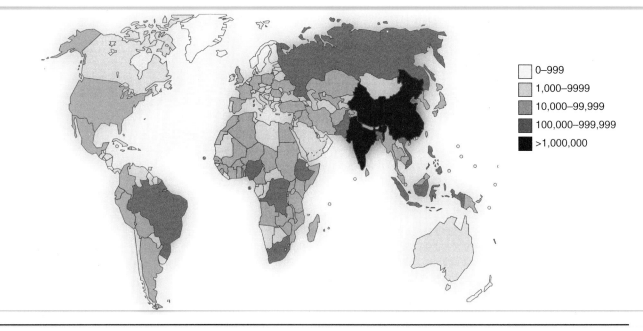

Figure 21.3
Estimated numbers of tuberculosis cases by country in 1997.

and HIV-infected patients. The incidence of tuberculosis in the United States has declined for many years, and is now at a historic low (Figure 21.5). Because transmission is facilitated by crowding and poor ventilation, individuals in nursing homes, homeless shelters, and prisons are among those particularly at risk. In contrast to the decline of tuberculosis in the West, the incidence of the disease in some Asian and sub-Saharan African nations has increased to more than 300 new cases per 100,000 people per year (compared to 6.8 per 100,000 in the United States). In some of these nations, nearly fifty percent of the HIV-infected population is co-infected with *M. tuberculosis*.

2. **Epidemiology:** Patients with active pulmonary tuberculosis shed large numbers of organisms by coughing, thus creating aerosol droplet nuclei. Because of resistance to dessication, the organisms can remain viable in the environment for a long time. The principal mode of contagion is person-to-person transmission by inhalation of the aerosol, and repeated or prolonged contact is usually required for transmission of infection. However, a single infected person can pass the organism to numerous people in an exposed group such as a family, a classroom, or a hospital ward. A large literature documents racial differences in susceptibility to tuberculosis. Dark-skinned races and groups that have come in contact with the organism in recent times (for example, Native Americans and Hawaiians) are more susceptible. Studies of disease frequency in twins demonstrate a genetic component as well. When one twin is infected, the attack rate in the other is 75 percent for identical pairs, but only 25 percent in fraternal twins.

3. **Pathogenicity:** After being inhaled, mycobacteria reach the alveoli, where they multiply in the pulmonary epithelium or in macrophages. Within two to four weeks, many bacilli are destroyed by the immune system, but some survive, and are spread by the blood to extrapulmonary sites. The virulence of *M. tuberculosis* rests with its ability to survive and grow within host cells (Figure 21.6). The organism produces no demonstrable toxins. However, when engulfed by macrophages, bacterial sulfolipids inhibit the fusion of phagocytic vesicles with lysosomes. The ability of the organism to grow even in immunologically activated macrophages, and to remain viable—although quiescent— within the host for decades, are keys to the unique character of tuberculosis.

4. **Immunity:** *M. tuberculosis* stimulates both a humoral and a cell-mediated immune response (see p. 59). Although circulating antibodies appear, they do not convey resistance to the organism. Instead, cellular immunity (CD4$^+$ T cells, see p. 68) and the accompanying delayed hypersensitivity, directed against a number of bacterial protein antigens, develop in the course of infection, and contribute to both the pathology of and immunity to the disease. Tubercle bacilli are excellent immunogens; their cell wall products, particularly a muramyl dipeptide fragment of the peptidoglycan, enhance immunologic responsiveness nonspecifically. Consequently, they have been used as experimental immunologic **adjuvants** (see p. 39).

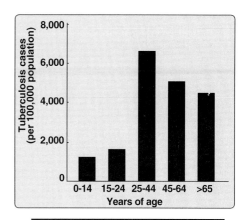

Figure 21.4
Incidence of new cases of tuberculosis, 1997, reported by age (United States).

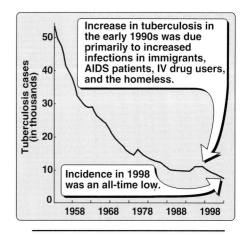

Figure 21.5
Incidence of new cases of tuberculosis (United States).

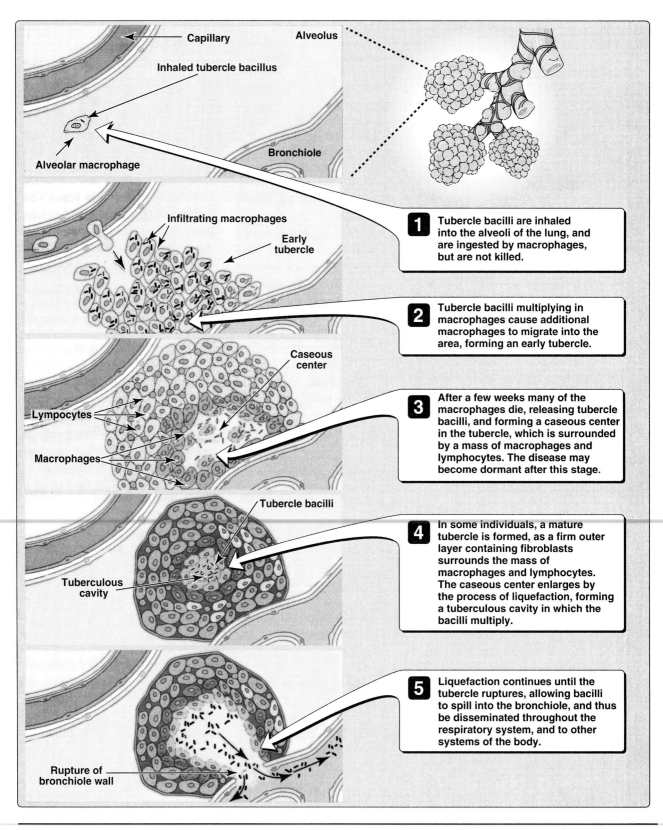

Figure 21.6
Progression of active tuberculosis infection.

5. Clinical significance: Primary tuberculosis occurs in a person who has had no previous contact with the organism. For the majority of cases (about 95 percent), the infection becomes arrested, and most people are unaware of this initial encounter. The only evidence of tuberculosis may be a positive tuberculin test (see p. 250). A chest X-ray sometimes shows the initial pulmonary nodule (a healing tubercle, see below), and some fibrosis—the classic **Ghon complex** (Figure 21.7). Approximately ten percent of those with an arrested primary infection develop clinical tuberculosis at some time later in their lives. Figure 21.6 illustrates the course of tuberculosis infection progressing to clinical disease.

a. **Primary disease—initial phase:** Primary tuberculosis is usually acquired via the respiratory tract; therefore, the initial lesion occurs in a small bronchiole or alveolus in the apical (mid-lung) periphery. The organisms are engulfed by local mononuclear phagocytes, and their presence initiates an inflammatory reaction. However, because tubercle bacilli grow well in phagocytic cells, the bacteria proliferate, and are carried by lymphatic drainage to the lymph nodes and beyond to set up additional foci. This initial phase of the infection is usually mild or asymptomatic, and results in exudative lesions where fluid and polymorphonuclear leukocytes accumulate around the bacilli. A specific immune response develops after about a month, and this changes the character of the lesions. Cell-mediated immunity to *M. tuberculosis*, and hypersensitivity to its antigens (tuberculoproteins), confer an enhanced ability to localize the infection and curb growth of the organism, but also cause a greater capacity to damage the host. Macrophages, activated by specific T lymphocytes, begin to accumulate and destroy the bacilli.

b. **Primary disease—tubercle formation:** The productive (granulomatous) lesion that develops is known as a **tubercle** (see Figure 21.6). It consists of a central area of large, multinucleate giant cells (macrophage syncytia) containing tubercle bacilli, a midzone of pale epithelioid cells, and a peripheral collar of fibroblasts and mononuclear cells. Tissue damage is produced by the destruction of both bacilli and phagocytes, which results in the release of degradative enzymes and reactive oxygen species, such as superoxide radicals and peroxide (see p. 56), accompanied by the interactions of various cytokines. The center of the lesion develops a characteristic expanding, caseous (cheesy) necrosis (Figure 21.8).

c. **Primary tuberculosis follows one of two courses:** If the lesion arrests, the tubercle undergoes fibrosis and calcification, although viable but nonproliferating organisms may persist (Figure 21.9). Alternatively, if the lesion breaks down, the caseous material is discharged, and a cavity is created that can facilitate spread of the infection. The organisms are dispersed by the lymph and the bloodstream, and can seed the lungs, the regional lymph nodes, or various distant tissues, such as liver, spleen, kidneys, bone, or meninges. In progres-

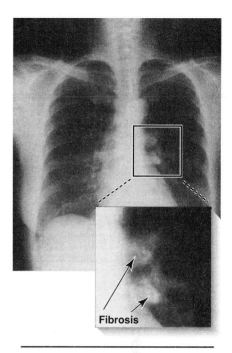

Fibrosis

Figure 21.7
A chest X-ray showing some fibrosis—the classic Ghon complex.

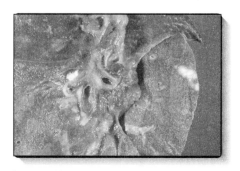

Figure 21.8
Lung with tuberculous lesion.

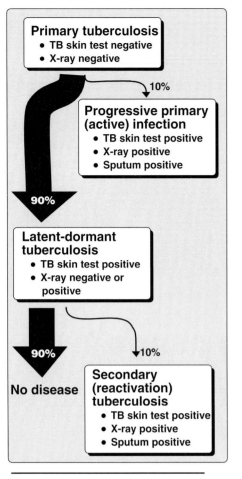

Figure 21.9
Stages in the pathogenesis of tuberculosis.

sive disease, one or more of the resulting tubercles may expand, leading to destruction of tissue and clinical illness, for example, **chronic pneumonitis**, **tuberculous osteomyelitis**, or **tuberculous meningitis**. In the extreme instance, active tubercles develop throughout the body, a serious condition known as **miliary (disseminated) tuberculosis**.

    d. Reactivation of tuberculosis: This is usually caused by *M. tuberculosis* that has survived in a dormant primary tubercle lesion (Figure 21.9). [Note: Resistance and hypersensitivity induced in the host by the first infection with tubercle bacilli normally prevent reinfection from external sources.] Any of the preexisting tubercles may be involved, but pulmonary sites are most common, particularly the lung apices where high oxygen tension favors mycobacterial growth. Bacterial populations in such lesions often become quite large, and many organisms are shed, for example, in sputum. The patient thus again becomes capable of exposing others to the disease. Reactivation is apparently due to an impairment in immune status, often associated with malnutrition, alcoholism, advanced age, or severe stress. Immunosuppressive medication, or diseases such as diabetes and, particularly, AIDS, are common preconditions.

6. Tuberculin reaction: The tuberculin reaction test is a manifestation of **delayed hypersensitivity** to protein antigens of *M. tuberculosis*. Whereas such tests can be used to document contact with the tubercle bacillus, they do not confirm that the patient currently has active disease.

    a. Mantoux test: Purified protein derivative (**PPD**) is prepared from culture filtrates of the organism, and is biologically standardized. Activity is expressed in **tuberculin units (TU)**. In the routine procedure, the so-called Mantoux test, a measured amount of PPD is injected intradermally in the forearm (Figure 21.10). It is read

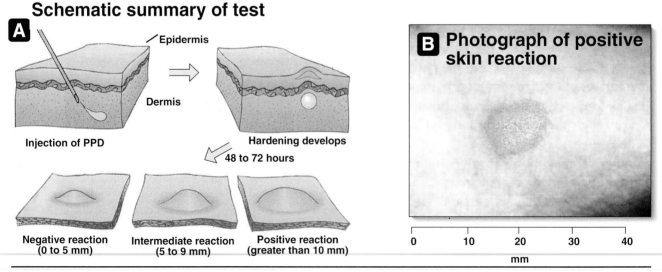

Figure 21.10
The Mantoux skin test for tuberculosis. [Note: For some people, determination of a positive reaction may be interpreted more stringently (see Figure 21.11).]

48 to 72 hours later for the presence and size of an area of induration (hardening) at the site of injection, which must be observed for the test to be positive (Figure 21.11). A positive reaction usually develops four to six weeks after initial contact with the organism. It remains positive for life, although it may wane after some years.

b. **Conditions affecting the tuberculin reaction:** Active tuberculosis is often associated with conditions of suppressed cell-mediated immunity. Under these circumstances, loss of delayed hypersensitivity and a state of anergy (absence of sensitivity), may develop; the tuberculin reaction will then be attenuated or negative. Finally, cross-reaction is occasionally observed with other pathogens in the genus *Mycobacterium*. [Note: Other techniques for tuberculin testing, such as the **Tine test**, are not quantitative, and are therefore useful for population screening, but not for individual diagnosis.]

7. **Laboratory identification:** Diagnosis of active pulmonary tuberculosis includes demonstration of clinical symptoms and abnormal chest X-rays, and confirmation by isolation of *M. tuberculosis* from relevant clinical material.

a. **Identification of *M. tuberculosis* in clinical specimens:** A microscopic search for acid-fast bacilli, using techniques such as the Ziehl-Neelsen stain, is the most rapid test for mycobacteria. Smears can be made from various specimens—sputum, bronchial washings, urine, spinal fluid sediment, biopsy material—either directly or after concentration procedures, and stained with fuchsin or a fluorescent acid-fast dye such as auramine. However, *M. tuberculosis* cannot be reliably distinguished on morphologic grounds from other occasional pathogens in the genus, from some saprophytic mycobacterial species that may contaminate glassware and reagents in the laboratory, or from those mycobacteria that may be part of the normal flora. Therefore, a definitive identification of *M. tuberculosis* can only be obtained by culturing the organism, or by using one of the newer molecular methods described below. Although two to eight weeks are required to culture the tubercle bacillus because of its slow growth on laboratory media, such cultures can detect small numbers of organisms in the original sample. Isolation of the organism is essential for determining its antibiotic sensitivity, in addition to confirming the specific identity of the bacillus by growth and biochemical characteristics. Figure 21.12 shows a culture of *M. tuberculosis*.

b. **Nucleic acid amplification:** Molecular techniques are increasingly important in the diagnosis of tuberculosis, because they have the potential to shorten the time required to detect and identify *M. tuberculosis* in clinical specimens. For example, the **amplified *M. tuberculosis* direct test** utilizes enzymes that rapidly make copies of *M. tuberculosis* 16S ribosomal RNA, which can be detected using genetic probes. The sensitivity of

---

An induration of >5 mm is interpreted as positive in the following populations:

- Persons who have had contact with infectious individuals
- Persons with an abnormal chest X-ray
- HIV-infected and other immuno-suppressed persons

An induration of >10 mm is interpreted as positive in the following populations:

- Foreign-born persons from high-prevalence countries
- Residents of prisons, nursing homes, and other institutions
- Health care workers
- Persons with other medical risk factors

An induration of >15 mm is interpreted as positive in the following populations:

- Persons with no risk factors

Figure 21.11
Interpretations of the Mantoux skin test for tuberculosis.

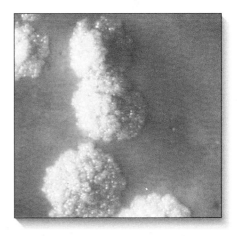

Figure 21.12
Mycobacterium tuberculosis coloniesgrown on Lowenstein-Jensen medium.

the test ranges from 75 to 100 percent, with a specificity of 95 to 100 percent (see p. 21), and is used for patients whose clinical smears are positive for acid-fast bacilli, and for which cultures are in progress. A second technique, the **polymerase chain reaction** (**PCR**), amplifies a small portion of a predetermined target region of the *M. tuberculosis* DNA. Using human sputum, commercial PCR kits can confirm the diagnosis of tuberculosis within eight hours, with a sensitivity and specificity that rivals culture techniques. In addition, PCR analysis facilitates DNA fingerprinting of specific strains, allowing studies of the progress of epidemics.

8. **Treatment:** Several chemotherapeutic agents are effective against *M. tuberculosis*. Because strains of the organism resistant to a particular agent emerge during treatment, multiple drug therapy is employed to delay or prevent their emergence. Isoniazid, rifampin, ethambutol, streptomycin, and pyrazinamide are the principal or so-called "first line" drugs because of their efficacy and acceptable degree of toxicity (Figure 21.13).

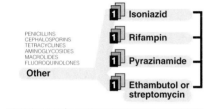

Figure 21.13
Some antimicrobial agents useful in treating infections caused by *Mycobacterium tuberculosis*.

a. **Drug resistance:** Mutants resistant to each of these agents have been isolated even prior to drug treatment. Therefore the standard procedure is to begin treatment with two or more drugs to prevent outgrowth of resistant strains. Sensitivity tests, administered as soon as sufficient cultured organisms are available, are an important guide to modifying treatment. In most parts of the United States, eight to fourteen percent of *M. tuberculosis* strains are resistant to one or more of the primary drugs, when initially isolated from new cases of tuberculosis. The higher incidence of **multiply drug-resistant strains** (**MDR-TB**) in some locations and patient populations (for example, in prisons) is obviously a cause for great concern.

b. **Course of treatment:** Clinical tuberculosis requires a long course of treatment due to characteristics of the organisms and the lesions they produce. For example, as intracellular pathogens, the bacilli are shielded from drugs that do not penetrate host cells, and large cavities with avascular centers are penetrated by drugs with difficulty. Further, in chronic or arrested tubercles, the organisms are nonproliferating, and therefore are not susceptible to many antimicrobial agents. Until recently, twelve to eighteen months of drug administration was thought to be required for a clinical cure. In recent years, short courses of six months, beginning with a daily dose of a combination of drugs, and later by twice weekly doses, have been successful in curing uncomplicated tuberculosis (Figure 21.14). If the drugs are effective in the pulmonary form of this disease, sputum acid-fast bacteria smears become negative, and the patient becomes noninfectious in two to three weeks. In general, treatment can be conducted on an outpatient basis, although this has made potential patient noncompliance with multiple drug schedules a major issue in management.

c. **Directly observed therapy:** Patient compliance is often low when multiple drug schedules last for six months or longer. One successful strategy for achieving better treatment completion rates is "directly observed therapy," in which patients take their medication while being supervised and observed. Some health care providers have embraced the concept of directly observed therapy; others regard the strategy as expensive and intrusive, suitable only for individuals who have a history of noncompliance.

9. **Prevention:** Public health measures such as tuberculin tests, chest X-rays, case registries, and contact tracing have done much to control tuberculosis at the population level. However, these measures were relaxed in the late 1980s, resulting in an increasing incidence of disease (see p. 246).

a. **Latent TB chemotherapy:** For individuals who are tuberculin-positive but asymptomatic, chemotherapy is indicated in several situations, usually with the single antibiotic, isoniazid. For example, people in whom a recent skin test conversion is documented, or tuberculin-positive patients who need immunosuppressive therapy for another illness, can be protected from active tuberculosis by this treatment.

b. **Vaccines:** A vaccine against tuberculosis has been available since early in the twentieth century. It is produced from **Bacille Calmette-Guerin (BCG)**, an attenuated strain of *Mycobacterium bovis*. When injected intradermally, it can confer tuberculin hypersensitivity, and an enhanced ability to activate macrophages that kill the pathogen. This vaccine is about eighty percent protective against serious forms of tuberculosis, such as meningitis in children, and has been used in mass immunization campaigns by the World Health Organization, and in several European countries. However, recommendations by public health officials in the United States suggest that vaccination be considered only for tuberculin-negative individuals under sustained heavy risk of infection, such as special groups of health care workers, or those at high risk in areas where multiply drug-resistant TB is common (Figure 21.15). The reason for its restricted use is that the vaccine causes a positive tuberculin reaction for several years after it is given, which greatly limits the usefulness of that diagnostic test in the event that the individual should later become infected with *M. tuberculosis*. BCG should also not be given to AIDS or other immunosuppressed individuals, because in such cases it has occasionally caused clinical disease. The use of genetically engineered BCG tailored for improved efficacy against tuberculosis is currently under investigation. [Note: Because BCG activates macrophages, it has also been used experimentally to stimulate cellular immune functions in the treatment of some malignancies, for example, cancer of the bladder.]

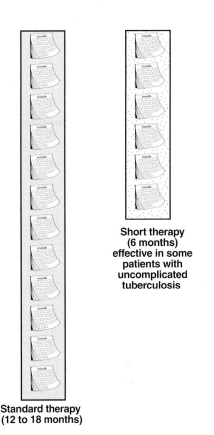

Short therapy
(6 months)
effective in some
patients with
uncomplicated
tuberculosis

Standard therapy
(12 to 18 months)

Figure 21.14
Duration of treatment for tuberculosis.

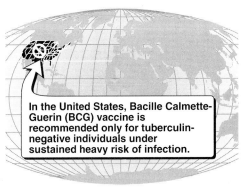

In the United States, Bacille Calmette-Guerin (BCG) vaccine is recommended only for tuberculin-negative individuals under sustained heavy risk of infection.

Figure 21.15
Bacille Calmette-Guerin (BCG) is used throughout the world, but seldom in the United States.

B. Mycobacterium bovis

There are tuberculosis-like illnesses in almost all vertebrates, caused by mycobacteria adapted to the particular species. The bovine organism, *Mycobacterium bovis*, is one of the few of the "other" mycobacteria capable of cross-infecting humans, and causes a clinical illness indistinguishable from that caused by *M. tuberculosis*. Milk is the common vehicle of transmission; therefore the primary lesion is often in cervical or intestinal lymph nodes rather than the lung. *M. bovis* infections are rare in the United States at present because of the pasteurization of milk, and because of the veterinary practice of sacrificing tuberculin reactors in cattle herds.

C. Atypical mycobacteria

Several other species of mycobacteria can be pathogenic in humans. Like *M. tuberculosis*, they are acid-fast bacilli that cause chronic granulomatous lesions and a delayed hypersensitivity reaction that may or may not cross-react with tuberculoprotein. These pathogens are often grouped together and referred to as "atypical mycobacteria", or "**mycobacteria other than tuberculosis (MOTT)**". When cultured, some species produce yellow to orange pigments if exposed to light (**photochromogens**), or under any conditions of illumination, including darkness (**scotochromogens**). [Note: Those species that do not produce pigment are termed **nonchromogens**.] These characteristics, together with other biochemical reactions, are used for identification. In general, these species are not transmitted from human to human. Most are found in the soil, although they may have mammalian or avian reservoirs. They are sensitive to the same range of chemotherapeutic agents as is *M. tuberculosis*, but, in some cases they require higher doses and more aggressive treatment schedules.

1. **Mycobacterium avium-intracellulare complex (MAC or MAI):** This is a complex of nonchromogenic organisms that can be divided into a number of serotypes with variable ecologies. For example, MACs are frequently recovered from soil and water. Some cause tuberculosis in birds (and grow best at 41°C) but do not infect humans, whereas others infect a variety of mammals including humans. In some geographic areas, such as in the southeastern United States, over fifty percent of healthy resident adults are skin test–positive to a PPD (see p. 250) prepared from MAC. In the United States, **disseminated (miliary) disease** caused by MAC is now recognized as a common opportunistic bacterial infection in AIDS patients (Figure 21.16; see also Figure 31.16, p. 369). Extensive pulmonary MAC infections are sometimes superimposed on **chronic bronchitis** or **emphysema**. **Cervical lymphadenitis**, **chronic osteomyelitis**, and **renal** or **skin infections** occur, usually following some compromise of the tissues. Diseases caused by the MAC complex are particularly refractory to chemotherapy. The usual practice is to treat with four or more drugs, regardless of sensitivity determinations. Relapses are common.

2. **Mycobacterium kansasii:** *M. kansasii* is a photochromogen that causes pulmonary, lymph node, and other systemic disease indistinguishable from tuberculosis. [Note: The organism causes three percent of the clinical illness known as tuberculosis.] The reservoir

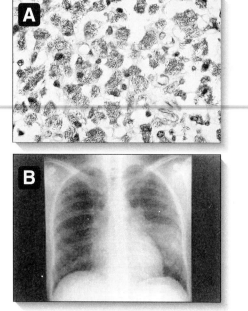

Figure 21.16
A. *Mycobacterium avium-intracellulare* infection of lymph node in patient with AIDS. Ziehl-Neelsen stain. Histopathology of lymph node shows tremendous numbers of acid-fast bacilli within plump histiocytes.
B. Chest radiograph of patient with AIDS and diffuse pulmonary MAC infection.

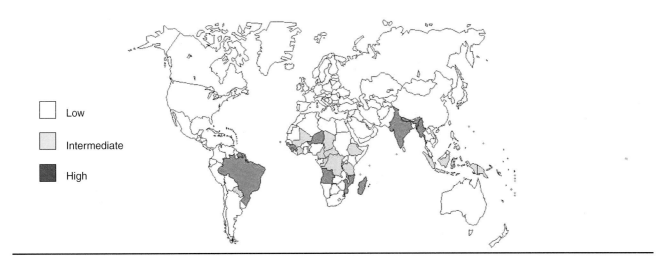

Figure 21.17
Worldwide distribution of leprosy.

of *M. kansasii* remains unknown. In the United States, infections by *M. kansasii* are most common in the central region and quite rare in the southeast. The delayed hypersensitivity that develops is strongly cross-reactive with standard PPD, and the organism is susceptible to standard antituberculous drugs, such as rifampin.

3. **Mycobacterium scrofulaceum:** This organism is a scotochromogen that is a common cause of chronic **cervical lymphadenitis** in children, and a rare cause of other granulomatous conditions. It can be recovered from environmental sources. It tends to be resistant to antituberculous drugs, but surgical excision of infected cervical nodes is curative.

D. Mycobacterium leprae

Leprosy, or, as it is specified by the United States Public Health Service, **Hansen's disease**, is rare in this country, but a small number of cases, both imported and domestically acquired, are reported each year. Worldwide, it is a much larger problem, with an estimated ten to twelve million cases (Figure 21.17).

1. **Pathogenicity:** *M. leprae* is transmitted from human to human through prolonged contact, for example, between exudates of a leprosy patient's skin lesions, and the abraded skin of another individual. The infectivity of *M. leprae* is low, and the incubation period protracted, so that clinical disease may develop years or even decades after initial contact with the organism.

2. **Clinical significance:** Leprosy is a chronic granulomatous condition of peripheral nerves and mucocutaneous tissues, particularly the nasal mucosa. It occurs as a continuum between two clinical extremes: tuberculoid and lepromatous leprosy (Figure 21.18). In **tuberculoid leprosy**, the lesions occur as large **maculae** (spots) in cooler body tissues such as skin (especially nose and outer ears, testicles), and in superficial nerve endings. Neuritis leads to patches of anesthesia in the skin. The lesions are heavily infiltrated by lymphocytes, and giant and epithelioid cells, but

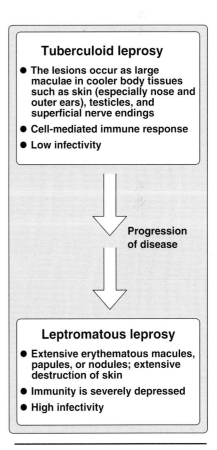

Figure 21.18
Classification of leprosy.

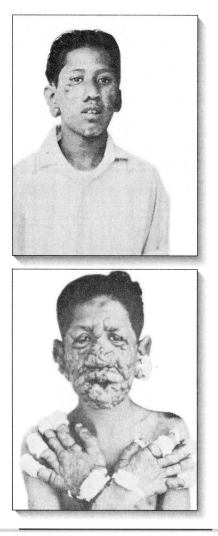

Figure 21.19
A. Leprosy in a 13-year-old Hawaiian boy in 1931. B. Same boy two years later. [Note: This patient had the misfortune of contracting leprosy before the era of effective antibiotics.]

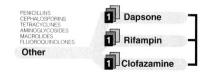

Figure 21.20
Some antimicrobial agents useful in treating infections caused by *Mycobacterium leprae*.

caseation does not occur. The patient mounts a strong cell-mediated immune response, and develops delayed hypersensitivity, which can be shown by skin test with **lepromin**, a tuberculin-like extract of lepromatous tissue. The course of **lepromatous leprosy** is slow but progressive (Figure 21.19). Large numbers of organisms are present in the lesions and reticuloendothelial system, and immunity is severely depressed.

3. **Laboratory identification:** *M. leprae* is an acid-fast bacillus. It has not been successfully maintained in artificial culture, but can be grown in the footpads of mice, and in the armadillo, which may also be a natural host although playing no role in human disease. Laboratory diagnosis of lepromatous leprosy, where organisms are numerous, involves acid-fast stains of specimens from nasal mucosa or other infected areas. In tuberculoid leprosy, organisms are extremely rare, and diagnosis depends on clinical findings and the histology of biopsy material.

4. **Treatment and prevention:** Several drugs are effective in the treatment of leprosy, including sulfones such as dapsone, rifampin, and clofazamine (Figure 21.20). Treatment is prolonged, and combined therapy is necessary to ensure the suppression of resistant mutants. The fact that vaccination with BCG (see p. 253) has shown some protective effect in leprosy has encouraged further interest in vaccine development. Thalidomide, an inhibitor of TNF-α (see p. 63), is being distributed under tight restrictions for use as a treatment for **erythema nodosum leprosum**, a serious and severe skin complication of leprosy. [Note: Thalidomide, originally marketed in the late 1950s as a sedative for pregnant women, was linked to severe limb deformities in their offspring, and was removed from the market.]

III. ACTINOMYCETES

Actinomycetes are a group of filamentous, branching, gram-positive organisms that easily fragment into slender rods (Figure 21.21). Although they superficially resemble fungi on morphologic grounds, they are prokaryotes of bacterial size. They are free-living, mostly soil organisms that are related to corynebacteria and mycobacteria, as well as to the streptomycetes that are sources of important antibiotics.

A. Actinomyces israelii, Arachnia propionica

Actinomyces israelii and *Arachnia propionica* are part of the normal oral and intestinal flora in humans. They are strict anaerobes.

1. **Clinical significance:** Actinomycosis is an opportunistic infection, in which a chronic suppurative abscess leads to scarring and disfigurement. The infection is probably initiated by accidental introduction of organisms into the underlying soft tissues during conditions of sufficient anaerobiasis to support their growth. About half of the cases have a cervicofacial location, and are associated with poor dental hygiene and/or tooth extraction. Other cases involve the lung and chest wall, the cecum, appendix, abdominal wall, and pelvic organs. The lesion (a **mycetoma**) begins as a

hard, red, relatively nontender swelling that develops slowly, becomes filled with liquid, and ruptures to the surface, discharging quantities of pus. It also spreads laterally, draining pus through several sinus tracts.

2. **Laboratory identification:** The most typical and diagnostic finding in actinomycosis is the presence of "sulfur granules" in the draining pus. These are small, firm, usually yellowish particles, which in fact do not contain sulfur. When examined under the microscope, these appear as microcolonies composed of filaments of the organism embedded in an amorphous, eosinophilic material thought to be antigen-antibody complexes. The organism can be grown anaerobically on enriched media such as thioglycollate broth or blood agar. Growth is slow, often requiring ten to fourteen days for visible colonies.

3. **Treatment:** Penicillin G is the treatment of choice for actinomycosis, although a number of antibiotics (clindamycin, erythromycin, and tetracycline) have been shown to have clinical effect (Figure 21.22). Treatment must be sustained for weeks to months, and may be accompanied by surgical debridement and/or drainage. No significant resistance to penicillin G has been reported. [Note: Good oral hygiene is an important preventive measure.]

B. Nocardia asteroides, Nocardia brasiliensis

Nocardiae are aerobic soil organisms. Infections of humans and domestic animals are opportunistic, and are not transmissible from person to person. Instead, nocardias are inhaled, or are acquired by contamination of skin wounds.

1. **Clinical significance:** The most common presentation of human **nocardiosis** is a pneumonia of rather chronic course with abscesses, extensive necrosis, and cavity formation. The organisms may metastasize, with the brain and kidneys as the most common secondary locations. Common predisposing conditions are the immunosuppression associated with lymphoma or other malignancy, or with drugs. In the United States, *N. asteroides* is the more common organism.

2. **Laboratory identification:** Nocardiae are gram-positive, but irregularly staining, branched filaments (Figure 21.23). They are usually numerous in clinical material, and do not form sulphur granules. They stain weakly acid-fast after decolorization with one percent sulfuric acid alcohol, but fully decolorize with the routine Ziehl-Neelsen procedure. Nocardiae are strictly aerobic. They grow slowly on a variety of simple media (such as fungal media without antibiotics) and on standard blood agar.

3. **Treatment:** The sulfonamides such as sulfamethoxazole, with or without trimethoprim, are the drugs of choice for treating nocardiosis (Figure 21.24). The nocardiae are relatively resistant to penicillin. Surgical drainage of the lesions is important, and prolonged therapy may be required to eliminate the infection.

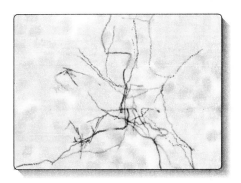

Figure 21.21
Actinomycete.

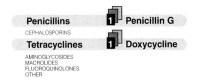

Figure 21.22
Antimicrobial agent useful in treating infections due to *Actinomyces*.

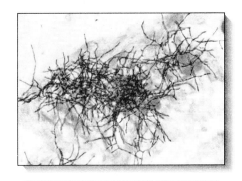

Figure 21.23
Nocardia

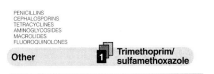

Figure 21.24
An antimicrobial agent useful in treating infections due to *Nocardia*.

Study Questions

Choose the ONE correct answer

21.1 Which one of the following is characteristic of mycobacteria?

    A. They contain mycolic acids.

    B. They are resistant to inactivation by heat.

    C. They grow extracellularly.

    D. They are anaerobic.

    E. They are spore-forming.

> Correct choice = A. Mycobacteria are unique in that their cell wall contains high concentrations of mycolic acids. Mycobacteria are not particularly heat resistant, as witness their susceptibility to pasteurization. They are aerobic, intracellular organisms that do not form spores.

21.2 Virulence in mycobacteria is most strongly correlated with:

    A. mycotoxin production.

    B. slow growth.

    C. composition of the cell envelope.

    D. small size of cells.

    E. dependence on oxygen for growth.

> Correct answer = C: Several cell wall components promote the intracellular growth of the organisms, and their dissemination in the infected host.)

21.3 An acid-fast smear on a patient's sputum is positive. The tuberculin test, however, is negative. A more definitive diagnosis could be obtained by:

    A. paying attention to the patient's history.

    B. a more extensive physical examination.

    C. a chest X-ray.

    D. repeat of the sputum smear.

    E. laboratory culture and speciation.

> Correct answer = E. Laboratory culture and speciation would best resolve the question, although any of the procedures listed might yield helpful information. The possibility of anergy could be investigated by skin-testing for delayed hypersensitivity to unrelated antigens, but the patient might be anergic and still be infected with a mycobacterium other than *M. tuberculosis* (MOTT).

21.4 Which of the following statements regarding *Actinomyces* and *Nocardia* is true?

    A. Both organisms have branching growth but are prokaryotes.

    B. Neither stains with Gram stain

    C. *Nocardia* infections are endogenous, and often initiated by trauma.

    D. *Actinomyces* usually causes infections in systemically compromised patients.

    E. Neither is sensitive to anti-bacterial drugs.

> Correct answer = B. Both species appear as gram-positive, filamentous rods or branching forms on Gram staining. *Actinomyces* are often seen in association with amorphous material from "sulfur granules" in such smears. *Nocardia* is weakly acid-fast, in addition to being gram-positive. *Actinomyces* infections are endogenous, and often initiated by trauma. *Nocardia* usually causes infections in systemically compromised patients.

21.5 The treatment of tuberculosis:

    A. is initiated with a single "first line" drug.

    B. is initiated after the results of sensitivity testing is available.

    C. is most effective in patients with chronic or arrested tubercles.

    D. may last two to three weeks.

    E. should be directly observed in individuals who have a history of noncompliance.

> Correct answer = E. The standard procedure is to begin treatment with two or more drugs to prevent outgrowth of resistant strains. Sensitivity tests are an important guide to modifying treatment, but sensitivity data are not required to initiate therapy. In chronic or arrested tubercles, the organisms are nonproliferating, and therefore are not susceptible to many antimicrobial agents. Therapy may last from six to eighteen months.

Rickettsiae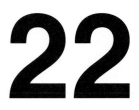

I. OVERVIEW

The group of organisms known as rickettsiae (family Rickettsiaceae) consists of three genera: *Rickettsia*, *Ehrlichia*, and *Coxiella* (Figure 22.1), which have a number of features in common. For example: 1) They grow only inside living host cells. [Note: Many pathogenic bacteria grow well inside particular cell types, but do not require this environment for multiplication; rickettsiae, like chlamydiae, are obligately intracellular parasites.] 2) Most rickettsial infections are transmitted by infected arthropods—lice, ticks, fleas, and/or mites. 3) Rickettsial diseases such as typhus, spotted fevers, human ehrlichiosis, and Q fever are generalized infections, with rash sometimes being a prominent feature. Mortality rates of these diseases are quite variable, but may be high in the absence of appropriate treatment.

II. RICKETTSIAE

Rickettsiae have the structural features of typical prokaryotic cells. They are small, rod-like or coccobacillary in shape (Figure 22.2), and have a typical double-layered, gram-negative cell wall. However, they stain poorly, and because of their usual occurrence inside host cells, are best visualized under the light microscope with one of the polychrome stains such as Giemsa or Macchiavello.

A. Physiology

The obligate requirement for an intracellular environment for rickettsial replication is not fully understood, but its plasma membrane is very leaky and therefore easily permeable to host cell nutrients and coenzymes. For example, rickettsiae appear to use host sources of essential nucleotide coenzymes such as NAD^+, coenzyme A, and ATP. [Note: *In vitro* suspensions of rickettsiae rapidly lose their pools of these and other essential compounds, and therefore survive poorly outside host cells.] Rickettsiae contain a number of antigens that convey both group and species specificity.

B. Pathogenesis

Rickettsia species parasitize endothelial cells throughout the circulatory system. They are transmitted to humans by arthropods such as fleas, ticks, mites, or lice, from reservoirs of infectious organisms.

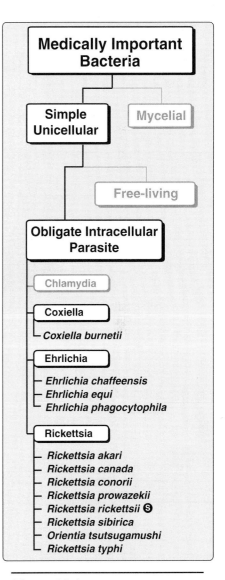

Figure 22.1
Classification of rickettsiae.
Ⓢ See pp. 417, 450 for a summary of this organism.

Lippincott's Illustrated Reviews: Microbiology,
by William A. Strohl, Harriet Rouse, Bruce D. Fisher.
Lippincott, Williams & Wilkins, Baltimore, MD © 2001

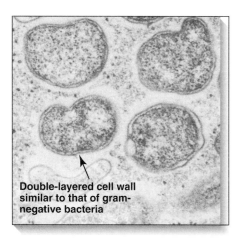

Figure 22.2
Electron micrograph of *Rickettsia prowazckii in experimentally infected tick tissue.*

Double-layered cell wall similar to that of gram-negative bacteria

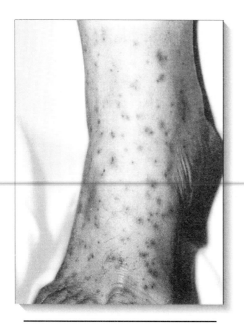

Figure 22.3
Rash caused by Rocky Mountain spotted fever.

Depending on the rickettsial species, rodents, humans, or arthropods themselves can serve as these reservoirs. Following introduction during the bite of an infected arthropod, the organisms are taken into cells by a process similar to phagocytosis. [Note: Only metabolically active organisms are engulfed. Rickettsiae produce a phospholipase that damages host cell membranes, a process that is thought to facilitate first cellular entry and then escape from phagosomes.] The organisms multiply directly in the cytoplasm by binary fission. They appear to mobilize host cell actin fibrils that facilitate their exit into adjacent cells in a manner similar to that of the genus *Listeria* (see p. 163). Ultimately host cells are killed, focal thrombi are formed in various organs including the skin (Figure 22.3), and a variety of small hemorrhages and hemodynamic disturbances create the symptoms of illness. [Note: Rickettsiae contain the characteristic gram-negative lipopolysaccharide (see p. 13), but a role for endotoxin has not been identified.]

C. **Clinical significance**

1. **Rocky Mountain spotted fever** is caused by *Rickettsia rickettsii*. Human infection is initiated by the bite of an infected wood or dog tick. Ticks transmit the organism via their ova intergenerationally (**transovarial transmission**, that is, vertically), and thereby the organism can be maintained without mammalian hosts in specific geographic regions for many years. Currently in the United States, such infected tick populations are prevalent in south central states and along the mid-Atlantic coast, and the disease usually occurs with highest frequency during the warmer months when tick activity is greatest. Symptoms begin to develop an average of seven days after infection. The disease is characterized by high fever and malaise, followed by a prominent rash, which is initially macular but may become petechial or frankly hemorrhagic (Figure 22.3). The rash typically begins on the extremities, involving the palms and soles, and develops rapidly to cover the body. In untreated cases, vascular disturbances and myocardial or renal failure may ensue. Rocky Mountain spotted fever occurs most frequently in children and teenagers, but mortality rates (five to thirty percent) are highest among individuals older than forty years of age.

2. **Other spotted fevers:** Tick-borne spotted fevers similar to Rocky Mountain spotted fever are found in several regions of the world. They vary in severity, and are caused by organisms such as *R. conorii*, *R. canada*, and *R. sibirica*, which may not represent biologically distinct species. A clinically different disease, **rickettsialpox**, is caused by *R. akari*. It has been reported in the United States and Japan. The vector for *R. akari* is a mite, and its reservoir is the common house mouse or similar small rodents. Rickettsialpox is characterized by a varicella-like rash with mild constitutional symptoms of a few days' duration. Figure 22.4 illustrates the spotted fevers caused by rickettsial organisms.

3. **Louse-borne (epidemic) typhus fever** is caused by *Rickettsia prowazekii*. [Note: Epidemic typhus fever is a different disease from salmonella-induced typhoid fever (see p. 180), but both were originally thought to be variations of the same disease, which was

called "typhus" after the Greek word that meant "stupor". When the two diseases were determined to be caused by different organisms, the salmonella-induced disease was named "typhoid", meaning "typhus-like."] *R. prowazekii* is transmitted from person to person by an infected human body louse that excretes organisms in its feces. The introduction of the pathogen through a bite wound is facilitated by scratching the louse bites. Infected lice are themselves eventually killed by the infecting bacterium. Thus this disease is not maintained in the louse population, but rather lice serve as vectors, transmitting the organism between humans. [Note: An organism indistinguishable from *R. prowazekii* has been recovered from flying squirrels and their ectoparasites in the southeastern United States. Sporadic human infections from squirrel flea bites have resulted.]

a. **Typhus epidemics:** Typhus occurs most typically in large epidemics under conditions of displacement of people, crowding, and poor sanitation. Currently a major focus of such outbreaks is found in northeast Africa. The epidemic form of typhus has not occurred in the United States since early in the twentieth century. Clinical symptoms of typhus develop an average of eight days after infection, and include high fever, chills, severe headache, and often a considerable degree of prostration and stupor. Rash may be observed. The disease lasts two weeks or longer, and tends to be more severe in older individuals. Complications of epidemic typhus may include CNS dysfunction and myocarditis. Mortality rates are variable in different outbreaks, but occasionally exceed fifty percent in the absence of treatment.

b. **Brill-Zinsser disease**, or **recrudescent typhus**, is a usually milder form of typhus that occurs in persons who previously recovered from primary infections (ten to forty years earlier). Latent infection is thought to be maintained in the reticuloendothelial system, and probably serves as a reservoir for the organism in interepidemic periods.

4. **Other forms of typhus-like fever: Murine (endemic) typhus**, caused by *Rickettsia typhi*, is a clinically similar, but usually milder disease than that caused by *R. prowazekii*. Human infections are initiated by the bites of infected rat fleas, and a worldwide reservoir for *R. typhi* exists in urban rodents. Murine typhus was endemic in rat-infested areas, particularly in the southeastern United States and in the Gulf region. However, with improving rodent control, it has become rare in this country. [Note: The cat flea, which also resides on skunks, opossums, and raccoons, is still a significant vector of murine typhus in the United States.] *Orientia tsutsugamushi* (formerly named *Rickettsia tsutsugamushi*), the cause of **scrub typhus**, occurs in Asia and the South Pacific. The disease is transmitted by mite larvae (chiggers) from a reservoir in common rodents.

D. **Laboratory identification**

A variety of serologic procedures have been developed, most of which rely on the demonstration of a rickettsia-specific antibody

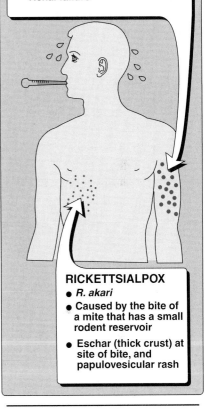

Figure 22.4
Spotted fevers caused by *Rickettsia*.

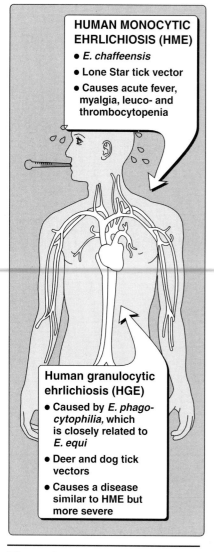

PENICILLINS
CEPHALOSPORINS

Tetracyclines **1** Doxycycline

AMINOGLYCOSIDES
MACROLIDES
FLUOROQUINOLONES

Other **2** Chloramphenicol

Figure 22.5
Some antimicrobial agents useful
in treating rickettsial infections.

**HUMAN MONOCYTIC
EHRLICHIOSIS (HME)**

• *E. chaffeensis*

• Lone Star tick vector

• Causes acute fever,
myalgia, leuco- and
thrombocytopenia

**Human granulocytic
ehrlichiosis (HGE)**

• Caused by *E. phago-
cytophilia,* which
is closely related to
E. equi

• Deer and dog tick
vectors

• Causes a disease
similar to HME but
more severe

Figure 22.6
Diseases caused by *Ehrlichia.*

response during the course of infection. Suspensions or soluble extracts of rickettsiae are used to demonstrate group- and species-specific antibodies by indirect immunofluorescence. Alternatively, although not widely available, infected cells can be detected by immunofluorescence or histochemical procedures on some clinical samples, such as punch biopsies from areas of rash. [Note: Because of their obligate intracellularity, rickettsiae are cultivated in tissue cultures of susceptible cells, and in the yolk sac of embryonated eggs. Such procedures are cumbersome, hazardous, and not useful for diagnostic purposes.]

E. Treatment

Tetracyclines (for example, doxycycline) and chloramphenicol have been shown to shorten the duration and improve chances for recovery in rickettsial infections, provided the drugs are administered early during the illness (Figure 22.5). Because the principal diagnostic methods await the demonstration of seroconversion, a decision to treat must be made on clinical grounds, together with a history or suspicion of contact with an appropriate arthropod vector, before the seroconversion data are available.

F. Prevention of infection

Prevention depends on vector control, for example, delousing, rodent-proofing buildings, or clearing brush in tick- or mite-infested areas as appropriate. Personal protection should include wearing clothes that cover exposed skin, use of tick repellents, and frequent inspection of the body and removal of attached ticks. It is of interest that infected ticks do not transmit the infection until several hours of feeding have elapsed. Vaccines have been developed for several rickettsial diseases. They have proved only moderately effective, and are not currently licensed for use in the United States.

III. EHRLICHIA

Ehrlichia resembles *Rickettsia* in appearance and behavior. However, these organisms parasitize leukocytes, and grow in cytoplasmic vacuoles creating characteristic inclusions called **morulae**. Human infection by *Ehrlichia* was not recognized in the United States until quite recently, although there were known pathogens of this group in some animals (for example, horses and dogs).

A. Clinical significance

Currently, two tick-borne forms of ehrlichiosis are known: **human monocytic ehrlichiosis (HME)** caused by *E. chaffeensis,* and **human granulocytic ehrlichiosis (HGE)** caused by the organism *E. phagocytophilia*, which is closely related to *E. equi* (Figure 22.6). The major clinical features of ehrlichiosis are acute fever, myalgia, and a moderate to severe leucopenia and thrombocytopenia. Rash is seldom seen for HME; deaths from HGE and HME have occurred. HME has been confirmed in some thirty states in the southeastern and south central United States, and has been most commonly associated with bites of the Lone Star tick. HGE has been associated with the bites of both deer ticks and dog ticks.

B. Laboratory identification

Antibody assays and a polymerase chain reaction method have been diagnostically useful in investigative laboratories. Occasionally the characteristic morulae can be seen in peripheral blood smears during acute illness.

C. Treatment

The treatment of choice is doxycycline (Figure 22.7).

IV. COXIELLA

Coxiella burnetii, the causal agent of **Q fever**, is found worldwide (the "Q" stands for "query" because the cause of the fever was unknown for many years). It has several features that distinguish it from other rickettsiae (Figure 22.8). For example: 1) It grows in cytoplasmic vacuoles and seems to be stimulated by the low pH of a phagolysosome, being resistant to the host degradative enzymes within that structure. 2) It is extremely resistant to heat and drying, and thus can persist outside its host for long periods. 3) It causes disease in livestock such as cattle, and in other mammals, but it does not seem to be transmitted to humans by arthropods. Although the organism has been reported to be recovered from ticks, human infection usually occurs following inhalation of infected dust in barnyards, slaughterhouses and such—a transmission route made possible because of the ability of *C. burnetii* to withstand drying. [Note: *C. burnetii* has also been known to enter the body via other mucous membranes, abrasions, and the gastrointestinal tract through consumption of milk from infected animals.]

A. Clinical significance

C. burnetii reproduces in the respiratory tract, and then (in the absence of treatment) is disseminated to other organs. Clinical illness takes several forms. Classic Q fever is an interstitial pneumonitis (not unlike some viral or mycoplasmal illnesses) that may be complicated by hepatitis, myocarditis, or encephalitis. *C. burnetii* should also be considered as a potential causative agent in culture-negative, subacute bacterial endocarditis. Infections are usually self-limiting, but in rare instances can become chronic.

B. Laboratory identification

Serologic assays are the principal means of specific diagnosis, and serologic surveys indicate that inapparent infections are quite common.

C. Treatment and prevention

Doxycycline is the drug of choice for treatment (Figure 22.9). A vaccine has been reported to be of limited use in occupationally exposed individuals, but is not readily available in the United States.

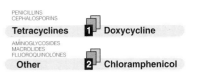

Figure 22.7
Some antimicrobial agents useful in treating *Ehrlichia chaffeensis* infections.

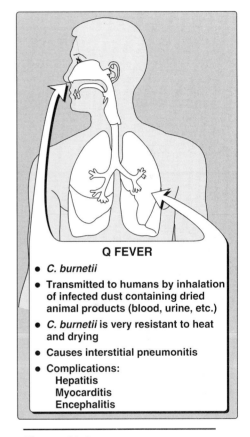

Figure 22.8
Disease caused by *Coxiella burnetii*.

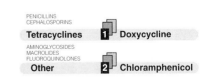

Figure 22.9
Some antimicrobial agents useful in treating *Coxiella burnetii* infections.

Study Questions

Choose the ONE correct answer

22.1 Rickettsiae:

  A. grow only extracellularly.

  B. have eukaryotic-type cell organization.

  C. cause contagious infections because they are disseminated by respiratory droplets.

  D. are clinically sensitive to penicillin.

  E. generally invade the endothelial lining of capillaries, causing small hemorrhages.

> Correct answer = E. Most rickettsiae cause rashes due to damage of the vascular system. They are obligate intracellular, prokaryotic parasites (A and B). With the exception of coxiella, which is transmitted by inhalation of infected dust, rickettsiae are transmitted by bite of an arthropod. They are sensitive to tetracyclines, but not to penicillin.

22.2 The vector of Rocky Mountain spotted fever is the:

  A. human body louse.

  B. rat flea.

  C. deer tick.

  D. dog tick.

  E. mosquito.

> Correct answer = D.

22.3 Ehrlichiosis and Rocky Mountain spotted fever have all but which of the following clinical features in common?

  A. Both involve parasitized blood cells.

  B. Both are acute fevers.

  C. Both are transmitted by the same vector.

  D. Both can be treated by doxycycline.

  E. Both are caused by members of the family *Rickettsiaceae*.

> Correct answer = A. *Ehrlichia* parasitizes leukocytes, whereas *R. rickettsii* invades capillary linings, causing the "spotted" rash of RMSF.

22.4 *Coxiella burnetii*:

  A. cannot survive outside its host.

  B. has no reservoir other than humans.

  C. causes a pneumonitis called Q fever.

  D. causes symptomatic disease only in the lower respiratory tract.

  E. is found only in the United States.

> Correct answer = C. Whereas lower respiratory tract disease is most characteristic, the organism fairly frequently causes hepatitis, myo- or endocarditis, and other visceral infections. It is quite resistant to drying, heat, etc., and infects a variety of animals (including ticks, but they play no role in human disease). Its distribution is worldwide.

22.5 Which one of the following most correctly describes *Rickettsia rickettsii*?

  A. Is sensitive to tetracyclines

  B. Infects red blood cells, resulting in hemolysis and production of rash.

  C. Is spread by aerosol droplets.

  D. Diagnosis is made by Gram stain of punch biopsies from areas of rash.

  E. Is found primarily on the west coast of the United States.

> Correct answer = A. Tetracyclines (for example, doxycycline) and chloramphenicol have been shown to shorten the duration and improve chances for recovery in rickettsial infections, provided the drugs are administered early during the illness. Rickettsia species parasitize endothelial cells, not red blood cells. The organisms multiply directly in the cytoplasm by binary fission. Ultimately host cells are killed, focal thrombi are formed in various organs including the skin, and a variety of small hemorrhages produce the characteristic rash. They are transmitted to humans by arthropods such as fleas, ticks, mites, or lice. Diagnosis relies on the demonstration of a rickettsia-specific antibody response during the course of infection. Currently in the United States, infected tick populations are prevalent in south central states and along the mid-Atlantic coast.

Fungi

23

I. OVERVIEW

The fungi are a diverse group of saprophytic (derives nourishment from dead organic matter) and parasitic eukaryotic organisms. Although formerly considered to be plants, they are now generally assigned their own kingdom, **Mycota**. Virtually all organisms are subject to fungal infection. Of the some 100,000 fungal species, only about 100 have pathogenic potential for humans, and of these only a few species account for most clinically important fungal infections (Figure 23.1). Human fungal diseases (**mycoses**) are classified by the location on or in the body where the infection occurs. They are called **cutaneous** when limited to the epidermis, **subcutaneous** when the infection penetrates significantly beneath the skin, and **systemic** when the infection is deep within the body or disseminated to internal organs. Systemic mycoses can be further divided into those that are caused by true pathogenic fungi capable of infecting healthy individuals, and those that are opportunistic, infecting primarily those individuals who have predisposing conditions such as immunodeficiency or debilitating diseases (for example, diabetes, leukemia, Hodgkin and other lymphomas). Fungi produce and secrete a variety of unusual metabolic products, some of which, when ingested, are highly toxic to animals, including humans. Thus fungi can cause poisonings as well as infections. Lastly, fungal spores are important as human allergenic agents.

II. CHARACTERISTICS OF MAJOR FUNGAL GROUPS

Fungi can be distinguished from other infectious organisms such as bacteria or viruses because they are eukaryotes (that is, they have a membrane-enclosed nucleus). Their characteristic structures, habitats, and modes of growth and reproduction are used to distinguish between different groups of fungi.

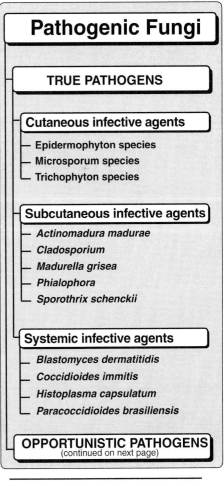

Pathogenic Fungi

TRUE PATHOGENS

Cutaneous infective agents
- Epidermophyton species
- Microsporum species
- Trichophyton species

Subcutaneous infective agents
- *Actinomadura madurae*
- *Cladosporium*
- *Madurella grisea*
- *Phialophora*
- *Sporothrix schenckii*

Systemic infective agents
- *Blastomyces dermatitidis*
- *Coccidioides immitis*
- *Histoplasma capsulatum*
- *Paracoccidioides brasiliensis*

OPPORTUNISTIC PATHOGENS
(continued on next page)

Figure 23.1
Classification of pathogenic fungi
(Figure continues on next page).

Lippincott's Illustrated Reviews: Microbiology,
by William A. Strohl, Harriet Rouse, Bruce D. Fisher.
Lippincott, Williams & Wilkins, Baltimore, MD © 2001 265

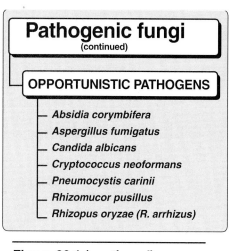

Pathogenic fungi
(continued)

OPPORTUNISTIC PATHOGENS

- *Absidia corymbifera*
- *Aspergillus fumigatus*
- *Candida albicans*
- *Cryptococcus neoformans*
- *Pneumocystis carinii*
- *Rhizomucor pusillus*
- *Rhizopus oryzae (R. arrhizus)*

Figure 23.1 (continued)
Classification of pathogenic fungi.

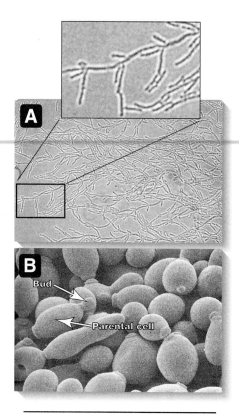

Figure 23.2
A. Filamentous (mold-like) fungi
(light micrograph). B. Budding
yeast-like fungi (scanning electron
micrograph).

A. Cell wall and membrane components

The fungal cell wall and cell membrane are fundamentally different from those of bacteria and other eukaryotes. Fungal cell walls are composed largely of **chitin**, a polymer of N-acetylglucosamine,[1] rather than peptidoglycan—a characteristic component of bacterial cell walls. Fungi are therefore unaffected by antibiotics (for example, penicillin) that inhibit peptidoglycan synthesis. The fungal membrane contains **ergosterol** rather than the cholesterol found in mammalian membranes. These chemical characteristics are useful in targeting chemotherapeutic agents against fungal infections. Many such agents interfere with fungal membrane synthesis or function. For example, **amphotericin B** and **nystatin** bind to ergosterol present in cell membranes of fungal cells. There they form pores that disrupt membrane function, resulting in cell death. The imidazole antifungal drugs (**clotrimazole**, **ketoconazole**, **miconazole**) and triazole antifungal agents (**fluconazole and itraconazole**) interact with C-14 α-demethylase to block demethylation of lanosterol to ergosterol. Ergosterol is a vital component of the cell membrane of fungi, and disruption in its biosynthesis results in cell death.

B. Habitat and nutrition

All fungi are **heterotrophs** (that is, they require some preformed organic carbon source for growth). Fungi do not ingest food particles as do organisms such as the protozoa (see p. 279), but instead, they depend upon transport of soluble nutrients across their cell membranes. To obtain these soluble nutrients, fungi secrete degradative enzymes (for example, cellulases, proteases, nucleases, etc.) into their immediate environment. It is this ability that enables fungi to live saprophytically on organic waste. Therefore, the natural habitat of almost all fungi is soil or water containing decaying organic matter. [Note: Some fungi can be parasitic on living organisms. However, these parasitic infections usually originate from the individual's contact with fungus-infested soil, an exception being *Candida*, which is part of the normal human mucosal flora (see p. 7).]

C. Modes of fungal growth

Most fungi exist in one of two basic morphologic forms (that is, either as a filamentous **mold** or a unicellular **yeast**). However, some fungi are **dimorphic** (that is, they switch between these two forms in response to environmental conditions).

1. **Filamentous (mold-like) fungi:** The vegetative body, or **thallus**, of the mold-like fungi is typically a mass of threads with many branches, resembling a cotton ball (Figure 23.2A). This mass is called a **mycelium**, which grows by branching and tip elongation. The threads, called **hyphae**, are actually tubular cells that, in some fungi, are partitioned into segments (**septate**), whereas in other fungi the hyphae are uninterrupted by crosswalls (**nonseptate**). Even in

[1]See p. 151 in *Lippincott's Illustrated Reviews: Biochemistry* (2nd ed.) for a discussion of N-acetylglucosamine.

septate fungi, however, the septae are perforated so that the cytoplasm of the hyphae is continuous. When hyphal filaments become very densely packed, the mycelium may have the appearance of a cohesive tissue. An example of this is the body of a mushroom.

2. **Yeast-like fungi:** These fungi exist as populations of single, unconnected, spheroid cells, not unlike many bacteria, although they are some ten times larger than a typical bacterial cell (Figure 23.2B). Yeast-like fungi generally reproduce by budding. [Note: Some fungal species, especially those that cause systemic mycoses, are **dimorphic**, being usually yeast-like in one environment and mold-like in another. Examples of conditions that affect the choice of morphology are temperature and carbon dioxide levels.]

D. Sporulation

Sporulation is the principal means by which fungi reproduce and spread through the environment. Fungal spores are metabolically dormant, protected cells, released by the mycelium in enormous numbers. They can be borne by air or water to new sites, where they germinate and establish colonies. Spores can be generated either asexually or sexually (Figure 23.3).

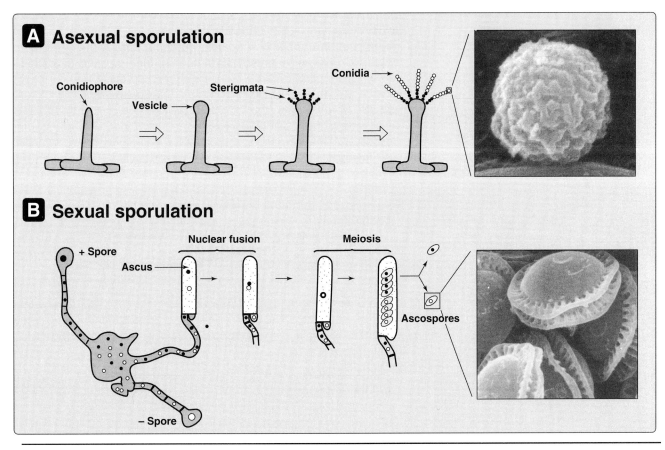

Figure 23.3
Examples of: A. Asexual sporulation. B. Sexual sporulation. Both spores are *Aspergillus nidulans*.

1. **Asexual sporulation:** Asexual spores, termed **conidia**, are formed by mitosis in or on specialized hyphae, the **conidiophores** (Figure 23.3A). The color of a typical fungal colony seen on bread, fruit, or culture plate is due to the conidia, which can number tens of millions per square cm of surface. Because they are easily detached from their underlying mycelial mats, conidia can become airborne, and are a major source of fungal infection (see p. 271).

2. **Sexual sporulation:** This process is initiated when a haploid nucleus from each of two compatible strains of the same species fuse to form a transient diploid (Figure 23.3B). The products of meiosis of this transient diploid become sexual spores (**ascospores**). Compared to asexual sporulation, sexual sporulation is relatively rare among human fungal pathogens. Spores, especially sexual spores, often have a characteristic shape and surface ornamentation pattern that may serve as the primary, or only means of identification of a species.

E. Laboratory identification

Most fungi can be propagated on any nutrient agar surface. The standard medium is Sabouraud's agar (a beef broth–dextrose mixture), which, because of its low pH (5.0), inhibits bacterial growth while allowing fungal colonies to form (Figure 23.4). Various antibacterial antibiotics can also be added to the medium to further inhibit bacterial colony formation. Cultures can be started from spores or hyphal fragments. Clinical samples may be pus, blood, spinal fluid, sputum, tissue biopsies, or skin scrapings. Identification is usually made on the basis of the microscopic morphology of conidial structures. If the organism displays sexual sporulation, which is rare among the pathogenic fungi, the morphology of the fruiting bodies and the sexual spores can also be useful. Serologic tests and immunofluorescent techniques are also useful in identification of fungi from clinical isolates. A simple and rapid office procedure for detecting fungal elements in clinical specimens is to examine a wet mount prepared in ten percent potassium hydroxide. The alkali partially degrades the obscuring proteinaceous components of host tissue, leaving fungal filaments intact and rendering them more visible.

III. CUTANEOUS MYCOSES

Also called **dermatophytoses**, these common diseases are caused by a group of related fungi, the dermatophytes. The dermatophytes fall into three genera, each with many species: *Trichophyton*, *Epidermophyton*, and *Microsporum*.

A. Epidemiology

The causative organisms of the dermatophytoses are often distinguished according to their natural habitats: **anthropophilic** (residing on human skin), **zoophilic** (residing on the skin of domestic and farm

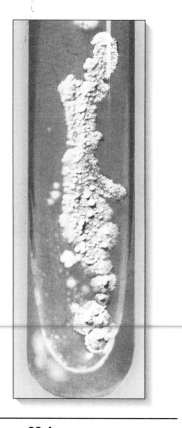

Figure 23.4
Colonies of *Nocardia asteroides* grown on Sabouraud's dextrolse agar.

animals), or **geophilic** (residing in the soil). Most human infections are by anthropophilic and zoophilic organisms. Transmission from human to human, or animal to human, is by infected skin scales.

B. Pathology

A defining characteristic of the dermatophytes is their ability to use keratin as a source of nutrition. This ability allows them to infect keratinized tissues and structures such as skin, hair, and nails. There is some specificity, however. Whereas all three organisms attack the skin, *Microsporum* does not infect nails, and *Epidermophyton* does not infect hair. They do not invade underlying, nonkeratinized tissues.

C. Clinical significance

Dermatophytoses are characterized by itching, scaling skin patches that can become inflamed and weeping. Specific diseases are usually identified according to affected tissues (for example, scalp, pubic area, or feet), but a given disease can be caused by any one of several organisms, and some organisms can cause more than one disease, depending on the site of infection, condition of the skin, etc. The following are the most commonly encountered dermatophytoses.

1. **Tinea pedis (athlete's foot):** Organisms most often isolated from infected tissues are *Trichophyton rubrum*, *Trichophyton mentagrophytes*, and *Epidermophyton floccosum*. The infected tissue is initially between the toes, but can spread to the nails, which become yellow and brittle. Skin fissures can lead to secondary bacterial infections, with consequent lymph node inflammation (Figure 23.5A). Another manifestation of tinia pedis is the **"id" reaction** (from dermatophyt<u>id</u>), in which skin lesions (vesicles) develop at sites distant from the infected area, for example, on the hands. It has been speculated the the id reaction is due to circulating fungal antigens.

2. **Tinea corporis (ringworm):** Organisms most often isolated are *Epidermophyton floccosum*, and several species of *Trichophyton* and *Microsporum*. Lesions appear as advancing annular rings with scaly centers (Figure 23.5B). The periphery of the ring, which is the site of active fungal growth, is usually inflamed and vesiculated. Although any site on the body can be affected, lesions most often occur on nonhairy areas of the trunk.

3. **Tinea capitis (scalp ringworm):** A number of species of *Trichophyton* and *Microsporum* have been isolated from scalp ringworm lesions, the predominant infecting species depending on the geographic location of the patient. For example, in the United States, the predominant infecting species is *Trichophyton tonsurans*. Disease manifestations range from small, scaling patches, to involvement of the entire scalp with extensive hair loss (Figure 23.5C). The hair shafts themselves can become invaded by *Microsporum* hyphae, as manifested by their green fluorescence in long-wave ultraviolet light (Wood's lamp).

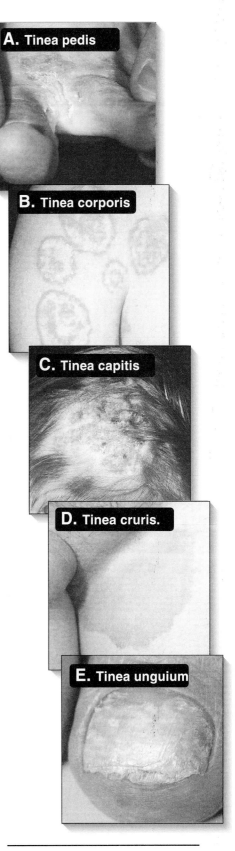

A. Tinea pedis

B. Tinea corporis

C. Tinea capitis

D. Tinea cruris.

E. Tinea unguium

Figure 23.5
Cutaneous mycoses.

4. Tinea cruris ("jock itch"): Causative organisms are *Epidermophyton floccosum*, and *Trichophyton rubrum*. Disease manifestations are similar to ringworm, except that lesions occur in the moist groin area, where they can spread from the upper thighs to the genitals (Figure 23.5D).

5. Tinea unguium (onychomycosis): The causative organism is most often *Trichophyton rubrum*. The nails are thickened, discolored, and brittle. Treatment must be continued for three to four months until all infected portions of the nail grow out and are trimmed off (Figure 23.5E).

D. Treatment

Removal of infected skin, followed by topical application of antifungal antibiotics such as miconazole or clotrimazole, is the first course of treatment. Refractory infections usually respond well to oral griseofulvin and itraconazole. [Note: Infections of the hair and nails usually require systemic (oral) therapy.]

IV. SUBCUTANEOUS MYCOSES

Subcutaneous mycoses are fungal infections of the dermis, subcutaneous tissues, and bone. The causative organisms reside in the soil and in decaying or live vegetation.

A. Epidemiology

Subcutaneous fungal infections are almost always acquired through traumatic lacerations or puncture wounds. **Sporotrichosis**, for example, is often acquired from the prick of a thorn. As expected, these infections are more common in individuals who have frequent contact with soil and vegetation, and who wear little protective clothing. The subcutaneous mycoses are not transmissible from human to human under ordinary conditions.

B. Clinical Significance

With the rare exception of sporotrichosis, which shows a broad geographic distribution in the United States, the common subcutaneous mycoses discussed below are confined to tropical and subtropical regions. [Note: *Candida* and *Aspergillus* species can colonize mucocutaneous surfaces of the normal host, but rarely produce invasive disease unless there is a lesion in the mucocutaneous surface, or the patient is immunocompromised. These organisms are discussed on pp. 274 to 275.]

1. Sporotrichosis: This infection is characterized by a granulomatous ulcer at the puncture site, and may produce secondary lesions along the draining lymphatics (Figure 23.6A). The causative organism, *Sporothrix schenckii*, is a dimorphic fungus that exhibits the yeast form in infected tissue (Figure 23.7) and the mycelial form upon laboratory culture. In most patients the dis-

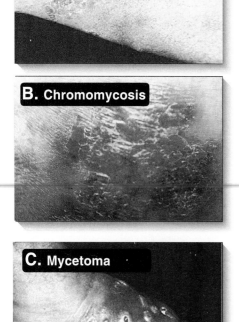

Figure 23.6
Subcutaneous mycoses.
A. Sporotrichosis. The forearm of a gardener exhibiting the cutaneous-lymphatic form of sporotrichosis.
B. Chromomycosis. Multiple plaques on the lower leg.
C. Mycetoma of the foot.

ease is self-limiting, but may persist in a chronic form. Oral itraconazole is the standard treatment.

2. **Chromomycosis (also called chromoblastomycosis):** This infection is characterized by warty nodules that spread slowly along the lymphatics, and develop crusty abscesses (Figure 23.6B). The pathogens causing this mycosis include several species of pigmented soil fungi, for example, *Phialophora* and *Cladosporium*. Treatment is difficult. Surgical removal of small lesions is effective, but must be performed cautiously and with wide margins to prevent dissemination. More advanced stages of the disease are treated with oral flucytosine combined with the antihelminthic drug, thiabendazole.

3. **Mycetoma (Madura foot):** Mycetoma appears as a localized abscess, usually on the feet, that discharges pus, serum, and blood through sinuses (in this usage, sinus means "abnormal channel"). The infection can spread to the underlying bone and result in crippling deformaties (Figure 23.6C). The pathogenic agents are various soil fungi or actinomycetes (see p. 256), depending on the climate of the geographic area. Most common are *Madurella grisea* and *Actinomadura madurae*. **Mycetomas** appear similar to the lesions of chromomycosis, but the defining characteristic of mycetoma is the presence of colored grains, composed of compacted hyphae, in the exudate. The color of the grains (black, white, red, or yellow) is characteristic of the causative organism, and is thus useful in identifying the particular pathogen. There is no effective chemotherapy for fungal mycetoma, and the treatment is usually surgical excision.

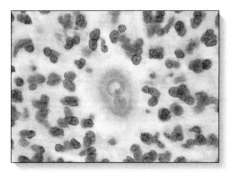

Figure 23.7
Tissue section showing the budding yeast *Sporothrix schenckii*.

V. SYSTEMIC MYCOSES

The organisms responsible for systemic mycoses fall into two general categories: 1) those that infect normal healthy individuals (the **true pathogens**), and 2) those that primarily infect debilitated, and/or immunocompromised individuals (the **opportunistic pathogens**, see p. 14). In the United States, **coccidioidomycosis**, **histoplasmosis**, and **blastomycosis** are the most common systemic mycotic infections in the immunocompetent host. These infections occur in defined geographic areas where the fungal pathogens are found in the soil and can be aerosolized. The clinical manifestations closely resemble those seen in tuberculosis in that asymptomatic primary pulmonary infection is common, whereas chronic pulmonary or disseminated infection is rare. The fungi causing these diseases are uniformly dimorphic, exhibiting the yeast form in infected tissue, and the mycelial form in culture or in their natural environment.

A. Epidemiology and pathology

Entry into the host is by inhalation of airborne spores, which germinate in the lungs. From the lungs, dissemination can occur to any organ of the body where the fungi can invade and destroy the tissue (Figure 23.8).

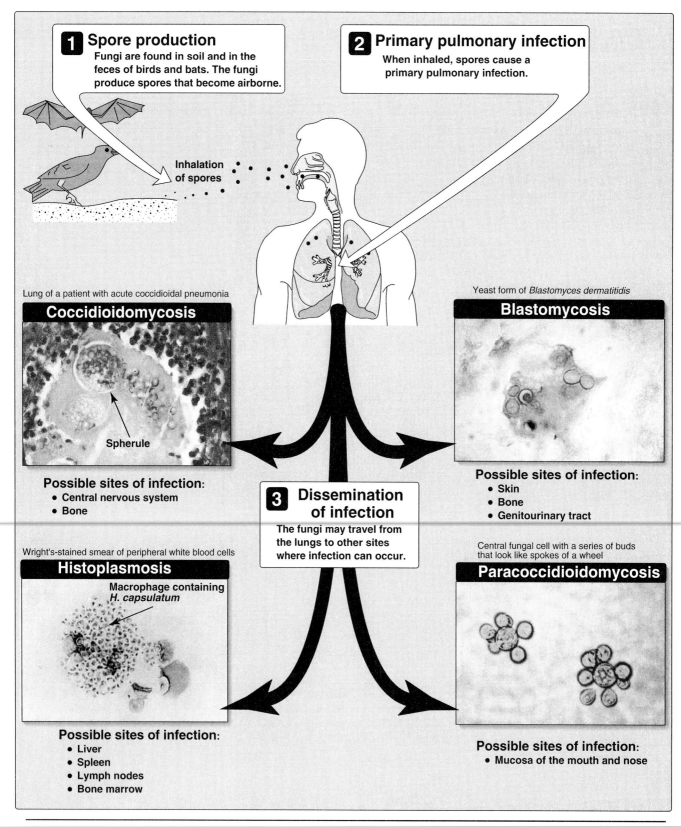

1 Spore production
Fungi are found in soil and in the feces of birds and bats. The fungi produce spores that become airborne.

2 Primary pulmonary infection
When inhaled, spores cause a primary pulmonary infection.

Inhalation of spores

Lung of a patient with acute coccidioidal pneumonia
Coccidioidomycosis
Spherule

Possible sites of infection:
- Central nervous system
- Bone

Yeast form of *Blastomyces dermatitidis*
Blastomycosis

Possible sites of infection:
- Skin
- Bone
- Genitourinary tract

3 Dissemination of infection
The fungi may travel from the lungs to other sites where infection can occur.

Wright's-stained smear of peripheral white blood cells
Histoplasmosis
Macrophage containing *H. capsulatum*

Possible sites of infection:
- Liver
- Spleen
- Lymph nodes
- Bone marrow

Central fungal cell with a series of buds that look like spokes of a wheel
Paracoccidioidomycosis

Possible sites of infection:
- Mucosa of the mouth and nose

Figure 23.8
Systemic mycoses.

B. Clinical significance

In spite of the seemingly grave nature of potentially systemic disease, most cases of coccidioidomycosis, histoplasmosis, and para-coccidioidomycosis in otherwise healthy patients present only mild symptoms and are self-limiting. In immunosuppressed patients, however, the same infections can be life-threatening.

1. **Coccidioidomycosis** is caused by *Coccidioides immitis*. Most cases of coccidioidomycosis occur in the arid areas of the southwestern United States (Figure 23.9), and Central and South America. In the soil, the fungus generates spores by septation of hyphal filaments (**arthrospores**). These spores become readily airborne, and enter the lungs, where they germinate and develop into large (twenty to forty μm) spherules filled with many endospores. Rupture of the spherule releases the endospores, each of which can form a new spherule. In cases of disseminated disease, lesions occur most often in the bones, and in the CNS, where they result in meningitis.

2. **Histoplasmosis** is caused by *Histoplasma capsulatum*. In the soil, the fungus generates conidia, which, when airborne, enter the lungs and germinate into yeast-like cells. These yeast cells become engulfed by macrophages in which they multiply. Pulmonary infections may be acute but relatively benign and self-limiting, or chronic, progressive, and fatal. Dissemination is rare. The disseminated disease results in invasion of cells of the reticuloendothelial system, which distinguishes this organism as the only fungus to exhibit **intracellular parasitism**. Definitive diagnosis is by isolation and culture of the organism, which is a slow process, taking four to six weeks, or by detection of exoantigen, which can be completed in several days. The disease occurs worldwide, but is most prevalent in central North America, especially the Ohio and Mississippi River Valley (Figure 23.10). Soils that are laden with bird, chicken, or bat droppings are a rich source of *H. capsulatum* spores. Local epidemics of the disease can occur, in fact, in areas where construction has disturbed bird, chicken, and bat roosts. AIDS patients who live in or travel through endemic areas are especially at risk. The wide range of clinical manifestations makes histoplasmosis a particularly complex disease, often resembling tuberculosis.

3. **Blastomycosis** is caused by *Blastomyces dermatitidis*. Like *Histoplasma,* the fungus produces microconidia, most often in the soil, which become airborne and enter the lungs. There they germinate into thick-walled yeast cells that often appear with buds. Initial pulmonary infections (Figure 23.11) rarely disseminate to other sites, but when dissemination occurs, the secondary sites are skin (seventy percent), bone (thirty percent), and the genitourinary tract (twenty percent), where they manifest as ulcerated granulomas. Definitive diagnosis is accomplished by isolation and culture of the organism. Identifiable colonies can be obtained in one to three weeks, but identity can be established more rapidly by subjecting the young mycelial colonies to an exoantigen test.

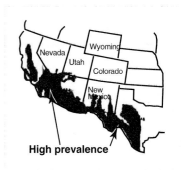

Figure 23.9
Geographical prevalence of coccidioidomycosis in the United States.

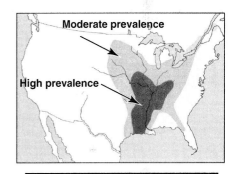

Figure 23.10
Endemic areas of histoplasmosis in North America.

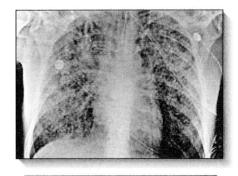

Figure 23.11
Chest radiograph showing a diffuse reticulonodular infiltrate of the lungs in a male landscaper. Broncho-alveolar lavage recovered *Blastomyces dermatitidis*.

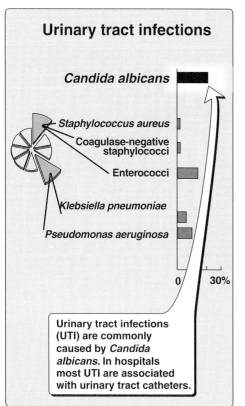

Urinary tract infections

Candida albicans

Staphylococcus aureus

Coagulase-negative staphylococci

Enterococci

Klebsiella pneumoniae

Pseudomonas aeruginosa

0   30%

Urinary tract infections (UTI) are commonly caused by *Candida albicans*. In hospitals most UTI are associated with urinary tract catheters.

Figure 23.12
Commonly reported pathogens from urinary tract infections in patients in adult medical intensive care units.

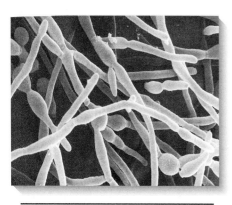

Figure 23.13
Candida albicans.

Infections are most common in the South Central and South Eastern United States, and are much more common in adult males than in females or children.

4. **Paracoccidioidomycosis**, also called **South American blastomycosis**, is caused by *Paracoccidioides brasiliensis*. The clinical presentation is much like that of histoplasmosis and blastomycosis except that the most common secondary site of infection is the mucosa of the mouth and nose, where painful, destructive lesions may develop. Like the other dimorphic pathogens, morphologic identification via conidia is slow, but the yeast form observed in infected tissue or exudates has a characteristic ship steering-wheel appearance due to the presence of multiple buds (see Figure 23.8). The disease is restricted to Central and South America, and over ninety percent of patients with symptomatic disease are mature males. It is speculated that female sex hormones may inhibit formation of the yeast form.

C. Laboratory identification

These diseases are not communicable from one person to another. However, laboratory cultures should be handled cautiously, especially those of *Coccidioides immitis*, because under culture conditions the fungi revert to their spore-bearing, infectious form. Because these organisms have slow growth rates, morphologic identification of the characteristic conidia can take several weeks. A rapid and simple method for identifying the four systemic pathogens discussed above is the exoantigen test in which cell-free antigens produced by young mycelial colonies (or liquid cultures) are detected by immunodiffusion assay. A recently developed, rapid and accurate diagnostic method uses nucleic acid probes that detect specific fungal sequences. Diagnostic probe kits are commercially available.

D. Treatment

Systemic mycoses are usually treated with amphotericin B, sometimes in combination with sulfadiazine in the case of paracoccidioidomycosis. Ketoconazole, fluconazole, and itraconazole are also used depending on the stage and site of the disease.

VI. OPPORTUNISTIC MYCOSES

The opportunistic mycoses are those that afflict debilitated and/or immunocompromised individuals, and which are rare in normal individuals. The use of immunosuppressive drugs for organ transplantation, the widespread use of chemotherapy in cancer treatment, and the high frequency of immunodeficient individuals due to the AIDS epidemic have resulted in significant expansion of the immunocompromised population, as well as increasing the spectrum of opportunistic fungal pathogens. For example, fungal infections represent approximately fifteen percent of all nosocomial infections in intensive care units in the United States, with candida species being the most commonly occurring fungal pathogen (Figure 23.12). The opportunistic mycoses most commonly encountered today include the following.

A. Candidiasis (candidosis) is caused by the yeast *Candida albicans*, and other *Candida* species, which are normal body flora found in the skin, mouth, vagina, and intestines. Although termed a yeast, *C. albicans* is dimorphic, and can form a true mycelium (Figure 23.13). Infections occur when competing bacterial flora are eliminated by, for example, antibacterial antibiotics, allowing the yeast to overgrow. *Candida* infections have various manifestations depending on the site. For example, **oral candidiasis (thrush)** presents as raised, white plaques on the oral mucosa, tongue, or gums (Figure 23.14). The plaques can become confluent and ulcerated, and can spread to the throat. Most HIV-positive individuals eventually develop oral candidiasis, which often spreads to the esophagus. The latter condition is considered an indicator of full-blown AIDS. **Vaginal candidiasis** presents as itching and burning pain of the vulva and vagina, accompanied by a thick or thin white discharge. HIV-positive females often suffer from recurrent vaginal candidiasis. Systemic candidiasis is a potentially life-threatening infection that occurs in debilitated individuals, cancer patients (with neutropenia secondary to chemotherapy), individuals on systemic corticosteroids, and patients being treated with broad-spectrum antibiotics. Systemic candidiasis may involve the gastrointestinal tract, kidneys, liver, and spleen. Both oral and vaginal infections are treated topically with nystatin or clotrimazole. Oral systemic antifungal agents such as ketoconazole, fluconazole, and itraconazole are preferred for ease of administration and increased efficacy. Amphotericin B by itself or in combination with flucytosine is used in systemic disease.

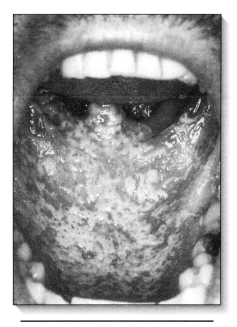

Figure 23.14
Oral candidiasis (thrush).

B. Cryptococcosis is caused by the yeast *Cryptococcus neoformans* (Figure 23.15), which is found world-wide. The organism is especially abundant in soil containing bird (especially pigeon) droppings, although the birds themselves are not infected. The organism has a characteristic thick capsule that surrounds the budding yeast cell, and is observable on a background of India ink. A positive India ink test on CSF can give a quick diagnosis of cryptococcal meningitis, but false negatives are common. The most common form of cryptococcosis is a mild, subclinical lung infection. In immunocompromised patients, the infection often disseminates to the brain and meninges, with fatal consequences. However, about half of the patients with cryptococcal meningitis have no obvious immunologic defect. In AIDS patients, cryptococcosis is the second most common fungal infection (after candidiasis) and is potentially the most serious. The antifungal drugs used to treat cryptococcosis are amphotericin B and flucytosine, the precise treatment regimen depending on the stage of the disease, the site of infection, and whether the patient has AIDS. Fluconazole is the drug of choice for prevention of cryptococcal meningitis in AIDS patients.

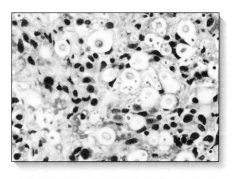

Figure 23.15
Cryptococcosis neoformans.

C. Aspergillosis is caused by several species of the genus *Aspergillus*, but primarily by *Aspergillus fumigatus*. *Aspergillus* is rarely pathogenic in the normal host, but can produce disease in immunosuppressed individuals, and patients treated with broad-spectrum antibiotics. The disease has a world-wide distribution. The aspergilli are ubiquitous, growing only as filamentous molds (Figure 23.16), and producing prodigious numbers of conidiospores. They reside in

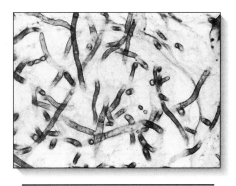

Figure 23.16
Aspergillus species.

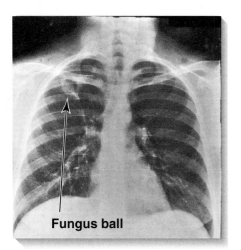

Figure 23.17
Fungus ball.

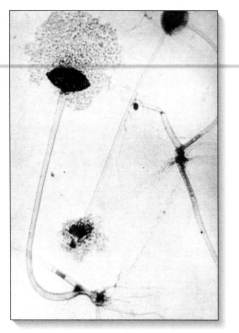

Figure 23.18
Rhizopus oryzae.

the soil, decomposing organic matter, and dust. In fact, hospital outbreaks affecting neutropenic patients (that is, those with a decreased number of neutrophils in their blood) have been traced to dust from neighboring construction work. Aspergillosis manifests itself in several forms, depending in part on the immunologic state of health of the patient.

1. **Acute aspergillus infections:** The most severe, and often fatal, form of aspergillosis is acute invasive infection of the lung, from which the infection can be disseminated to the brain, the gastrointestinal tract, and other organs. A less severe, noninvasive lung infection gives rise to a **fungus ball (aspergilloma)**, a mass of hyphal tissue that can form in lung cavities derived from prior diseases, such as tuberculosis (Figure 23.17). Although the lung is the most common primary site of infection, the eye, ear, nasal sinuses, and skin can also be primary sites.

2. **Allergic reaction to aspergillus:** A relatively rare condition, termed **allergic aspergillosis**, can arise from the mere inhalation of spores, without subsequent extensive spore germination or hyphal invasion. The allergic reaction results in the formation of mucus plugs that can block the bronchi.

3. **Diagnosis and treatment:** Definitive diagnosis of an aspergillus infection is afforded by detection of hyphal masses, and isolation of the organism from clinical samples. Aspergillus hyphae characteristically form V-shaped branches (septate hyphae that branch at a 45° angle, see Figure 23.16) that are distinguished from *Mucor* species, which form right-angle branches. Also, septae are present in aspergillus hyphae but are absent from mucor hypha. In culture, the spore-bearing structures of the aspergilli are unmistakable, but because these organisms are so ubiquitous, external contamination of clinical samples can give false positives. Treatment of aspergillus infections is almost always by amphotericin B, and surgical removal of fungal masses or infected tissue. The antifungal drugs miconazole, ketoconazole, and fluconazole have not proved useful, although itraconazole has been used with some effectiveness for aspergillus osteomyelitis.

D. **Mucormycosis** is caused most often by *Rhizopus oryzae* (also called *R. arrhizus,* Figure 23.18), and less often by other members of the Order Mucorales, such as *Absidia corymbifera,* and *Rhizomucor pusillus*. Like the aspergilli, these organisms are ubiquitous in nature, and their spores are found in great abundance on rotting fruit and old bread. *Mucor* infections occur worldwide, but are almost entirely restricted to individuals with some underlying predisposing condition such as burns, leukemias, or acidotic states such as diabetes mellitus. The most common form of the disease, which can be fatal within a week, is **rhinocerebral mucormycosis**, in which the infection begins in the nasal mucosa or sinuses, and progresses to the orbits, the palate, and the brain. Because the disease is so aggressive, many cases are not diagnosed until after death.

based on high-dose amphotericin B, but must be accompanied, when possible, by surgical debridement of necrotic tissue, and correction of the underlying predisposing condition. Antifungal drugs other than amphotericin have not proven useful. With early diagnosis and optimal treatment, about half of diabetic patients survive rhinocerebral mucormycosis, but for leukemic patients, prognosis is very poor.

E. **Pneumocystis carinii pneumonia (PCP)** is caused by the unicellular eukaryote, *Pneumocystis carinii*, whose taxonomic status and life cycle are still uncertain. Before the use of immunosuppressive drugs, and before the onset of the AIDS epidemic, PCP was a rare disease. It is currently one of the most common opportunistic diseases of individuals infected with HIV-1 (see Figure 31.16, p. 371), and is almost 100 percent fatal if untreated.

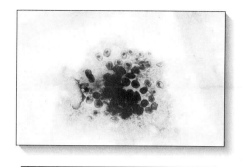

Figure 23.19
Pneumocystis carinii.

1. **Classification:** Previously, *P. carinii* had been considered a protozoan, but recent molecular homology studies of both protein and nucleic acid sequences strongly indicate that *P. carinii* is a fungus related to the ascomycetous yeasts. On the other hand, ergosterol, which is an essential component of most fungal membranes, is lacking in *P. carinii*. It has so far not been possible to cultivate *P. carinii* in culture, thus limiting understanding of its life cycle.

2. **Cellular forms:** Several cellular forms of *P. carinii* have been recognized, including encysted groups of dormant cells that release individual vegetative cells (the actively metabolizing trophozoite), Figure 23.19.

3. **Pathology:** The infectious form and the natural reservoir of this organism have not been identified, but they must be ubiquitous in nature, because almost 100 percent of children world-wide have antipneumocystis antibodies. The disease is not transmitted from person to person. Instead, the development of PCP in immunodeficient patients is thought to be by activation of preexisting dormant cells in the lungs. The encysted forms induce an inflammation of alveoli, resulting in an exudate that blocks gas exchange. Figure 23.20 shows typical radiographic findings in *Pneumocystis* pneumonia.

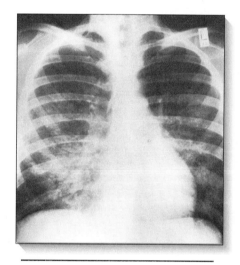

Figure 23.20
Pneumocystis pneumonia.

4. **Diagnosis and treatment:** Because *P. carinii* cannot be cultivated, diagnosis is based on microscopic examination of biopsied lung tissue, or lung washings. The most effective therapy is a combination of sulfamethoxazole and trimethoprim, which is also used prophylactically to prevent PCP in AIDS patients. Aggressive treatment can spare about half of the patients. [Note: Because the mechanism of action of many antifungal drugs, such as amphotericin, involves interfering with ergosterol synthesis or function, these drugs are useless for this ergosterol-lacking fungus.]

Study Questions

Choose the ONE correct answer

23.1 A component of the cell membrane of most fungi is

    A. cholesterol.

    B. chitin.

    C. ergosterol.

    D. peptidoglycan.

    E. keratin.

> Correct answer = C. Ergosterol in fungi is the functional equivalent of cholesterol in higher organisms. Peptidoglycan is a component of the bacterial cell wall, whereas chitin is a component of the cell wall of fungi. [Note: Chitin also comprises the exoskeletons of insects and crustacea.] Keratin is the major protein of hair and nails.

23.2 A common characteristic of fungi that causes systemic mycoses is that they

    A. are dimorphic.

    B. produce only asexual spores.

    C. produce motile spores.

    D. are carried by fowl.

    E. do not have chitin.

> Correct answer = A. The fungi of systemic mycoses exhibit the yeast form in infected tissue, and the mycelial form in laboratory culture or in their natural environment. Why this should be so is not entirely clear.

23.3 A physician visiting a rural Latin American village finds that many mature males, but few immature males or females of any age, are afflicted by a particular fungal disease. What is likely to be the diagnosis?

    A. Mycetoma

    B. Blastomycosis

    C. Paracoccidioidomycosis

    D. Mucormycosis

    E. Histoplasmosis

> Correct answer = C. For some reason, possibly hormonal, this disease favors mature males.

23.4 The asexual spores of many fungi are called

    A. endospores.

    B. conidiospores.

    C. ascospores.

    D. zygospores.

    E. basidiospores.

> Correct answer = B. Conidiospores (or conidia) are formed by mitosis, and are a major means of fungal propagation. Ascospores, zygospores, and basidiospores are the sexual spores of various genera that arise by a meiotic process. Endospores are bacterial spores.

23.5 A fungus that can attack hair is

    A. trichophyton.

    B. rhizopus.

    C. microsporum.

    D. sporothrix.

    E. epidermophyton.

> Correct answer = C. All attack skin, but only *Microsporum* attacks hair.

23.6 A farmer in Mississippi presents with a chronic cough. Chest x-ray reveals an opaque mass. Biopsy of the lung shows macrophages with multiple yeast forms. Which one of the following diagnoses is most likely?

    A. Coccidioidomycosis

    B. Histoplasmosis

    C. Blastomycosis

    D. Paracoccidioidomycosis

    E. Sporotrichosis

> Correct answer = B. Histoplasmosis is caused by *Histoplasma capsulatum*. In the soil, the fungus generates conidia, which, when airborne, enter the lungs and germinate into yeast-like cells. These yeast cells become engulfed by macrophages in which they multiply. Pulmonary infections may be acute but relatively benign and self-limiting, or chronic, progressive and fatal. Dissemination is rare. The disseminated disease results in invasion of cells of the reticuloendothelial system, which distinguishes this organism as the only fungus to exhibit intracellular parasitism. The disease occurs worldwide, but is most prevalent in central North America, especially the Ohio and Mississippi River Valley.

23.6 Sporotrichosis is most commonly acquired by

    A. consumption of contaminated food.

    B. an aerosol containing organisms.

    C. the bite of tick.

    D. a skin puncture by a thorn.

    E. by sexual contact.

> Correct answer = C. This infection is characterized by a granulomatous ulcer at the puncture site.

Protozoa

24

I. OVERVIEW

The protozoa are a diverse group of unicellular, eukaryotic organisms. Many have evolved structural features (**organelles**) that mimic the organs of multicellular organisms. Reproduction is generally by mitotic binary fission, although in some protozoal species, sexual (meiotic) reproduction with several variations occurs as well. Only a few of the many tens of thousands of protozoan species are pathogenic for humans. Those discussed in this chapter are listed in Figure 24.1. These pathogens are of two general kinds: those that parasitize the intestinal and urogenital tracts, and those that parasitize blood cells and tissues. Protozoal infections are common in developing tropical and subtropical regions where sanitary conditions and control of the vectors of transmission are poor. However, with increased world travel and immigration, protozoal diseases are no longer confined to specific geographic locales. Because they are eukaryotes, protozoa, like the fungi, have metabolic processes closer to those of the human host than to prokaryotic bacterial pathogens. Protozoal diseases are thus less easily treated than bacterial infections, because many antiprotozoal drugs are toxic to the human host.

II. CLINICALLY IMPORTANT PROTOZOA

Among the pathogenic protozoa, there are important common features that are clinically relevant. For example, many of these protozoa have both a dormant, immotile **cyst** stage that permits survival when environmental conditions are hostile, and a motile, actively feeding and reproducing vegetative (**trophozoite**) stage. For convenience, the protozoa are classified according to their mode of locomotion. The clinically relevant protozoa are thus divided into four groups (Figure 24.2).

A. Amebas

The amebas move by extending cytoplasmic projections (**pseudopodia**) outward from the main cell body. A single cell can have several pseudopodia projecting in the same general direction, with the remainder of the cytoplasm flowing into the pseudopodia. Amebas feed by engulfing food particles with their pseudopodia. [Note: Some amebas have flagella as well.]

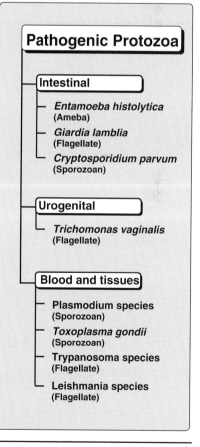

Figure 24.1
Clinically relevant protozoa, classified according to site of infection.

Lippincott's Illustrated Reviews: Microbiology,
by William A. Strohl, Harriet Rouse, Bruce D. Fisher.
Lippincott, Williams & Wilkins, Baltimore, MD © 2001

Pathogenic protozoa

Amebas
- Move by extending cytoplasmic projections.

Flagellates
- Move by rotating whip-like flagella.

Ciliates
- Move by synchronous beating of hair-like cilia.

Sporozoa
- Generally have non-motile adult forms.

Figure 24.2
The four major protozoal groups, classified according to their mode of locomotion.

B. Flagellates

The flagellates move by means of two or more whip-like projections (**flagella**) that rotate and propel the cells through their liquid environment. Some flagellates, for example the pathogen *Trichomonas vaginalis*, also have undulating membranes that assist in swimming. Flagellates ingest food particles through an oral groove called a **cytostome**.

C. Ciliates

The ciliates move by means of many hair-like projections (**cilia**) arranged in rows that cover the cell surface and beat in synchrony, propelling the cell much like an oar-driven galley. Most ciliates have **cytostomes** that pass food particles through a **cytopharynyx**, and finally into vacuoles where digestion takes place. Although there are some 7000 species of ciliates only one, *Balantidium coli*, is pathogenic for humans, and the disease, **balantidiasis**, is very rare.

D. Sporozoa

The sporozoans (also called the **apicomplexa**) are obligate, intracellular parasites. They generally have nonmotile adult forms, although in some species, the male gametes have flagella. An example of a sporozoan is *Plasmodium vivax* (see p. 283), which causes malaria. Sporozoans can have complex life cycles with more than one host.

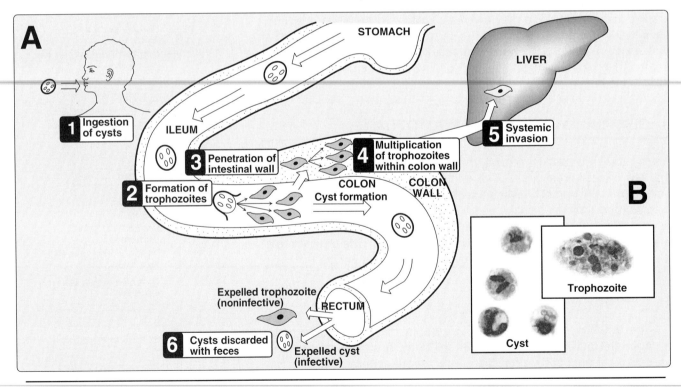

Figure 24.3
A. Life cycle of *Entamoeba histolytica*. B. Photomicrographs of tropozoite and cyst forms.

The **definitive host** is that which harbors the sexually reproducing stage, whereas the **intermediate host** provides the environment in which asexual reproduction occurs.

III. INTESTINAL INFECTIONS

There are three principal protozoal intestinal parasites: the ameba, *Entamoeba histolytica*, the flagellate, *Giardia lamblia*, and several varieties of the sporozoan, *Cryptosporidium*. Each causes a **dysentery**, which, although similar, differs in the site of infection, the severity, and secondary consequences.

A. Amebic dysentery (*Entamoeba histolytica*)

Ingested cysts from contaminated food or water form trophozoites in the small intestine (Figure 24.3). These pass to the colon, where they feed on intestinal bacteria, and may invade the epithelium, potentially inducing ulceration. [Note: One strategy for treating amebic dysentery is to administer antibiotics, such as tetracycline, to reduce the intestinal flora, the ameba's major food source.] The parasite can further spread to the liver and cause abscesses. In the colon, trophozoites form cysts that pass in the feces (amebic cysts are resistant to chlorine concentrations used in most water treatment facilities). Diagnosis is made by examination of fecal samples for motile trophozoites, or for cysts. Serologic test kits are useful when microscopic examination is negative. Liver abscesses should be biopsied from the abscess edge where the active amebas accumulate. Mild cases of amebic dysentery are treated with iodoquinol or diloxanide furoate. More severe cases, including liver infections, are treated with metronidazole (which also has antibacterial activity).

B. Giardiasis (*Giardia lamblia*)

Giardiasis is the most commonly diagnosed parasitic intestinal disease in the United States. Like *Entamoeba histolytica*, this protozoan has two life-cycle stages: the binucleate trophozoite that has four flagella, and the drug-resistant four-nucleate cyst. Ingested cysts form trophozoites in the duodenum where they attach to the wall but do not invade (Figure 24.4). *Giardia* infections are often clinically mild, although in some individuals, massive infection may inflame and damage the duodenal mucosa. Because the *Giardia* parasite preferentially inhabits the duodenum, fecal examination may be negative. A commercial immunologic ELISA test to measure *Giardia* antigen in fecal material has also proven to be useful. Metronidazole is a very effective treatment. Furazolidone is also useful for children. *G. lamblia* cysts are resistant to chlorine concentrations used in most water treatment facilities.

C. Cryptosporidiosis (*Cryptosporidium* species)

Cryptosporidium is an intracellular parasite that inhabits the epithelial cells of the villi of the lower small intestine. The source of infec-

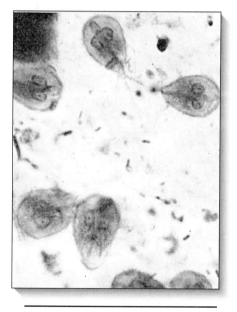

Figure 24.4
Giardia lamblia trophozoite in stool sample.

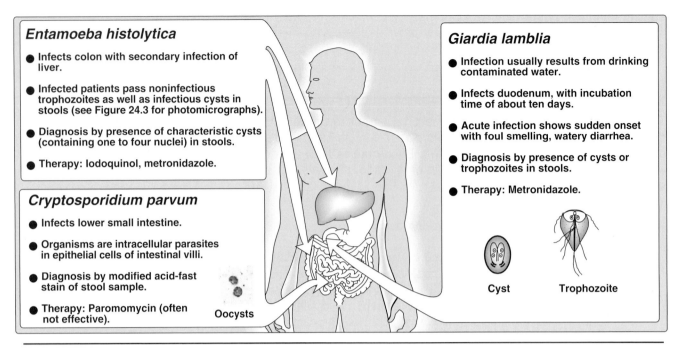

Figure 24.5
Summary of intestinal protozoal infections.

tion is often the feces of domestic animals, and farm run-off has been implicated as a source of *Cryptosporidium* contamination of drinking water. Asymptomatic to mild cases are very common. However, in immunocompromised individuals (for example, those with AIDS), infection may be severe and intractable. Diagnosis is made by the acid-fast staining of the tiny (four to six μm) oocysts in fresh stool samples. If the immune system of the patient is normal, the disease usually resolves without therapy. For immunocompromised patients, no treatment has proven completely effective, although paromomycin has provided some improvement. A summary of intestinal protozoal infections is shown in Figure 24.5.

IV. UROGENITAL TRACT INFECTIONS

Trichomoniasis, the most common protozoal urogenital tract infection of humans, is caused by *Trichomonas vaginalis*. The trichomonads are pear-shaped flagellates, with undulating membranes. Several nonpathogenic species, including *T. tenax* and *T. hominis*, can be found in the human mouth and intestines, respectively. In the living state, these species, which are part of the normal flora, are not easily distinguished morphologically from the pathogenic species, *T. vaginalis*.

A. Trichomoniasis (*Trichomonas vaginalis*)

T. vaginalis is responsible for the most common form of human trichomoniasis (Figure 24.6). In females, it causes inflammation of the mucosal tissue of the vagina, vulva, and cervix, accompanied by a copious, yellowish, malodorous discharge. Less commonly, it infects

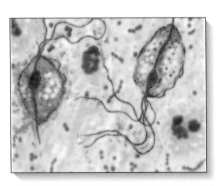

Figure 24.6
Trichomonas vaginalis.

the male urethra, prostate, and seminal vesicles, producing a white discharge. The disease is largely sexually transmitted, and both (or all) sexual partners should be treated. The optimum pH for growth of this organism is about 6.0; therefore *T. vaginalis* does not thrive in the normal, acidic vagina, which has a pH of about 4.0. Abnormal alkalinity of the vagina thus favors acquisition of the disease. Diagnosis is made by detection of motile trophozoites in vaginal or urethral secretions. If the concentration of parasites is too low to be observed directly, laboratory culture can be used to obtain observable organisms. Effective treatment is afforded by metronidazole. Figure 24.7 summarizes urogenital infections caused by *T. vaginalis*.

V. BLOOD AND TISSUE INFECTIONS

The major protozoal diseases that involve the blood and internal organs are malaria (*Plasmodium* species), toxoplasmosis (*Toxoplasma* species), trypanosomiasis (*Trypanosoma* species), and leishmaniasis (*Leishmania* species). *Plasmodium* and *Toxoplasma* are **sporozoans** (apicomplexa), whereas *Trypanosoma* and *Leishmania* are **flagellates**, sometimes referred to as **hemoflagellates**.

A. Malaria (*Plasmodium falciparum* and other plasmodial species)

Malaria is an acute infectious disease of the blood, caused by one of four species of the protozoal genus, *Plasmodium*, a sporozoan. *P. falciparum* accounts for some fifteen percent of all malaria cases, and *P. vivax* for eighty percent of malarial cases. The plasmodial parasite is transmitted to humans through the bite of a female *Anopheles* mosquito, or by use of an infected blood-contaminated needle. Sporozoans reproduce asexually in human cells by a process called **schizogony**, in which multiple nuclear divisions are followed by envelopment of the nuclei by cell walls producing **merozoites**. These in turn become **trophozoites**. Sexual reproduction occurs in the mosquito, where new **spores** (**sporozoites**) are formed.

1. **Pathology and clinical significance:** *Plasmodium* sporozoites are injected into the bloodstream, where they rapidly migrate to the liver. There they form cyst-like structures containing thousands of merozoites. Upon release, the merozoites invade red blood cells, using hemoglobin as a nutrient. Eventually, the infected red cells rupture, releasing merozoites that can invade other erythrocytes. [Note: If large numbers of red cells rupture at roughly the same time, a **paroxysm** (sudden onset) of fever can result due to the massive release of toxic substances. The paroxysms can be cyclic. The length of the period varies with different species of plasmodium.] *Plasmodium falciparum* is the most dangerous plasmodial species. It can cause a rapidly fulminating disease, characterized by persistent high fever and orthostatic hypotension. Infection can lead to capillary obstruction and death if treatment is not prompt. *P. malariae*, *P. vivax*, and *P. ovale* cause milder forms of the disease, probably because they invade either young or old red cells, but not both. This is in contrast to *P. falciparum*, which

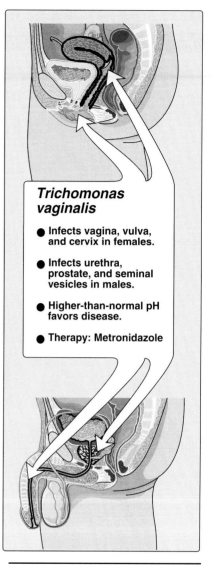

Trichomonas vaginalis

- Infects vagina, vulva, and cervix in females.

- Infects urethra, prostate, and seminal vesicles in males.

- Higher-than-normal pH favors disease.

- Therapy: Metronidazole

Figure 24.7
Summary of urogenital infections.

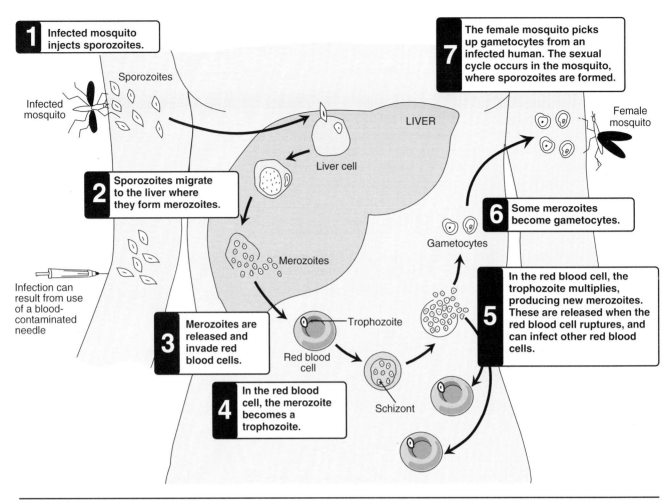

Figure 24.8
Life cycle of the malarial parasite, *Plasmodium falciparum.*

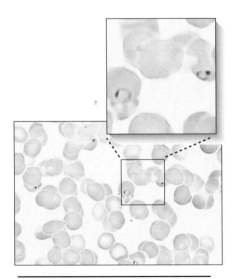

Figure 24.9
Ring form of *Plasmodium falciparum* in red blood cell.

invades cells of all ages. Even today, malarial infection is a common and serious disease, causing some 300 million cases per year, with a death rate of about one percent. A summary of the life cycle of *Plasmodium* is shown in Figure 24.8.

2. **Diagnosis and treatment:** Diagnosis depends on detection of the parasite inside red blood cells (Figure 24.9). Thick blood smears stained with Giemsa stain provide the most sensitive visual test. Thin blood smears, where more detail can be discerned, are used to determine the species involved, which is important in planning a course of therapy. [Note: Serologic tests are usually too slow for diagnosis of acute disease.] Drug treatment depends on the stage of the infection. Primaquine is effective against exoerythrocytic forms in the liver and bloodstream, but is inactive against parasites in red blood cells. Primaquine is thus administered in conjunction with a blood schizontocide such as chloroquine, quinine,

[1]See p. 115 in ***Lippincott's Illustrated Reviews: Biochemistry*** (2nd ed.) for a discussion of glucose 6-phosphate dehydrogenase

mefloquine, or pyrimethamine. All species may develop drug resistance. [Note: Patients with glucose 6-phosphate dehydrogenase deficiency[1] develop hemolytic anemia if they are treated with primaquine.]

B. Toxoplasmosis (*Toxoplasma gondii*)

Toxoplasma gondii is a sporozoan, distributed worldwide, that infects all vertebrate species, although the definitive host is the cat. Humans can become infected by the accidental ingestion of oocysts present in cat feces, by eating raw or undercooked meat, congenitally from an infected mother, or from a blood transfusion.

1. **Pathology and clinical significance:** There are two kinds of *Toxoplasma* trophozoites found in human infections: rapidly growing **tachyzoites** (tachy = rapid) that are seen in body fluids in early, acute infections, and slowly growing **bradyzoites** (brady = slow) that are contained in cysts in muscle and brain tissue, and in the eye. Tachyzoites directly destroy cells, particularly parenchymal and reticuloendothelial cells, whereas bradyzoites, released from ruptured tissue cysts, cause local inflammation with blockage of blood vessels and necrosis. Infections of normal human hosts are very common, and usually asymptomatic. However, they can be very severe in immunocompromised individuals, who may also suffer recrudescence (relapse) of the infection. Congenital infections can also be very severe, resulting in stillbirths, brain lesions, and hydrocephaly, and are a major cause of blindness in newborns.

2. **Diagnosis and treatment:** The initial diagnostic approach involves detection of parasites in tissue specimens, but this may often be inconclusive. With the recent availability of commercial diagnostic kits, serologic tests to identify toxoplasma are now routinely used. These include tests for *Toxoplasma*-specific IgG and IgM. The treatment of choice for this infection is the antifolate drug pyrimethamine, given in combination with sulfadiazine.

C. Trypanosomiasis (various trypanosome species)

Trypanosomiasis refers to two chronic, eventually fatal, diseases (African sleeping sickness, and American trypanosomiasis) caused by several trypanosome species. Some of the differences between these diseases, and the available chemotherapeutic agents, are summarized in Figure 24.10.

1. **Pathology and clinical significance: African sleeping sickness** is caused by the closely related flagellates, *Trypanosoma brucei gambiense* or *Trypanosoma brucei rhodesiense* (Figure 24.11). These parasites are injected into humans by the bite of the **tsetse fly**, producing a primary lesion or chancre. The organism then spreads to lymphoid tissues, and reproduces extracellularly in the blood. Later, the parasite invades the CNS, causing an inflammation of the brain and spinal cord, mediated by released toxins. This inflammation produces the characteristic lethargy, and even-

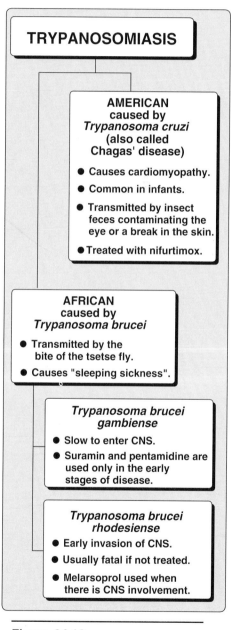

TRYPANOSOMIASIS

AMERICAN caused by *Trypanosoma cruzi* (also called Chagas' disease)
- Causes cardiomyopathy.
- Common in infants.
- Transmitted by insect feces contaminating the eye or a break in the skin.
- Treated with nifurtimox.

AFRICAN caused by *Trypanosoma brucei*
- Transmitted by the bite of the tsetse fly.
- Causes "sleeping sickness".

Trypanosoma brucei gambiense
- Slow to enter CNS.
- Suramin and pentamidine are used only in the early stages of disease.

Trypanosoma brucei rhodesiense
- Early invasion of CNS.
- Usually fatal if not treated.
- Melarsoprol used when there is CNS involvement.

Figure 24.10
Summary of trypanosomiasis.

tually, continuous sleep and death. **American trypanosomiasis (Chagas' disease)**, caused by *Trypanosoma cruzi*, occurs in Central and South America. Unlike the African forms of the disease, infection is not transmitted by an insect bite, but rather by insect feces contaminating the conjunctiva or a break in the skin.

2. **Diagnosis and treatment:** Diagnosis of African trypanosomiasis is made primarily by detection of motile trypanosomes in Giemsa-stained smears of body fluids, blood, cerebrospinal fluid, and lymph node aspirates. Highly specific serologic tests are also available, and are often used for diagnostic confirmation. Early-stage African trypanosomiasis is treated with suramin or pentamidine. Melarsoprol is used in late-stage disease when the CNS is involved. American trypanosomiasis is treated with nifurtimox, but the drug's effectiveness is limited.

D. Leishmaniasis (various *Leishmania* species)

Leishmaniasis refers to a group of infections caused by the flagellate protozoa of the genus *Leishmania*. About half a million new cases are reported each year, and it is estimated that 12,000,000 people are currently infected with this parasite. There are three clinical types of leishmaniasis: cutaneous, mucocutaneous, and visceral. The various infective organisms are indistinguishable morphologically, but can be differentiated by biochemical means. Two subgenera are recognized (*L. leishmania* and *L. viannia*), each with several species. Although in a given geographic locale one species usually is responsible for a single clinical manifestation, the causative species may be different in a different locale. Any species has the potential to cause

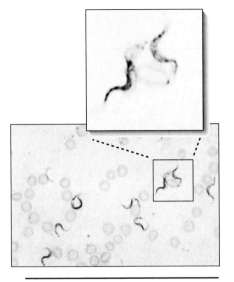

Figure 24.11
Trypanosoma brucei.

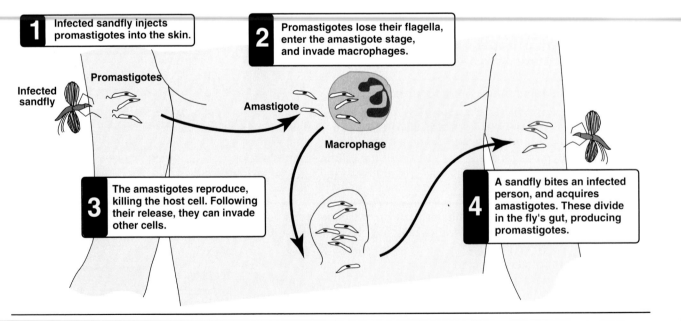

1 Infected sandfly injects promastigotes into the skin.

2 Promastigotes lose their flagella, enter the amastigote stage, and invade macrophages.

Infected sandfly

Promastigotes

Amastigote

Macrophage

3 The amastigotes reproduce, killing the host cell. Following their release, they can invade other cells.

4 A sandfly bites an infected person, and acquires amastigotes. These divide in the fly's gut, producing promastigotes.

Figure 24.12
Life cycle of *Leishmania.*

any one of the three clinical manifestations. The natural reservoir of the parasite varies with geography and species, but is usually wild rodents, dogs, and humans. Transmission to humans is by the bite of a sand fly of the genus *Phlebotomus* or *Lutzomyia*. The life cycle of *Leishmania* is shown in Figure 24.12.

1. **Cutaneous leishmaniasis (local name: oriental sore):** This disease is caused by *Leishmania tropica* in north and west Africa, Iran, and Iraq. The cutaneous form of the disease is characterized by ulcerating skin sores that can be single or multiple (Figure 24.13A). Most cases spontaneously heal, but the ulcers leave unsightly scars. In Mexico and Guatemala, the cutaneous form is due to *Leishmania mexicana*, which produces single lesions that rapidly heal.

2. **Mucocutaneous leishmaniasis (local name: espundia):** This disease is caused by *Leishmania viannia brasiliensis* in Central and South America, especially the Amazon regions. In this form of the disease, the parasite attacks tissue at the mucosal-dermal junctions of the nose and mouth, producing multiple lesions (Figure 24.13B). Extensive spreading into mucosal tissue can obliterate the nasal septum and the buccal cavity, ending in death from secondary infection.

3. **Visceral leishmaniasis (local name: kala-azar):** This disease is caused by *Leishmania donovani* in India, East Africa and China. In the visceral disease, the parasite initially infects macrophages, which in turn migrate to the spleen, liver, and bone marrow, where the parasite rapidly multiplies. The spleen and liver enlarge, and jaundice may develop. Most individuals have only minor symptoms, and the disease may resolve spontaneously. However, in some cases, complications due to secondary infection and emaciation result in death.

4. **Diagnosis and treatment:** Diagnosis is made by examination of Giemsa-stained tissue and fluid samples for the nonflagellated form (**amastigote**), which is the only form of the organism that occurs in humans and other mammals. Cutaneous and mucocutaneous disease can be diagnosed from tissue samples taken from the edges of lesions or lymph node aspirates. Visceral disease is more difficult to diagnose, requiring liver, spleen, or bone marrow biopsy. Serologic tests (for example, indirect fluorescent antibody, see p. 31, and complement fixation, see p. 29) are useful, and are used by the Centers for Disease Control and Prevention. The treatment of leishmaniasis is difficult because the available drugs have considerable toxicity and high failure rates. Pentavalent antimonials, such as sodium stibogluconate, are the conventional therapy, with pentamidine and amphotericin B as second-line agents.

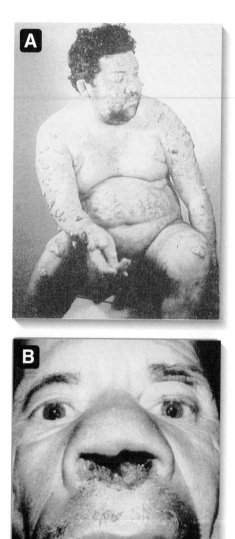

Figure 24.13
A. Diffuse cutaneous leishmaniasis.
B. Mucocutaneus leishmaniasis.

Study Questions

Choose the ONE correct answer

24.1 The protozoal trophozoite phase is characterized by

A. metabolic dormancy.

B. toxin production.

C. active feeding and reproduction.

D. flagellar locomotion.

E. residence in the intermediate host.

> Correct answer = C. The trophozoite is, generally speaking, the active phase, in contrast to the cyst, which is the dormant phase. In some species, several varieties of trophozoites are recognized, such as the tachyzoites and the bradyzoites of *Toxoplasma gondii*.

24.2 The definitive host of a parasite is the host

A. in which asexual reproduction occurs.

B. in which sexual reproduction occurs.

C. which is obligatory for the parasite.

D. that is capable of destroying the parasite.

E. that is the vector organism that transports a parasite from an uninfected to an infected host.

> Correct answer = B. Sexual reproduction occurs in the definitive host, whereas asexual reproduction occurs in the intermediate host. For example, in the case of the malarial *Plasmodium*, the definitive host is the mosquito and the intermediate host is the human. In most cases, both hosts are obligatory for propagation of the parasite.

24.3 *Plasmodium falciparum*, which causes malaria, is an example of

A. an ameboid protozoan.

B. a sporozoan.

C. a flagellate.

D. a ciliate.

E. a schizont.

> Correct answer = B. The sporozoans are also called apicomplexa, so named because of the presence of a complex of organelles at the cell tip that facilitate penetration of the parasite into host tissue. A schizont is not a taxonomic group but a mass of trophozoites.

24.4 Espundia and kala-azar are local names for two manifestations of the disease:

A. giardiasis.

B. toxoplasmosis.

C. trichomoniasis.

D. malaria.

E. leishmaniasis.

> Correct answer = E. Espundia and kala-azar refer respectively to the mucocutaneous and the visceral forms of leishmania.

24.5 A United States businessman who has recently returned home from Haiti suddenly develops a periodic high fever followed by orthostatic hypotension. What is the likely preliminary diagnosis?

A. Chagas' disease

B. Giardiasis

C. Syphilis

D. Malaria

E. Toxoplasmosis

> Correct answer = D. All of the signs point to malaria, especially the periodicity of the fever that results from the synchronous rupturing of large numbers of red blood cells.

Helminths

25

I. OVERVIEW

The helminths are worms, some of which are parasitic to humans. These parasites belong to one of three groups: **cestodes** (**tapeworms**), **trematodes** (**flukes**), or **nematodes** (**roundworms**) (Figure 25.1). Although individual species may have preferred primary sites of infestation—often the intestines where they generally do little damage—these organisms may disseminate to vital organs (for example, the brain, lungs, or liver) where they can cause severe damage. It is estimated that at least seventy percent of the world's population is infected with a parasitic helminth. The mode of transmission to humans varies from species to species, and includes ingestion of larvae in raw or undercooked pork, beef, or fish, and ingestion of helminth eggs in feces, by insect bites, or by direct skin penetration. In North America, helminthic diseases are becoming rare, whereas they are endemic in regions of the world where community sanitary conditions are poor, and human feces is used as fertilizer.

II. CESTODES

The cestodes (**tapeworms**) are ribbon-like, segmented worms that are primarily intestinal parasites. They totally lack a digestive system, and thus do not ingest particulate matter, but instead absorb soluble nutrients directly through their cuticle. In the small intestine some species, for example, the tapeworm *Diphyllobothrium latum*, can attain enormous lengths of up to fifteen meters. Cestodes cause clinical injury by sequestering the host's nutrients, by excreting toxic waste, and, in massive infestations, by causing mechanical blockage of the intestine. The anterior end of the worm consists of a **scolex**, a bulbous structure with hooks and suckers that functions to attach the worm to the intestinal wall (Figure 25.2). The body (**strobila**), is composed of many segments called **proglottids**, which form continuously in the region just behind the scolex. Each proglottid has a complete set of sexual organs—both male and female—that generate fertilized eggs. The mature, egg-filled proglottids are located at the posterior end of the organism. These can break off of the chain, and pass out of the body in the stool. Characteristics of infections by the four medically important cestodes are summarized in Figure 25.3. Note that *Taenia solium* has two different disease manifestations, depending on whether transmission is by ingestion of larvae from undercooked pork, or by ingestion of its eggs. In the former case, infestation is limited to the intestines, whereas in the latter case, the eggs develop into larvae that form cysts (**cysticerci**) in the brain and other tissues.

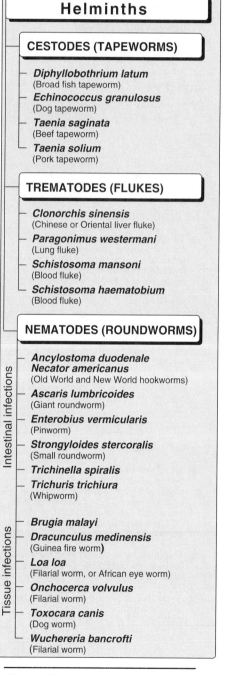

Helminths

CESTODES (TAPEWORMS)

- *Diphyllobothrium latum* (Broad fish tapeworm)
- *Echinococcus granulosus* (Dog tapeworm)
- *Taenia saginata* (Beef tapeworm)
- *Taenia solium* (Pork tapeworm)

TREMATODES (FLUKES)

- *Clonorchis sinensis* (Chinese or Oriental liver fluke)
- *Paragonimus westermani* (Lung fluke)
- *Schistosoma mansoni* (Blood fluke)
- *Schistosoma haematobium* (Blood fluke)

NEMATODES (ROUNDWORMS)

Intestinal infections
- *Ancylostoma duodenale* *Necator americanus* (Old World and New World hookworms)
- *Ascaris lumbricoides* (Giant roundworm)
- *Enterobius vermicularis* (Pinworm)
- *Strongyloides stercoralis* (Small roundworm)
- *Trichinella spiralis*
- *Trichuris trichiura* (Whipworm)

Tissue infections
- *Brugia malayi*
- *Dracunculus medinensis* (Guinea fire worm**)**
- *Loa loa* (Filarial worm, or African eye worm)
- *Onchocerca volvulus* (Filarial worm)
- *Toxocara canis* (Dog worm)
- *Wuchereria bancrofti* (Filarial worm)

Figure 25.1
Clinically important helminths.

Lippincott's Illustrated Reviews: Microbiology,
by William A. Strohl, Harriet Rouse, Bruce D. Fisher.
Lippincott, Williams & Wilkins, Baltimore, MD © 2001

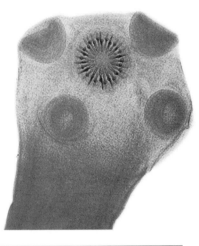

Figure 25.2
The scolex of *Taenia solium* is 1 mm in diameter and has four suckers.

III. TREMATODES

The trematodes, commonly called **flukes**, are small (about 1 cm), flat, leaf-like worms that, depending on the species, infest various organs of the human host (for example, intestinal veins, urinary bladder, liver, or lung). All parasitic trematodes use freshwater snails as an intermediate host.

A. Hermaphroditic flukes

Developmental events in the life cycle of a typical fluke begin when the adult fluke, which is hermaphroditic, produces eggs in the human (the definitive host). The eggs are then excreted into the environment. Inside of the eggs the first larval stage (the **miracidium**) develops. These larvae seek out and infect suitable snail species, which are the first intermediate host. In the snail, asexual reproduction occurs, during which several intermediate developmental forms can be distinguished, including **sporocyst**, **redia** (an early larval stage) and eventually large numbers of the final larval

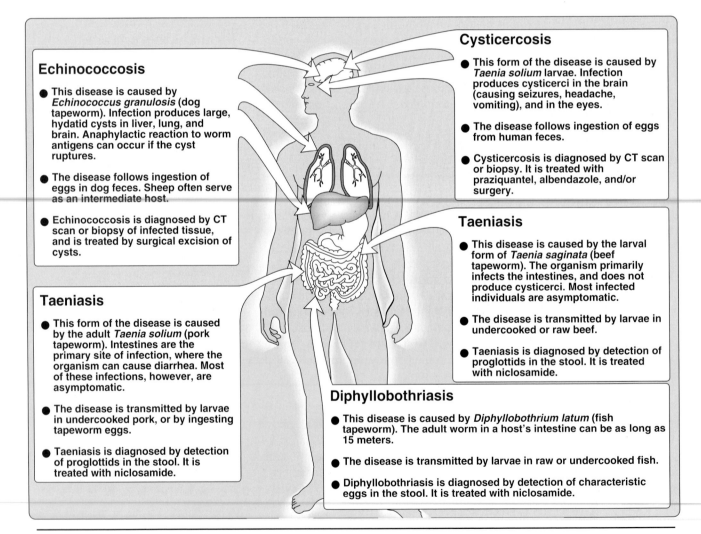

Echinococcosis

● This disease is caused by *Echinococcus granulosis* (dog tapeworm). Infection produces large, hydatid cysts in liver, lung, and brain. Anaphylactic reaction to worm antigens can occur if the cyst ruptures.

● The disease follows ingestion of eggs in dog feces. Sheep often serve as an intermediate host.

● Echinococcosis is diagnosed by CT scan or biopsy of infected tissue, and is treated by surgical excision of cysts.

Taeniasis

● This form of the disease is caused by the adult *Taenia solium* (pork tapeworm). Intestines are the primary site of infection, where the organism can cause diarrhea. Most of these infections, however, are asymptomatic.

● The disease is transmitted by larvae in undercooked pork, or by ingesting tapeworm eggs.

● Taeniasis is diagnosed by detection of proglottids in the stool. It is treated with niclosamide.

Cysticercosis

● This form of the disease is caused by *Taenia solium* larvae. Infection produces cysticerci in the brain (causing seizures, headache, vomiting), and in the eyes.

● The disease follows ingestion of eggs from human feces.

● Cysticercosis is diagnosed by CT scan or biopsy. It is treated with praziquantel, albendazole, and/or surgery.

Taeniasis

● This disease is caused by the larval form of *Taenia saginata* (beef tapeworm). The organism primarily infects the intestines, and does not produce cysticerci. Most infected individuals are asymptomatic.

● The disease is transmitted by larvae in undercooked or raw beef.

● Taeniasis is diagnosed by detection of proglottids in the stool. It is treated with niclosamide.

Diphyllobothriasis

● This disease is caused by *Diphyllobothrium latum* (fish tapeworm). The adult worm in a host's intestine can be as long as 15 meters.

● The disease is transmitted by larvae in raw or undercooked fish.

● Diphyllobothriasis is diagnosed by detection of characteristic eggs in the stool. It is treated with niclosamide.

Figure 25.3
Characteristics and therapy for commonly encountered cestode infections.

stage called **cercaria**, which leave the snail and seek out a second intermediate host (a fish or crustacean, depending on the species of fluke). In this second intermediate host the cercaria form cysts called **metacercaria** that can remain viable indefinitely. Finally, if the infected raw or undercooked fish or crustacean is eaten by a human, the metacercaria excysts, and the fluke invades tissues such as the lung or the liver and begins producing eggs, thus completing the life cycle.

B. Sexual flukes (schistosomes)

The life cycle of schistosomes is similar to that of the hermaphroditic flukes. One difference is that schistosomes have only one intermediate host, the snail. Another difference is that **schistosomiasis** is not acquired by ingestion of contaminated food, but rather from schistosome cercaria directly penetrating the skin of waders or swimmers in contaminated rivers and lakes. After dissemination and development in the human host, the adult schistosomes take up residence in various abdominal veins, depending on the species; they are therefore called "blood flukes". Also in contrast to the "typical" hermaphroditic flukes described above, the schistosomes have separate, distinctive sexes. A remarkable anatomical feature on the ventral surface of the large male is the long groove or **schist** in which the smaller female resides and continuously mates with the male (Figure 25.4). This mating takes place in the human liver.

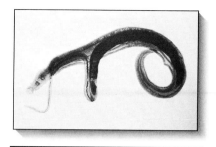

Figure 25.4
Male schistosome has long groove in which the smaller female resides and continuously mates with the male.

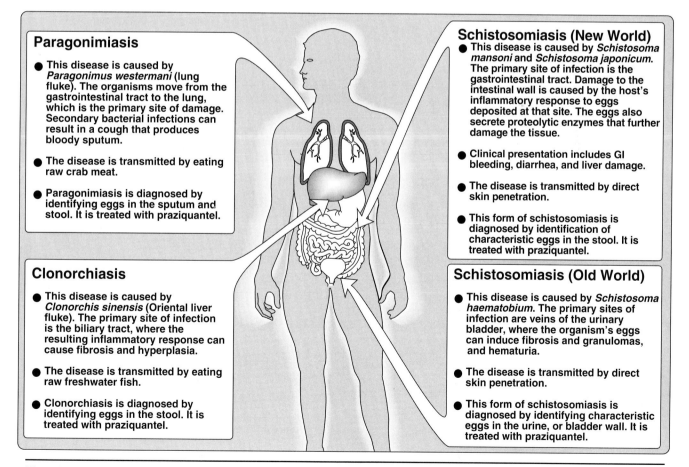

Figure 25.5
Characteristics and therapy for commonly encountered trematode infections.

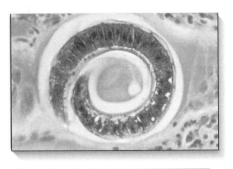

Figure 25.6
Coiled larva of *Trichinella spiralis* in skeletal muscle.

Fertilized eggs penetrate the human host's vascular walls, and enter the intestine or bladder, emerging from the body in feces or urine. In fresh water, the organisms infect snails in which they multiply, producing **cercaria** (the final, free-swimming larval stage), which are released into the fresh water to complete the cycle. Characteristics of clinically important trematodes are summarized in Figure 25.5.

IV. NEMATODES

The nematodes (roundworms) are elongated, nonsegmented worms that are tapered at both ends (Figure 25.6). Unlike other helminths, nematodes have a complete digestive system, including a mouth, an intestine that spans most of the body length, and an anus. The body is protected by a tough, noncellular cuticle. Most nematodes have separate, anatomi-

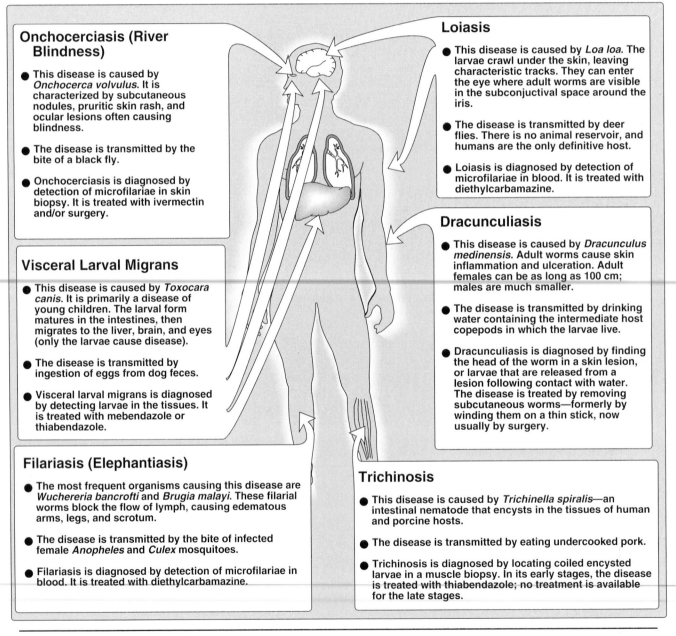

Onchocerciasis (River Blindness)

● This disease is caused by *Onchocerca volvulus*. It is characterized by subcutaneous nodules, pruritic skin rash, and ocular lesions often causing blindness.

● The disease is transmitted by the bite of a black fly.

● Onchocerciasis is diagnosed by detection of microfilariae in skin biopsy. It is treated with ivermectin and/or surgery.

Visceral Larval Migrans

● This disease is caused by *Toxocara canis*. It is primarily a disease of young children. The larval form matures in the intestines, then migrates to the liver, brain, and eyes (only the larvae cause disease).

● The disease is transmitted by ingestion of eggs from dog feces.

● Visceral larval migrans is diagnosed by detecting larvae in the tissues. It is treated with mebendazole or thiabendazole.

Filariasis (Elephantiasis)

● The most frequent organisms causing this disease are *Wuchereria bancrofti* and *Brugia malayi*. These filarial worms block the flow of lymph, causing edematous arms, legs, and scrotum.

● The disease is transmitted by the bite of infected female *Anopheles* and *Culex* mosquitoes.

● Filariasis is diagnosed by detection of microfilariae in blood. It is treated with diethylcarbamazine.

Loiasis

● This disease is caused by *Loa loa*. The larvae crawl under the skin, leaving characteristic tracks. They can enter the eye where adult worms are visible in the subconjuctival space around the iris.

● The disease is transmitted by deer flies. There is no animal reservoir, and humans are the only definitive host.

● Loiasis is diagnosed by detection of microfilariae in blood. It is treated with diethylcarbamazine.

Dracunculiasis

● This disease is caused by *Dracunculus medinensis*. Adult worms cause skin inflammation and ulceration. Adult females can be as long as 100 cm; males are much smaller.

● The disease is transmitted by drinking water containing the intermediate host copepods in which the larvae live.

● Dracunculiasis is diagnosed by finding the head of the worm in a skin lesion, or larvae that are released from a lesion following contact with water. The disease is treated by removing subcutaneous worms—formerly by winding them on a thin stick, now usually by surgery.

Trichinosis

● This disease is caused by *Trichinella spiralis*—an intestinal nematode that encysts in the tissues of human and porcine hosts.

● The disease is transmitted by eating undercooked pork.

● Trichinosis is diagnosed by locating coiled encysted larvae in a muscle biopsy. In its early stages, the disease is treated with thiabendazole; no treatment is available for the late stages.

Figure 25.7
Characteristics and therapy for commonly encountered nematode infections of tissues other than intestine.

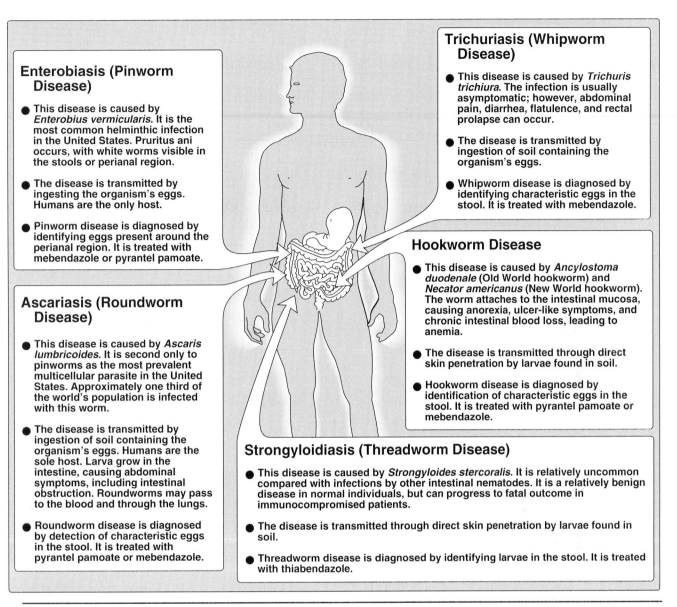

Enterobiasis (Pinworm Disease)

● This disease is caused by *Enterobius vermicularis*. It is the most common helminthic infection in the United States. Pruritus ani occurs, with white worms visible in the stools or perianal region.

● The disease is transmitted by ingesting the organism's eggs. Humans are the only host.

● Pinworm disease is diagnosed by identifying eggs present around the perianal region. It is treated with mebendazole or pyrantel pamoate.

Ascariasis (Roundworm Disease)

● This disease is caused by *Ascaris lumbricoides*. It is second only to pinworms as the most prevalent multicellular parasite in the United States. Approximately one third of the world's population is infected with this worm.

● The disease is transmitted by ingestion of soil containing the organism's eggs. Humans are the sole host. Larva grow in the intestine, causing abdominal symptoms, including intestinal obstruction. Roundworms may pass to the blood and through the lungs.

● Roundworm disease is diagnosed by detection of characteristic eggs in the stool. It is treated with pyrantel pamoate or mebendazole.

Trichuriasis (Whipworm Disease)

● This disease is caused by *Trichuris trichiura*. The infection is usually asymptomatic; however, abdominal pain, diarrhea, flatulence, and rectal prolapse can occur.

● The disease is transmitted by ingestion of soil containing the organism's eggs.

● Whipworm disease is diagnosed by identifying characteristic eggs in the stool. It is treated with mebendazole.

Hookworm Disease

● This disease is caused by *Ancylostoma duodenale* (Old World hookworm) and *Necator americanus* (New World hookworm). The worm attaches to the intestinal mucosa, causing anorexia, ulcer-like symptoms, and chronic intestinal blood loss, leading to anemia.

● The disease is transmitted through direct skin penetration by larvae found in soil.

● Hookworm disease is diagnosed by identification of characteristic eggs in the stool. It is treated with pyrantel pamoate or mebendazole.

Strongyloidiasis (Threadworm Disease)

● This disease is caused by *Strongyloides stercoralis*. It is relatively uncommon compared with infections by other intestinal nematodes. It is a relatively benign disease in normal individuals, but can progress to fatal outcome in immunocompromised patients.

● The disease is transmitted through direct skin penetration by larvae found in soil.

● Threadworm disease is diagnosed by identifying larvae in the stool. It is treated with thiabendazole.

Figure 25.8
Characteristics and therapy for commonly encountered intestinal nematode infections.

cally distinctive sexes. The mode of transmission varies widely, depending on the species, and includes direct skin penetration by infectious larvae, ingestion of contaminated soil, eating undercooked pork, and insect bites. The parasites can invade almost any part of the body: liver, kidneys, intestines, subcutaneous tissue, or eyes. Generally, nematodes are categorized by whether they infect the intestines or other tissues (Figures 25.7 and 25.8). Alternatively, they can be divided into those for which the eggs are infectious, and those for which the larvae are infectious. The most common nematode infection in the United States is **enterobiasis** (**pinworm disease**), which causes anal itching, but otherwise does little damage. A more serious disease of worldwide occurrence is **ascariasis**, caused by *Ascaris lumbricoides* (Figure 25.10).

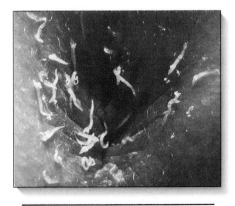

Figure 25.9
Female pinworms (*Enterobius vermicularis*) leaving the anus of a five-year-old child.

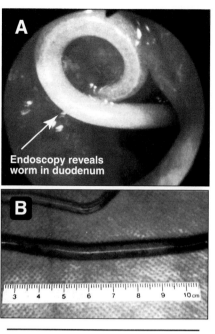

Figure 25.10
A. *Ascaris lumbricoides* in duodenum. B. Worms removed with biopsy forceps.

Study Questions

Choose the ONE correct answer

25.1 A proglottid is:

    A. the region anterior to the pharynx of trematodes.

    B. a fertile segment of a nematode.

    C. an egg-bearing segment of a cestode

    D. the dorsal surface of a trematode.

    E. a specialized cestode larva.

> Correct answer = C. A proglottid is a complete reproductive system, containing both male and female organs, unique to cestodes (tapeworms). Anatomically, proglottids form long chains, hundreds to thousands of units in length. Eggs develop in the more mature posterior segments, which are termed gravid proglottids.

25.2 A patient is diagnosed as having a trematode infection. Lacking a more specific identification of the causative organism, which of the following drugs would most likely be effective?

    A. Niclosamide

    B. Thiabendazole

    C. Praziquantel

    D. Diethylcarbamazine

    E. Tetracycline

> Correct answer = C. Praziquantel is the drug of choice for most trematode infections.

25.3 Which of the following is the most common helminthic infection in the United States?

    A. Schistosomiasis

    B. Diphyllothriasis

    C. Clonorchiasis

    D. Trichinosis

    E. Enterobiasis

> Correct answer = E. Enterobiasis is popularly known as pinworm disease.

25.4 Which of the following helminthic diseases is transmitted by the bite of a mosquito?

    A. Filariasis

    B. Onchocerciasis

    C. Taeniasis

    D. Schistosomiasis

    E. Visceral larval migrans

> Correct answer = A. Mosquitoes ingest filarial embryos (microfilariae) from infected blood. In the insect the embryos develop into the infective filariform larvae that are injected into the human host.

25.5 Which of the following helminthic diseases is transmitted by direct skin penetration by helminth larva?

    A. Filariasis

    B. Onchocerciasis

    C. Dracunculiasis

    D. Schistosomiasis

    E. Visceral larval migrans

> Correct answer = D. Schistosome cercaria released from snails in fresh water are capable of penetrating human skin.

Introduction to the Viruses

26

I. OVERVIEW

A virus is an infectious agent that is minimally constructed of two components: 1) a **genome** consisting of either RNA or DNA, but not both, and 2) a protein-containing structure (the **capsid**) designed to protect the genome (Figure 26.1A). Many viruses have additional structural features, for example, an **envelope** composed of a protein-containing lipid bilayer, whose presence or absence further distinguishes one virus group from another (Figure 26.1B). A complete virus particle combining these structural elements is called a **virion**. In functional terms, the primary characteristic of a virus is that replication is **obligately intracellular**. Similarities and differences in the basic modes of viral replication are further criteria contributing to the grouping of viruses with common properties. The potentials of different groups of viruses to cause disease depend on a great variety of structural and functional viral characteristics. Therefore, even within a closely related group of viruses, different species may produce significantly distinct clinical pathologies.

II. CHARACTERISTICS USED TO DEFINE VIRUS FAMILIES, GENERA, AND SPECIES

Similarities in virion structure, nature of the genome, and mechanism of replication provide the main determinants for dividing viruses into related groups, or **families**, and, sometimes, in more complex viral families [for example, the Herpesviridae (see p. 317), Paramyxoviridae (see p. 382), Parvoviridae (see p. 314), and Poxviridae (see p. 334)], families are subdivided into **subfamilies**. Within a virus family, differences in additional specific properties, such as host range, serologic reactions, amino acid sequences of viral proteins, degree of nucleic acid homology, among others, form the basis for division into **genera** (singular = **genus**) and **species**. [Note: The ending of the name of a virus **family** is "**-viridae**" (for example,

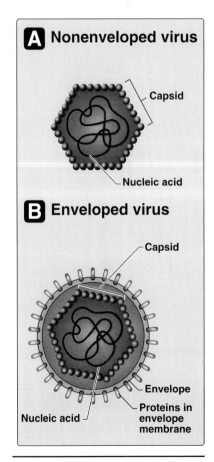

Figure 26.1
General structure: A. nonenveloped and B. enveloped

Lippincott's Illustrated Reviews: Microbiology,
by William A. Strohl, Harriet Rouse, Bruce D. Fisher.
Lippincott, Williams & Wilkins, Baltimore, MD © 2001

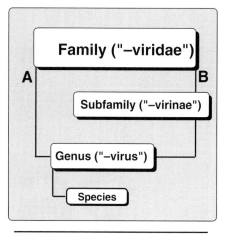

Figure 26.2
Classification of viruses: A. No subfamilies present. B. Subfamilies present.

Herpesviridae), the ending of the **genus** name is "**-virus**" (for example, *Herpesvirus*), and **subfamily** names end in "**-virinae**" (for example, *alpha-herpesvirinae*), (Figure 26.2).] Species of the same virus isolated from different geographic locations may differ from each other in nucleotide sequence. In this case they are referred to as **strains** of the same species.

A. Characteristics of viral families

Division of viruses into family groups is based largely on the type and polarity (negative or positive sense, see below) of the nucleic acid they contain, their mechanism of genome replication, and also the structural characteristics of the virus particles (Figure 26.3).

1. **Genome:** The type of nucleic acid found in the virus particle is perhaps the most fundamental and straightforward of viral properties. It may be **RNA** or **DNA**, either of which may be **single-stranded** (**ss**) or **double-stranded** (**ds**). The most common forms of viral genomes found in nature are ssRNA and dsDNA. However, both dsRNA and ssDNA genomes are found in viruses of medical importance. Single-stranded viral RNA genomes are further subdivided into those that are of "positive polarity" (that is, of messenger RNA sense, which can therefore be used as a template for protein synthesis), and those that are of "negative polarity", or are antisense. Viruses containing these two types of RNA genomes are commonly referred to as **positive strand** and **negative strand** RNA viruses, respectively.

2. **Capsid symmetry:** The protein shell enclosing the genome is, for most virus families, found in either of two geometric configurations (Figure 26.3): **helical** (rod shaped or coiled), or **icosahedral** (spherical or symmetric). The capsid is constructed of multiple copies of a single polypeptide type (found in helical capsids), or a small number of different polypeptides (found in icosahedral capsids), thus requiring only a limited amount of genetic information to code for these structural components.

   a. **Helical symmetry:** Capsids with helical symmetry, such as that of the paramyxoviridae (see p. 382), consist of repeated units

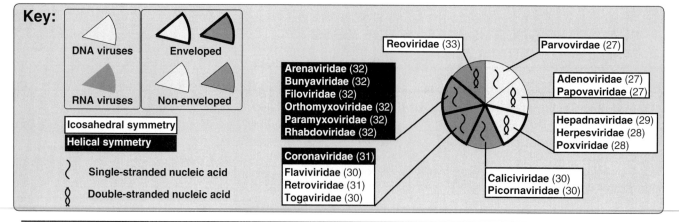

Figure 26.3
Viral families classified according to type of genome, capsid symmetry, and presence or absence of an envelope. [Note: Numbers indicate chapters where detailed information is presented].

of a single polypeptide species that—in association with the viral nucleic acid—self-assemble into a helical cylinder (Figure 26.4). Each polypeptide unit (called a **protomer**) is hydrogen-bonded to neighboring protomers. The nucleic acid is wound in a helical path by hydrogen bonding in an identical way to each successive protomer in the helix. The complex of protomers and nucleic acid is termed the **nucleocapsid**. Because the nucleic acid is surrounded by the capsid, it is protected from environmental damage. Because nucleocapsids form by the interaction of nucleic acids and protomers, these particles are never "empty" (that is, helical protein shells that do not contain nucleic acid do not naturally occur).

b. **Icosahedral symmetry:** An icosahedron is a structure with twelve vertices and twenty triangular faces (Figure 26.5). Capsids with icosahedral symmetry are more complex than those with helical symmetry, in that they consist of several different polypeptides grouped into structural subassemblies called **capsomers**. These, in turn, are hydrogen-bonded to each other to form an icosahedron. The nucleic acid genome is located within the empty space created by the rigid, icosahedral structure. [Note: Unlike helical particles, "empty" icosahedral particles can form, where the protein shell contains no nucleic acid.] The simplest (and smallest) icosahedral structure is composed of twelve capsomers, each of which consists of five polypeptides. All medically important viruses are larger than this, however. The increased size is achieved by adding additional identical capsomers. In the more complex viruses (for example, the adenoviruses, see p. 312), the vertex capsomers (called **pentons**) are composed of polypeptides that are different from the polypeptides making up all of the rest of the capsomers (called **hexons**).

3. **Envelope:** An important structural feature used in defining a viral family is the presence or absence of a lipid-containing membrane surrounding the nucleocapsid. This membrane is referred to as the **envelope**. A virus that is not enveloped is referred to as a **naked** virus. Among the viruses of medical importance, there are both naked and enveloped icosahedral viruses, but all the helical viruses of animals are enveloped. In the latter case, the nucleocapsid is flexible, and is coiled within the envelope, resulting in most such viruses appearing to be roughly spherical (Figure 26.6). The envelope is derived from host cell membranes. However, the cellular membrane proteins are replaced by virus-specific proteins, thus conferring virus-specific antigenicity upon the particle.

B. **Characteristics of viral genera and species.**

Criteria commonly used for distinguishing viral **genera** include, for example, degree of serologic relatedness, and structural/chemical differences between members of a virus family. **Speciation** may further include determination of the host species targeted by the specific virus, and whether the natural host class is plant, vertebrate, or invertebrate. In some cases, the nature of the disease produced, and the tissue

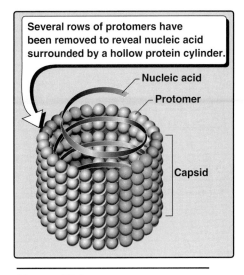

Figure 26.4
Nucleocapsid of a helical virus.

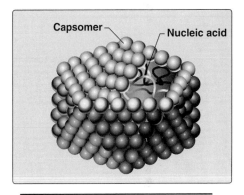

Figure 26.5
Structure of a nonenveloped virus showing icosahedral symmetry.

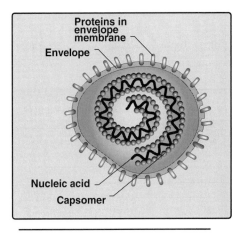

Figure 26.6
Structure of an enveloped helical virus.

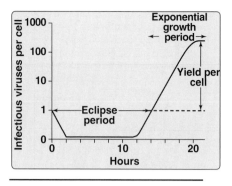

Figure 26.7
One-step growth curve of a single cell infected with a single virus particle. Initiation of infection is at zero time.

specificity of the infection, may also be considered in distinguishing species within a genus. Historically, serologic relationships have been important in defining species. However, species are increasingly being defined at the molecular level, for example, using the molecular weight and amino acid sequence of specific viral proteins, as well as differing degrees of variation in nucleotide sequences.

III. VIRAL REPLICATION: THE ONE-STEP GROWTH CURVE

The one-step growth curve is a representation of the overall change, with time, in the amount of infectious virus in a single cell that has been infected by a single virus particle. In practice, this is determined by following events in a large population of infected cells in which the infection is proceeding as nearly synchronously as can be achieved by manipulating the experimental conditions. Whereas the time scale and yield of progeny virus vary greatly among virus families, the basic features of the infectious cycle are similar for all viruses. The one-step growth curve begins with the eclipse period, which is followed by a period of exponential growth (Figure 26.7).

A. Eclipse period

Following initial attachment of a virus to the host cell, the ability of that virus to infect other cells disappears. This is the eclipse period, and represents the time elapsed from initial entry and disassembly of the parental virus to the assembly of the first progeny virion. During this period, active synthesis of virus components is occurring. The eclipse periods for most human viruses fall within a range of one to twenty hours.

B. Exponential growth

The number of progeny virus produced within the infected cell increases exponentially for a period of time, then reaches a plateau, after which no additional increase in virus yield occurs. The maximum **yield per cell** is characteristic for each virus-cell system, and reflects the balance between the rate at which virus components continue to be synthesized and assembled into virions, and the rate at which the cell loses the synthetic capacity and structural integrity needed to produce new virus particles. This may be from eight hours to 72 hours or longer, with yields of 100 to 10,000 virions per cell.

IV. STEPS IN THE REPLICATION CYCLES OF VIRUSES

The individual steps in the virus replication cycle are presented below in sequence, beginning with virus attachment to the host cell, leading to penetration and uncoating of the viral genome. Gene expression and replication are followed by assembly and release of viral progeny.

A. Adsorption

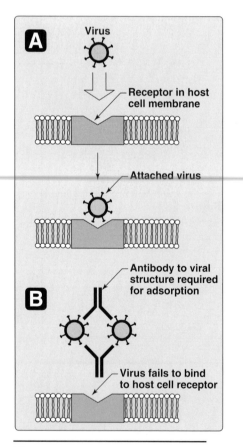

Figure 26.8
A. Attachment of virus to receptor on host cell membrane. B. Antibody prevents adsorption of virus.

The initial attachment of a virus particle to a host cell involves an interaction between specific molecular structures on the virion surface, and molecules in the host cell membrane that recognize these viral structures (Figure 26.8A).

1. **Attachment sites on the viral surface:** Some viruses have specialized attachment structures, such as the glycoprotein spikes found in viral envelopes (for example, rhabdoviruses, see p. 380), whereas for others, the unique folding of the capsid proteins forms the attachment sites (for example, picornaviruses, see p. 350). In both cases, multiple copies of these molecular attachment structures are distributed around the surface of the virion. [Note: In some cases, the mechanism by which antibodies neutralize viral infectivity is through antibody binding to the viral structures that are required for adsorption (Figure 26.8B).]

2. **Host cell receptor molecules:** The receptor molecules on the host cell membrane are specific for each virus family. Not surprisingly, these receptors have been found to be molecular structures that usually carry out normal cell functions. For example, cellular membrane receptors for compounds such as growth factors may also inadvertently serve as receptors for a particular virus. Many of the compounds that serve as virus receptors are present only on specifically differentiated cells, or are unique for one animal species. Therefore, the presence or absence of host cell receptors is one important determinant of tissue specificity within a susceptible host species, and also for the susceptibility or resistance of a species to a given virus. [Note: The detailed, three-dimensional structures of cell receptors and/or of the corresponding virus binding sites for a number of clinically significant viruses are currently being determined. This information is being used to design anti-viral drugs that specifically interact with these sites, thus blocking adsorption.]

B. Penetration

Penetration is the passage of the virion from the surface of the cell, across the cell membrane, and into the cytoplasm. There are two principal mechanisms by which viruses enter animal cells: **receptor-mediated endocytosis**, and direct **membrane fusion**.

1. **Receptor-mediated endocytosis:** This is basically the same process by which the cell internalizes compounds such as growth regulatory molecules and serum lipoproteins, but with the infecting virus particle bound to the host cell surface receptor in place of the normal ligand (Figure 26.9). The cell membrane invaginates, enclosing the virion in an endocytotic vesicle (endosome). Release of the virion into the cytoplasm occurs by various routes, depending on the virus, but in general it is facilitated by one or more viral molecules. In the case of an enveloped virus, its membrane may fuse with the membrane of the endosome, resulting in the release of the nucleocapsid into the cytoplasm. With the exception of the Reovirus family (see p. 394), failure to exit the endosome before fusion with a lysosome results in degradation of the virion by lysosomal enzymes. This is one reason why not all potentially infectious particles are successful in establishing infection.

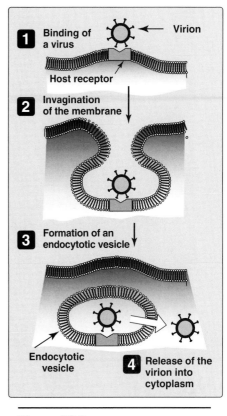

Figure 26.9
Receptor-mediated endocytosis of virus particle.

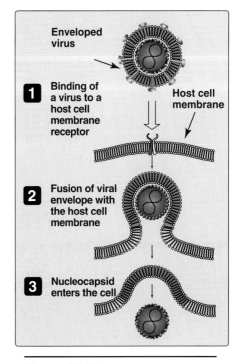

Figure 26.10
Fusion of viral envelope with membrane of host cell.

2. **Membrane fusion:** Some enveloped viruses (for example, human immunodeficiency virus, see p. 363) enter a host cell by fusion of their envelope with the plasma membrane of the cell (Figure 26.10). One or more of the glycoproteins in the envelope of these viruses promotes the fusion. The end result of this process is that the nucleocapsid is free in the cytoplasm, whereas the viral membrane remains associated with the plasma membrane of the host cell.

C. Uncoating

The term "uncoating" refers to the stepwise process of disassembly of the virion that enables the expression of the viral genes that carry out replication. For enveloped viruses, the penetration process itself is the first step in uncoating. In general, most steps of the uncoating process occur within the cell, and depend on cellular enzymes, but in some of the more complex viruses, newly synthesized viral proteins are required to complete the process. The loss of one or more structural components of the virion during uncoating predictably leads to a loss of the ability of that particle to infect other cells, and is the basis for the eclipse period of the growth curve. It is during this phase in the replication cycle that viral gene expression begins.

D. Mechanisms of DNA virus genome replication

Each virus family differs in significant ways from all others in terms of the details of the macromolecular events comprising the replication cycle. However, those with the same type of genome (that is, DNA or RNA) share many basic features of gene expression and mechanisms of genome replication. For example, the basic mechanisms of genome replication and gene expression by viruses with DNA genomes closely resemble those of eukaryotic cells. However, the wide range of molecular weights of these genomes (from approximately 2 to 250 x 10^6) gives rise to great differences in the

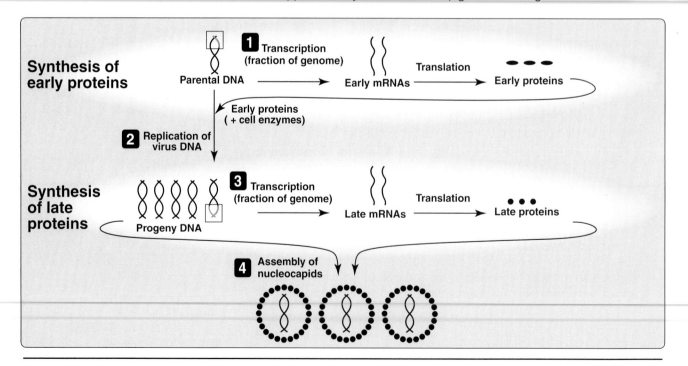

Figure 26.11
Replication of DNA viruses.

number of proteins for which the virus can code. In general, the smaller the viral genome, the more the virus must depend on the host cell to provide the functions needed for viral replication. For example, some small DNA viruses such as polyomavirus (see p. 311), produce only one or two replication-related gene products, which function to divert host cell processes to those of viral replication. Other larger DNA viruses, such as poxvirus (see p. 334), provide virtually all enzymatic and regulatory molecules needed for a complete replication cycle. Figure 26.11 outlines the essential features of gene expression and replication of DNA viruses. [Note: The detailed mechanism of viral DNA replication varies considerably among the families, but the general principle of synthesis of progeny DNA strands complementary to parental DNA templates applies to all except the Hepadnaviridae (see p, 338).] The parental DNA of these viruses is transcribed into an RNA intermediate, which is then "reverse transcribed" into double-stranded DNA progeny.

1. **Early genes:** The viral genes that are transcribed before DNA replication begins are referred to as **early genes**, the products of their transcription as **early mRNA**, and the resulting proteins as **early proteins**. The functions of the early proteins are primarily related to genome replication; they are not usually found as part of the physical virion structure.

2. **Late genes:** Genes that begin to be transcribed after initiation of viral genome replication are referred to as **late genes**, their transcription products as **late mRNA**, and the resulting proteins as **late proteins**. Transcription of the late genes usually occurs on the newly replicated viral DNA genomes. Most of the late proteins are incorporated into the progeny virus particles. [Note: Late proteins required for assembling the capsid, but that are not found in the virion, are produced by some of the more complex viruses.]

E. Mechanisms of RNA virus genome replication

Viruses with RNA genomes must overcome two specific problems that arise from the need to replicate the viral genome, and to produce a number of viral proteins in eukaryotic host cells. First, there is no host cell RNA polymerase that can use the viral parental RNA as a template for synthesis of complementary RNA strands. Second, translation of eukaryotic mRNAns begins at only a single initiation site, and they are therefore translated into only a single polypeptide. However, RNA viruses, which frequently contain only a single molecule of RNA, must express the genetic information for at least two proteins: an RNA-dependent RNA polymerase, and a minimum of one type of capsid protein. Although the replication of each RNA virus family has unique features, the mechanisms evolved to surmount these restrictions can be grouped into four broad patterns (or "types") of replication.

1. **Type I: Viruses with an ssRNA genome of (+) polarity that replicates via a complementary (–) strand intermediate:** In Type I viral replication, the infecting parental RNA molecule serves both as mRNA, and later as a template for synthesis of the complementary (–) strand (Figure 26.12).

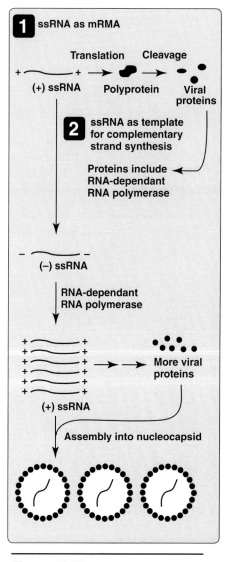

Figure 26.12
Type I virus with a ssRNA genome of (+) polarity replicates via a complementary (–) strand intermediate.

a. **Role of (+) ssRNA as mRNA:** Because the parental RNA genome is of (+), or messenger, polarity, it can be translated directly upon uncoating and associating with cellular ribosomes. The product is usually a single polyprotein from which individual polypeptides, such as the RNA-dependent RNA polymerase and the various proteins of the virion, are cleaved by a series of proteolytic processing events carried out by a protease domain of the polyprotein itself (see Figure 26.12).

b. **Role of (+) ssRNA as the template for complementary (–) strand synthesis:** The viral (+) ssRNA functions early in infection not only as mRNA for translation of polyproteins, but it also serves as a template for virus-encoded RNA-dependent RNA polymerase to synthesize complementary (–) ssRNA (see Figure 26.12). The progeny (–) strands, in turn, serve as templates for synthesis of progeny (+) strands, which can serve as additional mRNAs, thus amplifying the capacity to produce virion proteins for progeny virus. When a sufficient quantity of capsid proteins has accumulated later in the infection, progeny (+) ssRNAs begin to be assembled into newly formed nucleocapsids.

2. **Type II: Viruses with a ssRNA genome of (–) polarity that replicate via a complementary (+) strand intermediate:** Viral genomes with (–) polarity, like the (+) strand genomes, also have two functions: first, to provide information for protein synthesis, and second, to serve as templates for replication. Unlike (+) strand genomes, however, the (–) strand genomes cannot accomplish these goals without prior construction of a complementary (+) strand intermediate (Figure 26.13).

a. **Mechanism of replication of viral ssRNA with (–) polarity:** The replication problems for these viruses are two-fold. First, the (–) strand genome cannot be translated, and therefore the required viral RNA polymerase cannot be synthesized immediately following infection. Second, the host cell has no enzyme capable of transcribing the (–) strand RNA genome into (+) strand RNAs capable of being translated. The solution to these problems is for the infecting virus particle itself to contain viral **RNA-dependent RNA polymerase**, and to bring this enzyme into the host cell along with the viral genome. As a consequence, the first synthetic event after infection is transcription of (+) strand mRNAs from the parental viral (–) strand RNA template.

b. **Mechanisms for multiple viral protein synthesis in Type II viruses:** The synthesis of multiple proteins is achieved in one of two ways among the (–) strand virus families: 1) the viral genome may be a **polycistronic** molecule, from which transcription produces a number of mRNAs, each specifying a single polypeptide; 2) alternatively, the (–) strand viral genome may be **segmented** (that is, composed of a number of different RNA molecules, most of which code for a single polypeptide).

c. **Production of infectious virus particles:** Although the details differ, the flow of information in both segmented and unsegmented genome viruses is basically the same. In the Type II replication

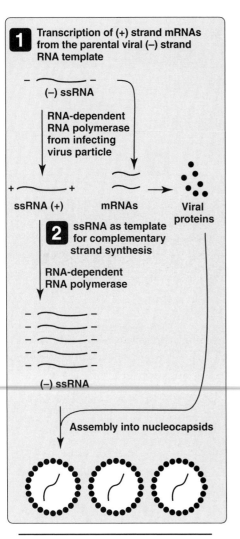

Figure 26.13
Type II virus with an ssRNA genome of (–) polarity that replicates via a complementary (+) strand intermediate.

scheme, an important control element is the shift from synthesis of (+) strand mRNAs to production of progeny (−) strand RNA molecules that can be packaged in the virions. This shift is not due to a different polymerase, but rather to the sequestering of (+) strand RNA molecules by interaction with one or more of the newly synthesized proteins. This makes the (+) strands available as templates for the synthesis of genomic (−) strands. Further, segmented genome viruses have the additional problem of assuring that all segments are incorporated into the progeny virions. The mechanism by which this occurs is not clear, and, in fact, is not perfect, because a rather high proportion of progeny viral particles with segmented genomes are often noninfectious due to the absence of one or more segments.

3. **Type III: Viruses with a dsRNA genome.** The dsRNA genome is segmented, with each segment coding for one polypeptide (Figure 26.14). However, eukaryotic cells do not have an enzyme capable of transcribing dsRNA. Type 3 viral mRNA transcripts are therefore produced by a virus-coded, RNA-dependent RNA polymerase (transcriptase) located in a **subviral core particle**. This particle consists of the dsRNA genome and associated virion proteins, including the transcriptase. The mechanism of replication of the dsRNA is unique, in that the (+) RNA transcripts are not only used for translation, but also as templates for complementary (−) strand synthesis, resulting in the formation of dsRNA progeny.

4. **Type IV: Viruses with a genome of ssRNA of (+) polarity that is replicated via a DNA intermediate.** The conversion of a (+) strand RNA to a double-stranded DNA is accomplished by an **RNA-dependent DNA polymerase**, commonly referred to as a "**reverse transcriptase**," that is contained in the virion. The resulting dsDNA becomes integrated into the cell genome by the action of a viral "**integrase**." Viral mRNAs and progeny (+) strand RNA genomes

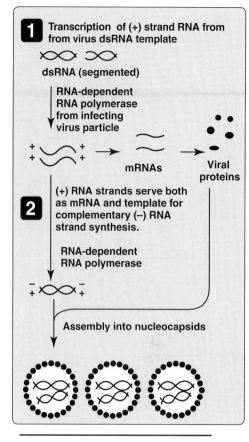

Figure 26.14
Type III virus with a dsRNA genome.

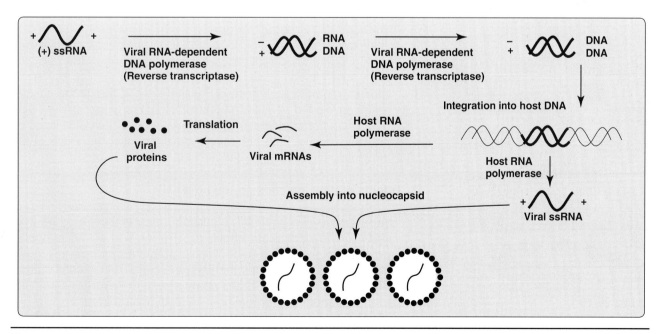

Figure 26.15
Type IV virus with a ssRNA genome of (+) polarity that replicates via a DNA intermediate.

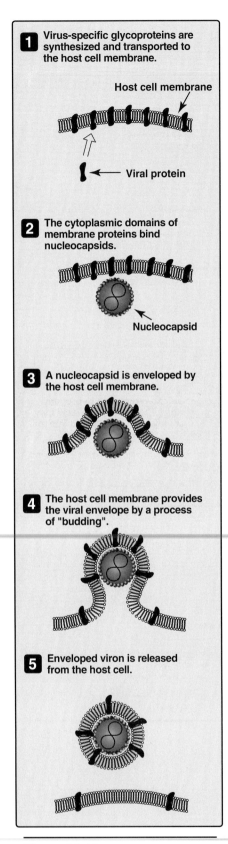

Figure 26.16
Release of enveloped virus from a
host cell by the process of "budding".

are transcribed from this integrated DNA by the host cell RNA polymerase (Figure 26.15). [Note: Only one family, the Retroviridae (see p. 361), is of this type. However, replication of the Hepadnaviruses (see p. 338), which have a DNA genome, also require an RNA to DNA step carried out by a "reverse transcriptase" that has homology to the retrovirus enzyme (see p. 362).]

F. Assembly and release of progeny viruses

Assembly of nucleocapsids generally takes place in the host cell compartment where the viral nucleic acid replication occurs, that is, in the cytoplasm for most RNA viruses, and in the nucleus for most DNA viruses. For DNA viruses, this requires that capsid proteins be transported from their site of synthesis, the cytoplasm, to the nucleus. The various capsid components accumulate in pools throughout the period of synthesis, and, when concentrations reach sufficient levels, begin to self-assemble. Capsid assembly is often a stepwise process, from protomers to capsomers to partial capsids; eventually association with the nucleic acid occurs, and the nucleocapsid is completed.

1. **Naked viruses:** In the case of a naked virus, the virion is complete at this point. Release of progeny is usually a passive event resulting from the disintegration of the dying cell, and therefore may be at a relatively late time after infection.

2. **Enveloped viruses:** In the case of enveloped viruses, virus-specific glycoproteins are synthesized and transported to the host cell membrane in the same manner as are cellular membrane proteins. When inserted into the membrane they displace the cellular glycoproteins, resulting in patches on the cell surface that have viral antigenic specificity. The cytoplasmic domains of these proteins associate specifically with one or more additional viral proteins (matrix proteins) to which the nucleocapsids bind. Final maturation then involves envelopment of the nucleocapsid by a process of "**budding**" (Figure 26.16). A consequence of this mechanism of viral replication is that progeny virus are released continuously while replication is proceeding within the cell, and ends when the cell loses its ability to maintain the integrity of the plasma membrane. A second consequence is that in the case of most enveloped viruses, all infectious progeny are extracellular. The exceptions are those viruses that acquire their envelopes by budding through internal cell membranes, such as those of the endoplasmic reticulum or the nucleus.

G. Effects of viral infection on the host cell

The response of a host cell to infection by a virus can range from 1) little or no detectable effect, to 2) alteration of the antigenic specificity of the cell surface due to presence of virus glycoproteins, to 3) latent infections that in some cases cause cell transformation, or ultimately, to 4) cell death due to the expression of viral genes that shut off essential host cell functions (Figure 26.17).

1. **Viral infections in which no progeny virus are produced:** In this case, the infection is referred to as **abortive**. An abortive response to infection is commonly due to: 1) a normal virus infecting cells that are lacking in enzymes, promoters, transcription factors, or other compounds required for complete viral replication, in which case the cells are referred to as **nonpermissive**; 2) infection by a defective virus of a cell that normally supports viral replication (that is, by a virus that itself has genetically lost the ability to replicate in that cell type); or 3) death of the cell as a consequence of the infection, before viral replication has been completed.

2. **Viral infections where the host cell may be altered antigenically but is not killed, although progeny virus are released:** In this case, the host cell is **permissive**, and the infection is **productive** (progeny virus are released from the cell), but viral replication and release does not kill the host cell, nor interfere with its ability to multiply and carry out differentiated functions. The infection is therefore said to be **persistent**. The antigenic specificity of the cell surface may be altered due to the insertion of viral glycoproteins. This type of response may be a characteristic of the virus itself; for example, it is seen for many retroviruses (see p. 364). In contrast, it may be characteristic of only certain virus/cell combinations but not others. For example, togaviruses reproduce in but do not kill arthropod cells, but togavirus infections do kill vertebrate cells (see p. 353).

3. **Viral infections that result in a latent viral state in the host cell:** Some viral infections result in the persistence of the viral genome inside a host cell with no production of progeny virus. Such **latent** viruses (for example, herpesvirus, see p. 322) can be **reactivated** months or years in the future, leading to a productive infection. [Note: In many cases, at the level of the whole organism, whether long-term presence of virus is due to reactivation of latent infection or is maintained as a persistent infection has not been determined.] Some latently infected cells contain viral genomes that are stably integrated into a host cell chromosome. This can cause alterations in the host cell surface, in cellular metabolic functions, and significantly, in cell growth and replication patterns. Such viruses may induce tumors in animals, in which case, they are said to be **tumor viruses**, and the cells they infect are **transformed**.

4. **Viral infections resulting in host cell death and production of progeny virus:** Eliminating host cell competition for synthetic enzymes and precursor molecules increases the efficiency with which virus constituents can be synthesized. Therefore, the typical result of a productive (progeny-yielding) infection by a **cytocidal virus** is the shut-off of much of the cell's macromolecular syntheses by one or more of the virus gene products, thereby causing the death of the cell. Such an infection is said to be **lytic**. The mechanism of the shut-off varies among the viral families.

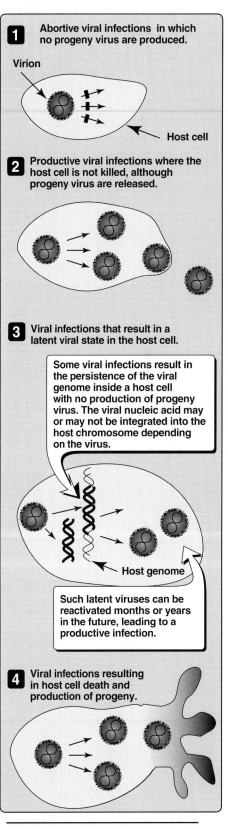

Figure 26.17
Effects of viral infection on a host cell.

Study Questions

Choose the ONE correct answer

26.1 The capsid of a virus with helical symmetry is composed of:

A. multiple identical copies of a single polypeptide molecule.

B. several polypeptides produced by sequential processing of a single large protein molecule.

C. several different polypeptides encoded by different open reading frames in the viral genome.

D. several different polypeptides generated by differential splicing of the same RNA transcript.

E. each of the above occurs, and is a characteristic of the specific virus family.

Correct answer = A. B, C, and D each do occur in families with icosahedral symmetry, but helical capsids are composed of only one species of polypeptide, encoded by a single gene. In contrast, none of those with icosahedral symmetry have only a single polypeptide species.

26.2 The term "eclipse period" refers to:

A. the period between epidemic outbreaks of diseases that occur in a cyclic pattern.

B. the period between recurrences of disease in individuals with latent virus infections.

C. the time between exposure of an individual to a virus and the first appearance of disease.

D. the time between infection of a susceptible cell by a cytocidal virus and the first appearance of cytopathic effects (CPE).

E. the time between entry into the cell and disassembly of the parental virus, and the appearance of the first progeny virion.

Correct answer = E. C: This time is referred to as the incubation period. There is no specific term applied to the time periods described by A, B, and D.

26.3 The early genes of DNA viruses code primarily for proteins whose functions are required for:

A. transcription of viral mRNA.

B. translation of the capsid proteins.

C. replication of the viral DNA.

D. final uncoating of the infecting virions.

E. processing of the mRNA precursors.

Correct answer = C. Depending on the virus family, this may consist of a DNA polymerase and other enzymes directly involved in DNA replication, or, alternatively, may be a product that stimulates the cell to produce all of the enzymes and precursors needed for DNA synthesis. A: Transcription for the most part is carried out by cellular RNA polymerase. B: Similarly, translation is done with the cell's translation system. D: The poxviruses do code for proteins that are involved in completion of uncoating, but this is an exception. E: mRNA processing is accomplished by cell enzymes.

26.4 An abortive infection is one in which:

A. the infected cells are not killed.

B. progeny virus is not produced.

C. transplacental infection of the fetus occurs.

D. episodes of virus multiplication alternate with periods when no infectious virus is present and no multiplication occurs.

E. cell multiplication is stopped.

Correct answer = B. A and E: Whether the infected cells are killed or multiplication is inhibited depends on the specific virus/cell combination in either productive or abortive infections. D: This is the definition of a latent infection.

Non-enveloped DNA Viruses

27

I. OVERVIEW

The DNA viruses discussed in this chapter—the Papovaviridae, the Adenoviridae, and the Parvoviridae (Figure 27.1)—share the properties of lacking an envelope, and having relatively simple structures and genome organization. However, the diseases commonly associated with these viruses, and their mechanisms of pathogenesis, are quite different, ranging from upper respiratory infections to tumors.

II. INTRODUCTION TO THE PAPOVAVIRIDAE

The papovaviruses are nonenveloped (naked), have icosahedral nucleocapsids, and contain supercoiled, double-stranded, circular DNA. However, basic differences in genome complexity and regulation of gene expression led to division of this family into two subfamilies: the Papillomavirinae and the Polyomavirinae. [Note: The name "papovavirus" was coined from the names of the three viruses originally included in this group, namely the papilloma, polyoma, and simian vacuolating viruses.] Papovaviruses induce both lytic infections, and either benign or malignant tumors, depending on the infected cell type.

III. PAPOVAVIRIDAE: SUBFAMILY PAPILLOMAVIRINAE

There are numerous papillomaviruses that infect animal species other than humans. All exhibit a high degree of species specificity, there being no known transmission between species, including to humans. All papillomaviruses induce **hyperplastic epithelial lesions** in their host species. Over seventy types (species) of human papillomaviruses (HPVs) are now recognized, based on differences in their DNA base sequences in certain well-characterized virus genes. The HPVs exhibit great tissue and cell specificity, infecting only surface epithelia of skin and mucous membranes. They can therefore also be grouped informally on the basis of their preferential infection of cutaneous (keratinizing) or mucosal epithelium. The HPVs within each of these tissue-specific groups have varying potentials to cause malignancies. For example, there are: 1) a small number of virus types that produce lesions having a high risk of progression to malignancy, such as in the case of **cervical carcinoma**; 2) other virus types produce mucosal lesions that progress to malignancy with lower frequency, causing, for example, **anogenital**

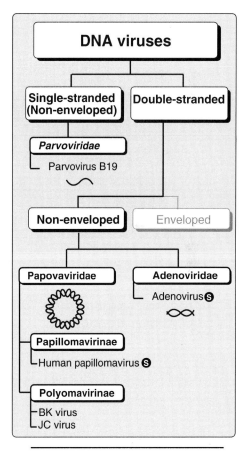

Figure 27.1
Classification of Non-enveloped DNA viruses. Ⓢ See p. 424, 433 for summaries of these viruses.

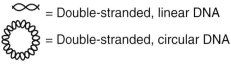

= Single-stranded, linear DNA

= Double-stranded, linear DNA

= Double-stranded, circular DNA

Lippincott's Illustrated Reviews: Microbiology,
by William A. Strohl, Harriet Rouse, Bruce D. Fisher.
Lippincott, Williams & Wilkins, Baltimore, MD © 2001

warts (**condyloma acuminata**, a common sexually transmitted disease) and **laryngeal papillomas** (the most common benign epithelial tumors of the larynx); and 3) still other virus types that are associated only with benign lesions, for example, **common**, **flat**, and **plantar warts**.

A. Epidemiology

Transmission of HPV infection requires direct contact with infected individuals (for example, sexual contact), or contaminated surfaces (such as communal bathroom floors). Because the initial phase, as well as the maintenance of infection, occur in cells of the basal layer of the skin, access to these cells is presumably via epithelial surface lesions such as abrasions.

B. Pathogenesis

The most striking characteristics of HPV multiplication and pathogenesis are its specificity for epithelial cells, and its dependence on the differentiation state of the epithelial host cell.

1. **Wart formation:** The development of a typical wart results from cell multiplication and delayed differentiation induced by certain of the papillomavirus early proteins. For example, in cutaneous tissues, infected cells leave the basal layer and migrate toward the surface of the skin. The virus replication cycle proceeds in parallel with the steps of keratinocyte differentiation, which end with the terminally differentiated cornified layer of the growing wart. An important function of two early viral proteins is the activation of host cells, causing them to divide. This activation involves interaction between these viral proteins and cellular proteins ("antioncoproteins") that normally

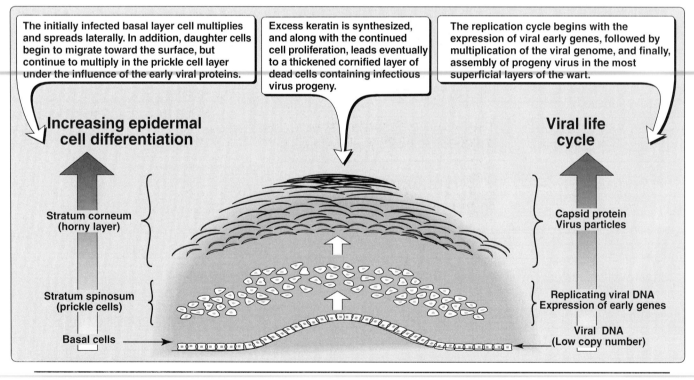

Figure 27.2
Relationship between steps in the development of a skin wart and the life cycle of papilloma virus.

function to regulate the cell cycle. Two of these antioncogenic cellular proteins are p53 (the cellular growth suppressor protein), and pRb (the retinoblastoma gene product). The viral genome is maintained in low copy numbers as a plasmid in the nuclei of multiplying basal cells. Another early gene regulates HPV replication so that a few copies of its genome are present in each daughter cell following cell division. Expression of only one early gene appears to be required for maintaining this balance between plasmid persistence and basal cell division. (See Figure 27.2 for a summary of papillomavirus replication and wart formation.)

2. **Development of malignancies:** Progression to malignancy occurs primarily in warts located on mucosal surfaces, particularly those of the genital tract, and is associated with a limited number of papillomavirus types. The affinity of binding between virus early proteins and the cellular anti-oncoproteins, p53 and pRb (which inactivates these cellular regulatory proteins), correlate with a high risk for malignant progression. However, it is clear that this interaction is only the first step in a multistep process involving alterations in expression of other cell onco- and anti-oncoproteins, and including at some point the non–site-specific integration of part of the viral genome into a host cell chromosome.

C. Clinical significance

HPVs cause diseases that cover the spectrum from simple warts to malignancies. Warts can occur on any part of the body, including both cutaneous and mucosal surfaces (Figure 27.3). Specific HPV types tend to be associated with specific wart morphology, although a wart's morphologic type is also related to its location (Figure 27.4).

1. **Cutaneous warts:** These warts may be classified as **common** (fingers and hands), **plantar** (sole of foot), or **flat** (arms, face, and knee). Another category of cutaneous lesion occurs in patients with what appears to be an inherited predisposition for multiple warts that do not regress, but instead spread to many body sites—a disease called **epidermodysplasia verruciformis**. Of particular interest is that these lesions give rise with high frequency to **squamous cell carcinomas** several years after initial appearance of the original warts, especially in areas of skin exposed to sunlight. The fact that the HPV types causing these lesions are not commonly found in warts of normal individuals suggests that the defect lies in a specific cell-mediated immune response that normally aids in resolving HPV infections.

2. **Mucosal infections:** HPV infections of the mucosal surfaces of greatest clinical importance are those of the genital tract. All of these are acquired primarily as sexually transmitted infections. Several types of HPV produce **anogenital warts** (**condyloma acuminata**), which are occasionally quite large but usually benign lesions that often regress spontaneously. Infections with other types of HPV do not lead to overt wart formation, but have a high risk of progressing to malignancy. In fact, HPV has been established as the primary cause of **cervical cancer** in the vast majority of cases (especially HPV types 16 and 18). Other mucosal sur-

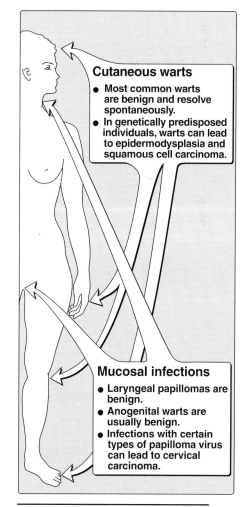

Cutaneous warts
- Most common warts are benign and resolve spontaneously.
- In genetically predisposed individuals, warts can lead to epidermodysplasia and squamous cell carcinoma.

Mucosal infections
- Laryngeal papillomas are benign.
- Anogenital warts are usually benign.
- Infections with certain types of papilloma virus can lead to cervical carcinoma.

Figure 27.3
Location and properties of papilloma infections.

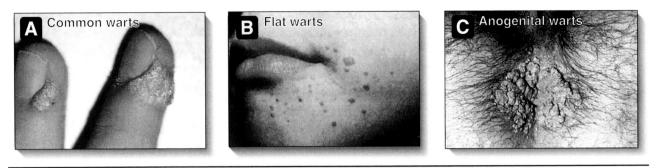

Figure 27.4
Some warts caused by papilloma virus.

faces are infected by some of these same HPV types, affecting such sites as the respiratory tract, the oral cavity, and the conjunctiva. Most of these infections result in benign papillomas.

D. Laboratory identification

Diagnosis of cutaneous warts generally involves no more than visual inspection. The major role of laboratory identification in papillomavirus infections is to determine, first, whether HPV is present in abnormal tissue recovered by biopsy or cervical swab, and second, whether the HPV type detected is one considered to present a high risk for progression to malignancy (the latter applying primarily to infections of the genital tract). Testing for HPV DNA as an alternative routine screening procedure is being evaluated. The lack of any tissue culture system for recovery of the virus, and the fact that HPV types are defined by molecular criteria, means that typing is done by DNA hybridization reactions using defined, type-specific nucleic acid probes (see 32).

E. Treatment and prevention

Treatment of warts generally involves the surgical removal or destruction of the wart tissue with liquid nitrogen, laser vaporization, or cytotoxic chemicals such as podophyllin or trichloroacetic acid (Figure 27.5). Such treatments remove the wart itself, but HPV often remains present in cells of the surrounding tissue, and recurrence rates of fifty percent have been reported. On the other hand, common warts regress spontaneously with high frequency, and removal is not usually warranted unless there is unusual pain due to the location, or for cosmetic reasons. Cidofovir, an inhibitor of DNA synthesis, appears to be effective when applied topically. Interferon, given orally, has been shown to be effective in causing regression of laryngeal papillomas, and when injected directly into genital warts, has given positive results in about half of the patients treated by this method. Because transmission of the infection is by direct inoculation, avoidance of the opportunity for contact with wart tissue is the primary means of prevention. In the case of genital tract warts, all of the procedures for prevention of sexually transmitted diseases are appropriate. Attempts to produce a vaccine against HPV are currently in progress.

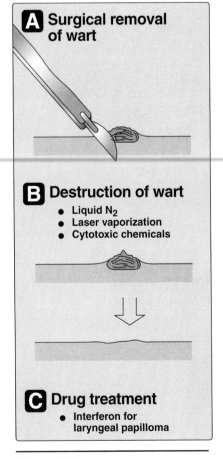

Figure 27.5
Treatment of papilloma.

IV. PAPOVAVIRIDAE: SUBFAMILY POLYOMAVIRINAE

All of the members of this virus subfamily have the capacity to transform normal cells in culture (see p. 305), and to induce tumors in species other than those in which they are normally found in nature. [Note: The name "polyoma" means many (poly-) tumor (-oma). However, polyomavirus has not yet been shown to cause tumors in humans.] The best studied viruses of this subfamily are of animal origin: the type species of this group, polyoma, which is an endemic virus of mice, and simian vacuolating virus 40 (SV40), a virus endemic in monkeys. There are also two human polyoma viruses, BK and JC viruses (BKV and JCV). JCV has been associated with the rare, fatal, demyelinating disease, progressive multifocal leukoencephalopathy (PML), which occurs only in patients with impaired immune function, for example those with AIDS. BKV can cause cystitis in this same population.

A. Epidemiology and pathogenesis

The human polyomaviruses, BKV and JCV, are transmitted by droplets from the upper respiratory tract of infected persons, and possibly through contact with their urine. Infection with these viruses usually occurs in childhood. Specific antibody to one or both human polyomaviruses is present in seventy to eighty percent of the adult population, and there is evidence that both BKV and JCV spread from the upper respiratory tract to the kidneys, where they may persist in an inactive state in the tubular epithelium of healthy individuals. The polyomaviruses follow the basic pattern of DNA virus genome replication and gene expression in the nucleus (see p. 300). The enzymes and precursors synthesized in preparation for cellular DNA synthesis are made available for synthesis of viral DNA. This productive cycle leads to viral multiplication, and ultimately to the death of the host cell.

B. Clinical significance

Immune compromise of various types can be associated with the development of **progressive multifocal leukoencephalopathy (PML)**, so called because the lesions are restricted to the white matter (Figure 27.6). PML is thought to be due to reactivated JCV that has entered the CNS via the blood, and occurs as a complication of a number of lymphoproliferative disorders and chronic diseases that affect immune competence. [Note: In recent years, PML has been seen especially in patients with AIDS.] In PML, JCV carries out a cytocidal infection of the brain, specifically of oligodendrocytes, thus leading to demyelination due to the loss of capacity of myelinated cells to maintain their myelin sheaths. Early development of impaired speech and mental capacity is rather rapidly followed by paralysis and sensory abnormalities, with death commonly occurring within three to six months of the initial symptoms. [Note: BKV is also found in the urine (Figure 27.7), but rarely has pathologic consequences except in immunocompromised patients, who may develop hemorrhagic cystitis.]

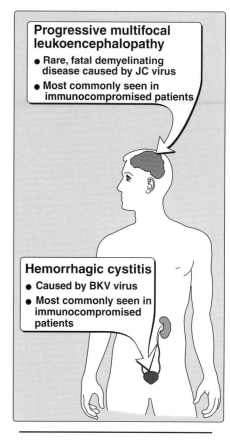

Figure 27.6
Location and properties of polyomavirus infections.

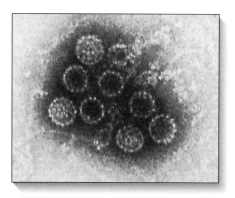

Figure 27.7
Electron micrograph of BK virons from urine of infected patient.

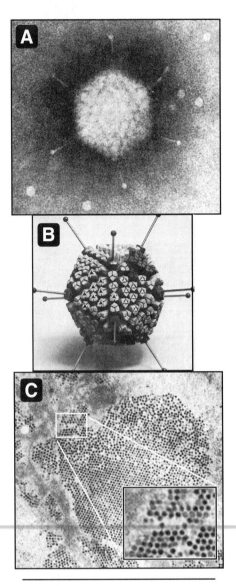

Figure 27.8
A. Electron micrograph of adenovirus virion with fibers. B. Model of adenovirus. C. Crystalline aggregate of adenovirus in nucleus of cell.

C. Laboratory identification

Because most people have antibodies to these viruses, serologic techniques are not generally useful in the diagnosis of acute infections. Identification by DNA hybridization of BKV in the urine or JCV in PML lesions in brain tissue are the most sensitive and specific techniques for diagnosis of these infections.

D. Treatment and prevention

No successful, specific, antiviral therapy is available. Because the infection with JCV and BKV is nearly universal and asymptomatic, and PML represents reactivation of "latent" virus, there are no viable preventive measures at present.

V. ADENOVIRIDAE

The adenoviruses are nonenveloped, icosahedral viruses containing double-stranded linear DNA (Figure 27.8). They commonly cause diseases such as respiratory tract infections, gastroenteritis, and conjunctivitis. Adenoviruses were first discovered during screenings of throat washings and cultures of adenoids and tonsils, performed in the search for the common cold virus. They are now recognized as a large group of related viruses commonly infecting humans, other mammals, and also birds. Over forty serotypes (species) of human adenoviruses are known, and antibody surveys have shown that most individuals have been infected by several different types of adenoviruses by adulthood. [Note: Although some human serotypes are highly oncogenic in experimental animals, none have been associated with human malignancies.]

A. Epidemiology and pathogenesis

The site of the clinical syndrome caused by an adenovirus infection is generally related to the mode of virus transmission. For example, most of the adenoviruses are primarily agents of respiratory disease, and are transmitted via the respiratory route. However, most of the adenoviruses also replicate efficiently and asymptomatically in the intestine, and can be isolated from the stool well after respiratory disease symptoms have ended, as well as from the stools of healthy persons. Two adenovirus serotypes associated specifically with gastrointestinal disease are presumably transmitted by the fecal-oral route. Similarly, ocular infections are transmitted by direct inoculation of the eye by virus-contaminated hands, ophthalmologic instruments, or bodies of water in which groups of children swim together.

B. Structure and replication

The capsid of adenoviruses is composed of hexon capsomers making up the triangular faces of the icosahedron, with a penton capsomer at each of the vertices (Figure 27.8). Unlike other naked viruses, the pentons of adenoviruses are composed of a penton base structure from which projects a glycoprotein fiber. Replication of adenoviruses essentially follows the general model for DNA viruses (see p. 300). Attachment to a host cell receptor occurs via knobs on the tips of the viral fibers, following which, entry into the cell occurs by receptor-mediated endocytosis. The viral genome is then progressively uncoated while it is transported to the nucleus, where all transcription of viral genes, genome replication, and assembly occurs.

Two early viral genes have the same function as the early proteins of the papovaviruses [that is, inactivating cellular regulatory proteins (including p53 and pRb) that normally prevent progression through the cell cycle (see p. 309)]. However, the considerably larger adenovirus genome encodes a number of additional early proteins, including a DNA polymerase, and others that affect transcription and replication of the viral genome. The productive cycle kills the host cell, as cellular DNA, RNA, and protein synthesis are all shut off during the course of the infection. Release of infectious virus from the cell occurs by the slow disintegration of the dying cell.

C. Clinical significance

The adenoviruses all replicate well in epithelial cells. The observed disease symptoms are related primarily to the killing of these cells; systemic infections are rare. Most adenovirus infections are asymptomatic, but certain types are more commonly associated with disease than others. These diseases can be conveniently grouped into those affecting 1) the respiratory tract, 2) the eye, and 3) the GI tract (Figure 27.9).

1. **Respiratory tract diseases:** The most common manifestation of adenovirus infection of infants and young children is **acute febrile pharyngitis**, characterized by a cough, sore throat, nasal congestion, and fever. Isolated cases may be indistinguishable from other common viral respiratory infections. Some adenovirus types tend in addition to produce a conjunctivitis, in which case the syndrome is referred to as **pharyngoconjunctival fever**. This entity is more prevalent in school-age children, and occurs both sporadically, and in outbreaks, often within family groups or in groups using the same swimming facility ("swimming pool conjunctivitis"). The syndrome referred to as **acute respiratory disease** occurs primarily in epidemics among new military recruits. It is thought to reflect the lowered resistance brought on by exposure to new strains, fatigue, and crowded conditions, promoting efficient spread of the infection. Lastly, the respiratory syndromes described above may progress to true **viral pneumonia**, which in infants has a mortality rate of about ten percent.

2. **Ocular diseases:** In addition to the conjunctivitis that sometimes accompanies the upper respiratory syndrome described above, a similar **follicular conjunctivitis** may occur as a separate disease. It is self-limiting, and has no permanent sequelae. A more serious infection is **epidemic keratoconjunctivitis** in which the corneal epithelium is also involved, and which may be followed by corneal opacity lasting several years. The epidemic nature of this disease arises in part from transmission via shared towels or ophthalmic solutions, person-to-person contact, or by improperly sterilized ophthalmologic instruments.

3. **Gastrointestinal diseases:** Most of the human adenoviruses multiply in the GI tract, and can be found in stools. However, these are generally asymptomatic infections. Two serotypes have been associated specifically with **infantile gastroenteritis**, and have been estimated to account for five to fifteen percent of all viral diarrheal disease in children.

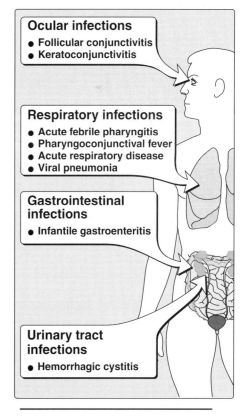

Figure 27.9
Adenovirus infections.

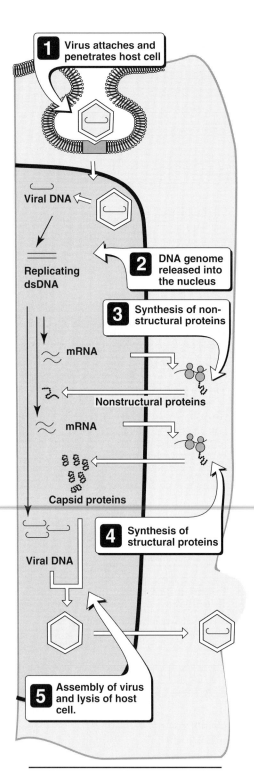

Figure 27.10
Replication of B19 parvovirus.

4. Less common diseases: Several adenovirus serotypes have been associated with an acute, self-limited, **hemorrhagic cystitis**, which occurs primarily in boys. It is characterized by hematuria, and virus can usually be recovered from the urine. Similarly, adenovirus infection of heart muscle has recently been shown to be one of the causes of left ventricular dysfunction in both children and adults. In immunocompromised patients, such as those with AIDS, the common respiratory adenovirus infections have a greater risk of proceeding to serious, often fatal, pneumonia. Other disseminated infections leading to a fatal outcome have been reported in patients with a compromised immune system, or who are immunosuppressed due to drug therapy.

D. Laboratory identification

Isolation of virus for identification is not done on a routine basis, but may be desirable in cases of epidemic disease or a nosocomial outbreak, especially in the nursery. Identification of the adenovirus serotype can be done by neutralization or hemagglutination inhibition using type-specific antisera. The enteric adenoviruses grow in only certain special human cell lines, and then, with difficulty. They are more commonly detected by direct test of stool specimens by ELISA (see p. 30).

E. Treatment and prevention

No antiviral agents are currently available for treating adenovirus infections. Prevention of epidemic respiratory disease by immunization has been used only for protection of the military population. A live, attenuated adenovirus vaccine is used for this purpose, and produces a good neutralizing antibody response. The oncogenic capacity of the adenoviruses in experimental animals has inhibited the use of vaccines on a wider scale.

VI. PARVOVIRIDAE

The parvoviruses are the smallest of the DNA viruses. They are nonenveloped and icosahedral, with single-stranded, linear DNA. A human parvovirus, B19, has been isolated and identified as the cause of transient aplastic crisis in patients with sickle cell disease. This virus is also the cause of the common childhood disease, erythema infectiosum, and is associated with fetal death in pregnant women experiencing a primary infection. The parvovirus family is divided into two genera, based on whether their ability to replicate requires coinfection with a helper DNA virus, or if they are capable of independent replication ("autonomous parvoviruses"). Members of the first group are referred to as adeno-associated viruses (AAV), because they are usually found in infected cells in combination with a helper adenovirus. [Note: In the absence of helper virus, AAV integrates into a cell's chromosome. AAV is thus being developed as a possible vector for gene therapy.]

A. Epidemiology and pathogenesis

Transmission of parvoviruses appears to be by the respiratory route. A very high-titered viremia lasting a few days follows about one week after infection, during which time virus is also present in throat secretions. A specific antibody response occurs rapidly, resulting in suppression of the viremia. Replication of parvoviruses requires a host cell in which DNA synthesis is in progress. Therefore, damage is limited primarily to specific tissues that are mitotically active. [Note: In the case of B19 virus, these are primarily tissues of erythroid origin.] Because of the single-stranded nature of the genome, conversion to a double stranded DNA molecule by a cellular DNA polymerase must occur before production of additional single-stranded viral DNA genomes or viral mRNA transcription can begin. In spite of the limited amount of genetic material, two or three capsid proteins and two nonstructural regulatory proteins are produced by a combination of alternative RNA splicing patterns and posttranslational processing. The parvovirus life cycle is summarized in Figure 27.10.

B. Clinical significance

The single human pathogen in this family is the autonomous parvovirus, B19. The spectrum of illnesses caused by this virus is related to its unique tropism for cycling erythroid progenitor cells. Although the initial isolation of B19 was from sickle cell disease patients undergoing a transient aplastic crisis, it has since been recognized that a **chronic**, **progressive bone marrow suppression** results from B19 infection of immunocompromised patients who are unable to mount an immune response capable of eliminating the virus.

1. **Erythema infectiosum:** The observation that thirty to sixty percent of some human populations have antibodies to B19 led eventually to the identification of this virus as the causative agent of the common childhood rash, **erythema infectiosum** (**fifth disease**, Figure 27.11). The characteristic rash ("face slap" appearance) occurs about two weeks after initial exposure, when virus is no longer detectable. It is apparently immune system–mediated. In addition to a rash, a complication accompanying B19 infection is an acute arthritis that usually involves joints symmetrically. This is considerably more frequent in adults than in children, and usually resolves within several weeks.

2. **Birth defects:** Based on previous experience with animal parvovirus diseases, a human parvovirus that caused birth defects was long considered a possibility. Studies to evaluate the risk to the fetus are ongoing, but there is evidence that the **spontaneous abortion** rate is elevated in women having a primary infection during the first trimester, and that primary infection during the second or third trimester is associated with some instances of **hydrops fetalis**.

C. Laboratory identification

Laboratory identification of B19 infection is not routinely done. The large amount of virus present during the viremic (usually asymptomatic) phase permits detection of viral proteins by immunologic methods, or of viral DNA by various hybridization techniques. Retrospective diagnosis can be made by any of the usual procedures used to demonstrate a specific antibody response (see p. 29).

D. Treatment and prevention

No antiviral agent or vaccine is available for treating B19 infections. Isolation of patients with signs of parvovirus disease is not a useful approach to control, because subclinical infections occur, and infected individuals shed virus before symptoms appear.

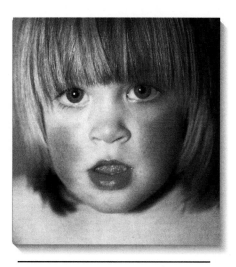

Figure 27.11
Typical "slapped cheek" appearance of a child infected with parvovirus B19 ("fifth disease").

Study Questions

Choose the ONE correct answer

27.1 An important step in the mechanism proposed for oncogenesis by human papillomaviruses is:

   A. inactivation of a cellular regulatory gene by HPV integration into the coding region of the gene.

   B. transactivation of a normally silent cellular oncogene by an HPV early protein.

   C. reversal of keratinocyte differentiation due to continued active replication and production of progeny HPV.

   D. specific binding of certain HPV early proteins to cellular anti-oncoproteins.

   E. induction of a specific chromosome translocation that results in activation of a cellular oncogene.

> Correct answer = D. The early proteins of both the adenoviruses and the papovaviruses required for immortalization and transformation of normal cells have been shown to bind specifically to the cellular proteins p53 and Rb, which are important in maintaining regulation of the mitotic cycle. Interaction with the viral proteins is believed to result in loss of their normal functions, as do the mutations that are commonly associated with spontaneously occurring cancers. A, B: Neither gene inactivation by integration nor transcriptional activation by an early protein has been observed. C: Virus replication occurs only in differentiated keratinocytes, but dedifferentiation does not occur. E: Multiple chromosome rearrangements are observed late in progression to malignancy, but none are specific for HPV-transformed cells.

27.2 The characteristic spectrum of diseases caused by the autonomous parvoviruses is related to the fact that they:

   A. integrate into a specific chromosomal site that disrupts an essential gene and leads to death of the cell.

   B. require host cells that are actively progressing through the mitotic cycle.

   C. infect only terminally differentiated cells.

   D. code for an early protein that shuts off cellular protein synthesis.

   E. increase the severity of the disease normally caused by their associated helper virus.

> Correct answer = B. The diseases caused by the autonomous parvoviruses all result from the effects of killing multiplying cells that are essential for normal functions, for example, B19 specifically infects erythroblasts, leading to anemia in the fetus or in immunodeficient patients. A,B,C: Parvoviruses are not observed to integrate during the replicative cycle, they cannot replicate in terminally differentiated cells, and they do not shut off cell syntheses. E: By definition, the autonomous parvoviruses do not require a helper virus for replication.

27.3 Which one of the following clinical entities is NOT associated with adenovirus infections?

   A. Epidemic keratoconjunctivitis

   B. Pharyngoconjunctival fever

   C. Infantile gastroenteritis

   D. Fetal death and birth defects

   E. Acute respiratory disease

> Correct answer = D. Transplacental transmission has not been observed. The most common sites of infection leading to illness are the respiratory tract, GI tract, eye, and urinary bladder.

27.4 The characteristic rash of erythema infectiosum is due to:

   A. virion/antibody immune complex formation.

   B. bone marrow suppression due to killing of erythrocyte precursors by B19 infection.

   C. damage to the liver.

   D. B19 infection of epithelial cells.

   E. the inflammatory response to B19 infection of capillary endothelium.

> Correct answer = A. The appearance of the rash coincides with production of antibodies to B19, which occurs several days after the peak of viremia. B: In immunodeficient individuals infection can lead to a chronic, progressive depletion of erythrocyte precursors and severe anemia, but not rash. C: The host range of B19 is restricted to erythroid precursors, including those found in the fetal liver. Whereas this may be a factor in causing hydrops fetalis due to B19 infection of a pregnant woman, it is not related to the rash. D and E: Again, B19 is not known to infect other than erythroid precursor cells.

Enveloped DNA Viruses

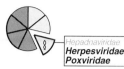

28

I. OVERVIEW

Two of the three enveloped DNA virus families—the Herpesviridae and the Poxviridae—are discussed in this chapter. [Note: Hepadnaviridae, the third enveloped DNA virus family, is discussed in Chapter 29.] The Herpesviridae and the Poxviridae are both structurally and genetically more complex than the DNA viruses discussed in Chapter 27. For example, there is less dependence on host cell-supplied functions, with a correspondingly greater number of virus-coded functions involved in viral replication. This latter fact is partly responsible for the greater success in developing antiviral drugs against these viruses, because there are more virus-specific enzymes that can serve as targets for inhibitors (in contrast to viruses that are more host cell function-dependent). Replication of herpes- and poxviruses is also independent of the host cell cycle. The herpesvirus family includes a number of very important human pathogens (Figure 28.1). The one highly virulent member of the poxvirus family, variola (the cause of smallpox), is the only human pathogen that has been successfully eradicated. This success serves as a model for attempts to control and potentially eradicate other infectious diseases.

II. HERPESVIRIDAE: STRUCTURE AND REPLICATION

Eight human herpesvirus species are known. All have the ability to enter a **latent state** following primary infection of their natural host, and to be reactivated at a later time. However, the exact molecular nature of the latency, and the frequency and manifestation of reactivation, vary with the species of herpesvirus.

A. Structure of herpesviruses

Herpesvirus virions consist of an **icosahedral capsid** enclosed in a lipoprotein **envelope** (Figure 28.2). [Note: Neutralizing antibody reacts with species-specific glycoprotein components of the envelope.] Between the envelope and the capsid lies an amorphous proteinaceous material, the **tegument**, which contains virus-coded enzymes and transcription factors that are essential for initiation of the infectious cycle, although none of these is a polymerase. The **genome** is a single molecule of **linear, double-stranded DNA**, encoding from 70 to 200 proteins, depending on the species. Although all members of the family have some genes with homolo-

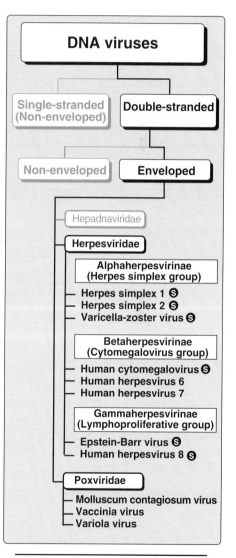

Figure 28.1
Classification of enveloped DNA viruses. [Note: Hepadnaviridae are discussed in Chapter 29.]
Ⓢ See p. 401 for summaries of these viruses.

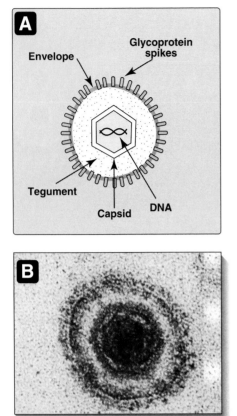

Figure 28.2
Structure of herpesvirus.
A. Schematic drawing.
B. Transmission electron micrograph.

gous functions, there is very little nucleotide sequence homology, and very little antigenic relatedness between species.

B. Classification of herpesviruses

The herpesviridae cannot readily be differentiated by their morphology in the electron microscope—they all have similar appearances. However, the Herpesviridae have been divided into three subfamilies, based primarily on their biologic characteristics (see Figure 28.1).

1. **Alphaherpesvirinae (herpes simplex virus group):** These viruses have a relatively rapid, cytocidal growth cycle, and establish latency in nerve ganglia. Herpes simplex virus types 1 and 2 (HSV-1 and HSV-2), and varicella-zoster virus (VZV) belong to this group. HSV-1 and HSV-2 share a significant amount of nucleotide homology, and therefore share many common features in replication and pathogenesis. VZV has a smaller genome than HSV, but the two viruses have many genes that are homologous.

2. **Betaherpesvirinae (cytomegalovirus group):** These viruses have a relatively slow replication cycle that results in the formation of characteristic, multinucleated, giant host cells, hence the name "cytomegalo-". Latency is established in nonneural tissues, primarily lymphoreticular cells and glandular tissues. Human cytomegalovirus (HCMV) and human herpesviruses types 6 and 7 (HHV-6 and HHV-7) are in this group.

3. **Gammaherpesvirinae (lymphoproliferative group):** These viruses replicate in mucosal epithelium, where they also establish latent infections. They induce cell proliferation in lymphoblastoid cells. Epstein-Barr virus (EBV) was previously the only well-characterized human gammaherpesvirus. However, genome analysis of a virus recovered from cells of Kaposi's sarcoma recently revealed it to also be a human member of the gammaherpesvirinae. It has been designated human herpesvirus type 8 (HHV-8).

C. Replication of the Herpesviruses

Herpesviruses replicate in the nucleus, following the basic pattern of DNA virus replication (see p. 300). Regulation of herpesvirus transcription is referred to as "cascade control," in that expression of a first set of genes is required for expression of a second set, which in turn is required for expression of the third set of genes. [Note: A similar pattern is found in some other DNA virus families where the genes are referred to as **immediate early**, **delayed early**, and **late genes**.] The general features of herpesvirus replication are summarized in Figure 28.3.

1. **Virus adsorption and penetration:** Herpesviruses adsorb to host cell receptors that can differ according to the virus species and the tissue type being infected. The viral envelope glycoproteins promote fusion of the envelope with the cell's plasma membrane, depositing the nucleocapsid and tegument proteins in the cytosol. One of the tegument proteins induces a cell RNase that degrades cellular mRNA, effectively shutting off host cell protein synthesis.

2. **Viral DNA replication and nucleocapsid assembly:** The nucleo-capsid is transported to a nuclear pore, through which the viral DNA is released into the nucleus. Another of the tegument pro-teins is a transactivator of cellular RNA polymerase, and causes that enzyme to initiate transcription of the set of viral **immediate early genes**, which code for a variety of regulatory functions, including initiation of further gene transcription. Next, the **delayed early genes** are expressed. They code primarily for enzymes that are required for replication of viral DNA, such as viral DNA poly-merase, helicase, and thymidine kinase. [Note: Because these enzymes are virus-specific, they provide excellent targets for anti-herpes agents, such as acyclovir, that are relatively nontoxic for the cell (see p. 333).] As is the case with other DNA viruses, the **late genes** code for the structural proteins of the virion, and for pro-teins involved in the assembly and maturation of the viral progeny. Although the genome of the virion is a linear molecule, it replicates after circularization, and unit length genomes are inserted into pre-formed empty capsids in the nucleus (see Figure 28.3).

3. **Acquisition of the viral envelope:** Unlike most other enveloped viruses, newly synthesized envelope proteins accumulate in patches on the **nuclear membrane**, and nucleocapsids that have been assembled in the nucleus acquire their envelopes by bud-ding through these patches. The completed virus is transported by a vacuole to the surface of the cell. Additional copies of the envelope glycoproteins are also transported to the plasma mem-brane, which thus acquires herpesvirus antigenic determinants. These glycoproteins may also cause the fusion of neighboring cells, in some cases producing characteristic multinucleated giant cells. The end result of this productive cycle is death of the cell, because most cellular synthetic pathways are turned off.

4. **Latency:** All herpesviruses can undergo an alternative infection cycle, entering a quiescent state (latency) from which they subse-quently can be reactivated. The cell type in which this occurs is usually not the same cell type in which the productive, cytocidal infection occurs. Because the mechanism of latency, the cells in which it is established, the frequency of reactivation, and the nature of the recurrent disease are characteristic for each of the herpesviruses, the topic of latency is discussed in this chapter in the context of the individual virus species.

III. HERPES SIMPLEX VIRUS, TYPES 1 AND 2

Herpes simplex viruses, types 1 and 2 (HSV-1 and HSV-2) are the only human herpesviruses that have a significant degree of nucleotide homology (about fifty percent). They therefore share many common fea-tures in replication, disease production, and latency.

A. Epidemiology and pathogenesis

Transmission of both HSV types is by direct contact with virus-con-taining secretions, or with lesions on mucosal or cutaneous sur-

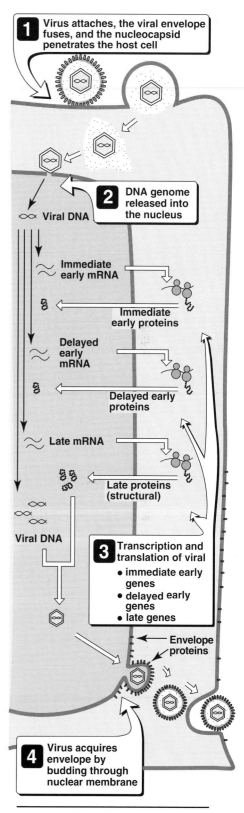

Figure 28.3
Replication of herpes viruses.

faces. Primary or recurrent infections in the oropharyngeal region, caused primarily by HSV-1, are accompanied by virus release into saliva; thus kissing or saliva-contaminated fingers are major modes of transmission. In genital tract infections, caused primarily by HSV-2, virus is present in the genital tract secretions. Consequently sexual intercourse and infections of newborns during passage through the birth canal are major modes of transmission. Both HSV-1 and HSV-2 multiply in the epithelial cells of the mucosal surface onto which they have been inoculated, resulting in production of vesicles or shallow ulcers containing infectious virus. In immunocompetent individuals, the epithelial infection remains localized due to cytotoxic T lymphocytes that recognize the HSV-specific antigens on the surface of infected cells, and kill these cells before progeny virus has been produced. A life-long latent infection is usually established in the regional ganglion as a result of entry of infectious virions into sensory neurons that terminate at the site of the infection.

B. Clinical significance

A useful generality is that HSV-1 is most commonly found in lesions of the upper body, and HSV-2 is the more common cause of genital tract lesions. Either can, however, infect and cause similar lesions at the opposite site.

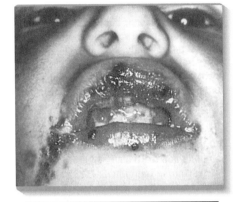

Figure 28.4
Herpes simplex gingivostomatitis.

1. **Primary infections of the upper body:** Many primary HSV infections are subclinical, but the most common symptomatic infections of the upper body are **gingivostomatitis** in young children (Figure 28.4), and **pharyngitis** or **tonsillitis** in adults. The lesions typically consist of vesicles and shallow ulcers, which are often accompanied by systemic symptoms such as fever, malaise, and myalgias. Another clinically important site of infection is the eye, in which **keratoconjunctivitis** can lead to corneal scarring and eventual blindness. [Note: HSV-1 infection of the eye is the second most common cause of corneal blindness in the United States (after trauma).] In Figure 28.6, HSV diseases of the eye are described along with other infectious eye diseases. If HSV infection spreads to the CNS it can cause **encephalitis**, which if untreated, has a mortality rate estimated to be seventy percent. Survivors are usually left with neurologic deficits. HSV infections of the CNS account for up to twenty percent of encephalitis viral infections in the United States.

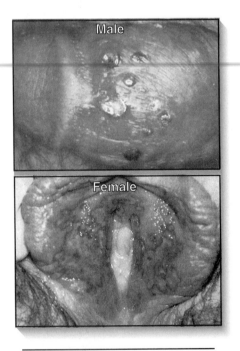

Figure 28.5
Genital herpes simplex infections.

2. **Primary infections of the genital tract:** Primary genital tract lesions are similar to those of the oropharynx, but based on the frequency of antibody in the population, the majority of these infections are asymptomatic. When symptomatic (**genital herpes**), local symptoms include painful vesiculoulcerative lesions on the female's vulva, cervix, and vagina, or the male's penis (Figure 28.5). Systemic symptoms of fever, malaise, and myalgias may also be more severe than those that accompany primary oral cavity infections. However, it should be noted that prior infection with one HSV type provides some degree of immunity to the second type, resulting in a milder symptomatic disease. In pregnant women with a primary genital HSV infection, the risk of infecting the newborn during birth is estimated to be thirty to forty percent (**neonatal herpes**). Because such infants have no protective

Disease Summary: Diseases of the Eye

Herpes Simplex Virus

● Herpes simplex virus types 1 and 2 are the most common causes of **infectious keratitis** (infection of the cornea leading to **corneal ulcers**) in developed countries. Symptoms include a red eye with moderately severe pain, tearing, decreased visual acuity, and photophobia. The infection usually involves only one eye. HSV keratitis may be **primary** (symptoms ranging from subclinical to conjunctivitis with vesicular eruption of the eyelid and potential corneal ulcers) or **recurrent** (more common than primary keratitis, especially in the immunocompromised, where symptoms generally include mild irritation and photophobia). [Note: The conjunctiva is a thin, translucent, mucus membrane that lines the eyelid and covers the white portion of the eyeball. Viral conjunctivitis is more common than bacterial conjunctivitis in developed countries.] Treatment involves application of topical antiherpes agents.

● Other herpesviruses also cause eye infections. For example, cytomegalovirus infection is particularly dangerous in AIDS patients, in whom it causes a variety of diseases (see Figure xxx, and p.xxx). One of these syndromes is **chorioretinitis**, which can cause blindness if untreated (for example, with ganciclovir or foscarnet). Varicella-zoster virus (VZV, see p.xxx) is also dangerous for AIDS patients, causing **acute retinal necrosis** that is treated with acyclovir. In non-AIDS patients, VZV reactivation can cause **herpes zoster**.

Adenovirus

● Adenovirus infection is a common cause of **acute conjunctivitis**, especially in children. This infection may occur while the child is experiencing acute febrile pharyngitis, in which case the syndrome is referred to as **pharyngoconjunctival fever**. Adenoviruses may be transmitted via the hands, contaminated eye drops, or insufficiently chlorinated swimming pools. Adenoviral conjunctivitis usually resolves after seven to ten days without therapy.

● A more serious infection is **epidemic keratoconjunctivitis**, which involves formation of a painful ulcer of the corneal epithelium. The ulcer may result in corneal opacity lasting several years. The epidemic nature of this disease arises in part from transmission by improperly sterilized ophthalmologic instruments. No antiviral agents are currently available for adenovirus infections. (See p. 312)

Staphylococcus aureus

● *S. aureus*, a member of the normal flora of the body (see p.xxx), is a major cause of infections of the eyelid and cornea. For example, *S. aureus* can infect the glands of the eyelid, resulting in the production of a **stye**—a painful red swelling on the margin of the eyelid. Treatment consists of warm compresses applied regularly, and topical antibiotic ointment (for example, bacitracin ointment).

Staphylococcus aureus (continued)

● *S. aureus* is an important cause of **chronic bacterial conjunctivitis** leading to **keratitis**. The organism invades the cornea following trauma that causes a break in the corneal epithelium. The resulting ulcers are very painful, and must be treated with antibiotic drops. (See p. 138)

Neisseria gonorrhoeae

● *N. gonorrhoeae* is the most common cause of **hyperacute bacterial conjunctivitis**—the most severe form of conjunctivitis. Untreated, it can lead to keratitis and corneal perforation. Ceftriaxone can be used to treat gonococcal conjunctivitis.

● The term **ophthalmia neonatorum** (ON) refers to any conjunctival inflammation of the newborn. It is acquired by the infant during its passage through the birth canal of a mother infected with gonococcus. [Note: Gonococci are the most serious infectious cause of ON, although chlamydia are the most common cause.] If untreated, acute conjunctivitis may lead to blindness. Treatment is with doxycycline or erythromycin—antibiotics that also eradicate *Chlamydia trachomatis*, if present. (See p. 165)

Chlamydia trachomatis

● *C. trachomatis*, serotypes A, B, Ba, and C cause a chronic keratoconjunctivitis (**trachoma**) that often results in blindness. Trachoma is a leading cause of blindness in endemic areas of northern India, the Middle East, and North Africa. Trachoma is transmitted by personal contact, for example, by eye to eye via droplets, by contaminated surfaces touched by hands and conveyed to the eye, or by flies. Because of persistent or repeated infection over several years, the inflammatory response with attendant scarring leads to permanent opacities of the cornea, and distortion of eyelids.

● Over 50 percent of infants born to women infected with *C. trachomatis* serotypes D–K will contract **ophthalmia neonatorum** (see *N. gonorrhoeae*, above) on passage through the birth canal. The most common presentation is **inclusion conjunctivitis of the newborn**. This acute, purulent conjunctivitis (named for the inclusion bodies seen in infected conjunctival epithelial cells) usually heals without permanent damage to the infant's eye. Treatment is with oral erythromycin. Individuals of any age may develop a **transient purulent inclusion conjunctivitis** due to *C. trachomatis* serotypes D–K. Such individuals are often found to be genitally infected as well. Treatment includes any of a number of broad-spectrum antibacterial agents, such as azithromycin, erythromycin, or tetracycline (in patients older than 8 years. (See p. 237)

Figure 28.6

Examples of bacteria and viruses that cause diseases of the eye.
Other viruses causing eye diseases include influenza virus and rubella virus. Other bacteria causing eye diseases include *S. pneumoniae* and *S. pyogenes*, haemophilus species, *Pseudomonas aeruginosa*, *Treponema pallidum*, and *Mycobacterium tuberculosis*.

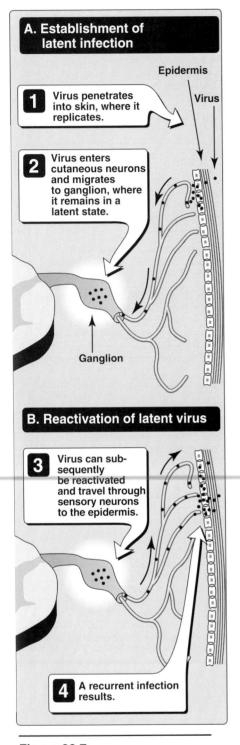

A. Establishment of latent infection

Epidermis

Virus

1 Virus penetrates into skin, where it replicates.

2 Virus enters cutaneous neurons and migrates to ganglion, where it remains in a latent state.

Ganglion

B. Reactivation of latent virus

3 Virus can subsequently be reactivated and travel through sensory neurons to the epidermis.

4 A recurrent infection results.

Figure 28.7
Primary and recurrent herpes simplex infections.

maternal antibody, a disseminated infection, often involving the CNS, results. There is a high mortality rate if untreated, and survivors are likely to have permanent neurologic sequelae. A newborn is also at risk of acquiring infection from an infected mother by transfer on contaminated fingers or in saliva. However, infection *in utero* appears to occur only rarely.

3. **Latency:** In latently infected cells of the ganglia—HSV-1 in trigeminal ganglia and HSV-2 in sacral or lumbar ganglia—from one to thousands of copies of the viral genome are present as nonintegrated, circular molecules of DNA in the nuclei (Figure 28.7). Expression of HSV genes is shut off in latently infected cells, although characteristic, nontranslated RNA transcripts are present in some cells. Their function has not been definitively established, but they may be involved in repression of gene expression.

4. **Reactivation:** Several factors, such as hormonal changes, fever, and physical damage to the neurons, are known to induce reactivation and replication of the latent virus (Figure 28.7). The newly synthesized virions are transported down the axon to the nerve endings, from which the virus is released, infecting the adjoining epithelial cells. Characteristic lesions are thus produced in the same general area as that of the primary lesions. [Note: Virus replication occurs in only a fraction of the latently infected neurons, and these nerve cells eventually die.] The presence of circulating antibody does not prevent this recurrence, but does limit the spread of virus to surrounding tissue. Sensory nerve symptoms such as pain and tingling often precede and accompany the appearance of lesions. In general, the severity of any systemic symptoms is considerably less than that of a primary infection, and many recurrences, in fact, are characterized by shedding of infectious virus in the absence of visible lesions.

   a. **HSV-1:** The frequency of oropharyngeal symptomatic recurrences is quite variable, ranging from none to several per year. The lesions occur as clusters of vesicles at the border of the lips (**herpes labialis**, "**cold sores**", "**fever blisters**") and heal without scarring in eight to ten days.

   b. **HSV-2:** Reactivation of HSV-2 genital infections can occur with considerably greater frequency, for example, monthly, and is often asymptomatic, but still results in viral shedding. Consequently, sexual partners or newborn infants may be at increased risk of becoming infected due to lack of precautions against transmission. The risk of transmission to the newborn is much less than in a primary infection, because considerably less virus is shed, and there is maternal anti-HSV antibody in the baby. This antibody also lessens the severity of the disease if infection does occur.

C. Laboratory identification

Laboratory identification is not required for diagnosis of characteristic HSV lesions in normal individuals. Identification is important, however, to prevent neonatal infection, and in HSV encephalitis and keratoconjunctivitis, where early initiation of therapy is essential but characteristic lesions are not present. Further, for purposes of therapy in the immunocompromised patient, HSV infection must be distinguished from that of varicella-zoster virus (VZV, see p. 324). It must also be distinguished from similar exanthems (skin eruptions) caused by other viruses, or in some cases by bacteria, or noninfectious, allergy-based reactions. Demonstration of HSV by inoculation of human cell tissue culture with a sample of vesicle scraping, fluid, or genital swab is the definitive method for demonstrating infection. Gross cytopathic changes may require several days to appear, but individual infected cells can be detected within 24 hours by use of immunofluorescence (see p. 31) or immunoperoxidase staining with antibodies directed against viral early proteins. Using these same techniques, infected cells can also be demonstrated directly in clinical specimens, although this approach is generally less sensitive than virus isolation in tissue culture. Direct detection of viral DNA by liquid or *in situ* hybridization complements these procedures, and, after amplification of the DNA by the polymerase chain reaction (see p. 32), is considerably more sensitive. For example, in patients with encephalitis, HSV etiology can be confirmed by demonstration of viral DNA in the CSF instead of by brain biopsy.

D. Treatment

The guanine analog, acycloguanosine (acyclovir), is selectively effective against HSV because it becomes an active inhibitor of DNA synthesis only after initially being phosphorylated by the HSV thymidine kinase (Figure 28.8). It is the drug of choice for any primary HSV infection, but is especially important in treating herpes encephalitis, neonatal herpes, and disseminated infections in immunocompromised patients. Other drugs effective in treating herpes simplex infection include famciclovir and topical penciclovir (Figure 28.9). Famciclovir is a prodrug that is metabolized to the active penciclovir. It provides more convenient dosing and greater bioavailability than does oral acyclovir. Penciclovir is active against herpes simplex virus types 1 and 2, and against varicella-zoster virus. None of these drugs can cure a latent infection, but they can minimize asymptomatic viral shedding, and recurrences of symptoms (Figure 28.10). Penciclovir is negligibly absorbed from topical application, and is well tolerated. Both healing and pain are shortened approximately one-half day in duration, compared to placebo-treated subjects. [Note: Resistance of HSV to these drugs due to mutations in the viral thymidine kinase and DNA polymerase genes is observed. However, inhibitors with different modes of action have been developed, for example, pyrophosphate analogs (foscarnet) and phosphonate analogs (cidofovir), that can be used to treat HSV strains resistant to conventional drugs.]

E. Prevention

Prevention of HSV transmission is enhanced by avoidance of contact with potential virus-shedding lesions, and by safe sexual practice. Prevention of neonatal HSV infections is of great importance, but genital infection of the mother is difficult to detect, because it is often asymptomatic. When overt genital tract lesions are detected at the

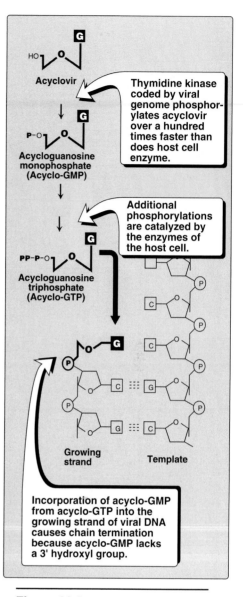

Thymidine kinase coded by viral genome phosphorylates acyclovir over a hundred times faster than does host cell enzyme.

Additional phosphorylations are catalyzed by the enzymes of the host cell.

Acyclovir

Acycloguanosine monophosphate (Acyclo-GMP)

Acycloguanosine triphosphate (Acyclo-GTP)

Growing strand   Template

Incorporation of acyclo-GMP from acyclo-GTP into the growing strand of viral DNA causes chain termination because acyclo-GMP lacks a 3' hydroxyl group.

Figure 28.8
Mechanism of action of acyclovir.

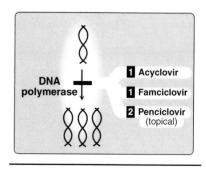

DNA polymerase

1 Acyclovir
1 Famciclovir
2 Penciclovir (topical)

Figure 28.9
Drug therapy for herpes simplex infection.

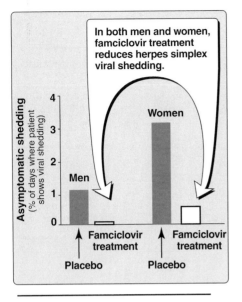

In both men and women, famciclovir treatment reduces herpes simplex viral shedding.

Figure 28.10
Chronic suppressive antiviral therapy reduces the frequency of asymptomatic herpes simplex virus shedding.

time of delivery, cesarean section is usually warranted. Prophylactic therapy of the mother and the newborn with acyclovir can be employed if the presence of HSV is detected just before or at the time of birth, and measures to prevent physical transmission following birth are also important. A vaccine is not currently available.

IV. VARICELLA-ZOSTER VIRUS

Varicella-zoster virus (VZV) has biologic and genetic similarities to HSV, and is classified along with the HSVs in the Alphaherpesvirinae subfamily. Among the biologic similarities between VZV and HSV are the facts that latency is established in sensory ganglia, and that infections are rapidly cytocidal. Primary infections with VZV cause **varicella ("chickenpox")**, whereas reactivation of the latent virus causes **herpes zoster ("shingles")**.

A. Epidemiology and pathogenesis

Transmission of VZV is usually via respiratory droplets, which results in initial infection of the respiratory mucosa, followed by spread to regional lymph nodes (Figure 28.11). Progeny virus enter the bloodstream, undergo a second round of multiplication in cells of the liver and spleen, and are disseminated throughout the body by infected mononuclear leukocytes. Endothelial cells of the capillaries, and ultimately skin epithelial cells, become infected, resulting in the characteristic, virus-containing vesicles of chickenpox, which appear from 14 to 21 days after exposure. The infected individual is contagious from one to two days before the appearance of the exanthema, implying that viruses reinfect cells of the respiratory mucosa near the end of the incubation period. Contact with vesicular fluid does not appear to be a common mode of transmission. The humoral response is of primary importance in providing lifelong immunity to reinfection. In individuals lacking a cell-mediated immune response, dissemination and virus replication at secondary sites (especially lungs, liver, and CNS) are not controlled, and extensive damage to these organs can occur. [Note: Whereas most VZV primary infections are symptomatic, rare asymptomatic infections do occur.]

B. Clinical significance

In contrast to HSV infections, the primary and recurrent diseases (varicella and zoster) due to VZV are quite distinct. Whereas neither is usually life-threatening in the normal, healthy individual, both can have severe complications in immunocompromised patients.

1. **Primary infection (varicella or chickenpox"):** In a normal, healthy child, the incubation period is most commonly from 14 to 16 days. The first appearance of **exanthem** is often preceded by one or two days of a prodrome of fever, malaise, headache, and abdominal pain. The exanthem begins on the scalp, face, or trunk as erythematous macules, which evolve into virus-containing vesicles that begin to crust over after about 48 hours (Figure 28.12). Itching is most severe during the early stage of vesicle development. While the first crop of lesions is evolving, new crops appear on the trunk and extremities. In older adults and the immunocompromised,

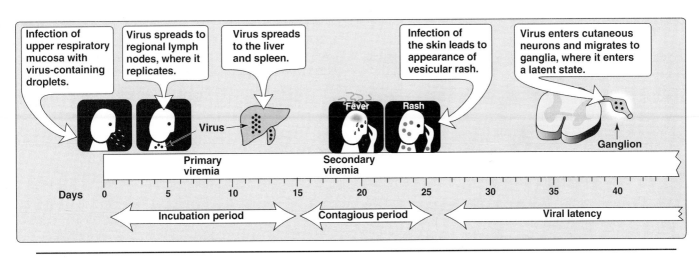

Figure 28.11
Time course of varicella (chickenpox) in children. In adults the disease shows a longer time course and is more severe.

lesions may also appear on mucous membranes, such as in the oropharynx, conjunctivae, and vagina. New lesions continue to appear over a period of up to six or seven days. Healing occurs without scarring. [Note: Reye's syndrome, an acute encephalopathy accompanied by fatty liver, is a complication of VZV and of influenza A and B infections of children. A possible relationship exists between the use of aspirin to control the child's pain and fever, and the manifestation of Reye's syndrome.] Varicella is a more serious disease in healthy adults and immunocompromised patients. **Varicella pneumonia** is the most common of the serious complications, but **fulminant hepatic failure** and **varicella encephalitis** may also result. Primary infection of a pregnant woman may cause her to contract the more severe adult form of varicella, and may affect the fetus or neonate as well. Fetal infection early in pregnancy is uncommon, but can result in multiple developmental anomalies. More commonly, a fetus infected near the time of delivery may exhibit typical varicella at birth or shortly thereafter. The severity of the disease depends on whether the mother has begun to produce anti-VZV IgG by the time of delivery.

2. **Recurrent infection (herpes zoster or "shingles"):** Due to the disseminated nature of the primary infection, latency is established in multiple sensory ganglia, the trigeminal and dorsal root ganglia being most common. Unlike most of the herpesviruses, asymptomatic virus shedding is a rare event. Herpes zoster results from reactivation of the latent virus, not from a new, exogenous exposure. Reactivation occurs in approximately fifteen percent of infected individuals. The most striking feature of herpes zoster is that distribution of the clustered vesicular lesions is dermatomal (affecting the area of skin that is supplied by cutaneous branches from a single spinal nerve, Figure 28.13). Roughly half of the recurrences affect the thoracic dermatomes, but cranial nerve and lumbosacral dermatome distributions are also quite common. Although appearance of new lesions ends in three to seven days, the lesions may become confluent, and take several weeks to heal completely. Another distinctive feature of herpes zoster is the sometimes debilitating postherpetic neuralgia and abnormal sen-

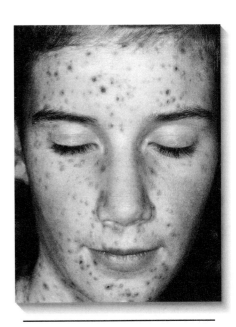

Figure 28.12
Appearance of chickenpox with lesions at all stages of development.

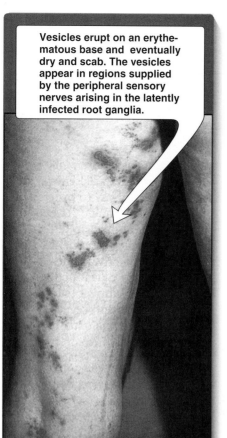

Vesicles erupt on an erythematous base and eventually dry and scab. The vesicles appear in regions supplied by the peripheral sensory nerves arising in the latently infected root ganglia.

Figure 28.13
Cutaneous manifestations of acute herpes zoster.

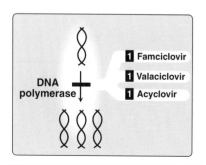

DNA polymerase
1 Famciclovir
1 Valaciclovir
1 Acyclovir

Figure 28.14
Drug therapy for varicella virus.

sory phenomena, which may last as long as several months. The likelihood of reactivation increases with age and with depressed cellular immune competence, probably due to depletion of VZV-specific cytotoxic T-cells. In immunocompromised patients, there is risk of varicella hepatitis, pneumonia, and encephalitis, as well as extension of cutaneous lesions outside of the initial dermatome.

C. Laboratory identification

Laboratory diagnosis of uncomplicated varicella or zoster is generally not necessary, and is not usually done because of the typical clinical appearance and distribution of the lesions. However, in the immunocompromised patient where therapy is warranted, it is important to distinguish VZV infection from other similar exanthems. Cell tissue cultures inoculated with a sample of vesicle fluid show gross cytopathic changes in several days; individual infected cells can be detected within 24 hours by use of immunofluorescence or immunoperoxidase staining with antibodies against viral early proteins. More rapid diagnosis can be made by reacting epithelial cells scraped from the base of vesicles with the stains described above, or by doing *in situ* hybridization with VZV-specific DNA probes.

D. Treatment

Treatment of primary varicella in immunocompromised patients, adults, and neonates is warranted by the severity of the disease (Figure 28.14). Acyclovir has been the drug of choice in such patients, but requires intravenous administration to achieve effective serum levels. Oral acyclovir reduces the time course and acute pain of zoster, but has little or no effect on the subsequent postherpetic neuralgia. Famciclovir and valacyclovir—base analogues similar to acyclovir—have greater activity against VZV. Given early in the acute phase of zoster they decrease acute pain and the time to resolution of lesions, and also reduce the risk and shorten the duration of postherpetic pain.

E. Prevention

A live, attenuated vaccine was approved in 1995 for use in the United States by children one year of age or older, and is now recommended as one of the routine childhood vaccines. It is also indicated for nonimmune adults who are at risk of being exposed to contagious individuals. Susceptible individuals (for example, neonates, nonimmune healthy adults, and immunocompromised children who have been exposed to chickenpox or to zoster lesion fluid) can be protected by administration of varicella-zoster immune globulin (VZIG). Administration of VZIG has no effect on the occurrence of zoster.

V. HUMAN CYTOMEGALOVIRUS

Human cytomegalovirus (HCMV) is a member of the Betaherpesvirinae subfamily, and as such, differs from HSV and VZV in a number of ways. Its replication cycle is significantly longer, and infected cells typically are greatly enlarged and multinucleated, thus the name, "cytomegalo-" (Figure 28.15). There is only one recognized human species of HCMV, but there are many distinct strains that can be distinguished by antigenic differences as well as by restriction fragment analysis of their genomes. In the United States, HCMV is the most common cause of intrauterine infections, and of congenital abnormalities. It also represents a serious threat to immunodeficient or immunosuppressed patients.

A. Epidemiology and pathogenesis

Initial infection with HCMV commonly occurs during childhood. Depending on geographic location and socioeconomic group, 35 to 90 percent of the population have antibody by adulthood.

1. **Transmission:** Infection in children is usually asymptomatic, and such children continue to shed virus for months in virtually all body fluids, including tears, urine, and saliva. Transmission is by intimate contact with these fluids, although saliva may be the most common source. In adults, the virus can also be transmitted: 1) by sexual means, because it is present in semen and vaginal secretions; 2) by organ transplants; and 3) by blood transfusions. Similarly, virus is present in breast milk, and thus neonates can be infected by this route. HCMV can also cross the placenta and infect a fetus *in utero*. Initial replication of the virus in epithelial cells of the respiratory and GI tracts is followed by viremia and infection of all organs of the body. In symptomatic cases, kidney tubule epithelium, liver, and CNS, in addition to the respiratory and GI tracts, are most commonly affected.

2. **Latency and reactivation:** A distinctive feature of HCMV latency is the phenomenon of repeated episodes of asymptomatic virus shedding over prolonged periods of time. Latency is probably established in monocytes and macrophages, but other cell types, such as those of the kidney, are also involved.

B. Clinical significance

In healthy individuals, primary HCMV infection is usually inapparent. Whereas most infections occur in childhood, primary infection as an adult may result in a mononucleosis syndrome that is clinically identical to that caused by Epstein-Barr virus (EBV, see p. 331). It is estimated that about eight percent of **infectious mononucleosis (IM)** cases are due to HCMV. The IM symptoms of persistent fever, muscle pain, and lymphadenopathy are characteristic, as are elevated levels of abnormal lymphocytes and liver enzymes. The major distinguishing feature of HCMV IM is the absence of the heterophile antibodies that characterize IM caused by EBV (see p. 331). Two specific situations have greater clinical significance, namely congenital infections and infection of immunocompromised patients.

1. **Congenital infections:** HCMV is the most common intrauterine viral infection. However, there is a great disparity in incidence of fetal infection and severity of outcome, depending on whether the mother is experiencing a primary or recurrent infection. In women experiencing their first HCMV infection during pregnancy (and who therefore have not yet produced antibodies against HCMV), 35 to 50 percent of fetuses will be infected, and ten percent of these will be symptomatic (Figure 28.16). The severity of the

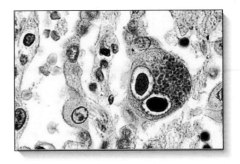

Figure 28.15
Cytomegalovirus infection. Lung section showing typical owl-eye inclusions.

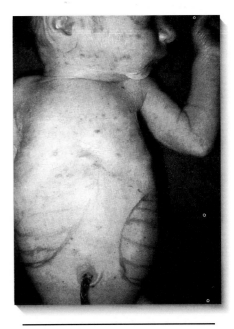

Figure 28.16
Newborn with congenital cytomegalovirus disease, showing hepatosplenomegaly and rash.

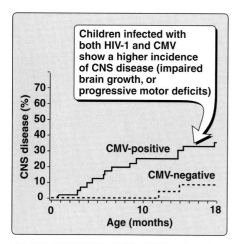

Figure 28.17
Incidence of central nervous system (CNS) disease in HIV-1-infected children with or without cyto-megalovirus infection.

symptoms is most pronounced when infection occurs during the first trimester. Referred to as **cytomegalic inclusion disease**, results caused by the infection range from fetal death to various degrees of damage to liver, spleen, blood-forming organs, and components of the nervous system. The latter is a common cause of hearing loss and mental retardation. Even in infants who are asymptomatic at birth, hearing deficits and ocular damage, for example, chorioretinitis, may appear later and continue to progress during the first few years of life. Whether symptomatic or not, congenitally and perinatally infected infants may continue to excrete virus for years after birth, thus serving as an important virus reservoir. Reactivation of virus shedding in a woman with anti-HCMV antibodies yields a much lower rate of fetal infection, and only rarely do symptoms or sequelae occur.

2. Infections of immunosuppressed and immunodeficient patients: Immunosuppressed transplant recipients are multiply at risk from: 1) HCMV present in the tissue being transplanted; 2) virus carried in leukocytes in the associated blood transfusions; and 3) reactivation of their own endogenous latent virus. Immune suppression for the transplant can negate any protective advantage of a seropositive recipient. Destruction of GI tract tissues, hepatitis, and pneumonia are common, the latter being a major cause of death in bone marrow transplant recipients. HCMV infection is also associated with decreased survival of solid tissue grafts (heart, liver, kidney). HCMV coinfection of patients with HIV infection occurs very frequently, probably because of their similar modes of transmission (see p. 364). As a common opportunistic infection in AIDS patients, invasive HCMV infections—arising from reactivation of latent virus— become increasingly important as CD4+ lymphocyte counts and immune competence decline (see p. 367). Any organ system can be affected, but pneumonia and blindness due to HCMV retinitis are especially common. Encephalitis and dementia, esophagitis, enterocolitis, and gastritis are other significant problems. In addition, coinfection with HCMV may accelerate the progression of the pathology of AIDS (Figure 28.17).

C. Laboratory identification

Because the incidence of HCMV infection in the population is so high, and periodic inapparent recurrent infections occur frequently, simple detection of virus or of anti-HCMV antibody is not generally useful. Recovery of virus is not usually done. Serologic diagnosis using ELISA techniques can distinguish primary from recurrent infection either by demonstrating IgG seroconversion, or the presence of HCMV-specific IgM. The use of purified HCMV antigens produced by recombinant DNA methods has improved the reliability of both IgG and IgM determinations. Direct determination of the presence and amount of viral DNA or proteins in white blood cells is useful as an indicator of invasive disease, whereas extracellular virus in urine or saliva may simply be due to an asymptomatic recurrence. Any of these techniques can be used in the screening of transplant donors and recipients to determine their HCMV status.

D. Treatment and prevention

Treatment of HCMV infections is indicated primarily in immunocompromised patients (Figure 28.18). Acyclovir is ineffective because HCMV lacks its own thymidine kinase. However, two inhibitors of the HCMV DNA polymerase are available: **ganciclovir**, a guanine analog that is phosphorylated by a virus-coded protein kinase, and, more recently, **cidofovir**, a deoxycytidine analog. Ganciclovir is used for invasive infections of transplant recipients and AIDS patients, but has considerable toxicity. For retinitis in AIDS patients, the toxic side effects can be avoided by direct intraocular inoculation. Unfortunately, recurrence of the infection occurs after these drugs are withdrawn, necessitating continuous maintenance therapy, eventually resulting in selection of resistant mutants. Due to differences in modes of action, most ganciclovir-resistant mutants are not resistant to cidofovir, which can then be substituted. However, mutants resistant to the new drug arise after several months. A third inhibitor of DNA polymerase, unrelated to the two just described, is **phosphonoformic acid (foscarnet)**. Although relatively selective for the virus enzyme, it does exhibit considerable renal toxicity. It can be used in combination with ganciclovir, or as an alternative when resistant mutants have appeared. After a period of maintenance therapy, however, foscarnet-resistant mutants appear. Additional analogs that inhibit HCMV are in various stages of clinical evaluation. Treatment of HIV-infected individuals with highly active antiretroviral therapy (HAART, or drug "cocktail"), along with specific anti-HCMV drugs, has significantly lessened the incidence and improved the outcome of HCMV infections in these patients. In some cases, improved immunologic status has permitted discontinuance of anti-HCMV therapy. Human immune globulin has been used in an attempt to prevent or reduce the severity of HCMV invasive disease in transplant recipients, but the efficacy of this approach has not been established. A vaccine for active immunization is not available.

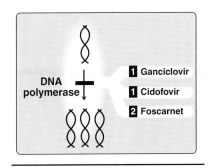

Figure 28.18
Drug therapy for cytomegalovirus.

VI. HUMAN HERPESVIRUS TYPES 6 AND 7

Human herpesvirus types 6 (HHV-6) and 7 (HHV-7) are classified as members of the Betaherpesvirinae, and have marked similarities in biologic and genome characteristics to HCMV. Both HHV-6 and HHV-7 are causative agents of **roseola infantum (exanthem subitum)**, although infection with HHV-7 is more frequently asymptomatic.

A. Epidemiology and pathogenesis

Most infections with HHV-6 and HHV-7 occur during the first three years of life, with overall incidence of antibody approaching ninety percent of the population by the age of three. Transmission is thought to be via oral secretions, because the viruses replicate in salivary glands and are secreted into saliva. HHV-7 in particular has been recovered frequently from saliva of healthy individuals. These viruses also infect peripheral blood lymphocytes and the cells of various solid organs including the central nervous system. HHV-6 infection of lymphoid cells induces a number of significant cell responses, including the synthesis of the CD4 glycoprotein, inter-

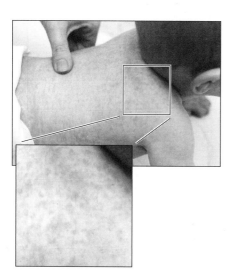

Figure 28.19
Roseola infantum.

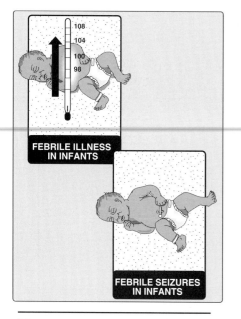

Figure 28.20
Some clinical signs of human herpesvirus 6 infection occurring without the characteristic rash.

feron–α, tumor necrosis factor α, and interleukin-1-β. The ability of HHV-6 to induce expression of CD4 in cells not normally expressing it has the consequence of extending the range of cells infectible by HIV. In addition, HHV-6 transactivates transcription of HIV, thereby accelerating the rate of cell death in coinfected cells. Latently infected cells are found among the peripheral blood lymphocyte population.

B. Clinical significance

HHV-6 infections resulting in disease are most common in infants and in individuals who are immunocompromised.

1. **Primary infections:** Symptomatic **roseola infantum (exanthem subitum)** occurs in roughly one third to one half of infants with a primary HHV-6 infection (Figure 28.19). It is characterized by a high fever of three to five days, after which a characteristic **erythematous macular rash** appears on the neck and trunk, resolving after several more days without sequelae. HHV-7 infection has been shown to produce an identical clinical picture. Of greater clinical significance is the fact that primary HHV-6 infection of infants is the cause of many **acute febrile illnesses** and **febrile seizures** in the absence of the characteristic rash (Figure 28.20). In some of these cases, HHV-7 has been shown to be the causative agent. In others, the patient was coinfected with both HHV-6 and HHV-7. In fact, over twenty percent of emergency room visits for febrile illness in infants, and one third of febrile seizures, are due to primary infection with HHV-6 and/or HHV-7. In the relatively rare cases of primary infection of adults, **prolonged lymphadenopathy**—a mononucleosis-like syndrome, hepatitis, and assorted other lymphoproliferative diseases may result.

2. **Recurrent infections:** Following immunosuppression for organ transplantation, or immunocompromise related to HIV infection, reactivation of latent HHV-6, frequently together with HCMV, has been associated with sometimes-fatal interstitial pneumonitis, fever, hepatitis, and encephalitis, as well as with transplant rejection. The relationship of HHV-6 to AIDS has not been completely elucidated, but the facts that: 1) HHV-6 broadens the range of cell types infectible by HIV by inducing CD4; 2) coinfected cells are killed more rapidly; and 3) extensive disseminated HHV-6 infection frequently occurs in terminal AIDS patients, all suggest that HHV-6 may be an important factor in accelerating the progression from early HIV infection to terminal AIDS). The most common clinical syndrome associated with HHV-6 in AIDS patients is encephalitis (Figure 28.21).

C. Laboratory identification

A simple diagnostic test for primary infection with HHV-6 is not available. PCR amplification has been used to demonstrate HHV-6 DNA in the CSF of patients with neurologic disease, and in serum of patients undergoing posttransplant reactivation of a latent infection. Serologically, there is considerable cross-reaction between HHV-6 and HHV-7, and cross-absorption steps must be included to permit specific determination of either HHV-6 or HHV-7 antibody. Cross-reaction with certain HCMV antigens also occurs, and must be excluded.

D. Treatment and prevention

Because of its genetic relationship to HCMV, HHV-6 is in general inhibited by the same drugs (see p. 329), but extensive clinical trials have not yet been done. In AIDS patients, treatment of the HIV infection appears to reduce the amount of HHV-6 as well. No vaccine for these viruses is currently available. Although there is considerable homology between both HHV-6 and HHV-7, there appears to be no cross-immunity between them.

VII. EPSTEIN-BARR VIRUS

Epstein-Barr virus (EBV) is most commonly known as the causative agent of infectious mononucleosis in young adults, but its initial discovery in association with the childhood disease Burkitt's lymphoma led to its recognition as the first human virus clearly related to a malignancy. More recently, EBV has been associated with a number of additional human neoplastic diseases.

A. Epidemiology and pathogenesis

Most transmission of EBV occurs by intimate contact with saliva that contains virus during both primary infection and in repeated episodes of asymptomatic shedding. The initial site of virus replication appears to be the oropharyngeal epithelium, following which some of the progeny viruses infect B lymphocytes (Figure 28.22). The B cell receptor for EBV is the complement component C3b receptor (see p. 92). The B cell infection is an abortive one, in that only a limited number of early proteins are synthesized. The infection also causes the induction of a number of cellular lymphokines, including B cell growth factors. In contrast to other herpesviruses, the early genes of EBV induce cell multiplication and immortalization, rather than cell death. Thus infection induces a polyclonal B cell proliferation, and an accompanying nonspecific increase in total IgM, IgG, and IgA. The IgM class contains "**heterophile antibodies**" that agglutinate sheep and horse red blood cells. These antibodies are the basis for the classic diagnostic test for EBV-associated infectious mononucleosis (see p. 333). During the first week of the primary infection, as high as ten to twenty percent of circulating B cells contain EBV genomes, and express the early proteins. Within weeks, an active cytotoxic T cell (CTL) response to the EBV antigens expressed by the infected B cells results in a rapid decrease of EBV-containing B cells to less than one percent. It is this CTL response that constitutes the characteristic "atypical lymphocytosis" of infectious mononucleosis. EBV can remain latent in B cells, with several molecules of its circular DNA present in the cytoplasm as well as copies of its genome integrated into host DNA. Reactivation results in initiation of the viral lytic cycle, with progeny EBVs infecting permissive epithelial cells, such as those of the oropharynx.

B. Clinical significance

As stated earlier, primary infection in infancy or childhood is usually asymptomatic, but as high as fifty percent of those infected later in life develop the disease **infectious mononucleosis**. Although B cells

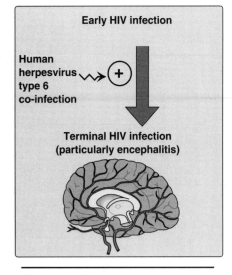

Figure 28.21
Coinfection with human herpesvirus type 6 accelerates the progesssion of HIV symptoms.

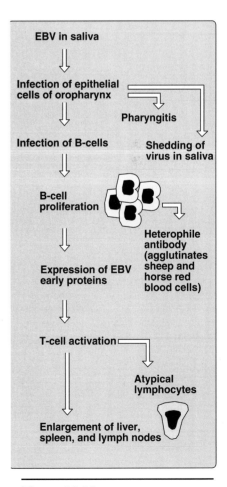

Figure 28.22
Pathogenesis of infectious mononucleosis due to Epstein-Barr virus.

are the primary target of infection due to the presence of the EBV receptor molecule, EBV has more recently been found to be associated with a small number of T cell malignancies as well. In patients who are immunodeficient or immunosuppressed, the lack of cell-mediated immune control increases the likelihood of lymphoproliferative disorders of various kinds. Throughout life, healthy EBV carriers continue to have episodes of asymptomatic virus shedding. The source of this virus is presumably productively infected oropharyngeal cells that acquire the virus from latently infected B cells in which the lytic cycle has been activated.

1. **Infectious mononucleosis (IM):** The manifestations and severity of primary EBV infection vary greatly, but the typical IM syndrome appears after an incubation period of four to seven weeks, and includes pharyngitis, lymphadenopathy, increased levels of liver enzymes in the blood, and fever (Figure 28.23). Headache and malaise often precede and accompany the disease, which may last several weeks. Complete recovery may take much longer.

2. **EBV and malignancies:** Since the initial discovery of EBV in association with Burkitt's lymphoma (BL), it has been shown to be associated with a number of other human neoplastic diseases.

   a. **Burkitt's lymphoma (BL):** BL was first described in 1958 as a rather unique malignancy of the jaw, found at an unusually high frequency in children in regions of equatorial Africa. The cells of Burkitt's lymphoma all contain one of three characteristic chromosome translocations. The breakpoints of these translocations are such that the c-myc proto-oncogene on chromosome eight is constitutively activated. Malarial infection and HIV infection are known risk factors for development of BL. Tumors with the same histologic and cytogenetic characteristics as BL have also been found at much lower frequencies ("sporadic") worldwide. These differ from the original African form, however, in that 1) only 15 to 25 percent contain the EBV genome, 2) they more frequently involve the bone marrow or abdomen as well as the jaw, and 3) they occur at an older age. They are still considered to be BL by virtue of the facts that they are histologically similar, and all contain one of the three distinctive chromosomal translocations.

   b. **EBV-associated nasopharyngeal carcinoma (NPC):** NPC is one of the most common cancers in southeast Asia, North Africa, and among the Eskimo population, but is less common elsewhere. NPC differs from BL in that there is no characteristic chromosomal alteration, and the cells involved are epithelial in origin. The role of EBV is indicated by the fact that all cells of the tumor contain cytoplasmic viral DNA molecules.

   c. **EBV infections in immunocompromised and immunosuppressed patients:** In BL and NPC, EBV infection appears to be only one step in a multi-step, disease-causing process, and its specific role is still not well defined. In contrast, EBV alone appears to be sufficient for induction of B-cell lymphomas in immunocompromised patients, such as transplant recipients and individuals with AIDS, who cannot control the cell multipli-

Classic clinical triad of infectious mononucleosis:

* **Fever**
* **Pharyngitis**
* **Lymphadenopathy** (usually enlargement of anterior and posterior cervical lymph nodes)

Note: Acute infection is often asymptomatic in children, whereas adolescents and young adults show the typical symptoms of infectious mononucleosis.

Transmission

* **Exposure to oropharyngeal secretions**

Clinical manifestations of Epstein-Barr-associated infectious mononucleosis by age-group.

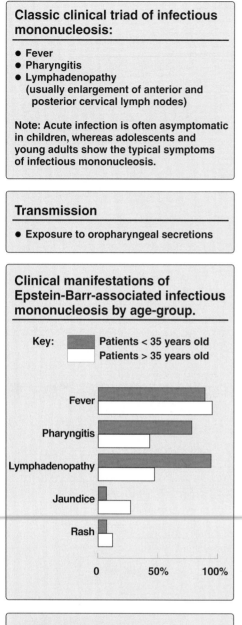

Incidence of Epstein-Barr-associated infectious mononucleosis

* Peak incidence occurs occurs between ages of 15 and 19.
* Incidence is 30 times higher in blacks than whites in the United States.
* No difference in incidence between sexes.
* 90% of general population shows evidence of previous infection with Epstein-Barr virus.

Figure 28.23
Some characteristics of infectious mononucleosis.

cation induced by the early proteins. For example, many AIDS patients develop a B cell malignancy of some type: BL of the sporadic type occurs with high frequency in the earlier stages of AIDS progression, whereas non–BL-type lymphoblastic lymphomas are more characteristic in late-stage AIDS patients. Not all of the HIV-associated BL cases contain the EBV genome. [Note: AIDS patients infected with EBV may also exhibit nonmalignant, white-gray lesions on the tongue ("hairy leukoplakia", Figure 28.24.]

C. Laboratory identification

Atypical lymphocytes (cytotoxic T cells) can be observed in the blood smear of a patient with IM (Figure 28.25). Detection of EBV DNA or RNA by hybridization, or of virus antigens using immunohistochemical techniques, can be done with cell homogenates or by *in situ* methods for visualization of individual infected cells. The "classic" test for infectious mononucleosis, the Paul-Bunnell-Davidsohn test, is based upon the fact that the polyclonal stimulation of B cells by EBV infection results in a nonspecific elevation of all immunoglobulins, among which is the population of **heterophile antibodies** that specifically agglutinate horse and sheep red blood cells. These heterophile antibodies are diagnostic for EBV-related IM, although they are not present in all cases of EBV IM. [Note: About ninety percent of adults with IM are positive, whereas the frequency is considerably less at younger ages.]

D. Treatment and prevention

Although acyclovir inhibits EBV replication, none of the antiherpes drugs have been effective in modifying the course or severity of IM due to EBV, or in preventing development of EBV-related B cell malignancies. Acyclovir has been used successfully in treating oral hairy leukoplakia, where the virus is actively replicating in the epithelial cells of the tongue. No vaccine for prevention of EBV infections is currently available. Some properties of the common herpesvirus infections are summarized in Figure 28.26.

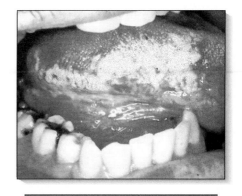

Figure 28.24
Hairy leukoplakia caused by Epstein-Barr virus infection.

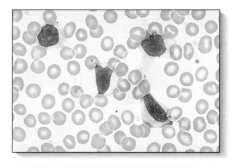

Figure 28.25
Abnormal mononuclear cells commonly seen in infectious mononucleosis.

VIRUS	VIRUS SUBFAMILY	CLINICAL MANIFESTATIONS OF PRIMARY INFECTION	CLINICAL MANIFESTATIONS OF RECURRENT INFECTION	SITE OF INITIAL INFECTION	SITE OF LATENCY
Herpes simplex-1	α	Keratoconjunctivitis, gingivostomatitis, pharyngitis, tonsilitis	Herpes labialis ("cold sores")	Mucoepithelial	Trigeminal sensory ganglia
Herpes simplex-2	α	Genital herpes; perinatal disseminated disease	Genital herpes	Mucoepithelial	Lumbar or sacral sensory ganglia
Varicella-zoster virus	α	Varicella ("chickenpox")	Herpes-Zoster ("shingles")	Mucoepithelial	Dorsal root ganglia
Cytomegalo-virus	β	Congenital infection (*in utero*); mononucleosis-like syndrome	Asymptomatic shedding of virus	Monocytes, lymphocytes, and epithelial cells	Monocytes, lymphocytes
Epstein-Barr virus	γ	Infectious mononucleosis; Burkitt's lymphoma	Asymptomatic shedding of virus	Mucosal epithelium, B lymphocytes	B lymphocytes

Figure 28.26
Properties of common herpesvirus infections.

VIII. HUMAN HERPESVIRUS TYPE 8

HHV-8 infection appears not to occur as frequently as the other human herpesviruses in the normal, healthy population. Yet the virus genome and/or viral proteins have been detected in over ninety percent of patients with **Kaposi's sarcoma** (KS), but in less than one percent of non-KS tissues. The notable feature of pathogenesis by HHV-8 is the finding that the viral genome encodes a number of cell-derived genes related to growth regulation. These include genes for several cytokines, cytokine receptors, growth factors that promote angiogenesis, and a factor that inhibits apoptosis. The primary method for detection of HHV-8 is by DNA hybridization following PCR amplification. Antibody status is evaluated by means of an immunofluorescence reaction with nuclei from a HHV-8 latently infected lymphoma cell line, or by ELISA, using one or more virion peptides as the antigen (see p. 30). Antibodies to HHV-8 antigens are found at elevated frequencies in the same populations that are at risk for HIV infection, leading to the conclusion that the primary mode of transmission is sexual, although other transmission modes have not been excluded. Therefore, the same approaches to prevention of sexually transmitted diseases, and of HIV infection in particular, should be applicable to HHV-8 as well.

IX. POXVIRIDAE

The poxviruses are a family of large, genetically complex viruses having no obvious symmetry. Members of this family are widely distributed in nature. The agent of previous medical importance to humans, **variola virus**, was the cause of **smallpox**, the first infectious disease to be declared eradicated from the earth. Among the factors that led to this success are: 1) the availability of a very effective, attenuated vaccine; 2) the fact that variola was antigenically stable and only a single antigenic type existed; 3) the absence of asymptomatic cases or persistent carriers; 4) the absence of an animal reservoir; and 5) the emotional effect of this highly lethal, disfiguring disease helping gain public cooperation in the eradication efforts. Currently, the highly effective vaccine poxvirus, **vaccinia virus**, is being used in attempts to construct vectors carrying immunizing genes from other infectious agents. Finally, the poxvirus, **molluscum contagiosum virus** (**MCV**), causes small, wartlike tumors (not to be confused with true warts caused by papilloma virus, see p. 308).

A. Structure and classification of the family

The genome is a single linear molecule of double-stranded DNA, with a coding capacity for over 200 polypeptides. The virion contains enzymes that are involved in the early steps of replication. The vertebrate poxviruses are related by a common nucleoprotein antigen, but are otherwise quite distinct. Humans are the natural host for variola and MCV, but monkeypox, cowpox, and a number of other animal poxviruses can also cause human disease. The structure of a typical poxvirus, vaccinia, is shown in Figure 28.27.

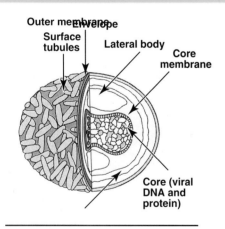

Outer membrane
Envelope
Surface tubules
Lateral body
Core membrane
Core (viral DNA and protein)

Figure 28.27
Structure of vaccinia virus.

B. Replication of the poxviruses

The poxviruses follow the basic replication pattern for DNA viruses (see p. 300), with a few notable exceptions. The most striking of these is the fact that the entire replication cycle takes place in the cytoplasm, the virus providing all of the enzymes (including a viral DNA-dependent RNA polymerase) necessary for DNA replication and gene expression. Final maturation by acquisition of a lipoprotein envelope occurs as the virus buds from the cell. The replication cycle is rapid, and results in early shut-off of all cell macromolecular syntheses, causing the death of the cell.

C. Epidemiology and clinical significance

The stages of the disease **smallpox** are illustrated in Figure 28.28. Whereas there is no longer the threat of naturally occurring smallpox, the mutation of one of the animal poxviruses to a form more virulent for humans has continued to be of some concern. Human infections with monkeypox are clinically similar to smallpox, and although somewhat less severe, still have a mortality rate of about eleven percent. Such infections have only been observed where the human population comes into close contact with infected monkeys; in its natural state monkeypox is not readily transmitted between humans. **Molluscum contagiosum** infection occurs only in humans, and causes benign wart-like tumors on various body surfaces. It is usually spread by direct contact, and is now recognized as a sexually transmitted disease.

D. Laboratory identification

The unique cellular localization of poxvirus replication has enabled rapid diagnosis to be made by the observation of DNA-containing intracytoplasmic inclusion bodies in cells scraped from skin lesions.

E. Treatment and prevention

Whereas immunization with vaccinia is no longer done routinely, it is still carried out in certain groups, such as the military and laboratory workers. Although one of the safest vaccines in healthy recipients, individuals with eczema may develop a generalized vaccinia rash covering the surface of the body, and immunocompromised patients are likely to develop progressive vaccinia, which has a high mortality rate. Postvaccinal encephalitis, with a mortality of forty percent, is a second hazard accompanying vaccination.

F. Smallpox as a biological weapon

Although the World Health Organization declared smallpox eradicated in 1980, stocks of the virus exist in the United States and Russia. It is feared that secret stocks of the virus may exist. Smallpox is potentially a devasting biological weapon because it is highly contagious and it has a high case fatality rate—more than thirty percent among unvaccinated persons. In 1972, the United States stopped routine vaccination of civilians against smallpox. As a result, more than forty percent of the population are now vulnerable to smallpox infection, with the percent increasing each year. Stores of vaccine and vaccinia immune globulin are currently inadequate to combat a massive outbreak of the disease.

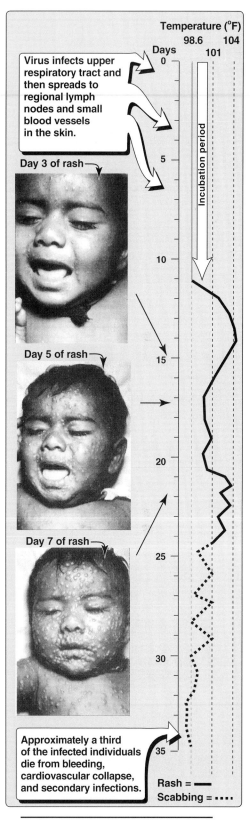

Figure 28.28
Time course of smallpox.

Study Questions

Choose the ONE correct answer

28.1 "For which one of the following viruses are recurrent episodes of asymptomatic (inapparent) virus shedding not an important factor in transmission of the virus?

   A. Herpes simplex virus

   B. Varicella-zoster virus

   C. Cytomegalovirus

   D. Epstein-Barr virus

   E. Human herpesvirus 6

> Correct answer = B. VZV is the only herpesvirus in which asymptomatic shedding does not appear to occur. All recurrences are evident as zoster. Asymptomatic recurrences are noted with all of the other herpes viruses, although the incidence of symptomatic vs. asymptomatic varies with the individual patient and the virus.

28.2 The initial infection with human cytomegalovirus most commonly occurs:

   A. during early childhood, by exchange of body fluids.

   B. *in utero*, by transplacental transmission from a latently infected pregnant woman.

   C. by transfer of saliva between young adults.

   D. by sexual intercourse.

   E. as a result of blood transfusion or organ transplantation.

> Correct answer = A. Depending on the population, up to ninety percent have antibody by adulthood. B: Among the most serious complications of infection are those resulting from transplacental transmission, but this is not the common mode of transmission. C and D: Transmission by kissing or sexual intercourse can occur, but most individuals have already been infected by this age. E: This mode of transmission has serious consequences in antibody-negative recipients, but most recipients had been infected at an earlier age. More common is reactivation of latent HCMV in recipients who have been immuno-suppressed for purposes of the transplantation.

28.3 The cellular response typical of infectious mononucleosis caused by Epstein-Barr virus is due to:

   A. stimulation of B cell proliferation by the EBV early proteins synthesized in the infected cells.

   B. proliferation of cytotoxic T cells responding to EBV antigens expressed on the surface of infected B cells.

   C. a primary humoral immune response to the EBV infection.

   D. macrophages responding to the death of EBV-infected cells.

   E. activation of an oncogene resulting from a chromosome translocation in EBV-infected lymphocytes.

> Correct answer = B. A: Polyclonal stimulation of B-cells by EBV infection does occur, and results in appearance of the characteristic "heterophile antibodies", but it is the CTL response that comprises the atypical lymphocytosis of IM. C: The EBV-specific humoral immune response is not related to the lymphocytosis. D: B cells are not killed by infection with EBV. E: Whereas this is the process that results in EBV-associated Burkitt's lymphoma, it occurs only years after the initial infection with the virus.

28.4 Acyclovir is largely ineffective in treatment of human cytomegalovirus infections because:

   A. HCMV exhibits a very high rate of mutation in the target enzyme.

   B. HCMV depends upon the host cell's DNA polymerase for replication of its DNA.

   C. HCMV lacks the thymidine kinase required for activation of acyclovir.

   D. The tissues in which HCMV multiplies are largely inaccessible to the drug.

   E. HCMV codes for an enzyme that inactivates the drug.

> Correct answer = C. The specificity of acyclovir derives from the fact that for it to be an active inhibitor of virus DNA synthesis, it must be phosphorylated by the HSV or VZV thymidine kinase. HCMV does not have a corresponding enzyme. A: HCMV does develop resistance to those drugs that are effective, such as ganciclovir and cidofovir, after long term therapy, but because their mechanisms of action are different, mutants resistant to one are usually not resistant to the other. B: All herpesviruses code for their own DNA polymerase. D: In those cases where access is a problem for treatment of herpesvirus infections, direct inoculation of the drug has been done. E: Resistance to antiherpesvirus drugs has generally involved mutation of the enzyme interacting with the drug, not inactivation of the drug.

28.5 Which one of the characteristics listed below is NOT associated with human herpesvirus 6?

   A. T-lymphocytes are the major host cell.

   B. It transactivates transcription of human immunodeficiency virus in coinfected cells.

   C. Infection induces the expression of the CD4 glycoprotein in cells not normally expressing it.

   D. Primary infection with HHV-6 usually occurs in parallel with initiation of sexual activity.

   E. Roseola is the most common clinical manifestation of primary infection.

> Correct answer = D. Most primary infections with HHV-6 occur during the first few years of life.

Hepatitis B and Hepatitis D (Delta) Viruses

29

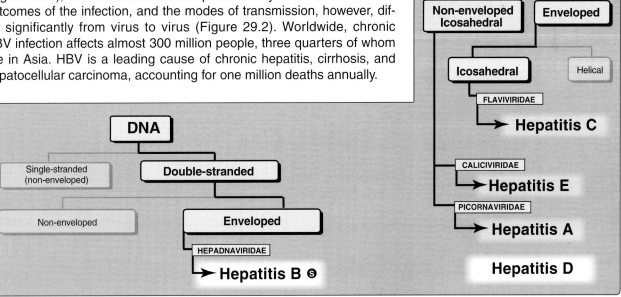

Hepadnaviridae
Herpesviridae
Poxviridae

I. OVERVIEW

Hepatitis (inflammation of the liver) can be caused by a variety of organisms and toxins. For example, there are many viral diseases that involve some degree of liver damage as a secondary effect (such as infectious mononucleosis caused by the Epstein-Barr virus, see p. 332). However, the viruses that are referred to as "hepatitis viruses" are those whose pathogenesis specifically involves replication in and destruction of hepatocytes. This chapter describes the only human hepatitis virus that has a DNA genome, hepatitis B virus (HBV, Figure 29.1). This chapter also discusses the defective agent that sometimes accompanies HBV during infections—the "delta agent," or hepatitis D virus (HDV). With the exception of HBV, the hepatitis viruses thus far identified—hepatitis A, C, D, and E viruses—contain RNA, and belong to several different families (Figure 29.1), but the acute disease produced by each is similar. The outcomes of the infection, and the modes of transmission, however, differ significantly from virus to virus (Figure 29.2). Worldwide, chronic HBV infection affects almost 300 million people, three quarters of whom are in Asia. HBV is a leading cause of chronic hepatitis, cirrhosis, and hepatocellular carcinoma, accounting for one million deaths annually.

Figure 29.1
Classification of major viral agents causing hepatitis. [Note: Hepatitis D is a defective virus and is classified in its own "floating" genus. Hepatitis A, C, and E are discussed in Chapter 30.] ⓢ See p. 426 for a summary of this virus.

Lippincott's Illustrated Reviews: Microbiology,
by William A. Strohl, Harriet Rouse, Bruce D. Fisher.
Lippincott, Williams & Wilkins, Baltimore, MD © 2001

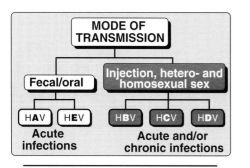

Figure 29.2
Classification of hepatitis viruses based on their mode of transmission.

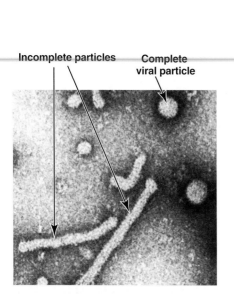

Figure 29.3
Electron micrograph of a fraction of serum from a patient with a severe case of hepatitis.

II. THE HEPADNAVIRIDAE

The family Hepadnaviridae (hepatotropic DNA viruses) consists of a group of hepatitis-causing viruses with DNA genomes. Each hepadnavirus has a very narrow host range in which it produces both acute infections and chronic, persistent infections; HBV is the only member of this family that infects humans. The presence of highly infectious virus in the blood of both symptomatic and asymptomatic, chronically infected individuals poses a serious threat to all health care workers, and immunization of such individuals is generally required. A highly effective vaccine produced in genetically engineered yeast cells is now available, and is included among the routine childhood immunizations (see p. 41). Biologically, HBV is unique among human disease agents in that replication of the DNA genome proceeds via an RNA intermediate, which in turn is "reverse transcribed" by a viral enzyme homologous to the retrovirus reverse transcriptase (see p. 362). However, whereas retroviruses package an RNA genome, Hepadnaviridae package a DNA genome.

A. Structure and replication of HBV

The virion of HBV, historically referred to as the **Dane particle**, consists of an icosahedral nucleocapsid enclosed in an envelope (Figure 29.3).

1. **Organization of the HBV genome:** The short HBV DNA genome is unusual in that it is a partly single-stranded, partly double-stranded, noncovalently closed, circular DNA molecule (that is, one strand is longer than the other, Figure 29.4). The short "plus" strand, which can vary in length, is only fifty to eighty percent as long as its mate, the "minus" strand. The circular structure of the genome is maintained by base-pairing of the strands at one end. The genome is organized into four overlapping genes. This allows the small DNA genome to code for four proteins, whose combined lengths would otherwise have required a significantly larger genome. A summary of HBV replication is shown in Figure 29.4.

2. **Viral proteins:** The four proteins encoded by the viral DNA are 1) the capsid protein [**hepatitis B capsid antigen (HBcAg)**], 2) the envelope protein [a glycoprotein referred to as the **hepatitis B surface antigen (HBsAg)**], 3) the multifunctional **reverse transcriptase/DNA polymerase**, which is complexed with the DNA genome within the capsid, and 4) a nonstructural regulatory protein designated the **X protein**. There is further complexity, in that two mRNA initiation sites in the capsid protein gene result in the translation of both the HBcAg itself, and a differently processed variant of this protein, the HBeAg, which is secreted by infected cells, and serves as a marker for active viral replication (see p. 340).

B. Transmission

Infectious HBV is present in all body fluids of an infected individual. Therefore, blood, semen, saliva, mother's milk, etc., serve as sources of infection. The titer of infectious virus in the blood of an acutely infected patient can be as high as 10^8 virus particles per ml, but generally is lower in other body fluids. In areas of high endemicity, for example, Southeast Asia, Africa, and the Middle East, the majority of the population becomes infected at or shortly after birth from a chronically infected mother or from infected siblings. [Note: A small percentage of infected newborns are thought to acquire the virus *in utero*.] Individuals infected at this young age have a significant chance of becoming chronic carriers (see p. 10), thus maintaining the high prevalence of virus in the population. In the United States and other western countries the carrier rate is much lower, and primary infection rarely occurs in newborns. Hepatitis B is therefore primarily a disease of infants in developing nations, whereas in Western countries it is mostly confined to adults who usually contract HBV infection through sexual intercourse or by IV drug use. [Note: This has been true only since methods for screening blood and organ donors for HBV antigens virtually eliminated these as sources of infection. Hepatitis C virus (HCV, see p. 356) is currently responsible for most cases of serum-transmitted hepatitis.] Health care and laboratory workers continue to be at risk, but this can be minimized by immunization, and by strict adherence to the universal precautions for working with blood and body fluids.

C. Pathogenesis

Fully differentiated hepatocytes are the primary cell type infected by HBV. However, viral genomes and RNA transcripts have been detected in a variety of extrahepatic tissues. This could account for the diverse symptoms sometimes observed in patients with HBV infection. The primary cause of hepatic cell destruction appears to be the cell-mediated immune response (see p. 72). The cells involved are HLA–I-restricted cytotoxic T cells (see p. 74), which react specifically with the fragments of nucleocapsid proteins, HBcAg and HBeAg, expressed on the surface of infected hepatocytes. This response also contributes to control of the infection by eliminating virus-producing cells. Enhanced natural killer cell activity (see p. 55), as well as production of interferon-α, also contribute to limiting the extent of the infection. Humoral anti-HBsAg antibody, which is the neutralizing Ab, does not appear until well into the convalescence period, when it may aid in clearing any remaining circulating free virus. Of greater importance, however, is that this antibody provides protection against reinfection. On the other hand, it is this same humoral antibody that is thought to be the source of the extrahepatic damage that is seen in ten to twenty percent of patients, through the formation and deposition of HBsAg/anti-HBs Ab immune complexes, and the consequent activation of complement (see p. 91).

D. Clinical significance: acute disease

HBV is of medical and public health importance, not only as the cause of acute liver disease, but especially as the cause of chronic, persistent infections that can result in the eventual death of the infected individual due to cirrhosis and liver cancer. Chronically infected people serve as the reservoir of transmissible virus in the population. In a majority of individuals, the primary infection is asymptomatic, and resolves as a result of an effective cell-mediated immune response (Figure 29.5).

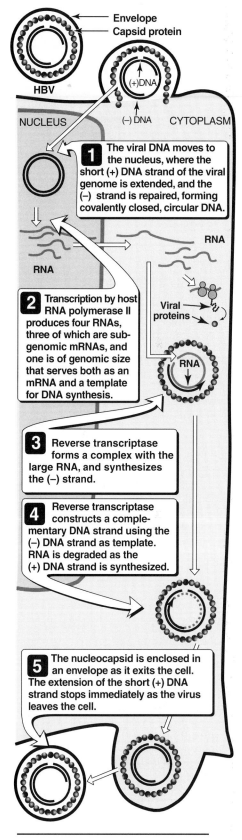

Figure 29.4
Replication of hepatitis B virus.

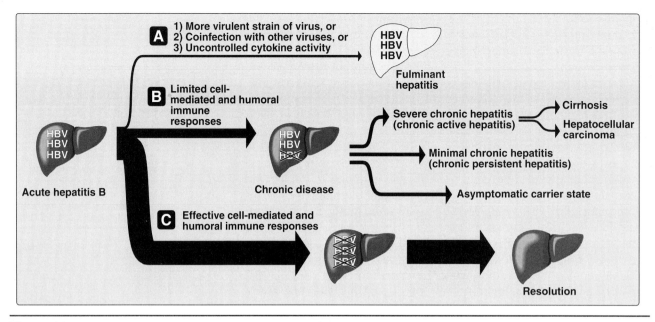

Figure 29.5
Clinical outcomes of acute hepatitis B infection.

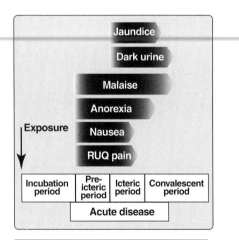

Figure 29.6
Symptoms of acute hepatitis B infection. RUQ = right upper quadrant.

1. **Phases in acute HBV infections:** Following infection, HBV has a long but variable incubation period of between 45 and 120 days. [Note: The size of the inoculum and route of infection are two of the factors that affect the length of the incubation period.] Following this period, a pre-icteric (pre-jaundice) phase occurs, lasting several days to a week. This is characterized by mild fever, malaise, anorexia, myalgia, and nausea. These rather nonspecific symptoms are likely due to the interferon-α synthesis induced by the infection. The acute, icteric phase then follows, and lasts for one to two months. It is during this phase that dark urine, due to bilirubinuria, and jaundice, seen as a yellowish coloration of mucous membranes, conjunctivae, and skin, are evident. There usually is an enlarged and tender liver as well. In eighty to ninety percent of adults, a convalescent period of several more months is followed by complete recovery (Figure 29.6).

2. **Monitoring the course of acute HBV infection:** Whereas liver-specific enzymes are important clinical determinants of all of the viral hepatitides, HBV infection is unusual in that the quantities of virions and virion components in the blood are so great that the time course of their appearance and clearance, along with that of the antibodies directed against them, serve as convenient markers of the stage of the disease, and of the likely future course (Figure 29.7A).

   a. **Appearance of viral antigens:** During the incubation period, HBsAg and HBeAg are the first indicators of HBV infection to appear in the blood. Their presence indicates an active infection, but does not distinguish between acute and chronic infections. Next, viral DNA, viral DNA polymerase, and complete virions become detectable. These continue to increase during the acute disease phase, when a patient's blood has the high-

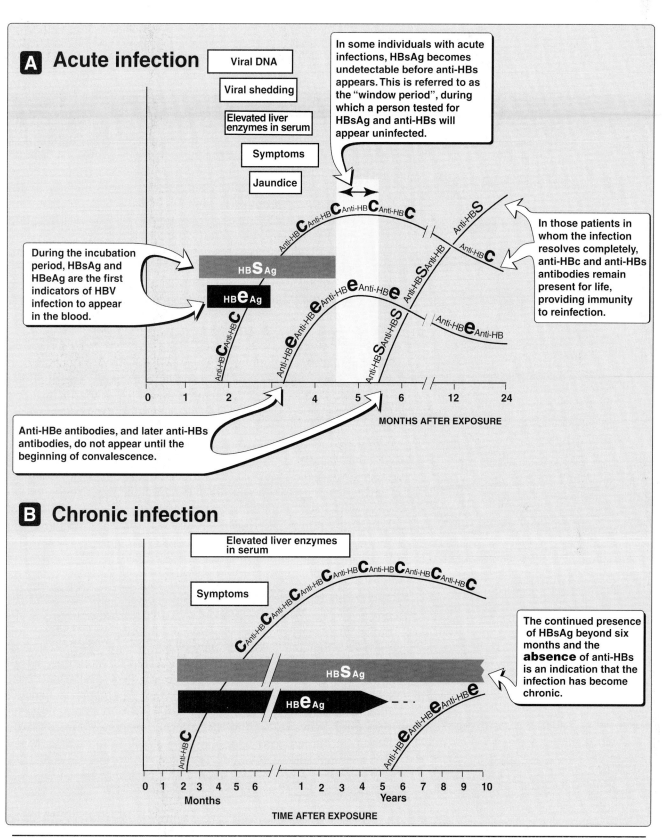

Figure 29.7
Typical course of hepatitis B virus infection. A. Acute infection. B. Chronic infection.

est titer of infectious virus. [Note: Liver damage, as evidenced by abnormalities in enzymes such as alanine aminotransferase (ALT[1]), and symptoms of hepatitis, appear after significant viral replication has already occurred.]

b. **Appearance of antiviral antibodies:** Antibodies to the HBcAg rise concurrently with liver enzymes, whereas anti-HBe antibodies, and still later anti-HBs antibodies, do not appear until the beginning of convalescence—generally after the respective antigens have disappeared from the blood. [Note: In some individuals with acute infections, HBsAg becomes undetectable before anti-HBs appears. This is referred to as the "window period", during which a person tested for HBsAg and anti-HBs appear uninfected. Anti-HBc antibody is, however, present.] In those patients in whom the infection resolves completely, anti-HBc and anti-HBs antibodies remain present for life, providing immunity to reinfection. On the other hand, the continued presence of HBsAg beyond six months and the absence of anti-HBs is an indication that the infection has become chronic (Figure 29.8).

3. **Fulminant hepatitis:** In one to two percent of acute symptomatic cases, much more extensive necrosis of the liver occurs during the first eight weeks of the acute illness. This is accompanied by high fever, abdominal pain, and eventual renal dysfunction, coma, and seizures. Termed fulminant hepatitis, this condition is fatal in roughly eight percent of cases. Whereas it is not clear why the acute disease takes this course, a more highly virulent strain of HBV, coinfection with HDV or another hepatitis virus (for example, HCV), and/or perhaps an uncontrolled immune response by the patient, are thought to play a role. [Note: The observed clinical outcome reflects the balance between elimination of virus and liver cell destruction, both mediated by the immune system.]

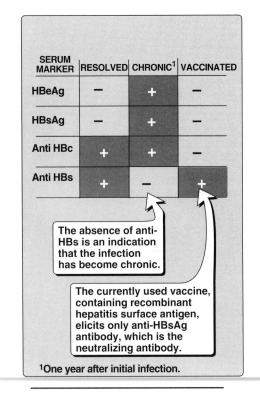

SERUM MARKER	RESOLVED	CHRONIC[1]	VACCINATED
HBeAg	−	+	−
HBsAg	−	+	−
Anti HBc	+	+	−
Anti HBs	+	−	+

The absence of anti-HBs is an indication that the infection has become chronic.

The currently used vaccine, containing recombinant hepatitis surface antigen, elicits only anti-HBsAg antibody, which is the neutralizing antibody.

[1]One year after initial infection.

Figure 29.8
Interpretation of serologic markers of HBV infection.

E. Clinical significance: chronic disease

The factors determining the eventual outcome of infection with HBV are not well understood. In about two thirds of individuals, the primary infection is asymptomatic, even though such patients may later develop symptomatic chronic liver disease, indicating persistence of the virus. Following resolution of the acute disease (or asymptomatic infection), about two to ten percent of adults, and over twenty five percent of young children, remain chronically infected (Figure 29.9). The very high rate of progression to chronic liver disease seen in infants born to HBV-infected mothers is thought to be related to the less competent immune status of newborns. Adults with immune deficiencies also have a considerably higher probability of developing a chronic infection than do individuals with normal immune systems.

1. **Types of chronic carriers:** The **asymptomatic carriers** of HBsAg are the most common type of persistently infected individuals. They usually have anti-HBe antibodies, and little or no infectious virus in their blood (see Figures 29.7B and 29.8). Later progres-

sion of liver damage or recurrence of acute episodes of hepatitis is rare in such patients. Those carriers with **minimal chronic hepatitis** (formerly termed "chronic persistent hepatitis") are asymptomatic most of the time, but have a higher risk of reactivation of disease, and a small fraction do progress to cirrhosis. [Note: The use of highly sensitive PCR amplification methods has revealed a type of asymptomatic infection referred to as "occult", in which no markers of HBV infection are present, but low levels of HBV DNA can be detected. Such **occult infections** have now been recognized to occur frequently as a coinfection in individuals with chronic HCV infection. These coinfected patients have a higher rate of cirrhosis, and a reduced response to interferon–α.] **Severe chronic hepatitis** (formerly called "chronic active hepatitis") results in more frequent exacerbations of acute symptoms including progressive liver damage, potentially leading to cirrhosis and/or hepatocellular carcinoma (see below), chronic fatigue, anorexia, malaise, and anxiety. These symptoms are accompanied by active virus replication, and the corresponding presence of HBeAg in the blood. Serum levels of liver enzymes and bilirubin are increased to varying degrees, reflecting the extent of necrosis that is occurring. The risk of developing cirrhosis is highest in those carriers with more frequent recurrences of acute disease, and in those in whom HBeAg is not cleared from the blood, indicating continuing virus replication. Overall life expectancy is significantly shorter in those individuals with cirrhosis. [Note: These carrier states are not static, and one may proceed into the other over a period of time.]

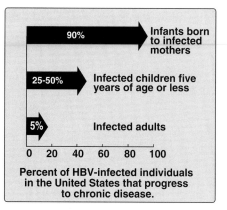

Figure 29.9
Effect of patient's age on the tendency of acute HBV infection to progress to chronic disease.

2. **Development of hepatocellular carcinoma (HCC, hepatoma):** This is one of the major causes of death due to malignancy worldwide, and its distribution parallels that of HBV incidence (approximately eighty percent of primary HCCs occur in HBV-infected individuals). Thus, in the United States, HCC is fairly uncommon, whereas it is ten to a hundred times more frequent in areas of high HBV endemicity. In all populations, males experience a higher rate of chronic HBV infections, a higher rate of progression to cirrhosis, and ultimately a higher rate of HCC, for which the male-to-female ratio is six to one. HCC typically appears many years after the primary HBV infection, and the tumor itself is rather slow growing, and only occasionally metastasizes. Clinically, a patient with HCC exhibits weight loss, right upper quadrant pain, fever, and intestinal bleeding. Although there is no doubt that chronic HBV infection greatly increases the risk of HCC, the mechanisms relating HBV and HCC are not understood. However, by causing continuing liver necrosis accompanied by continuing regeneration of the damaged tissue, chronic HBV infection provides the opportunity for chromosome rearrangements and mutations. The presence of environmental carcinogens could further contribute to the disease process.

F. Laboratory identification

The purposes of diagnostic laboratory studies of patients with clinical hepatitis are, first, to determine which hepatitis virus is the cause of the illness, and second, for HBV, to distinguish acute from chronic infections. The diagnosis of hepatitis is made on clinical grounds, coupled with biochemical tests that evaluate liver damage. Elevations of the aminotransferases, bilirubin, and the prothrombin time, all contribute to the initial evaluation of the hepatitis. ELISA (see p. 30) and other immunologic techniques for detection of viral antigens and antibodies are the primary means used to distinguish between HAV, HBV, HCV and HDV. In addition, identification of the presence or absence of specific antiviral antibodies and viral antigens permits differentiating between acute and chronic HBV infections (see Figure 29.7). When titers of infectious virus are high, HBV DNA can be demonstrated in the blood by DNA–DNA hybridization techniques. Use of PCR amplification of the DNA (see p. 32) can increase the sensitivity of hybridization assays to the extent that low levels of HBV DNA can also be demonstrated in serum, even when none of the other markers of replication, such as HBeAg, are detectable (the **occult state**).

G. Treatment

In the past, treatment for acute hepatitis was largely supportive, and not directed towards inhibiting virus replication. Prolonged (months) treatment with interferon-α has succeeded in reducing or eliminating indicators of HBV replication in about one third of patients, but in some of these, recurrence of indications of the infection occurs after discontinuance of the therapy. Antiviral analogs used in HIV therapy (see p. 374), and targeted especially against the reverse transcriptase, have been tested, and have had some success. In clinical trials, lamivudine, an oral nucleoside analog, has been shown to be an effective treatment in patients with previously untreated chronic hepatitis B (Figure 29.10). Treatment with lamivudine for one year was well tolerated. It decreased histologic liver abnormalities, and increased the rate of HBeAg seroconversion (defined as the loss of HBeAg in serum, undetectable HBV DNA levels, and the presence of antibodies against HBeAg). Most lamivudine-treated patients had undetectable serum HBV DNA during the one year of treatment, but four months after treatment was stopped, the median HBV DNA level had returned to about fifty percent of the pretreatment value. Initial reports show no greater benefits from combination therapy with interferon plus lamivudine than with lamivudine monotherapy.

H. Prevention

The purpose of controlling the spread of HBV infection is to prevent cases of acute hepatitis. An additional goal is to decrease the pool of chronically infected individuals who serve as the reservoir for infectious virus in the population, and who are at greatly increased risk for developing cirrhosis and liver cancer. The availability of a highly effective vaccine has led to a several-pronged approach: 1) protection of those adults who are at risk because of life-style or occupation; 2) protection of newborns from infection by transmission from HBV-positive mothers (important because of the high rate of resulting chronic infections, see p. 339); and 3) protection of siblings and other children from infection by chronically infected family members.

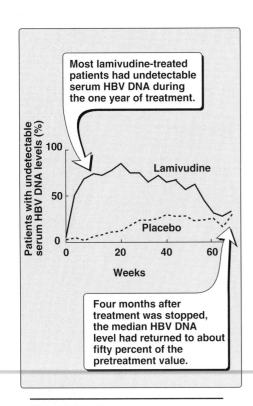

Figure 29.10
Effect of lamivudine therapy on the levels of serum HBV DNA (expressed as percentages of patients with undetectable HBV DNA).

1. **Active immunization:** The HBsAg is used to prepare vaccines conferring protection, because it is antibody to this virion component that neutralizes infectivity. Recombinant DNA techniques made it possible to clone the gene for HBsAg in yeast, and this is now the source of a virtually unlimited supply of vaccine. Thus immunization has become feasible on a population-wide scale. HBV vaccination is now recommended as one of the routine infant immunizations, as is the immunization of adolescents who were not given the vaccine as infants. An unusual feature of the recommended vaccination schedule (see Figure 5.8, p. 41) is to initiate an HBV vaccine series at birth. This is possible because infants have adequate antibody response to neonatal vaccination with the HBV vaccine. Early immunization is desirable because of the risk of vertical transmission in cases where the mother is infected or is at high risk for HBV infection. Similarly, adults in health care professions, or with lifestyles that present a high risk of infection, are also among the groups whose protection is recommended (Figure 29.11). Families of recent immigrants from regions of the world in which HBV is endemic are also targeted for immunization, because they represent a major reservoir of the virus in the United States.

2. **Passive immunization:** Hepatitis B immune globulin (HBIG) is prepared from the blood of donors having a high titer of anti-HBs antibody. Immediate administration of HBIG is recommended as the initial step in preventing infection of individuals accidentally exposed to HBV-contaminated blood by needle stick or other means, and of those exposed to infection by sexual contact with an HBV-positive partner. [Note: In such cases, this should be accompanied by a course of active immunization with the hepatitis B vaccine.] It is also strongly recommended that pregnant women should be screened for HBsAg. Infants born to mothers who are HBV-positive are given HBIG plus hepatitis B vaccine at birth, followed by additional doses of vaccine at one and six months. [Note: The two injections must be given at separate anatomical sites to prevent injected HBIG from neutralizing the injected vaccine.] The goal is to prevent the later chronic liver disease and HCC that occur with high frequency in individuals infected as infants.

III. HEPATITIS D VIRUS ("DELTA AGENT")

Hepatitis D virus (HDV) is found in nature only as a coinfection with HBV. Its significance lies in the fact that its presence results in more severe acute disease, with a greater risk of fulminant hepatitis, and, in chronically infected patients, a greater risk of cirrhosis and liver cancer.

A. Structure and replication

HDV does not fall into any of the other known groups of animal viruses. It has a circular, single-stranded RNA genome with negative polarity that codes for one protein, the **delta antigen**, with which the genome is complexed in the virion (Figure 29.12). In the infectious particle, the nucleoprotein complex is enclosed within an envelope

Routine immunization

- All infants and previously unvaccinated children by the age of 11 years

Increased risk of hepatitis B

- People with multiple sexual partners
- Sexual partner or household contacts of HBsAg-positive people
- Homosexually active men
- Users of illicit injection drugs
- Travelers to regions of endemic disease
- People occupationally exposed to blood or body fluids
- Hemodialysis patients
- Patients receiving clotting-factor concentrates

Figure 29.11
Candidates for hepatitis B virus immunization.

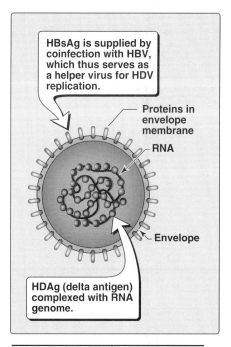

Figure 29.12
Structure of hepatitis D virus.

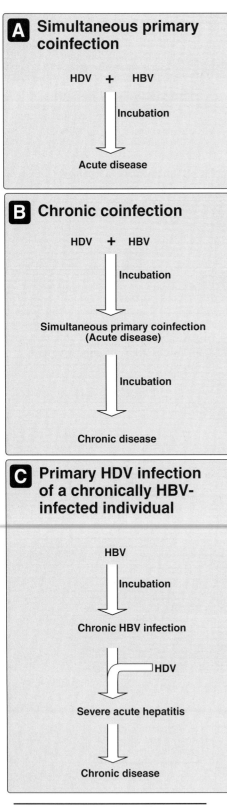

A Simultaneous primary coinfection

HDV + HBV

↓ Incubation

Acute disease

B Chronic coinfection

HDV + HBV

↓ Incubation

Simultaneous primary coinfection
(Acute disease)

↓ Incubation

Chronic disease

C Primary HDV infection of a chronically HBV-infected individual

HBV

↓ Incubation

Chronic HBV infection

HDV

↓

Severe acute hepatitis

↓

Chronic disease

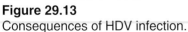

Figure 29.13
Consequences of HDV infection.

containing HBV-coded HBsAg. Thus HDV requires HBV to serve as a **helper virus** for infectious HDV production. The HDV RNA genome is replicated and transcribed in the nucleus by cellular enzymes, whose specificity is probably modified by complexing with the delta protein. [Note: This phase of HDV replication is independent of HBV, whose only helper function is to supply HBsAg for the envelope.]

B. Transmission and pathogenesis

Because HDV exists only in association with HBV, it can be transmitted by the same routes. However, it does not appear to be transmitted sexually as frequently as are HBV or HIV. Pathologically, liver damage is essentially the same as in other viral hepatitides, but the presence of HDV usually results in more extensive and severe damage.

C. Clinical significance

Disease due to HDV can occur in one of three variations (Figure 29.13). First, **simultaneous primary coinfection** with both HBV and HDV can cause an acute disease that is similar to that caused by HBV alone, except that, depending on the relative concentrations of the two agents, two successive episodes of acute hepatitis may occur. The risk of fatal fulminant hepatitis due to the presence of HDV is also considerably higher than with HBV alone. The likelihood of progression to the second variation of HDV disease, **chronic coinfection** with HBV, is greatly increased as well. In this case, cirrhosis and HCC, or death due to liver failure, also develop more frequently than with HBV infection alone. The third variation—**primary HDV infection of a chronically HBV-infected individual**—leads to an episode of severe acute hepatitis after a short incubation period, and develops into chronic HDV infection in over seventy percent of the cases. Again in this situation, the risk of the acute hepatitis becoming fulminant is greatly increased, and the persistent infection is often of the severe chronic type (see p. 342).

D. Laboratory identification

The immunologically based methods used to diagnosis HBV are also applied to HDV. The delta (or D) antigen in serum, and IgM antibodies to it, can be detected. The presence of HDV RNA in serum or in liver tissue, as detected by hybridization with or without the use of reverse transcriptase and PCR amplification, is an indicator of active infection.

E. Treatment and prevention

No specific treatment for HDV infection is available. Because HDV depends on coinfection with HBV, the approaches for preventing HBV infection are also effective in preventing HDV infection. There is no vaccine specifically for HDV. Therefore, those who are chronically infected with HBV can only be protected from HDV infection by limiting chances for exposure. Those who are protected against HBV infection through vaccination will not be affected by HDV.

A summary of the hepatitis viruses is presented in Figure 29.14.

Disease Summary: HEPATITIS

A Common pathogens[1]

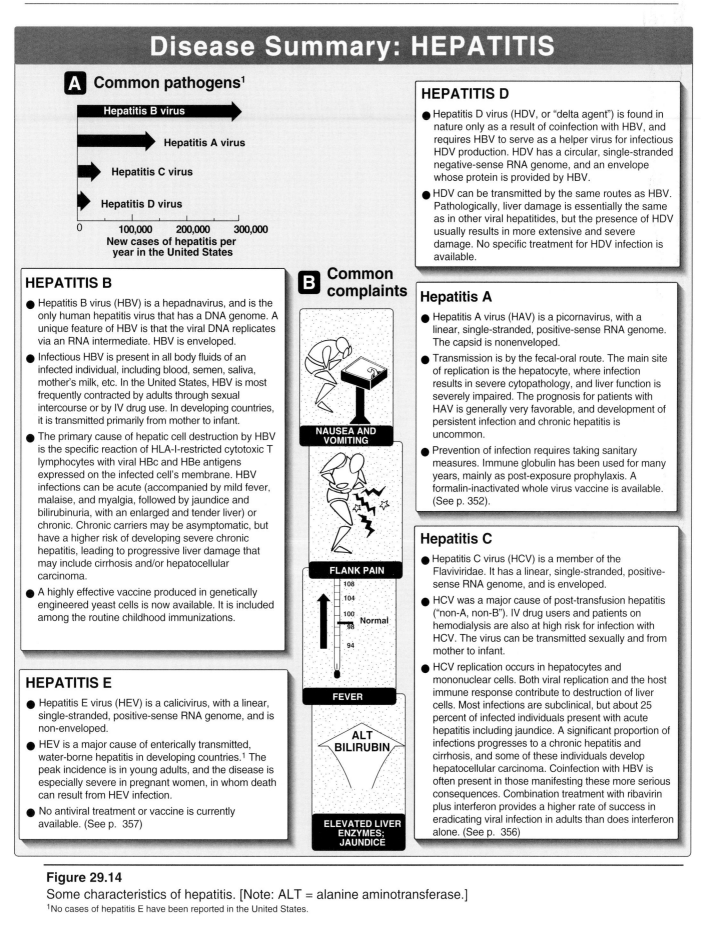

Hepatitis B virus

Hepatitis A virus

Hepatitis C virus

Hepatitis D virus

0   100,000   200,000   300,000
New cases of hepatitis per year in the United States

HEPATITIS D

- Hepatitis D virus (HDV, or "delta agent") is found in nature only as a result of coinfection with HBV, and requires HBV to serve as a helper virus for infectious HDV production. HDV has a circular, single-stranded negative-sense RNA genome, and an envelope whose protein is provided by HBV.

- HDV can be transmitted by the same routes as HBV. Pathologically, liver damage is essentially the same as in other viral hepatitides, but the presence of HDV usually results in more extensive and severe damage. No specific treatment for HDV infection is available.

HEPATITIS B

- Hepatitis B virus (HBV) is a hepadnavirus, and is the only human hepatitis virus that has a DNA genome. A unique feature of HBV is that the viral DNA replicates via an RNA intermediate. HBV is enveloped.

- Infectious HBV is present in all body fluids of an infected individual, including blood, semen, saliva, mother's milk, etc. In the United States, HBV is most frequently contracted by adults through sexual intercourse or by IV drug use. In developing countries, it is transmitted primarily from mother to infant.

- The primary cause of hepatic cell destruction by HBV is the specific reaction of HLA-I-restricted cytotoxic T lymphocytes with viral HBc and HBe antigens expressed on the infected cell's membrane. HBV infections can be acute (accompanied by mild fever, malaise, and myalgia, followed by jaundice and bilirubinuria, with an enlarged and tender liver) or chronic. Chronic carriers may be asymptomatic, but have a higher risk of developing severe chronic hepatitis, leading to progressive liver damage that may include cirrhosis and/or hepatocellular carcinoma.

- A highly effective vaccine produced in genetically engineered yeast cells is now available. It is included among the routine childhood immunizations.

B Common complaints

NAUSEA AND VOMITING

FLANK PAIN

108
104
100   Normal
98
94

FEVER

ALT
BILIRUBIN

ELEVATED LIVER ENZYMES; JAUNDICE

Hepatitis A

- Hepatitis A virus (HAV) is a picornavirus, with a linear, single-stranded, positive-sense RNA genome. The capsid is nonenveloped.

- Transmission is by the fecal-oral route. The main site of replication is the hepatocyte, where infection results in severe cytopathology, and liver function is severely impaired. The prognosis for patients with HAV is generally very favorable, and development of persistent infection and chronic hepatitis is uncommon.

- Prevention of infection requires taking sanitary measures. Immune globulin has been used for many years, mainly as post-exposure prophylaxis. A formalin-inactivated whole virus vaccine is available. (See p. 352).

Hepatitis C

- Hepatitis C virus (HCV) is a member of the Flaviviridae. It has a linear, single-stranded, positive-sense RNA genome, and is enveloped.

- HCV was a major cause of post-transfusion hepatitis ("non-A, non-B"). IV drug users and patients on hemodialysis are also at high risk for infection with HCV. The virus can be transmitted sexually and from mother to infant.

- HCV replication occurs in hepatocytes and mononuclear cells. Both viral replication and the host immune response contribute to destruction of liver cells. Most infections are subclinical, but about 25 percent of infected individuals present with acute hepatitis including jaundice. A significant proportion of infections progresses to a chronic hepatitis and cirrhosis, and some of these individuals develop hepatocellular carcinoma. Coinfection with HBV is often present in those manifesting these more serious consequences. Combination treatment with ribavirin plus interferon provides a higher rate of success in eradicating viral infection in adults than does interferon alone. (See p. 356)

HEPATITIS E

- Hepatitis E virus (HEV) is a calicivirus, with a linear, single-stranded, positive-sense RNA genome, and is non-enveloped.

- HEV is a major cause of enterically transmitted, water-borne hepatitis in developing countries.[1] The peak incidence is in young adults, and the disease is especially severe in pregnant women, in whom death can result from HEV infection.

- No antiviral treatment or vaccine is currently available. (See p. 357)

Figure 29.14

Some characteristics of hepatitis. [Note: ALT = alanine aminotransferase.]

[1]No cases of hepatitis E have been reported in the United States.

Study Questions

Choose the ONE correct answer

29.1 Killing of liver cells infected with hepatitis B virus is primarily due to:

A. shut-off of cellular protein synthesis.

B. intracytoplasmic accumulation of aggregates of HBV antigens.

C. degradation of cellular mRNA.

D. attack by cytotoxic T lymphocytes directed against HBV antigens.

E. virus-induced aberrant chromosome rearrangements and deletions.

> Correct answer = D. There is no evidence that HBV infection is itself cytocidal. Protein synthesis is not shut off, and mRNA is not degraded in infected cells. Accumulation of HBV proteins is not observed, rather they are actively exported. Whereas chromosome damage is observed in cells of primary hepatocellular carcinoma, it is not characteristic of nonmalignant infected liver cells.

29.2 The most common natural mode of transmission of infection with hepatitis B virus is via:

A. contaminated water supply.

B. body fluids, such as urine, semen, etc.

C. respiratory droplets.

D. direct contact.

E. infected insect vectors.

> Correct answer = B. HBV is found at high levels in all body fluids, which results in transmission from mother to newborn, from sibling to sibling, in sexual intercourse, and by infection by virus-containing blood. Contaminated water or food is the typical source of HAV and HEV infection.

29.3 Hepatitis delta virus is unique in that:

A. infectivity requires an envelope protein provided by a helper virus.

B. it has an RNA genome that is replicated by a replicase supplied by a coinfecting helper virus.

C. its mRNA is transcribed by a transcriptase supplied by a helper virus.

D. the virion contains a reverse transcriptase provided by a helper virus.

E. it encodes a protein (HDAg) that replaces helper virus glycoproteins in the envelopes of helper virus particles.

> Correct answer = A. The only function of the HBV helper is to supply the envelope. B: Genome replication requires a cell RNA polymerase, presumably modified by the HDV delta protein such that it can use the HDV RNA as a template. C: Transcription likewise depends on cell enzymes. D: The virion contains only the delta protein. E: The HDAg is complexed with the RNA genome in the HDV virion, and is not found in the HBV virion.

29.4 Which of the following lines of evidence implicate HBV as a cause of hepatocellular carcinoma (HCC)?

A. A specific HBV protein is present in all of the cells of a majority of HCCs.

B. The HBV genome contains a specific oncogene-related sequence that is found in all cells of a majority of HCCs.

C. Chromosomally integrated, complete HBV genomes are found in all cells of a majority of HCCs.

D. All HCCs occurring in HBV-infected individuals contain a unique chromosomal rearrangement not found in other liver malignancies.

E. Chronic HBV carriers have a much greater risk of developing HCC than do noncarriers.

> Correct answer = E. Although HBV DNA is found integrated in a high percent of HCCs, most are present only as partial genomes, and there is no single HBV sequence characteristic of all HCCs. Furthermore, none of the HBV genes show any relationship to known oncogenes. Lastly, although chromosome rearrangements and deletions are common in the cells of HCCs, there is no single change that is characteristic of HCC.

29.5 In a chronically infected individual, the most important indicator of active virus replication, and corresponding risk of HBV transmission from that individual, is the presence of which one of the following in the blood?

A. HBsAg

B. Anti-HBs antibody

C. HBeAg

D. Anti-HBe antibody

E. HBcAg

> Correct answer = C. A and D: HBsAg is indicative of infection, but if it is accompanied by the presence of anti-HBe antibody the level of infectious HBV is generally very low. In contrast, if it is accompanied by HBeAg, infectivity is usually very high. B: Antibody to HBsAg is an indicator of immunity to infection. E: The HBcAg is not found free in serum during acute or chronic infection.

Positive-strand RNA Viruses

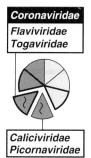
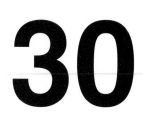

I. OVERVIEW

Viruses with a positive-strand RNA genome (that is, one that can serve as a messenger RNA in the infected cell) include the viral families Picorna-, Toga-, Flavi-, Calici-, and Coronaviridae. The viruses in these families cause a broad spectrum of diseases, but share the following features: 1) they replicate in the cytoplasm; 2) the genomic RNAs serve as messenger RNAs and are infectious; 3) the genomic RNAs are non-segmented; 4) the virions do not contain any enzymes; and 5) virus-specified proteins are synthesized as polyproteins that are processed in some cases by viral and in other cases by cellular proteases, giving rise to the individual viral proteins. Some positive-strand RNA viruses are enveloped; others are not. Figure 30.1 summarizes the positive-strand RNA viruses discussed in this chapter.

II. FAMILY PICORNAVIRIDAE

The picornaviruses are small, naked (nonenveloped), icosahedral viruses (Figure 30.2), which contain a single-stranded, non-segmented, RNA genome, and four structural proteins. The Picornaviridae are divided into five genera: the enteroviruses, rhinoviruses, cardioviruses, aphthoviruses, and hepatoviruses. The cardioviruses cause encephalitis and myocarditis in mice, whereas the genus aphthovirus is represented by the foot and mouth disease virus, which infects cattle. The entero-, rhino-, and hepatoviruses cause a wide variety of clinical syndromes in humans. [Note: The most intensively studied of the picornaviruses is poliovirus, but what has been learned about the structure and replication of polioviruses also applies in large measure to the other viruses in this family.]

A. Genus Enterovirus

Enteroviruses account for an estimated ten to fifteen million symptomatic infections per year in the United States. More than seventy enteroviruses have been identified. These include the three serotypes of **poliovirus**, 30 of **coxsackievirus**, and 34 of **echovirus**. The practice currently is that, as new enteroviruses are identified, they are not assigned to one of these groups, but are simply given numerical designations, for example, enterovirus 68, enterovirus 69, and so forth.

1. **Epidemiology:** Individuals are infected with enteroviruses by ingestion of contaminated food or water. Enteroviruses are stable at the

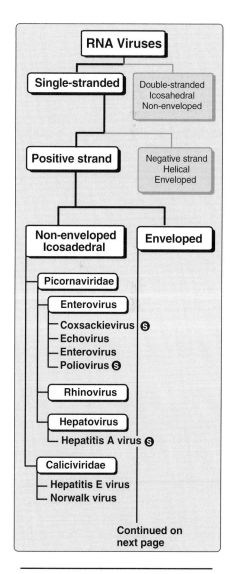

Figure 30.1
Classification of positive-strand RNA viruses (continued on next page). Ⓢ See p. 401 for summaries of these viruses.

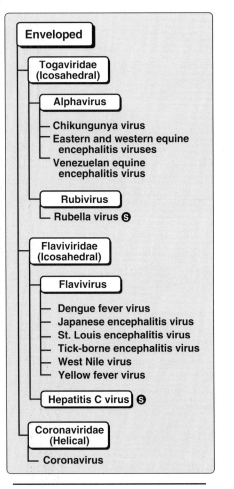

Figure 30.1 (continued)
Classification of positive-strand
RNA viruses. ❻ See p. 401
for summaries of these viruses.

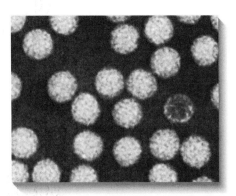

Figure 30.2
Poliovirus, a type of picornavirus,
is one of the simplest and smallest
viruses.

low pH of the stomach, replicate in the GI tract, and are excreted in the stool. Thus, these viruses are said to be transmitted by the **fecal-oral route**. After replicating in the oropharynx and intestinal tract lymphoid tissue, enteroviruses can leave the intestine by entering the bloodstream, and thus spread to various target organs (for example, poliovirus spreads to the CNS). Although the great majority of infections are asymptomatic, infection, whether clinical or subclinical, usually results in protective immunity.

2. **Viral replication:** Enteroviruses bind to specific receptors on host cell surfaces. For example, poliovirus binds to a receptor that is a member of the immunoglobulin supergene family of proteins (see p. 70). Cells lacking these specific receptors are not susceptible to infection.

   a. **Mechanism of genome replication:** This process is the same as that described for Type I RNA viruses (see p. 301), namely, the incoming parental RNA serves as the template for a genome-size, negative-strand RNA, and this in turn serves as a template for multiple copies of progeny positive-strand RNA. [Note: Unlike most mRNA molecules in animal cells, the RNA of picornaviruses does not have a 5' methylated guanine cap.[1] Instead, a long nucleotide sequence in the 5' untranslated region of the RNA forms a secondary structure to which ribosomes bind. This secondary structure is called an internal ribosomal entry site or IRES. A polyA sequence[1] is present at the 3' end of the viral RNA.]

   b. **Translation:** Enterovirus RNA contains a single, long, open reading frame. Translation of this message results in the synthesis of a single, long polyprotein, which is processed by viral proteases into structural proteins and nonstructural proteins, including the viral RNA polymerase needed to synthesize additional copies of the viral genome.

3. **General clinical significance of enterovirus infections:** All enteroviruses can cause CNS disease. For example, they are currently the major recognizable cause of **acute aseptic meningitis** syndrome—a term that refers to any meningitis (infectious or noninfectious) for which the cause is not clear after initial examination plus routine stains and cultures of the cerebrospinal fluid (CSF). Viral meningitis is a common infection in the United States, with an estimated 75,000 cases each year. Viral meningitis can usually be distinguished from bacterial meningitis because 1) the viral disease is milder; 2) there is an elevation of lymphocytes in the CSF, rather than the elevated neutrophils seen in bacterial meningitis; and 3) the glucose concentration in the CSF is not decreased. Viral meningitis occurs mainly in the summer and fall, affecting both children and adults. The treatment is symptomatic, and the course of the illness is usually benign. Viruses can be isolated from the stool, or from various target organs (CNS in fatal cases, or from conjunctival fluid in cases of conjunctivitis). Evidence of

[1]See p. 379 in *Lippincott's Illustrated Reviews: Biochemistry* (2nd ed.) for a discussion of the structure of mRNA.

infection can also be obtained by demonstration of a rise in antibody titer against a specific enterovirus. No antiviral drugs are available for treatment of enterovirus infections.

4. **Clinical significance of poliovirus infection:** Poliomyelitis is an acute illness in which the poliovirus selectively destroys the lower motor neurons of the spinal cord and brainstem, resulting in flaccid, asymmetrical weakness or paralysis. In the United States, no cases of paralytic poliomyelitis due to wild-type poliovirus have occurred in over twenty years. The few cases of polio that occur (less than ten per year) are all due to the reversion to virulence of the virus in the live-attenuated Sabin polio vaccine (see below). In countries with low immunization rates, paralytic polio continues to occur, with significant numbers of cases in sub-Saharan Africa and southern Asia. However, the World Health Organization has set the goal of eradicating polio from the world within the next decade.

a. **Transmission and pathogenesis:** Poliovirus infections may follow one of several courses: 1) asymptomatic infection, which occurs in 90 to 95 percent of cases and causes no disease and no sequelae; 2) abortive infection; 3) nonparalytic infection; or 4) paralytic poliomyelitis (Figure 30.3). The classic presentation of paralytic poliomyelitis is **flaccid paralysis**, most often affecting the lower limbs. This is due to viral replication in, and destruction of, the lower motor neurons in the anterior horn of the spinal cord (Figure 30.4). **Respiratory paralysis** may also occur, following infection of the brain stem. Poliomyelitis should be considered in any unimmunized person with the combination of fever, headache, neck and back pain, asymmetric flaccid paralysis without sensory loss, and pleocytosis (an increase in the number of lymphocytes in the spinal fluid).

b. **Prognosis:** Permanent weakness is observed in approximately two thirds of patients with paralytic poliomyelitis. Complete recovery is less likely when acute paralysis is severe, and patients requiring mechanical ventilation because of respiratory paralysis rarely recover without some permanent disability.

c. **Postpoliomyelitis syndrome:** Approximately twenty to thirty percent of patients who partially or fully recover from paralytic poliomyelitis experience a new onset of muscle weakness, pain, atrophy, and fatigue 25 to 35 years after the acute illness.

d. **Treatment and prevention:** Specific antiviral agents for the treatment of poliomyelitis are not available. Management, therefore, is supportive and symptomatic. Vaccination is the only effective method of preventing poliomyelitis (see p. 42). Poliomyelitis can be prevented by either **live-attenuated (Sabin)** or **killed (Salk) polio vaccines**. These vaccines have led to the elimination of wild-type polio from Western Europe, Japan, and the Americas. [Note: Killed polio vaccine has no adverse effects, whereas live polio vaccine may undergo reversion to a virulent form while it multiplies in the human intestinal

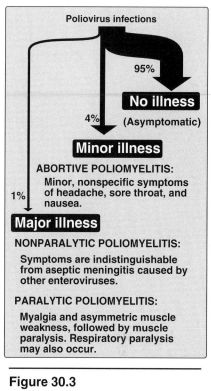

Figure 30.3
Clinical outcomes of infection with poliovirus.

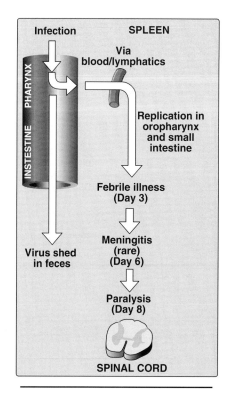

Figure 30.4
CNS invasion by poliovirus.

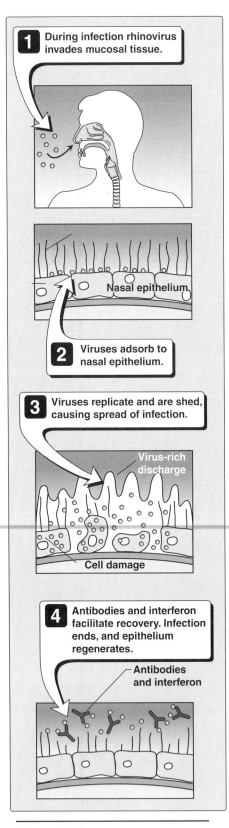

Figure 30.5
Pathogenesis of common cold showing stages from infection to recovery.

tract, and may cause vaccine-associated paralytic poliomyelitis in those receiving the vaccine. This risk is very low, but since 1979, vaccine-associated poliomyelitis has accounted for all of the four to eight cases per year of paralytic poliomyelitis that have occurred in the United States.]

5. **Clinical significance of coxsackievirus and echovirus infections:** These give rise to a large variety of clinical syndromes including meningitis, upper respiratory infections, gastroenteritis, herpangina (severe sore throat with vesiculoulcerative lesions), pleurisy, pericarditis, myocarditis, and myositis.

6. **Clinical significance of enteroviruses 70 and 71 infections:** These have been associated with severe CNS disease. A particularly acute form of extremely contagious hemorrhagic conjunctivitis has also been associated with enterovirus 70.

B. Genus rhinovirus

Rhinoviruses cause the **common-cold syndrome** (Figure 30.5). They differ in two important respects from enteroviruses. First, whereas enteroviruses are acid-stable (they must survive the acid environment of the stomach), rhinoviruses are acid-labile. Second, rhinoviruses, which replicate in the nasal passages, have an optimal temperature for replication that is lower than that of enteroviruses. [Note: This permits rhinovirus to replicate efficiently at temperatures several degrees below body temperature.] Rhinovirus replication is similar to that of the poliovirus (see p. 350). There are more than 100 serotypes of rhinoviruses; therefore development of a vaccine is impractical. Studies have shown that in addition to spread by respiratory droplets, rhinoviruses can also be spread by hand-to-hand contact. Thus washing of hands at appropriate intervals can be a useful preventive measure.

C. Genus hepatovirus

The sole member of this genus is **hepatitis A virus** (HAV). Although at one time HAV was also known as enterovirus 72, sufficient differences have been found between HAV and the enteroviruses to warrant placing HAV in a genus by itself. HAV, of which there is only one serotype, causes viral hepatitis (see Figure 29.2, p. 338). As with the enteroviruses, transmission is by the fecal-oral route, and the virus is shed in the feces. For example, a common mode of transmission of the virus is through eating uncooked shellfish harvested from sewage-contaminated water. The main site of replication is the hepatocyte. Viral replication results in severe cytopathology, and liver function is significantly impaired (Figure 30.6). In contrast to most of the other picornaviruses, HAV grows poorly in tissue culture. The prognosis for patients with hepatitis A is generally very favorable, and the development of persistent infection and chronic hepatitis is uncommon. Prevention depends on taking measures to avoid fecal contamination of food and water; therefore HAV infection is most common in underdeveloped countries with poor sanitation (Figure 30.7). Immune globulin has been used for many years, mainly as postexposure prophylaxis. Vaccines prepared from whole virus inactivated with formaldehyde are now available. See Figure 29.14, p. 347, for a comparison of HAV to the other hepatitis viruses.

III. FAMILY TOGAVIRIDAE

The togaviruses are enveloped, icosahedral viruses that contain a positive-sense, single-stranded RNA genome, and generally three structural proteins. The capsid (or C) protein encloses the viral RNA, forming the nucleocapsid; the two other proteins, E1 and E2, are glycoproteins that form the hemagglutinin-containing viral spikes that project from the lipid bilayer. The family Togaviridae is divided into two genera—alphavirus and rubivirus.

A. Genus alphavirus

The alphaviruses, of which there are approximately 26, are arthropod-borne viruses (**arboviruses**), and are transmitted to humans and domestic animals by mosquitoes. All alphaviruses share a common group antigen. [Note: Some arboviruses were initially isolated from horses, hence the word "equine" in their names (see below).]

1. **Epidemiology and pathogenesis:** Alphaviruses have a broad host range, being able to replicate in organisms that are widely separated phylogenetically, such as mosquitoes and humans. Following inoculation of an alphavirus by a mosquito, the patient is observed to have a viremia, following which the virus may be seeded in various target organs, for example, the CNS in the case of the encephalitis viruses. [Note: Togaviruses reproduce in but do not kill arthropod cells; they do kill vertebrate cells.]

2. **Viral replication:** Following attachment to the cell surface, the virus is internalized by receptor-mediated endocytosis. Like the picornaviruses, genome replication is as described for Type I RNA viruses (see p. 301). However, cells infected with alphaviruses contain not one but two viral mRNA species: the genome-length RNA that serves as the messenger RNA for translation of the nonstructural proteins, and a subgenomic RNA that serves as the messenger RNA for the structural proteins. The genome-length, negative-strand RNA serves as the template for both mRNA species. Both viral mRNA species resemble typical mRNAs in animal cells, having a methylated cap at their 5' end and a polyA tail at their 3' end.The envelope proteins, E1 and E2, are membrane proteins that are transported through the endoplasmic reticulum and Golgi system to the cell surface. Nucleocapsids move to areas of the plasma membrane that have been modified by insertion of the envelope proteins. There they bud through the plasma membrane, thus acquiring an envelope (see Figure 26.16, 304).

3. **Clinical significance:** Several different clinical syndromes are associated with alphavirus infections of humans. These include 1) acute encephalitis (**eastern and western equine encephalitis viruses**), 2) acute arthropathy (**Chikungunya virus**), and 3) a febrile illness with a flu-like syndrome (**Venezuelan equine encephalitis virus**). The great majority of infections, however, are subclinical, and can be diagnosed only by the demonstration of an immune response.

4. **Laboratory identification:** This is generally accomplished by the demonstration of a rise in antibody titer (that is, comparing acute

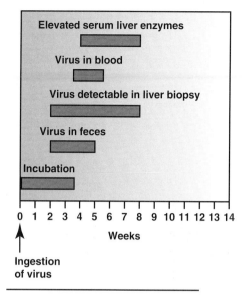

Figure 30.6
Time course of hepatitis A infection.

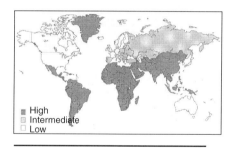

Figure 30.7
Distribution of hepatitis A virus infection worldwide.

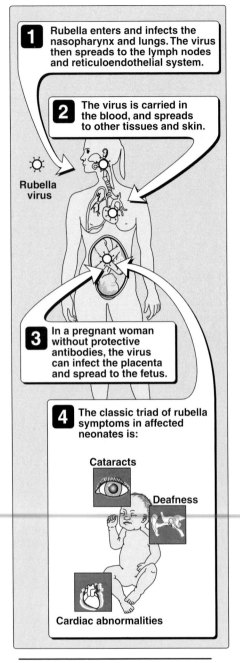

1 Rubella enters and infects the nasopharynx and lungs. The virus then spreads to the lymph nodes and reticuloendothelial system.

2 The virus is carried in the blood, and spreads to other tissues and skin.

Rubella virus

3 In a pregnant woman without protective antibodies, the virus can infect the placenta and spread to the fetus.

4 The classic triad of rubella symptoms in affected neonates is:

Cataracts

Deafness

Cardiac abnormalities

Figure 30.8
Pathology of rubella virus infection.

and convalescent sera). In fatal cases of encephalitis, the virus may be isolated from the CNS.

5. **Prevention:** The most important measure for prevention of alphavirus infection is control of the mosquito vector population. A Venezuelan equine encephalitis vaccine is available.

B. Genus rubivirus

The sole member of the rubivirus genus is **rubella virus**. The structure and replication of rubella virus are basically as described for the alphaviruses (see p. 353). Respiratory secretions of an infected person are the primary vehicles for rubella virus transmission. Rubella causes a very mild clinical syndrome that is characterized by a generalized maculopapular rash, and occipital lymphadenopathy ["**German measles**", not to be confused with "measles" (rubeola), caused by the measles virus, see p. 383]. In most cases, these symptoms may be hardly noticeable, and the infection remains subclinical. For this reason, the only reliable evidence for a prior infection with rubella virus is the demonstration of antirubella antibodies. The clinical significance of rubella lies not in the primary infection described above, but rather in the fact that when a woman is infected during pregnancy, there can be severe damage to the developing fetus, especially in the first trimester (**congenital rubella**). This damage can include congenital heart disease, cataracts, hepatitis, or abnormalities related to the CNS such as mental retardation, motor dysfunction, and deafness (Figure 30.8). Fetal damage due to rubella infection is preventable by use of the live attenuated rubella vaccine (see p. 43) that is included with the routine childhood vaccinations. This vaccine, which has few complications, is effective in preventing congenital rubella because it reduces the reservoir of the virus in the childhood populations, and also ensures that when women reach childbearing age, they are immune to rubella infection. [Note: The vaccine should not be given to women who are already pregnant, or to immunocompromised patients, including babies.] In the United States rubella outbreaks often begin among infected persons from countries where rubella is not included in routine immunizations.

IV. FAMILY FLAVIVIRIDAE

The members of this family are enveloped viruses that contain a single-stranded RNA genome, and three structural proteins. The capsid (or C) protein and the viral RNA form the icosahedral nucleocapsid; the other two proteins are envelope-associated. At the present time, the family Flaviviridae is divided into three genera: **flavivirus**, **hepatitis C virus**, and **pestivirus**. [Note: The viruses in the genus pestivirus (classical swine fever virus and bovine viral diarrhea virus) are of veterinary interest only.]

A. Genus flavivirus

The genus flavivirus is composed of more than sixty viruses. These include many viruses of medical importance such as **yellow fever**, **St. Louis encephalitis**, **Japanese encephalitis**, **dengue fever viruses**, and **West Nile virus**, all of which are mosquito-transmitted. **Tick-borne encephalitis virus** is, of course, transmitted by ticks. [Note: Like the viruses in the alphavirus genus of the family Togaviridae (see p. 353), most of the viruses in this genus are thus arboviruses.] All of the viruses in the genus flavivirus share a common group antigen.

1. **Epidemiology and pathogenesis:** As arboviruses, the medically important members of this genus are transmitted to humans by the bite of an infected mosquito or tick. These viruses are maintained in nature by replicating alternately in an arthropod vector and in a vertebrate host. In some cases (for example, St. Louis encephalitis virus) the usual vertebrate host is a bird, and the human is only an accidental host. In contrast, humans are the usual vertebrate hosts for yellow fever and dengue viruses. Figure 30.9 shows the global distributions of yellow fever and dengue fever.

2. **Replication:** Following attachment to the cell surface, the virus is taken up by receptor-mediated endocytosis (see Figure 26.9, p. 299). The viral RNA has a 5' methylated cap, but is not polyadenylated at the 3' terminus. Replication of the viral RNA is as described for Type I RNA viruses (see p. 301). Only one species of viral mRNA—the genomic RNA—is found in infected cells. It is translated into a single, long polyprotein, which is processed by virus-coded and cellular proteases, giving rise to three structural and seven nonstructural proteins. Nucleocapsids are formed in the cytoplasm, and maturation of the viral particle occurs by envelopment of the nucleocapsid, not at the plasma membrane as with viruses in the family Togaviridae, but instead, at cytoplasmic golgi membranes. Virus particles then accumulate in vesicles, and are extruded when the vesicles move to the cell surface.

3. **Clinical significance:** Viruses in the genus flavivirus are associated with several different clinical syndromes. These include: encephalitis (St. Louis encephalitis, Japanese encephalitis, and tick-borne encephalitis viruses), hemorrhagic fever (yellow fever virus), and fever, myalgia, and rash (the dengue viruses). [Note: Although there is little mortality associated with classic dengue fever, in certain parts of the world, such as Southeast Asia, a severe form of dengue infection occurs particularly in infants and young children. This is termed **dengue hemorrhagic fever**, or **dengue shock syndrome**, and is associated with a significant mortality (ten percent or higher) if untreated.] Like dengue fever, **West Nile fever** is a mosquito-transmitted, acute, usually self-limited illness that presents chiefly with fever, malaise, lymphadenopathy, and rash. Infection may also result in aseptic meningitis or meningoencephalitis, especially in the elderly. The first outbreak of West Nile encephalitis in the United States occurred in the New York City area in the summer of 1999, and has occurred in other northeastern states in subsequent years.

4. **Laboratory identification:** A specific diagnosis is most often made by serologic means (that is, by demonstrating at least a four-fold rise in antibody titer, when comparing acute and convalescent sera). In some cases, virus isolation or demonstration of specific viral antigens is also feasible.

5. **Prevention:** A safe, highly effective, live attenuated vaccine for yellow fever has been available for many years (see p.xxx). In China and Japan, a formalin-inactivated Japanese encephalitis virus vac-

■ **Areas most commonly at risk**

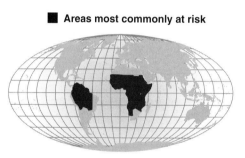

Yellow Fever

Roughly 15,000 cases occur yearly in the tropical regions of South America and Africa. Symptoms include fever, headache, chills, nausea, vomiting, and occasionally jaundice. Serious cases can also affect the liver and kidneys.

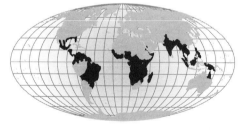

Dengue Fever

Approximately 50 million to 100 million cases occur each year. Characterized by sudden onset of fever, headache, severe myalgia. Severe dengue may lead to shock and hemorrhaging, and death.

Figure 30.9
Global distribution of yellow fever and dengue fever.

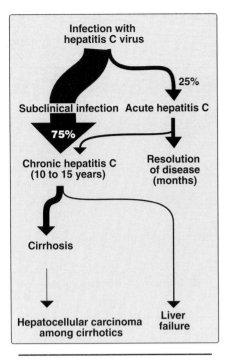

Figure 30.10
Natural history of infection with hepatitis C virus.

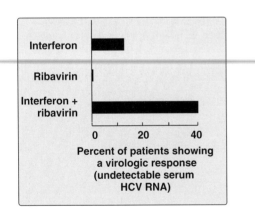

Figure 30.11
Combination treatment with interferon and ribavirin for chronic hepatitis C. [Note: Patients receiving ribavirin alone showed a biologic and histologic response, but no decrease in circulating virus.]

cine is used; and in central Europe, a formalin-inactivated vaccine is widely used to prevent tick-borne encephalitis. Another important method of prevention is vector control. In urban areas, elimination of breeding sites can dramatically reduce the population of *Aedes aegypti* mosquitoes, which serve as the vector for both yellow fever and dengue viruses.

B. Hepatitis C viruses

Hepatitis C virus (HCV) was discovered in 1988 in the course of searching for the cause of non-A, non-B, transfusion-associated hepatitis. At that time, HCV accounted for ninety percent of the cases of non-A, non-B hepatitis. The hepatitis C viruses are quite heterogeneous, and on the basis of their nucleotide sequences, can be divided into six types. It has not been possible thus far to grow HCV efficiently in tissue culture; therefore most of what has been learned about the virus and viral proteins has been by the use of recombinant DNA techniques.

1. **Transmission and pathogenesis:** Although HCV was initially identified as a major cause of posttransfusion hepatitis, intravenous drug users and patients on hemodialysis are also at high risk for infection with HCV. Tattoos are also a leading cause of HCV infection. In addition, there is evidence for sexual transmission of HCV, as well as for transmission from mother to infant. In the infected individual, viral replication occurs in the hepatocyte, and probably also in mononuclear cells (lymphocytes and macrophages). Destruction of liver cells may result both from a direct effect of viral replication and from the host immune response.

2. **Clinical significance:** The majority of infections with HCV are subclinical, but about 25 percent of infected individuals present with acute hepatitis including jaundice (Figure 30.10). More important, a significant proportion of infections progress to a chronic hepatitis and cirrhosis. Finally, some of these individuals go on to develop hepatocellular carcinoma (see p. 343) many years after the primary infection. Thus HCV bears many clinical and epidemiologic similarities to HBV in spite of the distinct molecular differences between the two. Figure 30.12 presents a summary comparison of HAV, HBC, and HCV.

3. **Laboratory identification:** A specific diagnosis can be made by demonstration of antibodies that react with a combination of recombinant viral proteins. Sensitive tests are also now available for detection of the viral nucleic acid by RT-PCR (PCR that amplifies a DNA copy—synthesized using **r**everse **t**ranscriptase—of the viral RNA, see p. 32).

4. **Treatment and prevention:** Tests to screen blood for HCV have been available for several years, so that HCV as a cause of transfusion-associated hepatitis is now unusual. Treatment of patients with chronic hepatitis by interferon–α is sometimes of benefit, but in most cases, only for the period during which the patient is receiving the interferon. Treatment with α-interferon plus ribavirin provides a significantly improved response, and combination therapy is the treatment of choice (Figure 30.11). Chronic hepatitis resulting in severe liver damage may be an indication for a liver transplant.

V. FAMILY CALICIVIRIDAE

Caliciviruses are small, non-enveloped, spherical particles. Each contains a single-stranded, nonsegmented RNA genome, and a single species of capsid protein. In contrast to the picornaviruses, the caliciviruses genome contains three open reading frames. Norwalk virus is the prototype human calicivirus. There are at least four strains of human caliciviruses.

A. Caliciviruses

Norwalk virus replicates in the gastrointestinal tract, and is shed in the stool. Infection by the Norwalk virus is by the fecal-oral route, following the ingestion of contaminated food or water. Norwalk virus is a major cause of epidemic acute gastroenteritis, particularly at schools, camps, military bases, prisons, and similar settings. It affects primarily adults and school-age children, but not infants. The clinical presentation is characterized generally by nausea, vomiting, and diarrhea. Symptoms last 24 to 48 hours, and the disease is self-limited. Radioimmunoassays and ELISA tests are available for the detection of antiviral antibodies (see p. 30). No specific antiviral treatment is available. Careful attention to hand washing, and measures to prevent contamination of food and water supplies, should reduce the incidence of these infections.

B. Hepatitis E virus (HEV)

HEV is a non-enveloped, single-stranded RNA virus. It is a major cause of enterically transmitted, water-borne hepatitis in developing countries. The peak incidence is in young adults, and the disease is especially severe in pregnant women, in whom death can result from HEV infection. Viral RNA can be detected in the feces of infected individuals by RT-PCR (see p. 32), and nearly all serologically confirmed epidemics of HEV can be attributed to fecally contaminated water. Apart from epidemic situations, the diagnosis of HEV cannot be made in an infected individual solely on clinical grounds. However, specific tests are available to detect antibodies to HEV. The signs and symptoms are similar to those seen with other forms of acute viral hepatitis, but like hepatitis A, progression to chronic hepatitis is not seen. Interestingly, in regions of the world where HEV is rarely, if ever, diagnosed, antibodies to HEV can still be found. No antiviral treatment nor vaccine is currently available. (See Figure 29.14, p. 347 for a summary of viral hepatitis.)

VI. FAMILY CORONAVIRIDAE

Coronaviruses are large, enveloped, pleomorphic particles, with a distinctive arrangement of spikes (peplomers) projecting from their surfaces. [Note: These projections have the appearance of a solar corona, hence the name of the virus.] Coronavirus RNA is the largest described thus far for any RNA virus genome. Virus budding is observed in association with intracytoplasmic membranes, specifically with vesicles located between the rough endoplasmic reticulum and the Golgi system. Human coronaviruses have been most commonly implicated in upper respiratory infections, such as the common cold syndrome.

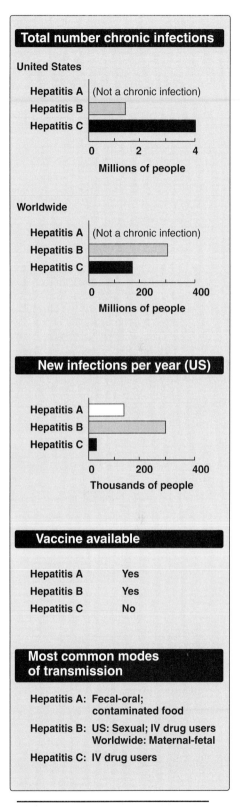

Figure 30.12
Summary of hepatitis A, B, and C.

Study Questions

Questions 30.1 to 30.5:

Match the appropriate virus from the following list with the statement to which it most closely corresponds. Each virus can match one, more than one, or none of the statements.

A. Hepatitis A virus (HAV)
B. Coxsackie viruses
C. Hepatitis C virus (HCV)
D. Hepatitis E virus (HEV)
E. Yellow fever virus
F. Rubella virus

30.1 Intravenous drug users are at high risk

Correct answer = C. Until the recent development of tests for the presence of HCV in blood, HCV was an important cause of transfusion-associated hepatitis. IV drug users are one of several groups still at high risk for infection with this virus.

30.2 Infection caused by bite of an infected mosquito

Correct answer = E. Yellow fever virus is an arthropod-borne virus and is transmitted by the bite of an infected *Aedes aegypti* mosquito. The virus does not spread from person to person.

30.3 Predisposes to hepatocellular carcinoma

Correct answer = C. Unlike HAV, HCV infection has a strong tendency to lead to a chronic hepatitis and cirrhosis, often resulting after many years in hepatocellular carcinoma.

30.4 Causes congenital malformations

Correct answer = F. Infection with rubella virus is generally of little consequence to the adult. The exception is the pregnant woman, in whom rubella virus infection can result in congenital malformations in the fetus. The risk is highest in the first trimester. These malformations can affect the CNS, the liver, the heart, and the eye.

Choose the ONE correct answer

30.5 A company held an elaborate holiday dinner party for its 42 employees. Within three to four weeks, many of the banquet attendees complained of experiencing fatigue, fever, nausea, and dark urine, and were observed to be jaundiced. The group exhibited no bacterial infections in common. The employees who became ill had all eaten raw oysters at the party. The company doctor assayed a sample of the employees' blood for anti-hepatitis B antibodies, but all samples were negative for anti-HBsAg IgM. The causative agent consistent with this history is most likely:

A. hepatitis A virus.
B. hepatitis B virus..
C. hepatitis C virus.
D. hepatitis D virus.
E. hepatitis E virus.

Correct answer = A. Hepatitis A is transmitted by the fecal/oral route, and is most frequently acquired by eating contaminated shellfish, or by contact with a carrier. The symptoms that were exhibited by the party-goers are consistent with liver damage due, for example, to hepatitis. Hepatitis B infection is excluded because of the negative test for antibodies. Hepatitis C infection is acquired most commonly by IV drug users, patients on dialysis, and individuals obtaining tattoos. Hepatitis D infection occurs only in combination with hepatitis B infection. Hepatitis E is a major cause of enterically transmitted, water-borne hepatitis in developing countries.

30.6 Norwalk virus

A. is a major cause of severe diarrhea in infants in the developing countries.
B. is an important cause of epidemic gastroenteritis in the United States.
C. contains an RNA genome with a single open reading frame.
D. is diagnosed by isolation and then growth of the virus in tissue culture.
E. generally causes a severe chronic gastroenteritis with diarrhea that may persist for several weeks.

Correct answer = B. In the United States, Norwalk virus (Family Caliciviridae) tends to infect older children and young adults rather than infants. Rotaviruses are one of the major causes of severe diarrhea in infants in the third world. The RNA genomes of viruses in the Calicivirus family have three open reading frames. Norwalk virus has still not been grown in tissue culture. Norwalk virus does cause gastroenteritis, but the disease is usually acute and self-limited, with signs and symptoms resolving after 24 to 48 hours.

Retroviruses and AIDS

Retroviridae

31

I. OVERVIEW

The family Retroviridae includes a large number of disease-producing animal viruses, several of which are of clinical importance to humans (Figure 31.1). Retroviridae are distinguished from all other RNA viruses by the presence of an unusual enzyme, reverse transcriptase, which converts a single-stranded RNA viral genome into double-stranded viral DNA (see p. 303). Because these viruses reverse the order of information transfer (RNA serving as a template for DNA synthesis, rather than the almost universal DNA serving as a template for RNA synthesis), they are are termed **retro**viruses. [Note: **Retro** is Latin for reversal.] Retroviridae are divided into seven genera on the basis of nucleotide sequence similarity and genome structure. The two genera of human interest are the genus **Lentivirus**, which includes the **human immuno-deficiency viruses 1** and **2** (**HIV-1** and **-2**), and the **human T-cell lymphotropic virus–bovine leukemia virus group** (**HTLV-BLV group**), which contains the **human T-cell leukemia viruses 1** and **2** (**HTLV-1** and **-2**). The lentiviruses cause neurologic and immunologic diseases, but do not have the oncogenic properties of the HTLV-BLV group. The oncogenic capacity of the animal retroviruses, and the hope of identifying one or more of them as a cause of human cancer, were reasons for their initial investigation. The discovery that **acquired immunodeficiency syndrome** (**AIDS**) is also caused by a retrovirus (HIV) greatly increased the attention given to this family of viruses. In this chapter, a consideration of the features common to all retroviruses is presented, following which HIV and HTLV are discussed in detail.

II. RETROVIRUS STRUCTURE

Despite their wide range of disease manifestations, all retroviruses are similar in structure, genome organization, and mode of replication. Retroviruses are enveloped particles (Figure 31.2). The viral envelope, formed from the host cell membrane, contains 72 spiked knobs. These consist of a transmembrane protein, TM (fusion protein, also called gp41), which is linked to a surface protein, SU (attachment protein, gp120), that binds to a cell receptor during infection. Host cell proteins, including the major histocompatibility complex class II proteins, are also

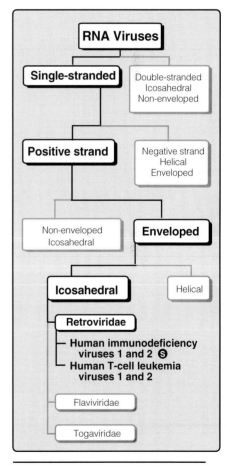

Figure 31.1
Classification of retroviruses that cause disease in humans. ◉ See p. 430 for a summary of this virus.

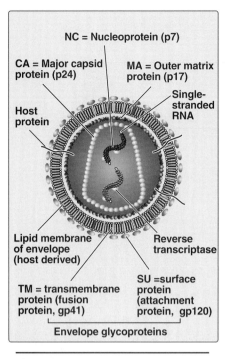

Figure 31.2
Structure of the human
immunodeficiency virus.

found in the envelope. The virion has a cone-shaped, icosahedral core containing the major capsid protein, CA (also called p24). Between the capsid and the envelope is an outer matrix protein, MA (p17), which directs entry of the double-stranded DNA provirus into the nucleus, and is later essential for the process of virus assembly. There are two identical copies of the positive sense, single-stranded RNA genome in the capsid (that is, unlike other viruses, retroviruses are diploid). The RNA is tightly complexed with a basic protein, NC (p7), in a nucleocapsid structure that differs in morphology among the different retrovirus genera. [Note: The designation "gp41" refers to the structure of the molecule, which is a **g**lyco**p**rotein with an originally determined molecular weight of 41,000. "p24" refers to a **p**rotein (nonglycosylated) with a molecular weight of 24,000.] Also found within the capsid are the enzymes reverse transcriptase and integrase (which are required for viral DNA synthesis and integration into the host cell chromosome), and protease (essential for virus assembly). A host cellular tRNA is hydrogen-bonded at the 5' end of each viral RNA molecule, where it functions as a primer for initiation of reverse transcription.

III. HUMAN IMMUNODEFICIENCY VIRUS (HIV)

Acquired immune deficiency syndrome (AIDS) was first reported in the United States in 1981. The earliest cases of AIDS were seen in large urban centers, such as Los Angeles, San Francisco, and New York City. Clusters of young, male homosexual patients exhibited a puzzling complex of symptoms, including severe pneumonia caused by *Pneumocystis carinii* (ordinarily a harmless eukaryotic organism), Kaposi's sarcoma (ordinarily an extremely rare form of cancer), sudden weight loss, swollen lymph nodes, and general suppression of immune function. This constellation of signs and symptoms associated with illness came to be known as acquired immune deficiency syndrome (AIDS). Early attempts at understanding the disease focused on the possibility of immune suppression induced by chronic injecting drug use (IDU) or infection. Soon, however, cases were reported in nonhomosexual, non-IDU patients who had received blood or blood products by transfusion. By 1984, AIDS was recognized as an infectious disease caused by a virus, and eventually HIV was isolated from AIDS patients. In the decade after this initial recognition, AIDS killed more United States citizens than the Korean and Vietnam wars combined. At the beginning of the year 2000, more than 34,000,000 people worldwide were known to be infected with HIV, with three-fourths of these infections occurring in sub-Saharan Africa (Figure 31.3). New infections were occurring at a rate of 16,000/day (6,000,000 per year), a majority of these occurring in individuals under 25 years of age. Worldwide, new infections are almost equally distributed between men and women, with heterosexual activity accounting for the vast majority of the cases. In the United States, the estimated prevalence of HIV has remained steady at 900,000, and the incidence of new cases was 40,000 in 1999 (Figure 31.4). Although the United States and other developed countries have identified combinations of drugs that significantly slow the progression of AIDS, 95 percent of HIV-infected people live in developing countries where, for logistic and financial reasons, few have access to these drugs. The social and economic impact of AIDS is and will continue to be enormous for some time.

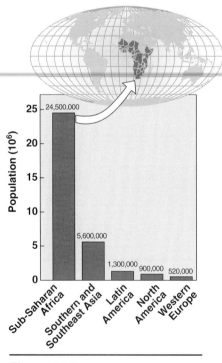

Figure 31.3
Estimated numbers of current HIV infections or AIDS cases as of December 1999, according to the CDC.

A. Organization of the HIV genome

The HIV RNA genome contains three major genes: the *gag* gene that codes for CA, MA, and NC (core and matrix proteins), the *pol* gene that codes for reverse transcriptase, protease, integrase, and ribonuclease, and the *env* gene that codes for TM and SU (transmembrane and surface proteins). Genes for additional regulatory and accessory proteins of diverse function are located between the *pol* and *env* genes. At the 5' end of the viral RNA is a unique sequence, U5, which contains part of the site required for viral integration into the host cell chromosome, and also contains the tRNA primer binding site for initiation of reverse transcription. At the 3' end of the viral RNA is the nucleotide sequence U3, which contains sequences that are important in the control of transcription of the DNA provirus. As with cellular mRNAs synthesized by RNA polymerase II, the 5' end of the viral RNA synthesized from proviral DNA has a methylated cap, and the 3' end has a poly-A tail.[1] At either end of the viral genome is a repeated sequence, R, which is involved in reverse transcription. Synthesis of the double-stranded DNA provirus results in duplication of the R and U sequences, producing two identical repeat units designated **long terminal repeats** (LTR). The genomic organization of the DNA provirus is illustrated in Figure 31.5. [Note: A brief overview of retrovirus replication is presented in Chapter 26 (see Figure 26.15, p. 303); additional details of some steps in the cycle are discussed below.]

B. HIV Replication

The first phase of HIV replication, which includes viral entry, reverse transcription, and integration of the virus into the host genome, is accomplished by proteins provided by the virus. The second phase of replication, which includes the synthesis and processing of viral genomes, mRNAs, and structural proteins, uses the host cell machinery for transcription and protein synthesis. The end result of HIV replication in most cell types is cell death. To facilitate the synthesis of more than nine distinct protein products from a genome shorter than ten kilobases, HIV uses a complicated process of differential mRNA splicing.

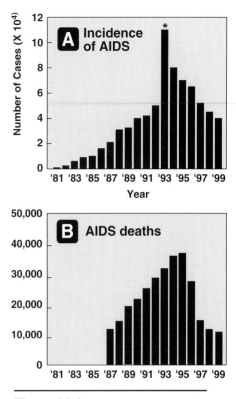

Figure 31.4
A. Incidence of AIDS in the United States, 1981 to1999. *Increase in 1993 was due to several changes introduced in January 1993 in the case definition of AIDS.
B. Deaths due to AIDS in the United States. Data on deaths were unreliable until 1987.

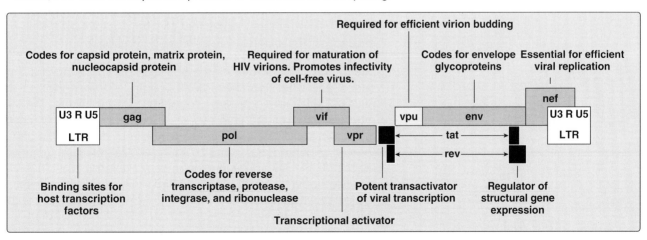

Figure 31.5
HIV proviral genome. The *rev* and *tat* genes are divided into noncontiguous pieces, and the gene segments are spliced together in the RNA transcript.

[1]See p. 386 in *Lippincott's Illustrated Reviews: Biochemistry* (2nd ed.) for a discussion of the poly-A tail of mRNA.

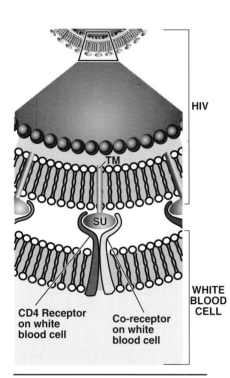

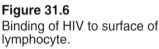

Figure 31.6
Binding of HIV to surface of lymphocyte.

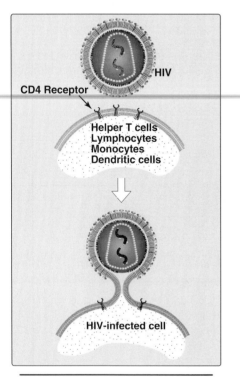

Figure 31.7
Attachement and entry of HIV virus.

1. **Attachment to a specific cell surface receptor:** Attachment is accomplished via the SU fragment of the *env* gene product on the surface of the HIV, which preferentially binds to a CD4 molecule (Figure 31.6; also see p. 72). Thus the virus infects helper T cells, lymphocytes, monocytes, and dendritic cells, which contain this protein in their cell membranes (Figure 31.7).

2. **Entry of virus into the cell:** An additional coreceptor—a chemokine receptor—is required for entry of the viral core into the cell (see Figure 31.6). [Note: A chemokine is a cytokine with chemotactic properties, produced by lymphocytes and macrophages.] Macrophages and T cells express different chemokine receptors that fulfill this function. Binding to a coreceptor activates the viral **TM** (fusion) glycoprotein, triggering fusion between the viral envelope and the cell membrane (Figure 31.8). [Note: A number of factors influencing the variable longevity among those infected with HIV have been identified. For example, mutations or deletions in the chemokine receptor genes have been found to correlate with decreased susceptibility to HIV infection, or the rate of progression of the disease. A further complication is that different strains of HIV occur, which preferentially use different chemokine receptors.]

3. **Reverse transcription of viral RNA:** After entering the host cell, the HIV RNA is not translated. Instead, it is transcribed into DNA by **reverse transcriptase**—an RNA-directed DNA polymerase that enters host cells as part of the viral nucleocapsid (see Figure 31.8). A host cellular transfer RNA (tRNA) is hydrogen-bonded to a specific site on each viral RNA molecule, where it functions as a primer for initiation of reverse transcription. This process takes place in the cytoplasm, within the core structure. The viral reverse transcriptase first synthesizes a DNA-RNA hybrid molecule, then its RNase activity degrades the parental RNA molecule while synthesizing the second strand of DNA. This process results in duplication of the ends to form the long terminal repeats (LTR). The resulting linear molecule of double-stranded DNA is termed the **provirus**. The LTRs at either end of the provirus contain promoter and enhancer sequences[2] that control expression of the viral DNA.

4. **Integration of the provirus into host cell DNA:** The provirus, still associated with virion core components, is transported to the nucleus with the aid of MA (the matrix protein). There, the viral **integrase** cleaves the chromosomal DNA, and covalently inserts the provirus; the integrated provirus thus becomes a stable part of the cell genome (see Figure 31.8). The insertion is random with respect to the site of integration in the recipient DNA. Thus HIV has two genomic forms, namely single-stranded RNA present in the extracellular virus, and proviral double-stranded DNA within the cell.

[2]See p. 384 in *Lippincott's Illustrated Reviews: Biochemistry* (2nd ed.) for a discussion of the enhancer in gene regulation.

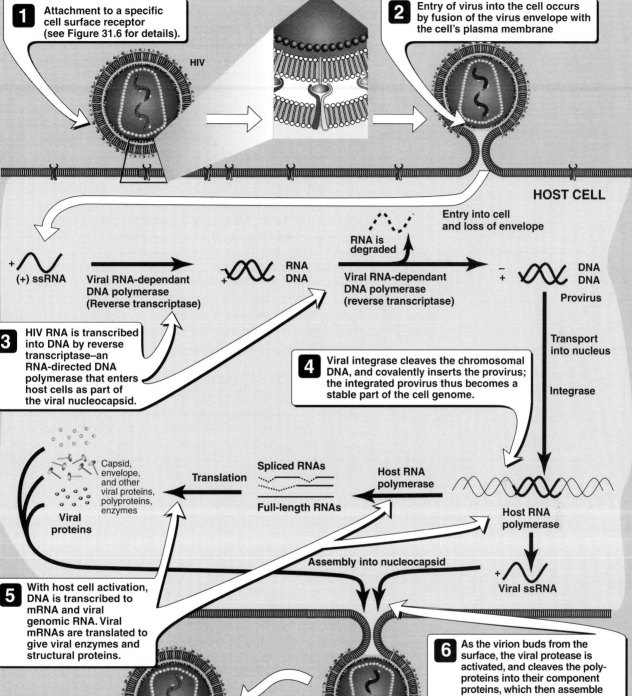

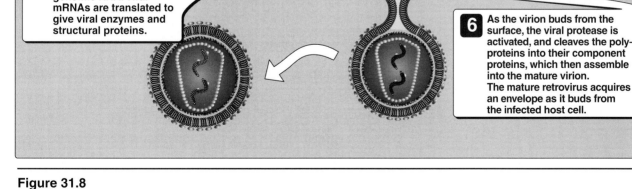

1 Attachment to a specific cell surface receptor (see Figure 31.6 for details).

HIV

2 Entry of virus into the cell occurs by fusion of the virus envelope with the cell's plasma membrane

HOST CELL

Entry into cell and loss of envelope

RNA is degraded

+ (+) ssRNA

Viral RNA-dependant DNA polymerase (Reverse transcriptase)

RNA DNA

Viral RNA-dependant DNA polymerase (reverse transcriptase)

DNA DNA

Provirus

3 HIV RNA is transcribed into DNA by reverse transcriptase–an RNA-directed DNA polymerase that enters host cells as part of the viral nucleocapsid.

4 Viral integrase cleaves the chromosomal DNA, and covalently inserts the provirus; the integrated provirus thus becomes a stable part of the cell genome.

Transport into nucleus

Integrase

Capsid, envelope, and other viral proteins, polyproteins, enzymes

Viral proteins

Translation

Spliced RNAs

Full-length RNAs

Host RNA polymerase

Host RNA polymerase

+ Viral ssRNA

Assembly into nucleocapsid

5 With host cell activation, DNA is transcribed to mRNA and viral genomic RNA. Viral mRNAs are translated to give viral enzymes and structural proteins.

6 As the virion buds from the surface, the viral protease is activated, and cleaves the poly-proteins into their component proteins, which then assemble into the mature virion. The mature retrovirus acquires an envelope as it buds from the infected host cell.

Figure 31.8
The HIV replication cycle.

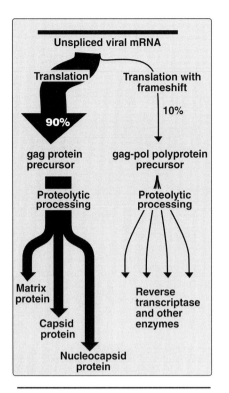

Figure 31.9
Processing of gag and gag-pol polyprotein precursor proteins by the viral protease.

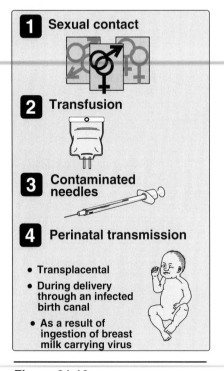

Figure 31.10
Common modes of transmission of HIV.

5. **Transcription and translation of integrated viral DNA sequences:** The provirus is transcribed into a **full-length mRNA** by the cell RNA polymerase II. The genome-length mRNA has at least three functions: 1) Some copies will be the genomes of progeny virus, and are transported to the cytoplasm in preparation for viral assembly. 2) Some copies are translated to produce the virion gag proteins. Further, by reading past the stop codon at the end of the *gag* gene about one time out of twenty, a gag-pol polyprotein is produced. This is the source of the viral reverse transcriptase and integrase that will be incorporated into the virion. 3) Still other copies of viral RNA are spliced, creating new translatable sequences (see Figure 31.8). In all retroviruses, one of the spliced mRNAs is translated into the envelope proteins. In the complex viruses, such as HIV and HTLV, additional spliced molecules produce accessory proteins that are important in regulating transcription and other aspects of replication.

6. **Assembly and maturation of infectious progeny:** These pathways differ from most other enveloped viruses. The env polyprotein is processed and transported to the plasma membrane by the usual cellular route through the Golgi, and is cleaved into the SU and TM molecules by a host cell protease. Assembly begins as the genomes and uncleaved gag and gag-pol polyproteins associate with the TM-modified plasma membrane. As the virion buds from the surface, the viral protease is activated, and cleaves the polyproteins into their component proteins, which then assemble into the mature virion (Figure 31.9). [Note: The enzymes of the gag-pol polyprotein are inactive until the proteolytic processing occurs within the budding virion. Thus, there is no infectious intracellular virus, and assembled virion structures are visible only as they bud from the cell surface, or as free, extracellular particles.] In lymphocytes, this replication and release of mature virions results in death of the cells. In contrast, macrophages can release infectious virus without cell death.

C. Transmission of HIV

It is unclear how and where HIV originated. The virus was shown to be related to simian (monkey) immunodeficiency virus, and it is speculated that the emergence of HIV began in the early 1950s, after the monkey virus mutated and began infecting humans. The first documented case of AIDS was in an African man in 1959. The initial infections were presumably sporadic and isolated until mutations produced a more virulent strain that was readily transmitted from human to human. Today, transmission of HIV generally occurs by one of four routes listed below (Figure 31.10). There has been no firm evidence for transmission by saliva, urine, nonsexual contact where blood is not exchanged, or by an insect bite.

1. **Sexual contact:** HIV is present in both semen and vaginal secretions, and is transmitted primarily as cell-associated virus in the course of either homosexual or heterosexual contact. Disruption of mucosal surfaces by sexually transmitted diseases, particularly those such as syphilis and chancroid that result in genital ulcerations, may greatly facilitate HIV-1 infection.

2. **Transfusions:** HIV has been transmitted by transfusion with whole blood, plasma, clotting factors, or cellular fractions of blood.

3. **Contaminated needles:** Transmission can occur by inoculation with HIV-contaminated needles—either accidentally, or through use of shared needles or syringes by drug users.

4. **Perinatal transmission:** An HIV-infected woman has a fifteen to forty percent chance of transmitting the infection to her newborn, either transplacentally, during passage of the baby through the birth canal, or via breast feeding. Because of the high rates of HIV-1 infection in women of childbearing age in developing countries, perinatally acquired HIV-1 infection is responsible for approximately twenty percent of all AIDS cases in these areas. Figure 31.11 compares the modes of transmission worldwide with those occurring in the United States.

D. Pathogenesis and clinical significance of HIV infection

The pathology of HIV disease results from either tissue destruction by the virus itself, or the host's response to virus-infected cells. In addition, HIV can induce an immunodeficient state that leads to opportunistic diseases that are rare in the absence of HIV infection. The progression from HIV infection to AIDS develops in fifty percent of HIV-infected individuals in an average of ten years, and if untreated, is itself uniformly fatal—generally within two years of the diagnosis. However, there is a significant fraction (about ten percent) of HIV-infected individuals who have not developed AIDS after twenty years. Development from HIV infection to end-stage AIDS progresses through several phases (Figure 31.12).

1. **Initial infection:** After the acquisition of HIV, the initially infected cells are generally macrophages within the genital tract. From this initial localized infection, HIV disseminates via the blood, and virus may then localize in dendritic cells throughout the lymphoid tissue. From the surface of follicular dendritic cells, HIV can then infect CD4+ lymphocytes moving through the germinal centers of lymph nodes. This process creates a reservoir of chronically HIV-infected cells within the lymphatic tissues of body.

2. **Acute phase viremia:** Several weeks after the initial infection with HIV, one third to two thirds of individuals experience an **acute disease syndrome** (also referred to as the **primary infection**) similar to infectious mononucleosis. During this period there is a very high level of virus replication occurring in CD4+ cells. Large amounts of virus and capsid protein (CA antigen) are present in the blood, and circulating antibody appears in one to ten weeks after the initial infection (**seroconversion**). A constant level of virus and virus-infected cells is maintained by a combination of replacement of the CD4+ cells killed by HIV infection with cells newly produced in lymphoid organs, and the subsequent infection of these new cells with progeny virus. Lymph nodes also become infected during this time; they later serve as the sites of virus persistence during the asymptomatic period.

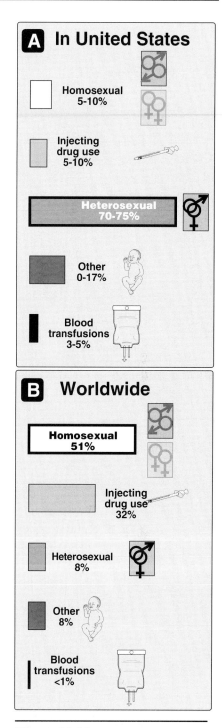

Figure 31.11
Modes of HIV transmission in the United States compared with those world-wide. (A) In the United States, the primary mode of HIV transmission is homosexual sex. Transmission in western Europe is similar to that in the United States. [Note: Segment labeled "Other" includes perinatal transmission.] (B) In most of the world, transmission is primarily by heterosexual sex.

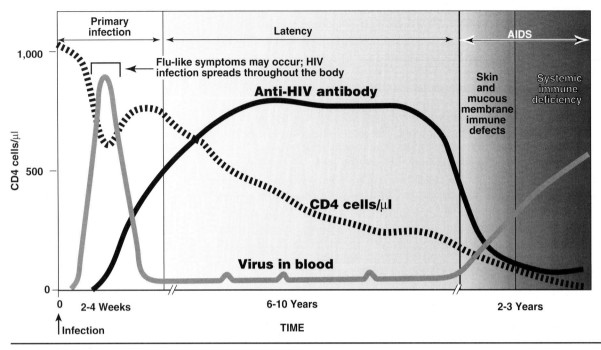

Figure 31.12
Typical time course of HIV infection.

3. **Latent period:** The acute phase viremia is eventually reduced significantly with the appearance of a HIV-specific cytotoxic T lymphocyte response, followed by a humoral antibody response (see p. 19). A clinically asymptomatic or "latent" period lasting from months to many years follows the acute infection. During this latent period, the majority (ninety percent) of the HIV proviruses are transcriptionally silent, so that only ten percent of the cells containing integrated HIV DNA also contain viral mRNA or viral proteins. There are transient peaks of viremia that are often correlated with stimulation of the immune system by infection with other pathogens, or by immunization. Although there is continuous loss of those CD4+ cells in which HIV is replicating, active replacement through stem cell multiplication compensates for this loss, and the CD4+ count declines only very slowly over a period of years. In addition, the host immune response is still sufficiently effective to maintain a relatively stable, low level of virus production. It has been estimated that 10^{11} virions and 10^9 CD4 T cells are produced each day. Virus isolated during this period is also less cytopathic for CD4+ cells, and replicates more slowly than does that isolated later during symptomatic AIDS. Despite the nearly normal levels of CD4+ cells, however, impairment of T cell responses to specific antigens is evident. The infection remains relatively clinically asymptomatic as long as the immune system is functional. [Note: The actual level of virus replication in peripheral blood cells varies greatly in different patients, and those with a higher steady-state viral load progress more rapidly to symptomatic AIDS and death.]

4. **Clinical complications of HIV infection during the latent period:** During this period—whose length is very variable, but lasts on average about ten years—there are multiple, nonspecific conditions,

such as persistent, generalized lymphadenopathy (swollen lymph nodes), diarrhea, chronic fevers, night sweats, and weight loss. The more common opportunistic infections such as herpes zoster and candidiasis may occur repeatedly during this period, as well as when patients progress to AIDS. The CD4+ cell count remains normal or gradually declines, but is greater than 200 per μl. Thus the progression from asymptomatic infection to AIDS is not sudden, but in fact occurs as a continuum of clinical states.

5. Progression to AIDS: A number of virologic and immunologic changes occur that affect the rate of this progression. For example, coinfection with a number of the herpesviruses, such as human herpesvirus type 6 (see p. 300), can transactivate transcription from the silent HIV provirus, thereby increasing HIV replication. Any stimulation of an immune response causing activation of resting T cells also activates HIV replication. Not only does this increase the number of infected CD4+ cells, but it also increases the opportunity to create generations of virus mutants. Eventually, a more highly cytocidal, more rapidly multiplying variant appears. In addition, these variants are often highly syncytium-inducing, promoting fusion between infected and previously uninfected cells. T-cell precursors in the lymphoid organs are also infected and killed, so the capacity to generate new CD4+ cells is gradually lost. The capacity to contain the infection is further compromised by the appearance of HIV mutants with altered antigenic specificity, which are not recognized by the existing humoral antibody or cytotoxic T lymphocytes. The eventual result of these accumulating, interacting factors is an increasingly rapid decline in CD4+ count, accompanied by loss of immune capacity. With the CD4+ count falling below 200/μl and the appearance of increasingly frequent and serious diseases and opportunistic infections (termed the "AIDS-defining illnesses"), the patient is said to have AIDS.

6. End-stage AIDS: Nearly all systems of the body can be affected as a result of HIV infection, either by HIV itself or by opportunistic organisms. The weakening immune system leads to many complications including malignancies.

    a. Spread of HIV to additional body sites: Cell types other than CD4+ lymphocytes can be infected by HIV. Infection of these cells produces some of the additional manifestations of the end stage of the disease. Chief among these are infected cells of the monocyte-macrophage lineage, which are not killed as rapidly as CD4+ T cells, and can transport the virus into other organs (Figure 31.13). For example, macrophages are the HIV-infected cells present in brains of patients with AIDS encephalopathy, which typically evolves over a period of a year with gradual deterioration resulting in severe dementia. This appears to be unrelated to CD4+ depletion, but rather to an expanded host range of variant HIV. The basis for damage to neuronal cells is, however, not known. Similarly, the wasting syndrome seen in late stages of AIDS is probably related to HIV-infected macrophages induced to produce various cytokines, especially tumor necrosis factor. Virus has also been found in Langerhans cells in the skin,

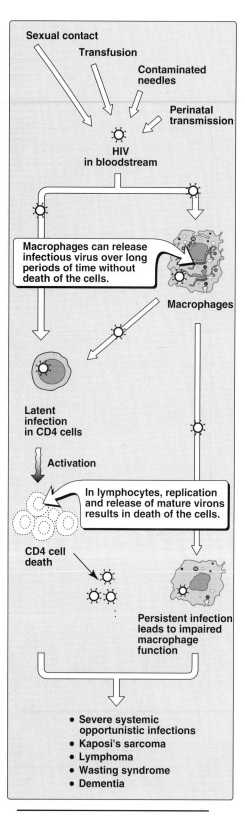

Figure 31.13
Pathogenesis of HIV.

dendritic cells in lymph nodes, and in monocytes in bone marrow, but their significance in the disease process is not clear. The eye is another site affected by HIV infection itself, which produces focal areas of ischemia in the retina. HIV infection of blood cell progenitors in the bone marrow leads to the anemia seen in most AIDS patients.

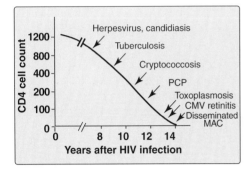

Figure 31.14
Pattern of opportunistic infections associated with declining CD4+ cell counts. CMV = Cytomegalovirus; MAC = *Mycobacterium avium* complex; PCP = *Pneumocystis carinii* pneumonia.

b. **Opportunistic infections in AIDS:** Multiple recurrent bouts of infections with fungi, bacteria, and viruses occur as the CD4+ cell count declines (Figure 31.14). For example, the nervous system can be the site of opportunistic infections with *Toxoplasma*, *Cryptococcus*, JC virus, and *Mycobacteria*. The eye can not only be infected with HIV, but also with opportunistic agents, the most prominent of which is cytomegalovirus (CMV)—a cause of retinal destruction. The lungs are also primarily affected by opportunistic infections, *Pneumocystis carinii* pneumonia being one of the most common. Mycobacterial infections are also a common problem in the lung; for example, currently thirty percent of AIDS patients die from tuberculosis (see p. 246). Serious gastrointestinal tract illnesses are due to opportunistic pathogens, but these may be in concert with HIV infection. CMV colitis is a common problem, but HIV is often present as well. Protozoal parasitic diseases, as well as infections with gram-negative enteric bacteria are other sources of gastrointestinal disorders. The immune deficiency also provides the opportunity for latent herpesvirus infections to recur repeatedly or become chronic, and to spread extensively. Mucocutaneous candidiasis (for example, oral, esophageal, or vaginal) is an ongoing problem in AIDS patients as well. In fact, vaginal candidiasis is the most frequent reason HIV-infected females seek medical attention. (See Figure 31.16 for a summary of common AIDS-defining opportunistic infections.)

c. **Malignancies associated with AIDS:** A number of malignancies commonly arise in HIV-infected patients. The most characteristic neoplasm present in AIDS patients is Kaposi's sarcoma (KS), which involves skin, mucous membranes, and deep viscera. Various lymphomas, including those of the CNS, are also common. These are probably the result of the immune compromise and not HIV itself. KS has been associated with human herpesvirus, type 8 (HHV-8, Figure 31.15). In AIDS patients, body cavity lymphomas are also usually associated with HHV-8 infection (see p. 334), whereas many other lymphomas are EBV-associated (see p. 332).

E. **Laboratory identification**

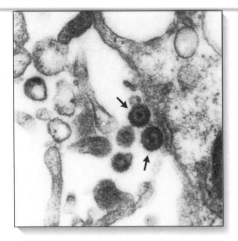

Figure 31.15
Herpesvirus 8 virions (arrows) associated with Kaposi's sarcoma.

1. **Demonstration of virus or virus components:** Amplification of viral RNA or DNA proviruses by the PCR technique (see p. 32) is the most sensitive method for early detection of virus in blood or tissue specimens. Recent adaptation of the technique to obtain quantitative estimates of viral load (measured, for example, as the amount of viral RNA per milliliter of blood plasma) now permit evaluation of the stage of the disease, effectiveness of a drug regimen, and prognosis. For purposes of screening the blood supply, ELISA testing (see p. 30) for the CA (p20) antigen in serum can

Disease Summary: OPPORTUNISTIC INFECTIONS OF HIV

A Bacteria

Mycobacterium avium complex

- *Mycobacterium avium-intracellulare complex* (MAC) is a complex of acid-fast bacilli, serotypes of which infect birds and a variety of mammals. MAC is ubiquitous, thus individuals can easily acquire a MAC infection.

- In the United States, **disseminated (miliary) disease** caused by MAC is the most common systemic bacterial infection in AIDS patients, and is responsible for significant morbidity. Serious pulmonary diseases include **chronic bronchitis** and **pneumonia**. **Cervical lymphadenitis**, **chronic osteomyelitis**, and **renal or skin infections** can occur. Clinical presentation usually includes fevers, night sweats, chills, and weight loss. In AIDS patients undergoing HAART treatment, cases of MAC-caused disease have sharply declined.

- Diseases caused by the MAC complex are particularly refractory to chemotherapy. Because of the large number of resistant variants, treatment of disease and prevention of reinfections requires two to four drugs given simultaneously. Current regimens include azithromycin or clarithromycin with or without rifabutin. Relapses are common. (See p. 254)

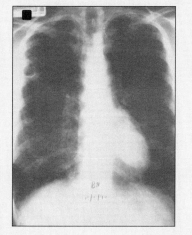

Pulmonary disease (A)

Streptococcus pneumoniae

- *S. pneumoniae* (pneumococci) are gram-positive, non-motile, encapsulated cocci that tend to occur in pairs (diplococci). They can be found in the nasopharynx of many healthy individuals. *S. pneumoniae* can be spread endogenously (if the carrier develops impaired resistance to the organism), or exogenously (by droplets from the nose of a carrier).

- *S. pneumoniae* is the most common bacterial respiratory pathogen in HIV-positive patients. The *S. pneumoniae* cell-associated virulence factors autolysin and pneumolysin contribute to its pathogenicity. The organism causes acute bacterial pneumonia, and is a leading cause of death. *S. pneumoniae* also causes bacteremia/sepsis, and meningitis.

- Most *S. pneumoniae* strains that are resistant to penicillin G remain sensitive to third generation cephalosporins and vancomycin. (See p.150)

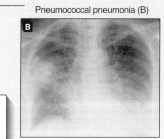

Pneumococcal pneumonia (B)

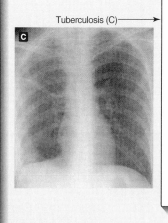

Tuberculosis (C)

Mycobacterium tuberculosis

- Once a disease mainly of the elderly, clinical tuberculosis has become more prevalent among younger individuals (25 to 44 years old) and among children. In the United States, the increase is attributed to the very high prevalence of mycobacterial disease in AIDS patients (for whom it is a major health threat), and to the increase in the number of immigrants, particularly from southeast Asia.

- Transmission occurs when patients with active pulmonary tuberculosis shed large numbers of organisms by coughing. The organisms are resistant to desiccation, and can remain viable in the surroundings for a long time. Individuals with a depressed immune system—especially those who are HIV positive—are particularly susceptible to infection.

- In the primary disease, *M. tuberculosis* survives and grows within host cells such as macrophages, which can carry the organisms to additional sites. Productive (granulomatous) lesions known as tubercles can develop at those sites. In AIDS patients, as their immunity wanes, the primary infection is generally progressive, and one or more of the tubercles may expand, leading to destruction of tissue and clinical illness, for example, **chronic pneumonitis**, **tuberculous osteomyelitis**, or **tuberculous meningitis**. If active tubercles develop throughout the body, the condition is known as **miliary (disseminated) tuberculosis**. Reactivation of preexisting tubercles is due to an impairment in immune status, such as that seen in AIDS.

- Because of the large number of drug-resistant strains of *M. tuberculosis*, treatment includes two or more drugs to prevent outgrowth of resistant strains. Principal drugs used include isoniazid, ethambutol, and/or pyrazinamide. The BCG anti-tuberculosis vaccine should not be given to AIDS or other immuno-suppressed individuals, because it contains live organisms, and in such cases it has occasionally appeared to become virulent. (See p. 246)

Figure 31.16 (continued on next page)
Organisms causing opportunistic infections in patients infected with human immunodeficiency virus (HIV). [Note: Other opportunistic bacterial species include *Haemophilus influenzae* (pneumonia), *Campylobacter* species (diarrhea), *Shigella* species (diarrhea and bacteremia).] HAART = highly active antiviral therapy.

Disease Summary: OPPORTUNISTIC INFECTIONS OF HIV

A Bacteria (continued)

Salmonella species

● Salmonella are flagellated, motile, gram-negative bacilli, routinely found in the gastrointestinal tract of humans and other animals. Salmonella are transmitted most frequently by the fecal/oral route—often with food as an intermediary—but can also be transmitted to humans by pets such as turtles. *S. typhimurium* is of particular concern because it is increasingly drug-resistant.

● *Salmonella* invade epithelial cells of the small intestine. In immunocompromised hosts, the infection can become systemic with disseminated foci. In HIV-infected individuals, a high-grade bacteremia can occur, in which salmonella seeds distant organs, and in older patients, promotes atherosclerotic plaque. Fever can persist for one to two weeks. Salmonella infections also cause severe gastroenteritis, characterized by nausea, vomiting, and diarrhea.

● The treatment for *Salmonella* infections in an immunocompromised host is typically ciprofloxacin. Alternative treatments (depending on drug-resistance) include ampicillin or trimethoprim-sulfamethoxazole. In patients with AIDS, relapse is a major problem. Therefore months of therapy are required. (See p.179)

← *Salmonella* species (D)

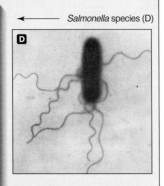

Pulmonary histoplasmosis (E) →

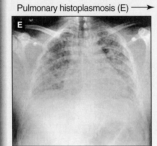

Histoplasma capsulatum

● *H. capsulatum* is a soil fungus that is found worldwide, but is most prevalent in central North America. The organism produces spores that, when airborne, enter the lungs and germinate into yeast-like cells. These yeast cells are engulfed by macrophages in which they multiply.

● In healthy individuals, pulmonary infections with *H. capsulatum* may be acute but self-limiting. In HIV-infected persons, nearly all cases are disseminated at the time of diagnosis. Dissemination results from invasion of cells of the reticuloendothelial system, which distinguishes this organism as the only fungus to exhibit intracellular parasitism. **Disseminated histoplasmosis** causes fever, weight loss, hypertension, and pulmonary distress. If untreated, it can lead to respiratory and liver failure.

● *H. capsulatum* infection is treated with itraconazole, with amphotericin B as an alternative. Life-long maintenance therapy may be required to prevent reoccurrence of the disease. (See p. 273)

B Fungi

Candida species

● *Candida albicans* and other candida species are part of the normal body flora. They are found in the skin, mouth, vagina, and intestines. **Candidiasis** is the most common fungal infection of HIV-positive individuals. The presence of esophageal candidiasis is a hallmark of the progression from HIV infection to AIDS.

● Candidiasis is generally limited to the oral, esophageal, or vaginal mucosa. **Oral candidiasis (thrush)** presents as raised, white plaques on the oral mucosa, tongue, or gums. The plaques can become confluent and ulcerated, and can spread to the esophagus (an indicator of full-blown AIDS). **Vaginal candidiasis** presents as itching and burning pain of the vulva and vagina, accompanied by a thick or thin white discharge. Vaginal candidiasis frequently reoccurs. **Systemic candidiasis** is rare.

● Candidiasis is treated with fluconazole or itraconazole. However, azole-resistant strains of candida require alternative treatment, for example, with amphotericin B. (See p. 274)

Cryptococcus neoformans

● *C. neoformans* is a yeast that is found worldwide. It is especially abundant in soil containing bird droppings. Its spores are inhaled.

● In healthy persons, cryptococcosis is generally a mild, subclinical lung infection. In AIDS patients, **cryptococcosis** is the second most common fungal infection, and is potentially the most serious. In these individuals, the infection often disseminates to the brain and meninges, causing **meningitis**—frequently with fatal consequences. Presenting symptoms include fever, headache, and malaise. Patients are often forgetful and lethargic.

● Cryptococcal meningitis is treated with fluconazole, with amphotericin B as an alternative. This therapy should be continued lifelong to prevent reoccurrence of the infection. (See p. 275).

← Oral candidiasis (F)

Cutaneous cryptococcosis (G)

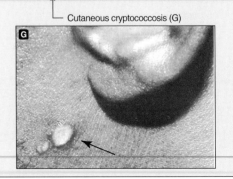

Figure 31.16 (continued on next page)
Organisms causing opportunistic infections in patients infected with human immunodeficiency virus (HIV).
[Note: Other opportunistic fungal infections include aspergillosis and coccidioidomycosis.]

Disease Summary: OPPORTUNISTIC INFECTIONS OF HIV

C Other

Pneumocystis carinii

- *P. carinii* is a unicellular eukaryote whose taxonomic status and life cycle are still uncertain. It is the most common opportunistic pathogen in AIDS patients.

- *P. carinii* causes frequently fatal **pneumonia (PCP)**. Before the use of immunosuppressive drugs, and before the AIDS epidemic, PCP was a rare disease. It is almost 100 percent fatal if untreated.

- Prophylaxis with trimethoprim-sulfamethoxazole is recommended for HIV-infected patients with fewer than 200 CD4+ cells/μl. However, individuals infected with HIV who are undergoing treatment with HAART have shown a significant decrease in incidence of PCP. (See p. 277)

Cryptosporidium species

- *Cryptosporidium* is an intracellular parasite that inhabits the epithelial cells of the villi of the lower small intestine. The source of infection is often the feces of domestic animals, and farm run-off has been implicated as a source of cryptosporidium contamination of drinking water.

- Infection of healthy individuals may be asymptomatic or may cause mild cases of diarrhea, which are generally self-limiting. However, in AIDS patients, the infection may be severe and intractable. **Cryptosporidiosis** causes diarrhea that varies from mild to a fulminant, persistent cholera-like illness. Patients experience nausea, vomiting, abdominal pain, and weight loss.

- In AIDS patients, no treatment for cryptosporidiosis has proven completely effective, although paramomycin has provided some improvement. (See p. 281)

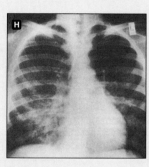
Pneumocystis pneumonia

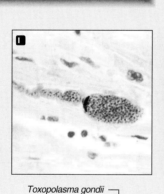
Toxopolasma gondii

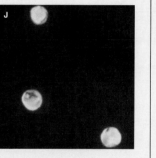
Cryptosporidium species

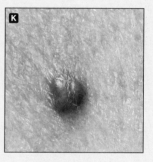
Kaposi's sarcoma

D Parasites

Toxoplasma gondii

- *T. gondii* is a sporozoan, distributed worldwide, which infects all vertebrate species, although the definitive host is the cat. Transmission is by accidental ingestion of oocysts present in cat feces, by eating raw or undercooked meat, congenitally from an infected mother, or from a blood transfusion. Rapidly growing *T. gondii* trophozoites establish early, acute infections. Slowly growing trophozoites encyst in muscle and brain tissue, and in the eye.

- *T. gondii* infections of healthy humans are asymptomatic and very common, but they are the most common cause of **focal encephalitis** in AIDS patients. **Toxoplasmosis** in this population is usually due to reemergence of encysted organisms, rather than from new, exogenous infection. Clinical presentation of the encephalitis can include weakness, confusion, seizures, or coma. Disseminated toxoplasmosis can involve the heart, skeletal muscle, lung, colon, and other organs.

- *T. gondii* infection is treated with a combination of sulfadiazine and pyrimethamine. Lifelong secondary prophylaxis involves sulfadiazine plus pyrimethamine. (See p. 285)

E Viruses

Human herpesvirus type 8

- Human herpesvirus type 8 (HHV-8) (also known as Kaposi's sarcoma-associated herpesvirus) is a member of the Herpesviridae family. It is enveloped, with a double-stranded DNA genome. Interestingly, its genome encodes a number of human cell-derived genes related to growth regulation, for example, cytokines, cytokine receptors, growth factors, and a factor that inhibits apoptosis.

- In the United States, antibodies to HHV-8 antigens are found primarily in the same populations that are at risk for HIV infection, leading to the conclusion that the primary mode of transmission is sexual. The frequency of perinatal transmission of HHV-8 appears low.

- HHV-8 has been detected in over ninety percent of patients with Kaposi's sarcoma (KS), but in less than one percent of non-KS tissues. KS was the most common neoplasm in AIDS patients, but has essentially disappeared from those HIV-infected individuals with access to HAART treatment. There is no established independent drug treatment for HHV-8 infected individuals. (See p. 334)

Figure 31.16 (continued on next page)
Organisms causing opportunistic infections in patients infected with human immuodeficiency virus (HIV).

Disease Summary: OPPORTUNISTIC INFECTIONS OF HIV

E Viruses (continued)

Herpes simplex virus

● Herpes simplex virus (HSV) types 1 and 2 are members of the Herpesviridae family. They are enveloped, with a double-stranded DNA genome. Initial infection with HSV is by direct contact with virus-containing secretions, or with lesions on mucosal surfaces. HSV can also be transmitted during a baby's journey down the birth canal. HSV coinfection of patients with HIV infection occurs very frequently, probably because of their similar modes of transmission. For example, 95 percent of homosexual men with AIDS are seropositive for HSV.

● Initial replication of the virus is in epithelial cells of the mucosal surface onto which they have been inoculated. In individuals with depressed immune systems, the virus reproduces, and can be transported to various sites in the body. It also establishes life-long latent infections in the regional ganglia.

● Reactivation of latent virus leading to invasive HSV infections in AIDS patients becomes increasingly important as CD4+ lymphocyte counts decline. Herpetic ulcers on the face, hand, or genitals, and oral ulcers occur. Recurrence of genital herpes can be more frequent and severe in HIV-infected persons.

● If primary or recurrent herpes episodes are particularly frequent and/or severe, acyclovir, or alternatively famciclovir can be administered. (See p. 319)

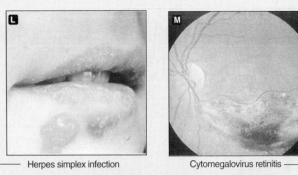

Herpes simplex infection — Cytomegalovirus retinitis

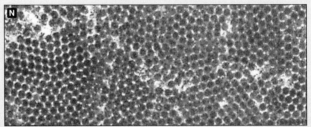

JC virus particles from an infected oligodendrocyte nucleus

JC virus

● JC virus (JCV) is a member of the Papovaviridae family, Polyomavirinae subfamily. It is a nonenveloped virus containing supercoiled, double-stranded, circular DNA.

● As HIV-infected individuals become increasingly immunocompromised, approximately five percent of them will develop **progressive multifocal leukoencephalopathy (PML)**—so called because the lesions are restricted to the white matter of the brain. In PML, reactivated JCV carries out a cytocidal infection of the brain's oligodendrocytes. This leads to demyelination due to the loss of capacity of myelinated cells to maintain their sheaths. Early development of impaired speech and mental capacity is rather rapidly followed by paralysis and sensory abnormalities, with death commonly occurring within three to six months of the initial symptoms.

● JCV is transmitted by droplets from the upper respiratory tract of infected persons, and possibly through contact with their urine. The virus spreads from the upper respiratory tract to the kidneys, where it may persist in an inactive state in the tubular epithelium of healthy individuals.

● A regimen of HAART plus cidofovir is currently showing some promise in patients suffering from PML. Since infection with JCV is nearly universal and asymptomatic, and PML represents reactivation of latent virus in the immunocompromised host, there are no viable preventive measures at present. (See p. 311)

Human cytomegalovirus

● Human cytomegalovirus (HCMV) is a member of the Herpesviridae family. It is enveloped, with a double-stranded DNA genome. Initial infection with HCMV commonly occurs during childhood. Transmission is via body fluids such as tears, urine, saliva, or milk, by semen and vaginal secretions, by organ transplants, and by blood transfusions. HCMV can also be transmitted transplacentally. HCMV coinfection of patients with HIV infection occurs very frequently, probably because of their similar modes of transmission.

● Initial replication of the virus in epithelial cells of the respiratory and GI tracts is followed by viremia and infection of all organs of the body, including the kidney tubule epithelium, liver, CNS, and respiratory and GI tracts. The virus establishes latency, predominantly in the monocytes and macrophages, among other cells.

● Reactivation of latent virus leading to invasive HCMV infections in AIDS patients becomes increasingly frequent as CD4+ lymphocyte counts decline. Any organ system can be affected, but blindness due to HCMV chorioretinitis is especially common, developing in more than twenty percent of AIDS patients whose CD4+ count is less than 50/µl. Encephalitis and dementia, esophagitis, enterocolitis, and gastritis are other significant problems caused by HCMV. In addition, coinfection with HCMV may accelerate the progression of AIDS. At autopsy, ninety percent of AIDS patients are shown to be infected with HCMV. However, the incidence of HCMV chorioretinitis has been significantly decreased in HIV-infected individuals being treated with HAART.

● The drug regimen for both primary prophylaxis (when recommended) and prevention of recurrence of HCMV infections in AIDS patients includes ganciclovir, cidofovir, and/or foscarnet. Oral valganciclovir is currently undergoing successful clinical trials for the treatment of HCMV chorioretinitis. (See p. 326)

Figure 31.16 (continued)
Organisms causing opportunistic infections in patients infected with human immunodeficiency virus (HIV).
[Note: Other opportunistic viral infections include shingles and oral hairy leukoplakia.]

detect infection about a week earlier than tests for antibody, and thus can identify those individuals who are infectious but undetectable by screening for anti-HIV antibodies.

2. **Demonstration of immune response:** The usual screening procedure for HIV infection is a two-step process, used both for purposes of diagnosing individuals who may be infected, and for protection of the blood supply. The first step in screening is an ELISA procedure (see p. 30) in which the serum sample is reacted with whole virus lysates or synthetic HIV peptides. The latter can detect antibody much earlier than the former, and is now standard. At its most sensitive, there is still a 25-day window between the time that virus is first present in the blood and antibody can be detected. Although the ELISA test is highly specific, there are false positives, so any positive result is confirmed using the Western blot technique. For this step, known HIV proteins are separated by electrophoresis and transferred to nitrocellulose, where they are reacted with the patient's serum. The serum must react with at least two known HIV proteins to be considered positive.

F. Treatment

Because of the progressive nature of the disease, it is the HIV infection that is treated as the clinical problem, rather than focusing on the end stage—AIDS—alone. Virtually every step in the HIV replication cycle is a potential target for an antiviral drug, but only those directed against the reverse transcriptase and the viral protease have thus far been used successfully (Figure 31.17). It should be noted that the reverse transcriptase inhibitors theoretically have the potential to prevent establishment of infection, whereas protease inhibitors act on the synthesis of progeny virus, but do not cure a cell with an integrated provirus. Used early in the infection, a combination of three different drugs administered together can reduce the plasma viral load to undetectable levels—at least temporarily. Effect on long-term survival is not yet known.

1. **Strategy for multiple-drug therapy in treating HIV infections:** Unlike DNA polymerase, which makes very few mistakes in the replication of DNA because of its proofreading activity, reverse transcriptase has no ability to proofread. Therefore DNA synthesis by the viral reverse transcriptase produces many errors (about one per cycle of synthesis). This results in mutations in all of the HIV genes, and accumulation of a pool of mutant viruses in any individual patient. In the presence of an antiviral drug, there is strong selection for mutations that confer resistance to that drug, and the high mutation rate ensures that such mutations will occur. The answer to this therapeutic dilemma has been to use multiple drugs that act on different steps in the viral replication cycle, because the probability of several different mutations occurring simultaneously in the appropriate genes in the same genome is very low. In addition, certain of the drug combinations are synergistic, the effect on reducing viral load being considerably greater than merely the sum of the individual drug effects. The use of potent combination regimens can limit viral replication and dissemination to lymphoid tissue, thus creating a smaller reservoir of chronically infected cells, and limiting the potential for viral mutations (acquired during the

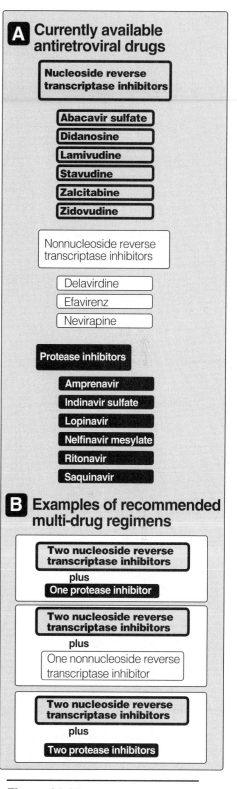

Figure 31.17
Highly active antiretroviral therapy (HAART). [Note: Lopinavir is co-formulated with ritonavir; ritonavir inhibits the metabolism of lopinavir, thereby increasing its level in the plasma.]

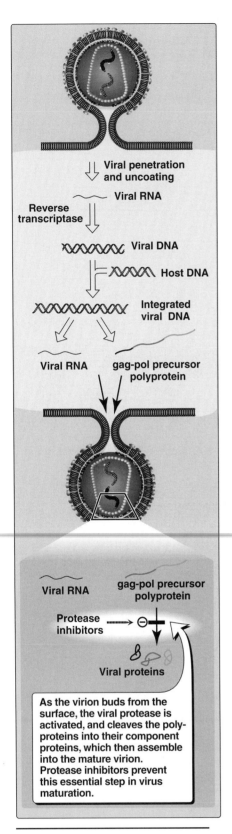

Figure 31.18
Role of HIV protease in viral replication.

replicative process) that could lead to acquisition of drug resistance. However, even this approach is not entirely effective, because HIV also exhibits a relatively high rate of recombination, enabling mutations from two different genomes to be combined into one virus particle. One approach to a more rational choice of drugs to overcome resistance is to sequence the regions of a patient's HIV genome where mutations to resistance are known to occur, and to choose that combination of drugs that is most likely to overcome those specific resistance mutations.

2. **Early therapy:** Approaches to therapy are evolving as more is learned about the nature of the disease. For example, it has been determined that the steady-state level of replicating virus in the plasma—the "**viral load**"—is a prognostic indicator of the rate of progression to AIDS. This has led to the principle that HIV infection should be treated as aggressively and as early as possible, thus minimizing the initial spread of the virus. Not only does this approach yield a lower steady-state level of virus, but it has the additional advantage of drugs being administered at a time when mutants are still rare, so that the drugs are more effective than they would be if given later in the infection.

3. **Highly active antiretroviral therapy:** Currently, combinations of various drugs described below that are given three at a time are being evaluated for efficacy, both in short-term reduction of viral load and/or increase in CD4+ cell count, and in long-term survival. Choice of a drug regimen is individualized based on criteria such as tolerability, drug-drug interactions, convenience/adherence, and possible baseline resistance. [Note: All such multiple drug therapies are commonly referred to as "**highly active antiretroviral therapy**" or **HAART** (see Figure 31.17).] Unfortunately, whereas such multidrug therapies can lower the viral load to undetectable levels, virus re-emerges if HAART is stopped, indicating that the HIV has not been eradicated. Therefore, with current drug therapy, HIV continues to exist in sanctuaries, such as the central nervous system, semen, or nonreplicating T-lymphocyte reservoirs. Thus HIV infection is currently both chronic and incurable.

   a. **Nucleoside analog reverse transcriptase inhibitors:** Reverse transcriptase inhibitors prevent the copying of the HIV RNA genome into a proviral DNA genome. There are both nucleoside analogs and nonnucleoside inhibitors of the viral reverse transcriptase. **Nucleoside analogs** inhibit primarily by serving as chain terminators after insertion into the growing DNA chain by the reverse transcriptase.[3] **Zidovudine** (AZT), which is a pyrimidine analog, is an example of such a drug. Other examples include **didanosine** (ddI), **zalcitabine** (ddC), **lamivudine** (3TC), **stavudine**, and **abacavir**. Resistant mutants inevitably arise after long-term treatment with any one of these drugs, but because cross-resistance is incomplete, AZT in combination with one of the other drugs has been quite successful in minimizing the effect of mutation. Significant side effects accompany use of these drugs, for example, macrocytic anemia with AZT, and peripheral neuropathy with ddI and ddC.

 [3]See p. 407 in *Lippincott's Illustrated Reviews: Biochemistry* (2nd ed.) for a discussion of reverse transcriptase.

The use of combined therapy in some cases permits less toxic doses to be administered.

b. **The nonnucleoside reverse transcriptase inhibitors** act by targeting the reverse transcriptase itself. They bind in a non-competitive, reversible manner to a unique site on the enzyme, thus altering its ability to function. Their major advantage is their lack of effect on the host blood-forming elements, and lack of cross-resistance with nucleoside analog reverse transcriptase inhibitors. A number of these drugs have been developed, including **efavirenz**, **delaviridine**, and **nevirapine**. Resistance to these compounds develops much more rapidly than that against the nucleoside analogs.

c. **Protease inhibitors:** The products of the *gag* and *pol* genes are translated initially into large polyprotein precursors that must be cleaved by the viral protease to yield the mature proteins. Protease inhibitors, which include **ritonavir**, **nelfinavir**, **saquinavir**, **amprenavir**, **indinavir**, and **lopinavir** interfere with the processing of the polyproteins in the budding virion, and result in noninfectious particles (Figure 31.18). However, viral resistance develops if protease inhibitors alone are used. Further, **lipodystrophy (**redistribution of fat, so that the limbs become skinny, and the fat is deposited along the abdomen and the upper back) and **hyperglycemia** can occur with these drugs.

4. **Effect of HAART on the incidence of opportunistic infections:** The incidence of opportunistic infections in AIDS patients is decreasing in response to widespread use of aggressive multidrug treatment. This is true for virtually all opportunistic infections (Figure 31.19).

5. **Perinatal treatment:** Zidovudine when administered to HIV-1–infected pregnant women during the second and third trimesters of pregnancy, followed by administration to the infants during the first six weeks of life, reduces risk of maternal-infant transmission of HIV-1 from approximately 23 percent to 8 percent. The availability of this effective intervention, which decreases perinatal transmission of HIV-1 has led to increased efforts to screen all pregnant women (with their consent) for the presence of HIV-1 infection. [Note: Post-natal transmission of HIV via breast milk can, however, occur.]

G. Prevention

Due to lower availability of antiretroviral drugs in developing countries, and lack of a vaccine, education concerning methods for preventing transmission of HIV is currently the primary means of preventing spread of the virus.

1. **Attempts to produce a vaccine:** An effective vaccine is not yet available in spite of intensive efforts to produce one. HIV has a high mutation rate, and antigenically distinct strains exist worldwide. There is also a lack of knowledge as to what type of immune response (humoral and/or cell-mediated), targeted to

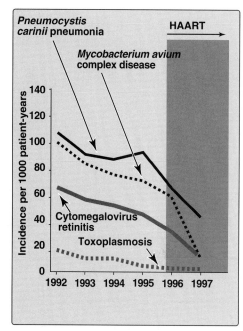

Figure 31.19
Incidence of selected opportunistic infections in patients with HIV infection. [Note: The shaded area labeled "HAART" indicates the period of wide availability of highly active anti-retorviral therapy (HAART). The decline in opportunistic infections after 1995 reflects in large part the effect of HAART.]

which antigens, would be most effective. Stimulation of a cell-mediated immune reaction is likely to be an essential component of the immune response, and trials are being done to address these issues. An early approach has been the use of synthetically-produced viral SU (gp120)—the envelope glycoprotein with which neutralizing antibody reacts. Other approaches to producing a vaccine include inserting HIV genes into various vectors (for example, vaccinia virus, herpes simplex virus, or plasmids), or using killed or attenuated intact virus.

2. **Other measures:** Screening of the blood supply has nearly eliminated transmission by that route. Perinatal transmission can be reduced by nearly seventy percent with AZT therapy of the pregnant woman, followed by several weeks of AZT to the newborn. Strict adherence to standard precautions by health care workers can minimize risk in that setting.

IV. HUMAN T-CELL LEUKEMIA VIRUSES, TYPES 1, 2

HTLV-1 and -2 share about 65 percent nucleotide sequence homology, and thus are genetically and biologically similar. However, their worldwide distribution is different. HTLV-1 has definitively been associated with a human malignant disease, **adult T-cell leukemia** (**ATL**), and a less common neurologic condition, **HTLV-associated myelopathy** (**HAM**). HTLV-2 infection causes a rare form of cancer, **hairy cell leukemia.**

A. Transmission of HTLV

The distribution of HTLV infection varies greatly with geographic area and socioeconomic group. For example, the overall incidence of antibody in United States blood donors is about 1 in 2500, whereas about 25 percent of New York City intravenous drug users are infected with either HTLV-1 or -2. HTLV-2 infection is also high among the Native American population of the southwestern United States. HTLV transmission occurs primarily by cell-associated virus, via one of three routes. First, in highly endemic regions, mother to fetus or newborn is the most common mode of transmission. This is accomplished via infected lymphocytes either transplacentally or in breast milk. Second, infection can be transmitted sexually by infected lymphocytes contained in semen. Third, any blood products containing intact cells are also a potential source of infection. There is very little evidence for transmission by cell-free fluids.

B. Pathogenesis and clinical significance of adult T-cell leukemia

HTLV-1 infection both stimulates mitosis and immortalizes T-lymphocytes, which acquire an "antigen-activated" phenotype. Following infection, the virus becomes integrated in the host cell as a provirus, and transforms a polyclonal population of T cells. Although these cells all have an integrated provirus, there is no common integration site in different tumors. No HTLV mRNA is transcribed, and no recognized oncogene is activated. However, in the course of continued multiplication over a period of many years, the infected T-cells accumulate many chromosomal aberrations, leading to selection of monoclonal populations of cells that have an increasingly malignant phenotype (Figure 31.20). The majority of infected individuals are

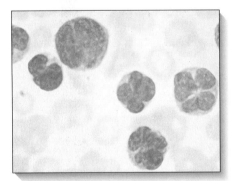

Figure 31.20
Typical "clover leaf" appearance of nuclei of HTLV-1 infected adult T cell leukemic cells.

asymptomatic carriers who have an estimated one percent chance of developing adult T-cell leukemia (ATL) within their lifetime. ATL typically appears twenty to thirty years after initial infection, when an increasingly larger population of monoclonal malignant ATL cells develops, and infiltration of various visceral organs by these cells occurs. There are accompanying serum chemistry abnormalities, and impairment of the immune system leads to opportunistic infections, for example, by human cytomegalovirus (see p. 328), *Pneumocystis carinii* (see p. 277), and/or various disseminated fungal and bacterial infections. Median survival after appearance of acute ATL is about six months.

C. Pathogenesis and clinical significance of HTLV-associated myelopathy

HTLV-associated myelopathy (HAM) is distinctly different from ATL in that it usually appears only a few years after infection. CNS involvement is indicated by 1) the presence of anti-HTLV-1 antibody in the CSF; 2) lymphocytic infiltration and demyelination of the thoracic spinal cord; and 3) brain lesions. The lymphocyte count is normal, although there is a polyclonal nonmalignant fraction with integrated HTLV. HAM occurs with lower frequency than ATL among HTLV-infected populations. It is characterized by progressive spasticity and weakness of the extremities, urinary and fecal incontinence, hyperreflexia, and some peripheral sensory loss.

D. Pathogenesis and clinical significance of hairy cell leukemia

This disease, caused by HTLV-2, is a rare, lymphocytic leukemia that is usually of B cell origin. It is characterized by malignant cells that look ciliated (Figure 31.21). These cells replace bone marrow and infiltrate the spleen, causing splenomegaly.

E. Laboratory identification

Screening of blood donors is done by ELISA (see p. 30) or agglutination tests (see p. 30), but the existence of false positives necessitates confirmatory testing by Western blotting[4]. Test sensitivity is also a problem due to the low and variable antibody titers in infected individuals. Routine screening does not distinguish HTLV-1 from -2. More definitive and sensitive diagnosis can be made by detecting HTLV genomes in lymphocytes. In ATL, sufficient numbers of lymphocytes contain the genome to permit detection by Southern blotting[5], but the small numbers of infected cells in asymptomatic carriers require use of PCR for amplification. Nucleotide sequencing can then be done to distinguish HTLV-1 from -2.

F. Treatment and prevention

The usual agents used in cancer chemotherapy have proven to be ineffective in treating ATL, and attempts to treat HAM have for the most part been equally unsuccessful. An estimated ten to twenty million people worldwide are infected with HTLV-1 or -2, and five percent of these will eventually develop either ATL or HAM. Screening of blood donors can effectively prevent transmission by transfusions, but the other modes of transmission could best be controlled by use of a vaccine. None is currently available for human use, but trials of experimental vaccines are in progress.

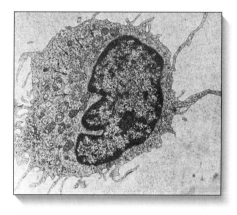

Figure 31.21
Appearance of hairy cell leukemia, a neoplasm of B lymphocytes caused by HTLV-2.

[4,5]See p. 411 in *Lippincott's Illustrated Reviews: Biochemistry* (2nd ed.) for a discussion of Western and Southern blotting.

Study Questions

Choose the ONE correct answer

31.1 Current approaches to therapy of AIDS involve the use of multiple drugs because:

  A. it is not known which one will be effective.

  B. mutants resistant to any one drug appear rapidly, but the chance for appearance of mutants resistant to all of them is small.

  C. all inhibit the same step in replication, thereby increasing their effectiveness.

  D. this is the most effective means of curing cells of integrated HIV genomes.

  E. each tends to neutralize the toxicity of the others.

Correct answer = B. The major problem with chemotherapy of AIDS is the high mutation rate of the virus, leading to rapid appearance of mutants resistant to any single drug. By choosing drugs that act at different steps in the replication cycle, or with different mechanisms of action, mutations in each of the affected proteins would have to occur in the same virus genome. The chance for this to occur is considerably lower than for either one individually. D: There is no way known to cure cells of their integrated genomes. E: Whereas these drugs do not neutralize each other's toxicity, it is possible in some cases to use a lower dose of each of the drugs, thereby decreasing the toxic side effects.

31.2 The "asymptomatic period" following the initial acute disease due to HIV infection is characterized by:

  A. high levels of HIV replication in lymphoid tissue.

  B. high levels of HIV replication in circulating T lymphocytes.

  C. inability of the immune system to respond to antigenic stimuli.

  D. absence of detectable HIV genomes or mRNA in circulating lymphocytes.

  E. high titers of free virus in the blood.

Correct answer = A. During this period a relatively large fraction of circulating lymphocytes can be shown to contain integrated HIV genomes, but a considerably smaller fraction have HIV mRNA, and virus replication occurs in relatively few cells. Infectious virus is largely confined to the lymphoid organs, although occasional bursts of viremia do occur, usually as the result of antigenic stimulation. The immune system retains its ability to respond to mitogenic stimuli generally, but there is some impairment of responses to specific antigens.

31.3 After infection of a cell by a retrovirus, synthesis of progeny genomes is carried out by:

  A. the DNA-dependent RNA polymerase activity of viral reverse transcriptase.

  B. the retrovirus RNA-dependent RNA polymerase.

  C. the host-cell DNA polymerase.

  D. a host-cell RNA polymerase.

  E. a complex of reverse transcriptase and a second virus protein that enables it to synthesize RNA rather than DNA.

Correct answer = D. Progeny virus RNA is synthesized by the same transcription process as that of cellular genes. A and E: Reverse transcriptase is involved only in the initial step converting the infecting parental RNA genome into dsDNA. B: Unlike other RNA viruses, retroviruses do not encode an RNA-dependent RNA polymerase. C: The host cell DNA polymerase replicates the integrated provirus, but plays no role in synthesis of progeny.

31.4 Oncogenesis associated with human T-cell lymphotropic virus (HTLV) differs from that caused by the leukemogenic retroviruses in that:

  A. HTLV does not integrate into its host cell's genome.

  B. HTLV does not interact with a known cell oncogene or anti-oncogene.

  C. an oncogene is present in the HTLV genome.

  D. leukemia appears only a few months after infection with HTLV.

  E. the resulting malignant cells are polyclonal with respect to the chromosomal site of HTLV integration.

Correct answer = B. There is no indication of activation of an oncogene or disruption of a cellular anti-oncogene. A: HTLV does integrate, as do all retroviruses. C: There is no recognized oncogene in either the HTLV genome or in that of the leukemogenic retroviruses. D: The malignant disease, ATL, appears twenty to thirty years after infection. E: The malignant cells of both HTLV and the leukemogenic retroviruses are usually monoclonal with respect to integration site.

Negative-strand RNA Viruses

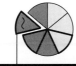

Arenaviridae
Bunyaviridae
Filoviridae
Orthomyxoviridae
Paramyxoviridae
Rhabdoviridae

32

I. OVERVIEW

The medically important negative-strand RNA viruses are shown in Figure 32.1. They have in common that 1) they are all enveloped; 2) their virions contain an RNA-dependent RNA transcriptase that synthesizes viral mRNAs using the genomic negative-strand RNA as a template; 3) the genomic negative-strand viral RNAs are not infectious, in contrast to the genomic RNAs of positive-strand viruses (see p. 349); and 4) following entry and penetration, the first step in the replication of negative-strand RNA viruses is the synthesis of mRNAs, whereas with positive-strand RNA viruses, the first step in replication is translation of the incoming genomic RNA (see p. 301). Some negative-strand RNA viruses have segmented genomes, whereas others have nonsegmented genomes. Although most of these viruses replicate in the cytoplasm, the replication of influenza virus RNA (an orthomyxovirus) occurs in the nucleus.

II. FAMILY RHABDOVIRIDAE

The rhabdoviruses are enveloped, bullet-shaped viruses (Figure 32.2). Each contains a helical nucleocapsid (see p. 296). The viruses in the family Rhabdoviridae known to infect mammals are divided into two genera: lyssavirus (**rabies virus**, the rhabdovirus of greatest medical importance to humans), and vesiculovirus [**vesicular stomatitis virus** (VSV), a virus of horses and cattle, and the best studied virus in this family]. Other rhabdoviruses infect invertebrates, plants, or other vertebrates.

A. Epidemiology

A wide variety of wildlife, such as raccoons, skunks, squirrels, foxes, and bats, provide a reservoir for the rabies virus (Figure 32.3B). In third-world countries, domestic dogs and cats also constitute an important reservoir for rabies. [Note: Laws in developed countries such as the United States mandate that domestic dogs must be vaccinated against the virus, causing the urban form of rabies to be almost unknown in these countries, although sylvatic rabies (that is, wildlife rabies) is widespread.] Cases of human rabies in the United States are rare. In contrast, in developing countries such as India, it is estimated that there are 15,000 deaths per year due to rabies.

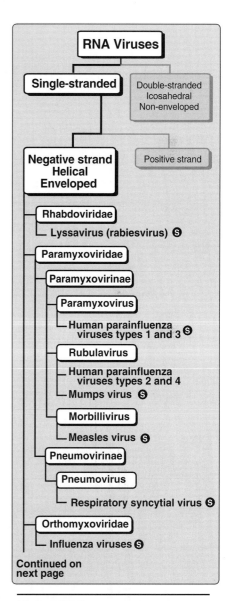

Figure 32.1
Classification of negative-strand RNA viruses (continued on next page). ⑤ See p. 401 for summaries of these viruses.

Lippincott's Illustrated Reviews: Microbiology, by William A. Strohl, Harriet Rouse, Bruce D. Fisher. Lippincott, Williams & Wilkins, Baltimore, MD © 2001

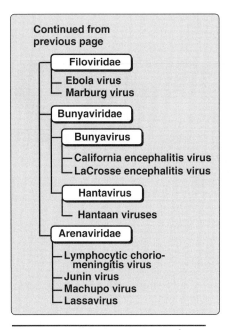

Figure 32.1 (continued)
Classification of negative-strand RNA viruses.

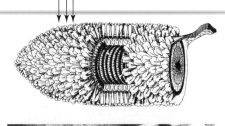

A Surface glycoproteins (G proteins) extending from the lipid envelope. The G protein is antigenic, resulting in host production of neutralizing antibodies.

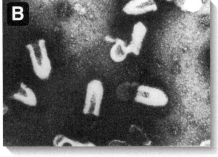

Figure 32.2
Rabies virus. A. Schematic drawing. B. Electron micrograph.

Humans are usually infected by the bite of an animal, but in some cases, infection is via an aerosol, for example, of droppings from infected bats. It is noteworthy that in about half of the cases of rabies reported in the United States during recent years, it has not been possible to get a definite history of exposure to an infected animal. However, sequence analysis of the viral RNA has shown that most human cases in the United States are now due to a bat strain of rabies virus.

B. Viral replication

The genomic negative-strand RNA is nonsegmented. The virion contains five proteins, one of which, the G (for glyco-) protein, is an envelope protein that comprises the viral spikes (see Figure 32.2). [Note: The G protein is antigenic, resulting in host production of neutralizing and hemagglutination-inhibiting antibodies.] The rabies virion attaches via its glycoprotein spikes to cell-surface receptors. Entry into the cell is by receptor-mediated endocytosis, following which the viral envelope fuses with the endocytotic vesicle's membrane, releasing the viral nucleocapsid into the cytoplasm where replication occurs. Five different mRNAs are transcribed from the genomic RNA template by the virion's RNA-dependent RNA polymerase (transcriptase function), and each encodes one of the five viral proteins. [Note: The polymerase that produces the mRNA also synthesizes positive-strand copies of the viral RNA template (replicase function), from which new negative-strand RNA genomic molecules can be transcribed.] This process is an example of the Type II virus genome replication described on p. 302. Viral structural proteins plus the negative-strand viral RNA form new helical nucleocapsids, which move to the cell surface. There, each nucleocapsid acquires its envelope by budding through a region of virus-modified plasma membrane (see Figure 26.16, p. 304).

C. Pathology

Following inoculation, the virus may replicate locally, but then travels via the axoplasm of peripheral neurons to the brain, where it replicates primarily in the gray matter (Figure 32.3A). From the brain, the rabies virus can travel along autonomic nerves, leading to infection of the lungs, kidney, adrenal medulla, and salivary glands. [Note: Contamination of saliva potentially leads to further transmission of the disease, for example, through a bite from an infected animal.] The incubation period is extremely variable, depending on the host's resistance, the amount of virus transferred, and the distance of the site of initial infection from the CNS. Incubation generally lasts one to eight weeks, but may range up to several months or, in unusual cases, as long as several years following exposure. Clinical illness may begin with an abnormal sensation at the site of the bite, then progress to a fatal encephalitis, with neuronal degeneration of the brain and spinal cord. Symptoms include hallucinations, seizures, weakness, mental dysfunction, paralysis, coma, and finally death. Many, but not all, patients show the classic rabid sign of hydrophobia (in this case, "hydrophobia" refers to an infected individual's painful inability to swallow liquids, leading to their avoidance). Once symptoms begin, death is inevitable.

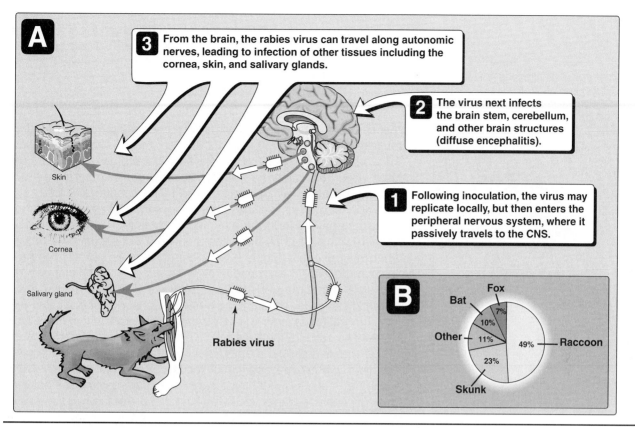

Figure 32.3
A. Schematic representation of pathogenesis of rabies infection. B. Wildlife rabies in the United States.

D. Laboratory identification

Clinically, diagnosis rests on a history of exposure, and signs and symptoms characteristic of rabies. However, a reliable history of exposure is often not obtainable, and the clinical presentation, especially in the initial stages, may not be characteristic. Therefore, a clinical diagnosis may be difficult. Postmortem, in approximately eighty percent of cases, characteristic eosinophilic cytoplasmic inclusions (**Negri bodies**) may be identified in certain regions of the brain, such as the hippocampus; these inclusion bodies are diagnostic of rabies (Figure 32.4). Prior to death, the diagnosis can be made by identification of viral antigens in biopsies of skin from the back of the neck or from corneal cells, or by demonstration of the viral nucleic acid by RT-PCR (see p. 356).

E. Treatment and prevention

Once an individual has clinical symptoms of rabies, there is no effective treatment. However, a killed rabies virus vaccine is available for prophylaxis. In the United States, this is generally the **human diploid cell vaccine** (**HDCV**). **Preexposure prophylaxis** is indicated for individuals at high risk because of the work they do, for example, for veterinarians. **Postexposure prophylaxis** refers to treatment instituted after an animal bite or exposure to an animal (or human) suspected of being rabid, and consists of thorough cleaning

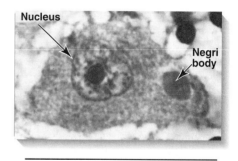

Figure 32.4
An oval Negri body in a brain cell from a human rabies case.

of the wound, passive immunization with antirabies immunoglobulin, and active immunization with the rabies vaccine (HDCV). Prevention of initial exposure is, however, clearly the most important mechanism for controlling human rabies.

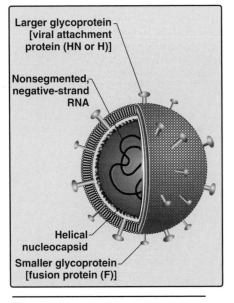

Figure 32.5
Model of paramyxovirus.

III. FAMILY PARAMYXOVIRIDAE

The members of the paramyxovirus family have recently been subdivided into two subfamilies (see Figure 32.1). First, the Paramyxovirinae, whose three genera include the **paramyxovirus (parainfluenza viruses**, which cause upper respiratory tract infections), the **rubulavirus (mumps virus)**, and the **morbillivirus (measles virus)**. The second subfamily is the Pneumovirinae, which includes **respiratory syncytial virus**, a major respiratory tract pathogen in the pediatric population. Paramyxoviruses are spherical, enveloped particles that contain a nonsegmented, negative-strand RNA genome (Figure 32.5). Paramyxoviridae typically consist of a helical nucleocapsid, surrounded by an envelope that contains two types of integral membrane or envelope proteins. The first, the HN protein (where H stands for hemagglutinin, and N for neuraminidase), is involved in the binding of the virus to a cell; measles virus lacks the neuraminidase activity. The second, the F protein (where F stands for fusion), functions to fuse viral and cellular membranes, thus facilitating virus entry into the cytoplasm where viral replication occurs (see Figure 26.10, p. 299). [Note: This mechanism of infection, whereby paramyxoviruses enter cells via a fusion process that occurs at a neutral pH at the cell surface, is in contrast to the entry mechanism of nearly all other enveloped viruses, which gain entry by receptor-mediated endocytosis (see Figure 26.9, p. 299).] Paramyxovirus mRNA transcription, genome replication, and viral assembly and release, resemble those of the rhabdoviruses (see p. 380).

A. Genus paramyxovirus

The clinically important viruses in this genus are type 1 and type 3 human parainfluenza viruses (hPIV). They cause croup, pneumonia and bronchiolitis, mainly in infants and children. The term "parainfluenza" was first coined because infected individuals may present with influenza-like symptoms, and, like influenza virus, these viruses have both hemagglutinating and neuraminidase activities.

B. Genus rubulavirus

This genus contains hPIV type 2 and type 4, and mumps virus. [Note: The separation of the four hPIV's into two separate genera is based on molecular features of their proteins and RNA genomes.]

1. **Type 2 and type 4 human parainfluenza viruses:** The clinical features of infection with parainfluenza virus type 2 are similar to those of the types 1 and 3 viruses. Type 4 hPIV has been associated only with a mild upper respiratory tract illness, affecting both children and adults.

2. **Mumps virus:** Mumps used to be one of the commonly acquired childhood infections. Adults who escape the disease in childhood could also be infected. In the prevaccine period, mumps was the most common cause of viral encephalitis. Complete recovery, how-

ever, was almost always the rule. The virus is spread by respiratory droplets. Although about one third of the infections are subclinical, the classic clinical presentation and diagnosis center on infection and swelling of the salivary glands, primarily the parotid glands (Figure 32.6). However, infection is widespread in the body, and may involve not only the salivary glands, but also the pancreas, CNS, and testes. [Note: Orchitis (inflammation of the testis) caused by mumps virus may cause sterility.] Virus may be recoverable from saliva, blood, CSF, or urine. If the clinical presentation is unusual, for example, if there is CNS infection without parotid gland involvement, the diagnosis may depend on virus isolation or, more commonly, on the demonstration of a rise in the titer of antiviral antibody in the blood or, if need be, in the CSF. A live, attenuated vaccine has been available for many years; this has resulted in a dramatic drop in the number of cases of mumps. [Note: Individuals who have had the disease develop life-long immunity.]

C. Genus morbillivirus

Measles virus (MV) is the only virus in this genus that causes disease in humans. Other viruses in the genus morbillivirus are responsible for disease in animals, for example, canine distemper virus. Measles virus differs in several ways from the other viruses in the family Paramyxoviridae.

1. **Viral replication:** The cellular receptor for measles virus is the CD46 molecule, a protein whose normal function is to bind certain components of complement (see p. 90). Although the viral attachment protein has hemagglutinating activity, it lacks neuraminidase activity. Hence, it is referred to as the H protein, rather than HN protein. A fusion (F) protein facilitates uptake of the virion. Measles virus replication in tissue culture, and in certain organs of the intact organism, is characterized by the formation of giant multinucleate cells (**syncytium** formation), resulting from the action of the viral spike F protein.

2. **Pathology:** Measles virus is transmitted by sneeze- or cough-produced respiratory droplets. The virus is extremely infectious, and almost all infected individuals develop a clinical illness. Measles virus replicates initially in the respiratory epithelium, and then in various lymphoid organs. Classically, **measles** (referred to in the past as **rubeola**) begins with a prodromal period of fever, upper respiratory tract symptoms, and conjunctivitis. Two to three days later, specific diagnostic signs develop; first, **Koplik spots** (small white spots on bright red mucous membranes of the mouth and throat (Figure 32.7), and then a generalized macular rash, beginning at the head and traveling slowly to the lower extremities (Figure 32.8). Soon after the rash appears, the patient is no longer infectious. The major morbidity and mortality due to measles are associated with various complications of infection, especially those affecting the CNS. The most important of these is **postinfectious encephalomyelitis**, which is estimated to affect one in 1,000 cases of measles, usually occurring within two weeks after the onset of the rash. This is an autoimmune disease, and is associated with an immune response to myelin basic protein. Children are particu-

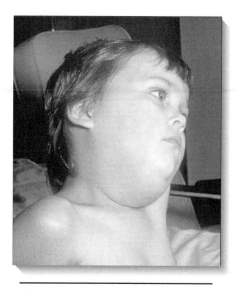

Figure 32.6
Child with mumps showing swollen parotid gland.

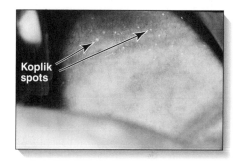

Figure 32.7
Koplik spots in the mouth caused by measles virus.

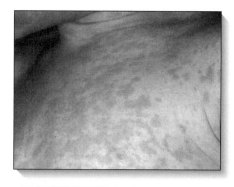

Figure 32.8
The measles rash consists of large, slightly raised lesions called maculopapules. These run into each other to form irregular blotches.

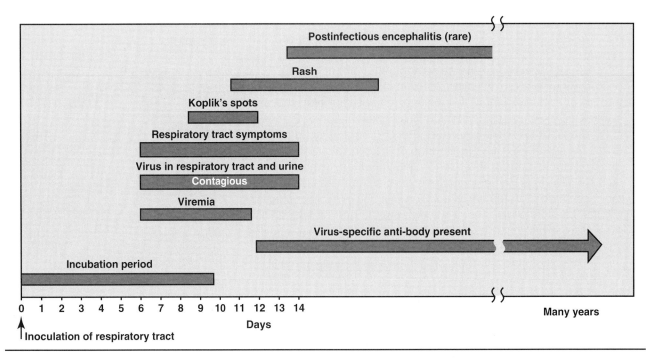

Figure 32.9
Time course of measles virus infection.

larly susceptible, especially those weakened by other diseases or malnutrition, and measles is thus an important cause of childhood mortality in developing countries. Figure 32.9 shows the time course of measles virus infection.

3. **Diagnosis:** In most cases, there is little difficulty in making a diagnosis of measles on clinical grounds, especially in an epidemic situation. The presence of Koplik's spots provides a definitive diagnosis. If a laboratory diagnosis is necessary, it is usually made by demonstrating an increase in the titer of antiviral antibodies.

4. **Prevention:** Measles is usually a disease of childhood, and is followed by life-long immunity. A live, attenuated measles vaccine, which has been available for many years, has greatly reduced the incidence of the disease. Nevertheless, occasional outbreaks of measles continue to occur, especially in older children and young adults, possibly due to waning immunity. Thus, two doses of the vaccine, in the form of the measles-mumps-rubella (MMR) vaccine (see p. 43), are now recommended, the first at twelve to eighteen months, the second at four to twelve years.

D. Genus pneumovirus

The one virus in this genus that is of medical importance is **respiratory syncytial virus** (RSV). RSV is the major viral respiratory tract pathogen in the pediatric population, and the most important cause of bronchiolitis in infants. It may also cause pneumonia in young children, an influenza-like syndrome in adults, and severe bronchitis with pneumonia in the elderly and organ transplant recipients. The viruses in the subfamily Pneumovirinae, genus pneumovirus, are set apart from those in the other three genera in the Paromyxovirus family by a somewhat more complex genome, and a larger number of virus-specific proteins. Nevertheless, the basic strategy of replication is as described for the other viruses in this family (see p. 382). RSV has one envelope protein that functions as an attachment protein, and another that functions as a fusion protein, but, like measles virus, RSV lacks neuraminidase activity. RSV is transmitted by respiratory droplets or by contaminated hands carrying the virus to the nose or mouth. Repeated infections are common. A definitive diagnosis of RSV infection can be made only on the basis of laboratory findings, such as a rise in the titer of serum antibody, or the demonstration of viral antigens in respiratory secretions. The only specific treatment is ribavirin, administered by aerosol, and this is only of moderate benefit. Much effort has been spent on vaccine development, but thus far, without success. Hand-washing and avoidance of others with the infection are the major preventive measures.

IV. FAMILY ORTHOMYXOVIRIDAE

The orthomyxoviruses are spherical, enveloped viruses containing a segmented, negative-strand RNA genome. Viruses in this family infect humans, horses, pigs, as well as nondomestic water fowl, and are the cause of **influenza**. Orthomyxoviruses are divided into 3 types: influenza A, B, and C. Only influenza virus types A and B are of medical importance. Type A influenza viruses differ from type B viruses in that they have an animal reservoir, and are divided into subtypes.

A. Structure

Influenza virions are spherical, enveloped, pleomorphic particles (Figure 32.10). Two types of spikes project from the surface: one is composed of hemagglutinin (H protein), and the second of neuraminidase (N protein). [Note: This is in contrast to the paramyxoviruses, where the H and N activities reside in the same spike protein.] Both the H and N influenza proteins are integral membrane proteins. The M (matrix) proteins underlie the viral lipid membrane. The RNA genome is located in a helical nucleocapsid, and is composed of eight distinct segments of RNA, six of which code for a single protein. Each nucleocapsid segment contains not only the viral RNA, but also four proteins (NP, the major nucleocapsid protein, and three P proteins that are present in much smaller amounts than NP, and are involved in the synthesis and replication of the viral RNA).

B. Viral replication

There are two unusual features associated with the synthesis and replication of influenza viral RNAs that distinguish the influenza viruses from the other RNA viruses discussed up to this point. First, the synthesis of influenza virus mRNAs, and the replication of the viral genome, occur in the **nucleus**. This is in contrast to the replication of other RNA viruses, which occurs completely in the cytoplasm. [Note: The retroviruses are an exception to this generalization (see p. 362).] Second, compounds such as actinomycin D and α-amanitin, which inhibit the synthesis of eukaryotic RNA polymerase II[1] (Pol II) transcripts (the messenger RNAs), inhibit the replication of influenza virus.

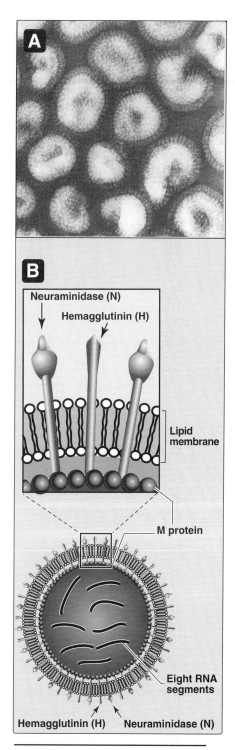

Figure 32.10
Influenza virus. A. Electron micrograph. B. Schematic drawing showing envelope proteins—called H and N spikes —that protrude from the surface.

[1]See p. 383 in *Lippincott's Illustrated Reviews: Biochemistry* (2nd ed.) for a discussion of RNA polymerase II.

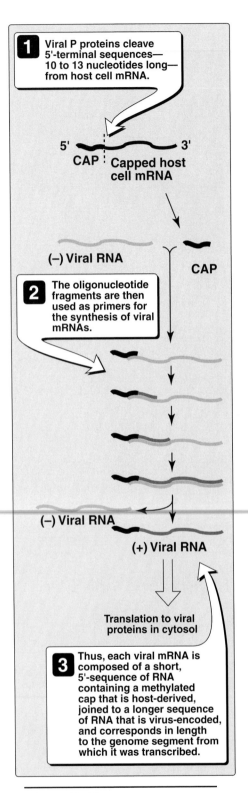

1. Viral entry into the cell: Influenza virus attaches to sialic acid residues on host cell glycoproteins or glycolipids. Entry then occurs via receptor-mediated endocytosis (see Figure 26.9, p. 299). [Note: This is in contrast to the Paramyxoviridae, which enter the cell by fusion at the plasma membrane (see Figure 26.10, p. 299).] Both the attachment and the fusion functions are associated with the H protein.

2. Synthesis and translation of viral mRNAs: The nucleocapsid segments are released into the cytosol, and, as with the other negative-strand RNA viruses, the viral genomic RNA serves as the template for synthesis of the viral mRNAs. Each of the eight genome segments directs the synthesis of one positive-strand mRNA. However, influenza virus is distinguished from the other negative-strand viruses in that, although the virions contain proteins that can transcribe mRNAs, these enzymes lack the ability to cap and methylate the viral mRNAs. The synthesis of influenza virus mRNA therefore begins with "cap snatching," in which the viral P proteins cleave 5'-terminal sequences (ten to thirteen nucleotides long) from nascent host cellular Pol II transcripts that had previously been synthesized, capped, and methylated in the nucleus. The oligonucleotide fragments are then used as primers for the synthesis of the viral mRNAs (Figure 32.11). Thus, each viral mRNA is composed of a short, 5'-sequence of RNA containing a methylated cap that is host-derived, joined to a longer sequence of RNA that is virus-encoded, and corresponds in length to the genome segment from which it was transcribed.

3. Assembly and release of influenza virus particles: Once the viral mRNAs are made and translated, the NP and the three P proteins move into the nucleus, whereupon replication of the eight genomic segments begins, and progeny nucleocapsids are assembled. Meanwhile certain regions of the plasma membrane become virus-modified by insertion of the H and N proteins and the alignment of the M protein on the inner side of the plasma membrane. The nucleocapsids move from the nucleus to the cytoplasm, and finally to virus-modified regions of the plasma membrane, which they bud through, giving rise to extracellular viral particles (Figure 32.12). [Note: Viral release is facilitated by the N protein, which cleaves neuraminic acid on the cell surface.]

C. Pathology and clinical significance

In humans, influenza is spread by respiratory droplets, and is an infection solely of the respiratory tract (Figure 32.13). There is rarely a viremia, or spread to other organ systems. Destruction of respiratory epithelial cells is attributed to the host immune response, specifically cytotoxic T cells (see p. 73). Typically, influenza has an acute onset characterized by chills, followed by a high fever, muscle aches (caused by circulating cytokines, see p. 63), and extreme drowsiness. The disease runs its course in four to five days, after which there is a gradual recovery. The most serious problems, such as development of pneumonia, occur in the very young, the elderly, and people with chronic cardiac or pulmonary disease, or who are immunodeficient. [Note: Reye's syndrome is a rare and serious

Figure 32.11
"Cap snatching" by influenza virus prior to viral mRNA translation.

complication of viral infections in children, especially in those who have had chickenpox or influenza B. Aspirin, used to lower the virus-induced fever, contributes to the appearance of this syndrome. Therefore, acetaminophen is usually recommended for fevers of unknown origin in children.]

D. The immunology of influenza viruses

When individuals are infected with influenza virus, antibodies are made against the various viral proteins. However, it is the antibodies made against the H protein that are neutralizing, and are the best index of protection. The antigenic properties of the influenza virus proteins are also important because they serve as the basis for the classification of influenza viruses.

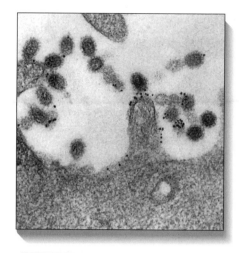

Figure 32.12
Influenza virus budding from the surface of an infected cell. Electron micrograph.

1. **Types and subtypes:** Influenza viruses are classified as types A, B, and C, depending on their inner proteins, mainly the M and NP proteins. Thus, all type A viruses share common internal antigens that are distinct from those shared by all type B viruses. Only the type A viruses are broken down into subtypes. The classification into subtypes depends on antigens associated with the outer viral proteins, H and N. Taking into consideration animal as well as human influenza viruses, 14 H and 9 N subtypes have been described. However, among human influenza viruses, only three H (H1, H2, and H3) and two N (N1 and N2) subtypes are found. Human influenza viruses are therefore designated, for example, as subtype H1N1, H2N2, H3N2, etc.

2. **Antigenic variability of influenza viruses:** In contrast to viruses such as polio or measles virus that have maintained antigenic stability since they were first isolated, the influenza viruses have shown marked variation over the years in their antigenic properties, specifically of the H and N proteins. Two distinct phenomena account for this observation: antigenic drift, and antigenic shift.

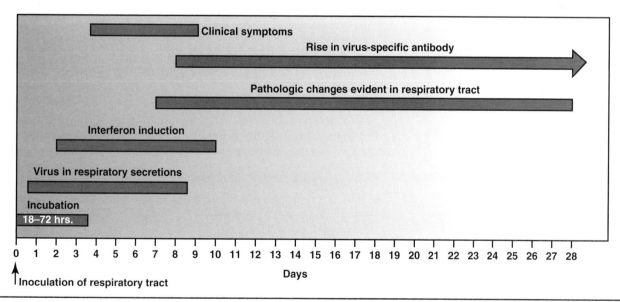

Figure 32.13
Time course of influenza A virus infection. The classic "flu syndrome" occurs early. Later, pneumonia may result from ascending bacterial infection.

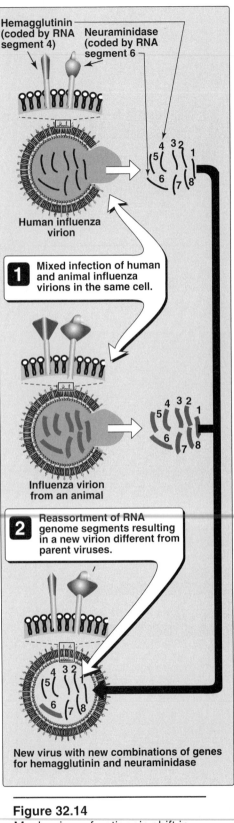

Figure 32.14
Mechanism of antigenic shift in
influenza virus.

a. Antigenic drift: This refers to minor antigenic changes in the H and N proteins that occur each year. Antigenic drift does not involve a change in the viral subtype. This phenomenon can be easily explained by random mutations in the viral RNA, and single or a small number of amino acid substitutions in the H and N proteins.

b. Antigenic shift: This phenomenon involves a much more dramatic change in the antigenic properties of the H and/or N proteins (Figure 32.14), and does involve a change in subtype, for example, from H1N1 to H3N2. Antigenic shift occurs only infrequently, perhaps every ten or twenty years. For example, the appearance of a new, extremely virulent H1N1 virus, due presumably to antigenic shift, probably accounted for the pandemic of 1918–1919 that resulted in the death of an estimated twenty million people worldwide, and more than 500,000 in the United States (Figure 32.15). In 1957, antigenic shift again occurred, and H1N1 virus was replaced by subtype H2N2, and in 1968, H2N2 was replaced by H3N2. Since 1977, multiple subtypes of influenza A have been circulating around the world. [Note: In most years, both type A and type B influenza viruses can be isolated from patients. Both type A and B viruses undergo antigenic drift, but only type A viruses show antigenic shift.] Currently, approximately 110,000 people are hospitalized, and 20,000 people die in the United States each year from influenza and its complications.

c. Consequences of antigenic variation: When antigenic shift occurs and a new subtype of virus appears that has not been in circulation for many years, the immune systems of a large proportion of the population have never encountered that virus, and these individuals are therefore immunologically unprotected. Thus, the conditions are set for an influenza epidemic or even pandemic (Figure 32.15). Antigenic shift also means that the vaccine that was in use before the antigenic shift will not be effective in protecting against the new subtype of virus. Thus, it becomes necessary to develop a new vaccine as quickly as possible, incorporating the new virus subtype.

d. The molecular basis of antigenic variation: The dramatic changes associated with antigenic shift result from reassortment of viral RNA segments, a process observed with all RNA viruses having a segmented genome. Reassortment results when a cell is infected with two genetically distinct influenza viruses; the genomic RNAs of both parental viruses are replicated, and progeny viruses are assembled that contain some genomic RNA segments from one of the parental viruses, and other genomic segments from the second parent (see Figure 32.14). In this way, new viruses can be generated that differ from both of the parents. Although all eight of the influenza virus RNA genome segments undergo reassortment, for antigenic shift to occur, it is the reassortment of the RNA segments that specify the mRNAs for the H and N proteins (the proteins that define the antigenic subtypes) that is most critical. Where do the genes for the new viral subtypes come from? We know

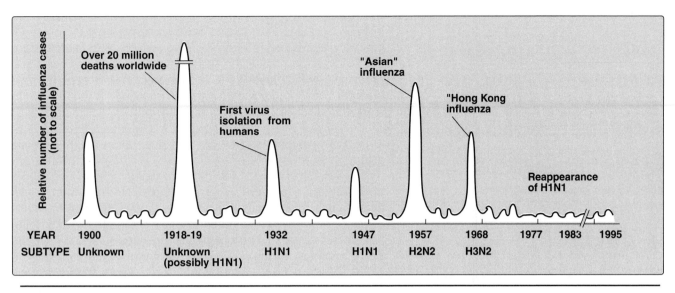

Figure 32.15
Time line showing the occurrence of some of the major outbreaks and antigenic shifts associated with type A influenza during the 1900s.

that influenza type A viruses are found in many different animals including horses, pigs, and wild migrating water fowl. Furthermore, it has been demonstrated that reassortment can occur between influenza A viruses from different animal species, and between different avian species, including between mammalian and avian viruses. For example, in situations where humans live in proximity to farm animals, there is opportunity for the generation of new, reassorted viral subtypes. [Note: Whether a new subtype will spread depends both on the efficiency with which it replicates, and the prevalence of antibody to that subtype in the population it encounters.]

E. Diagnosis

The collection of influenza-like symptoms described above can also be caused by other viruses, for example, respiratory syncytial virus (see p. 384). Therefore, a definitive diagnosis cannot be made on clinical grounds except in an epidemic situation. In most cases it is not practical to make a specific laboratory diagnosis. However, if needed, for example, for surveillance purposes, a widely performed and specific test is the quantitation of HI (hemagglutination inhibition) antibodies. This has the added advantage of identifying the subtype of the virus (see below). A more rapid diagnosis can be made by the demonstration of viral antigens in respiratory tract secretions.

F. Treatment and prevention

1. **Amantadine and rimantadine:** First-generation antiviral agents effective against influenza A include two related drugs, amantadine and rimantadine. Both drugs stop viral uncoating by inhibition of the viral M2 membrane protein. These agents reduce both the duration and the severity of flu symptoms, but only if given early in infection. Given before the onset of symptoms, these drugs can also prevent disease, and are useful for treating high-risk groups.

For example, if there are one or two cases of influenza in the elderly population of a nursing home, rimantadine can be used to prevent disease in the rest of the population. The usefulness of amantadine and rimantidine has been limited by a combination of problems: 1) lack of efficacy against influenza B virus, 2) rapid emergence of drug-resistant variants of the virus, and 3) neurologic side effects (especially for amantadine).

2. **Zanamivir and oseltamivir:** Second-generation antiviral agents effective against influenza A and B include zanamivir and oseltamivir. They inhibit viral neuraminidase, which is present in both influenza A and B viruses. [Note: Neuraminidase—an enzyme essential for viral replication—cleaves terminal sialic acid residues from glycoconjugates to allow the release of the virus from infected cells.] The drugs are indicated for uncomplicated acute illness in adults and adolescents twelve years of age and older who have been symptomatic for no more than two days. Zanamivir must be taken by inhalation. In contrast, oseltamivir is well absorbed when administered orally, and has proven to be effective for symptomatic patients as well as for prophylaxis (for example, to prevent the spread of influenza in nursing homes). For maximum benefit, therapy should begin within two days of symptom onset. For example, oseltamivir taken within 24 hours of symptom onset shortened the duration of illness by about two days, with patients reporting feeling better within a day of starting treatment (Figure 32.16).

3. **Vaccine:** As useful as new therapies are, they are not a substitute for the vaccine. A vaccine consisting of formalin-inactivated influenza virus has been available for many years. It is recommended for the elderly, and for people in high-risk groups, such as patients with chronic pulmonary or cardiac disease. [Note: It is of critical importance that the vaccine contain the specific subtypes of influenza virus that are in circulation at any given time. Therefore, the circulating strains worldwide are monitored each season, and the following year's vaccine includes the principal strains recovered during the previous year—usually one type B influenza and two type A influenza strains.]

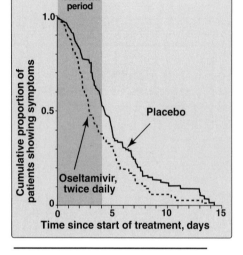

Figure 32.16
Time to alleviation of all symptoms in influenza-infected patients.

V. FAMILY FILOVIRIDAE

Filoviruses are pleomorphic viruses with unusual morphologies (Figure 32.17). They are generally seen as long, filamentous, enveloped particles that may be branched. **Marburg virus** was initially isolated in Germany and Yugoslavia from lab workers who became severely ill while preparing primary cell cultures from African green monkeys. **Ebola virus** was isolated from patients with hemorrhagic fever in Zaire and the Sudan. The two viruses are not related antigenically. Marburg and Ebola viruses cause severe hemorrhagic fever, characterized by widespread bleeding into the skin, mucous membranes, visceral organs, and the GI tract. The mortality rate is high, often greater than fifty percent. Although the natural reservoir for these viruses is unknown, they can be transmitted to humans from infected monkeys and probably other animals, or by exposure to the blood or other body

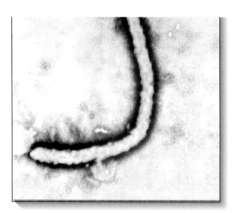

Figure 32.17
Electron micrograph of Ebola Zaire virus.

fluids from an infected patient. Outbreaks of hemorrhagic fever due to these viruses continue to occur at irregular intervals. Laboratory identification is made by the demonstration of antiviral antibodies, for example, by ELISA assays (see p. 30). If virus can be recovered, the morphology of the particles is quite characteristic. There is no specific treatment for infections due to these viruses. Strict barrier nursing techniques are essential when caring for infected individuals. Because of the hazards of working with filoviruses, they are studied only in a few reference laboratories around the world.

VI. FAMILY BUNYAVIRIDAE

About 320 serologically distinct viruses have been assigned to the family Bunyaviridae. These have been grouped into five genera, four of which contain viruses that infect animals or humans. In the United States, the clinically most important viruses in this family are **California encephalitis** and **LaCrosse viruses** (genus Bunyavirus), which cause meningitis and encephalitis, and the **Hantaan viruses** (genus Hantavirus), which are associated with hemorrhagic fever with or without renal syndrome, and hantavirus pulmonary syndrome, a condition associated with high mortality. The viruses in this family are spherical, enveloped particles, with spikes projecting from the surface of the virions. Because the RNA genome is divided into three segments, reassortment of RNA segments between closely related viruses is possible. The RNA genome is present in the virions in the form of helical nucleocapsids. Virus particles mature by budding into intracytoplasmic vesicles associated with the Golgi system. Arthropods serve as vectors for most of the viruses in the family Bunyaviridae that are transmitted to humans (Figure 32.18). However, viruses in the genus Hantavirus do not have an arthropod vector, and are transmitted to humans by rodents via aerosols formed from their dried excretions. No effective antiviral agent is currently available.

VII. FAMILY ARENAVIRIDAE

Arenaviruses are enveloped, spherical particles with a bipartite (two segment) RNA genome that exists in virions as helical nucleocapsids. Both RNAs have an ambisense organization, which means that coding information is contained in both the genomic and antigenomic viral RNAs. Viral particles mature by budding from the plasma membrane. Viruses in this family are associated with chronic infections of rodents, and humans are infected by inhaling contaminated aerosols or eating food containing viral particles, or by exposure of open wounds to dirt. Lymphocytic choriomeningitis (LCM) virus is a cause of viral meningitis, and is a relatively benign infection with little mortality. In Latin America, Junin and Machupo viruses are associated with Argentine and Bolivian hemorrhagic fevers, respectively; these are diseases with mortality rates of 25 to thirty percent. In Africa, Lassa fever caused by lassa virus is a severe infection that can be associated with bleeding, and has an expected mortality rate of about fifteen percent. Ribavirin appears to be of benefit both in Lassa fever and the hemorrhagic fevers. The most important measure in prevention, however, is rodent control.

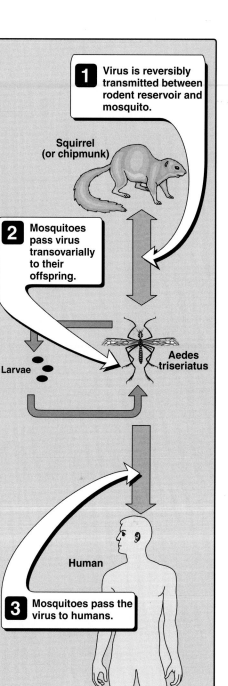

Figure 32.18
Transmission of California encephalitis virus.

Study Questions

Questions 32.1 to 32.4: Match the appropriate virus from the following list with the statement to which it most closely corresponds. Each virus can match one, more than one, or none of the statements.

A. Influenza virus
B. California encephalitis virus
C. Mumps virus
D. Parainfluenza virus
E. Hantavirus
F. Measles virus
G. Rabies virus
H. Respiratory syncytial virus

32.1 Negri bodies

Correct answer = G. Negri bodies are cytoplasmic inclusion bodies found in certain neurons in the brain, and are diagnostic of rabies. There are now more rapid methods of diagnosis of rabies that often make the diagnosis possible antemortem. Rabies virus is in the Family Rhabdoviridae.

32.2 Pulmonary syndrome with high mortality

Correct answer = E. The hantaviruses (Family Bunyaviridae) cause several different clinical syndromes, including hemorrhagic fever with or without renal syndrome, and a pulmonary syndrome. The latter, which has been associated with a high mortality, was first diagnosed in the southwestern United States, but subsequently has been found in other regions of the country.

32.3 Acute bronchiolitis in infants

Correct answer = H. Respiratory syncytial virus (Family Paramyxoviridae) is the most common cause of this syndrome.

32.4 Encephalitis that is invariably fatal

Correct answer = G. Once someone infected with rabies virus develops clinical signs and symptoms, death due to encephalitis is invariably the outcome. The prognosis of encephalitis due to California encephalitis virus (Family Bunyaviridae) is much better, the severity of the encephalitis varying from mild to severe. Measles virus (Family Paramyxoviridae) can cause a postinfectious encephalitis that can result in long-standing CNS sequelae, but which has a relatively low mortality rate.

Choose the ONE correct answer

32.5 An ornithologist was on a three-month trip to study several species of birds living in a rain forest in South America. On the tenth day of her trip, she was bitten on the hand by an unusually aggressive bat. The scientist applied a topical antibiotic ointment and continued her research. Four weeks later, the scientist lost feeling in her hand. She shortly began experiencing a high fever, periods of rigidity, difficulty in swallowing liquids, drooling, and disorientation. Death followed rapidly. A postmortem biopsy of her brain showed the presence of Negri bodies. These symptoms are consistent with the woman having died of:

A. California encephalitis virus.
B. hantaan virus.
C. ebola virus.
D, rabies virus.
E. lymphocytic choriomeningitis virus.

Correct answer = D. Rabies virus is usually transmitted via the bite of an infected animal, and the symptoms the woman experienced are consistent with those of rabies. California encephalitis virus is transmitted by arthropods, and causes meningitis and encephalitis. Hantaan virus is transmitted through aerosols formed from dried rodent excretions. This virus causes hemorrhagic fever and severe pulmonary infections. Ebola virus can be transmitted by an animal, but infection causes severe hemorrhagic fever. Lymphocytic choriomeningitis virus is a cause of viral meningitis, and is a relatively benign infection with little mortality. Humans are infected by inhaling contaminated aerosols or eating food containing viral particles, or by exposure of open wounds to dirt.

32.6 From 1918 until 1956 the only subtype of influenza that was seen in humans was H1N1. In 1957 H1N1 was replaced by H2N2. This is an example of

A. viral interference.
B. phenotypic mixing.
C. antigenic shift.
D. antigenic drift.
E. viral transformation.

Correct answer = C. A marked antigenic change in the N protein, the H protein, or both, as described above, is termed antigenic shift. In antigenic drift, there is also an antigenic change in one or both of these proteins, but the change is much less significant. Thus with antigenic drift, although the H protein does change antigenically, H1 remains H1, for example.

Double-stranded RNA Viruses: the Reoviridae

Reoviridae

33

I. OVERVIEW

The Reovirus family is divided into nine genera, and includes viruses that replicate in plants and insects as well as in mammals. The single genus in the family that is of medical importance is the genus Rotavirus, which causes severe viral gastroenteritis, primarily in infants and young children (Figure 33.1). Viruses in the family Reoviridae are spherical, non-enveloped particles that have an icosahedral structure. The viral genome consists of ten to twelve segments of double-stranded (ds) RNA. The virions contain all the enzymes needed to make positive strand RNA transcripts, which are capped and methylated.[1] Reoviruses replicate completely in the cytoplasm. The name "reovirus" stands for **r**espiratory and **e**nteric **o**rphan virus. [Note: An orphan virus is a virus not known to be the cause of any disease, although that is no longer the case for the reoviruses. Echoviruses were also initially considered orphan viruses (**e**nteric **c**ytopathic **h**uman **o**rphan viruses, see p. 349), but were soon discovered to cause a large number of clinical syndromes. Thus, as far as viruses are concerned, being an orphan may be only a temporary state.]

II. GENUS ROTAVIRUS

Rotaviruses are found in many mammalian species, and often have a fairly broad host range. Rotaviruses have a characteristic morphology that distinguishes them from other reoviruses, namely, they have the appearance of wheels with spokes radiating from the center, and a smooth outer rim (Figure 33.2). The particles also have a large number of channels connecting the outer surface of the virion to the inner core. It has been suggested that these channels are involved in the import of substrates needed for RNA transcription, and the extrusion of newly synthesized RNA transcripts.

A. Epidemiology

Rotaviruses are divided into seven serogroups, A through G, of which group A is the most important cause of outbreaks of disease in humans. Rotavirus infections account for about forty percent of cases of severe diarrhea in infants and young children (up to two

[1]See p. 379 in *Lippincott's Illustrated Reviews: Biochemistry* (2nd ed.) for a discussion of the structure of mRNA.

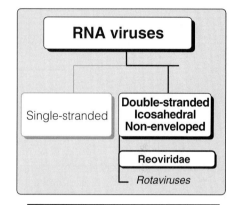

Figure 33.1
Classification of double-stranded, nonenveloped RNA viruses.

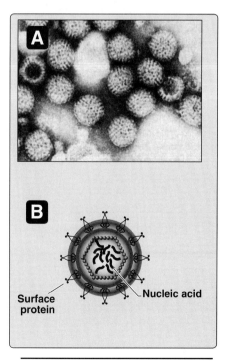

Surface protein
Nucleic acid

Figure 33.2
Structure of rotavirus. A. Electron micrograph. B. Schematic drawing.

Lippincott's Illustrated Reviews: Microbiology,
by William A. Strohl, Harriet Rouse, Bruce D. Fisher.
Lippincott, Williams & Wilkins, Baltimore, MD © 2001

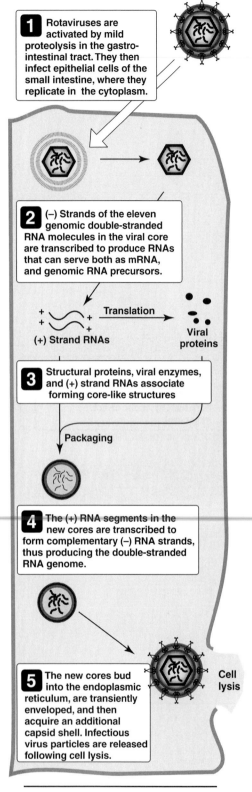

1 Rotaviruses are activated by mild proteolysis in the gastro-intestinal tract. They then infect epithelial cells of the small intestine, where they replicate in the cytoplasm.

2 (–) Strands of the eleven genomic double-stranded RNA molecules in the viral core are transcribed to produce RNAs that can serve both as mRNA, and genomic RNA precursors.

Translation

(+) Strand RNAs

Viral proteins

3 Structural proteins, viral enzymes, and (+) strand RNAs associate forming core-like structures

Packaging

4 The (+) RNA segments in the new cores are transcribed to form complementary (–) RNA strands, thus producing the double-stranded RNA genome.

5 The new cores bud into the endoplasmic reticulum, are transiently enveloped, and then acquire an additional capsid shell. Infectious virus particles are released following cell lysis.

Cell lysis

Figure 33.3
Replication of rotavirus.

years of age). Transmission of rotaviruses is via the fecal/oral route. There is a marked seasonal incidence associated with rotavirus infections, the peak months in the United States being January through March. Because infectious particles are relatively stable, they can survive for extended periods on various surfaces.

B. Viral replication

After attachment to and uptake by the host cell, rotaviruses become partially uncoated in a lysosome. The rotavirus genome has eleven segments of linear, double-stranded RNA, each of which codes for a single protein. Reassortment of the RNA segments can occur when a cell is infected with two different rotaviruses. The viral particles contain enzymes (such as RNA-dependent RNA polymerase) that are needed to synthesize positive sense RNA transcripts with a 5' cap. These positive RNA strands function not only as mRNA, but also as templates for the synthesis of negative strand RNA (see Figure 26.14, p. 303). After the negative-strand RNA is made, it stays associated with its positive strand template, giving rise to a double-stranded RNA segment that is packaged in the virion. Rotaviruses are released following cell lysis rather than by budding through the membrane, thus accounting for the lack of a viral envelope. Figure 33.3 illustrates some additional details of rotavirus replication.

C. Clinical significance

Following ingestion, rotaviruses infect the epithelial cells of the small intestine, primarily the jejunum. [Note: Rotaviruses are able to reach the small intestine because they are resistant to the acid pH of the stomach.] Observed histologic changes include shortening and atrophy of the villi, flattening of epithelial cells, and denuding of microvilli, thus decreasing the surface area of the small intestine, and limiting production of digestive enzymes such as the disaccharidases that are normally synthesized by the brush border (Figure 33.4). As a result, the patient suffers from a malabsorptive state in which dietary nutrients such as sugars are not absorbed by the small intestine, leading to a hyperosmotic effect that causes diarrhea. The incubation period is usually 48 hours or less. Infection can be subclinical, or may result in symptoms ranging from mild diarrhea and vomiting, to severe, nonbloody, watery diarrhea with dehydration and loss of electrolytes. Although rotavirus infections are probably equally widespread around the world, the outcomes of infection vary significantly in different regions of the world. In spite of the fact that more than ninety percent of children in the United States may have antibodies to rotaviruses by the age of three or four, mortality is very low, because patients who are severely ill are generally hospitalized and their fluid and electrolyte losses rapidly corrected. In contrast, in developing countries, or where medical facilities or personnel may be lacking, the mortality is quite significant. For example, it is estimated that there may be up to a million deaths per year worldwide due to rotavirus infection. Patients who are immunosuppressed are at particular risk.

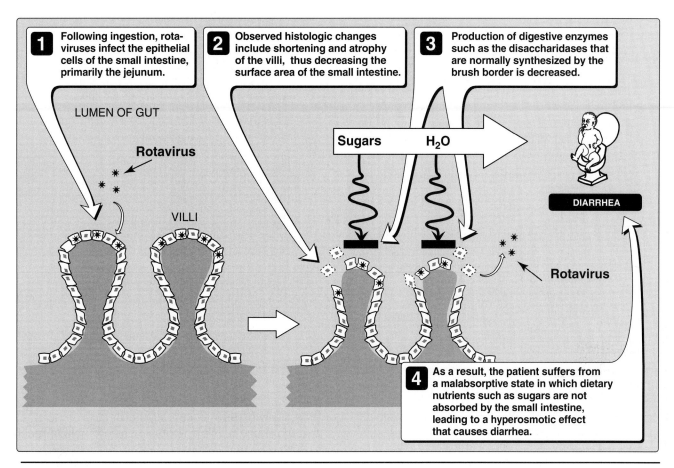

1. Following ingestion, rotaviruses infect the epithelial cells of the small intestine, primarily the jejunum.

2. Observed histologic changes include shortening and atrophy of the villi, thus decreasing the surface area of the small intestine.

3. Production of digestive enzymes such as the disaccharidases that are normally synthesized by the brush border is decreased.

LUMEN OF GUT

Rotavirus

VILLI

Sugars   H$_2$O

DIARRHEA

Rotavirus

4. As a result, the patient suffers from a malabsorptive state in which dietary nutrients such as sugars are not absorbed by the small intestine, leading to a hyperosmotic effect that causes diarrhea.

Figure 33.4
Mechanism of rotavirus diarrhea.

D. Laboratory identification

Severe diarrhea, dehydration, and electrolyte loss can be due to a variety of causes. Accordingly, a definitive diagnosis cannot be made on clinical grounds alone. As with many other viral infections, the identification can be made by using an ELISA test (see p. 30), or by recognition of an increase in the titer of antiviral antibody in a patient's serum. Electron microscopy of stool specimens, although not a routine diagnostic measure, can aid in the identification of the virus, because rotaviruses have a very distinctive appearance (see Figure 33.2).

E. Treatment and prevention

There is no specific antiviral drug appropriate for treatment of rotavirus infections. The most important clinical intervention is the rapid and efficient replacement of fluids and electrolytes, usually intravenously. Formulations are also being produced that can be used in developing countries so that fluids and electrolytes can be replaced orally. A vaccine was approved but later withdrawn because of severe side effects in a small number of infants. Prevention of rotavirus infections requires improved sanitation measures.

Study Questions

Choose the ONE correct answer

33.1 The typical clinical syndrome associated with rotavirus infection is

  A. acute gastroenteritis of young adults.

  B. acute bronchiolitis of infants.

  C. acute hepatitis.

  D. nausea, vomiting, and diarrhea in infants and very young children.

  E. acute paralytic syndrome.

> Correct answer = D. Rotaviruses infect and replicate in the gastrointestinal tract, and typically affect infants and very young children. Although rotavirus infections are seen all around the world, there is significant mortality only in developing countries, or in situations where good medical treatment, for example, fluid and electrolyte replacement, is not available.

33.2 Rotaviruses differ from polioviruses in that rotaviruses

  A. infect via the fecal-oral route.

  B. lack an envelope.

  C. can undergo genetic reassortment.

  D. do not contain any enzymes.

  E. have an icosahedral structure.

> Correct answer = C. Because rotaviruses contain a segmented genome, infection of a single cell with two different rotaviruses can result in genetic reassortment, and the emergence of a new viral strain with some genomic segments from one parent and the remaining genomic segments from the other parent. Rotaviruses do contain the enzymes required to synthesize the viral mRNAs. With respect to the other points, there are no differences between polioviruses and rotaviruses.

33.3 Rotaviruses can be distinguished from other viruses in the Reovirus family

  A. by their appearance.

  B. in that they contain the enzymes needed to transcribe functional messenger RNA molecules.

  C. in that they infect only humans.

  D. in that they replicate completely in the nucleus.

  E. in that they have a segmented genome.

> Correct answer = A. Rotaviruses have a characteristic appearance suggestive of a wheel with prominent spokes. Rotaviruses are found in many other mammalian species. With respect to the other points, there are no differences between rotaviruses and other viruses in the Reovirus family.

33.4 The diagnosis of a rotavirus infection

  A. can, in most cases, be made on the basis of the clinical presentation.

  B. can be made on the basis of an increase in antibody titer.

  C. is routinely made by electron microscopy of suitably treated stool samples.

  D. can only be made on epidemiologic grounds (for example, if there is an epidemic).

  E. must be made rapidly so that specific antiviral therapy is initiated as soon as possible.

> Correct answer = B. The diagnosis of rotavirus infection is readily made by serology (that is, by demonstrating a rise in antibody titer). There are also available several tests by which rotavirus antigens can be demonstrated in the stool. Although the diagnosis can be made by electron microscopy, it is not a routine procedure. The clinical presentation is not sufficiently distinctive to make the diagnosis, and there is no specific antiviral treatment for rotavirus infections.

Unconventional Infectious Agents

34

I. OVERVIEW

The designation "unconventional infectious agent" refers to a distinctive, transmissible, infectious agent that, while having some properties in common with viruses, does not fit the classic definition of a virus (Figure 34.1). One such highly unconventional infectious agent, the **prion**, has been strongly implicated as the causative agent of the **transmissible spongiform encephalopathies** (**TSEs**) of animals and humans. The TSEs occurring in humans are designated as **kuru, Creutzfeldt-Jakob disease** (**CJD**), **Gerstmann-Straussler syndrome** (**GSS**), and **fatal familial insomnia** (**FFI**). The most important TSEs of animals are **scrapie** in sheep, and the **bovine spongiform encephalopathy** (**BSE**) in cattle (popularly called "**mad cow disease**"). Histologically, all of these diseases are characterized by spongiform vacuolation of neuronal processes and gray matter, the accumulation of a unique protein (referred to as prion protein, or PrP, Figure 34.2), and in certain cases, the deposition in the brain of extracellular amyloid plaques composed of PrP. [Note: Such diseases are sometimes referred to as transmissible amyloidoses.]

II. PRIONS

After an extensive series of purification procedures, scientists were astonished to find that the infectivity of the agent causing scrapie in sheep was associated with a single protein species, with no detectable associated nucleic acid. This infectious protein is designated the **prion protein**. It is relatively resistant to proteolytic degradation, and, when infectious, tends to form insoluble aggregates of fibrils, similar to the amyloid found in some other diseases of the brain.

A. Presence of prion protein (PrP) in normal mammalian brain

A noninfectious form of PrP, having the same amino acid and gene sequences as the infectious agent, is present in normal mammalian brains on the surface of neurons and glial cells. Thus PrP is a host protein. The function of noninfectious PrP is unknown, but it is highly conserved in nature, the amino acid and gene sequences differing very little in divergent mammalian species. No primary structure or posttranslational covalent differences between the normal and the infectious forms of the protein have been found, although specific mutational changes of single amino acids at a few sites appear to be determinants of susceptibility to exogenous infection, and of the probability for spontaneous conversion of the normal PrP to the infectious form. The key to becoming infectious apparently lies in the

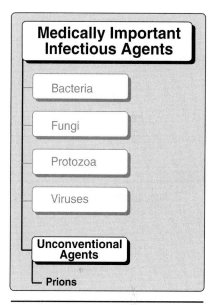

Figure 34.1
Classification of unconventional infectious agents.

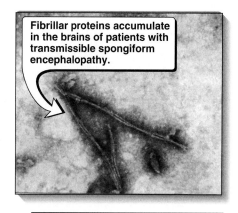

Fibrillar proteins accumulate in the brains of patients with transmissible spongiform encephalopathy.

Figure 34.2
Electron micrograph of fibrillar prion proteins.

Lippincott's Illustrated Reviews: Microbiology,
by William A. Strohl, Harriet Rouse, Bruce D. Fisher.
Lippincott, Williams & Wilkins, Baltimore, MD © 2001

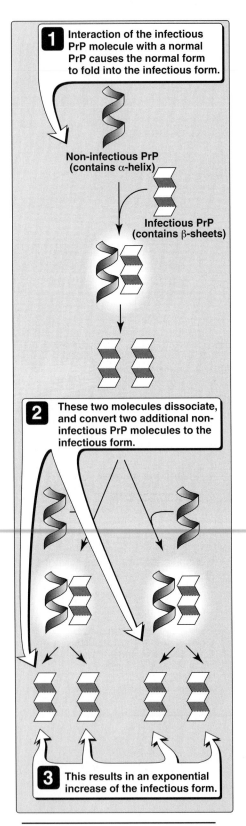

1 Interaction of the infectious PrP molecule with a normal PrP causes the normal form to fold into the infectious form.

Non-infectious PrP (contains α-helix)

Infectious PrP (contains β-sheets)

2 These two molecules dissociate, and convert two additional non-infectious PrP molecules to the infectious form.

3 This results in an exponential increase of the infectious form.

Figure 34.3
One proposed mechanism for multiplication of the infectious prion agents.

three-dimensional conformation of the prion protein. It has been observed that a number of α-helices[1] present in noninfectious PrP are replaced by β-sheets[2] in the infectious form. It is presumably this conformational difference that confers on infectious prions relative resistance to proteolytic degradation, and permits them to be distinguished from the normal PrP in infected tissues. One model for multiplication of the agent is shown in Figure 34.3.

B. Epidemiology

The normal mode of transmission among animals, for example, among sheep in a flock infected with scrapie, has not been elucidated. It is clear, however, that several diseases of domestic animals have been transmitted via feed prepared from other diseased animals.

1. **Bovine spongiform encephalopathy:** BSE, commonly called "**mad cow disease**," arose in British cattle presumably due to their feeding with processed animal parts prepared from diseased sheep and cattle. The obvious question raised by this occurrence is whether the BSE from infected cattle can be transmitted to humans. This was originally thought to carry negligible risk, but a study of infectious material from a cluster of histologically distinctive British CJD cases in unusually young patients (now referred to as "new variant", or nvCJD), indicated that animal-to-human transmission very likely did take place. Because the incubation time for symptoms to appear varies from four to forty years, the extent of a potential epidemic due to BSE is unknown.

2. **Kuru:** An example of human-to-human transmission of a TSE is found in the disease kuru, in which the infectious agent is acquired by an individual's exposure to diseased brain tissue in the course of ritualistic cannibalism among members of a tribe in New Guinea. Infection occurs by consumption of contaminated brain tissue, or by inoculation through breaks in the skin following handling of the diseased tissue. With the cessation of cannibalism in the late 1950s, the disease is disappearing.

3. **Creutzfeldt-Jakob disease:** Of more general significance are the documented cases of iatrogenic (done unintentionally by a physician) transmission of Creutzfeldt-Jakob disease, for example, by use of prion-contaminated human pituitary-derived growth hormone prepared from individuals who died from CJD. Thus far there has been no evidence of transplacental transmission, infection from blood products, or transmission by person-to-person contact. In about fifteen percent of CJD, the condition is inherited as a mutation in the PrP gene. However, the majority of CJD cases are sporadic and have an unknown etiology (that is, they occur with no known exposure or mutational change). The incidence of sporadic CJD is very low—about one per million population—but in those families with a PrP mutation, an attack rate of fifty to one hundred percent is seen in those carrying the mutation. In contrast to CJD, all cases classified as GSS or FFI have involved inheritance of specific PrP mutations. However, in spite of the inherited nature of the disease, brain tissues from these patients are infectious.

[1,2]See pp. 18-19 in *Lippincott's Illustrated Reviews: Biochemistry* (2nd ed.) for a discussion of the α-helix and β-sheet.

C. Pathology

Extracerebral exposure to prions results in significant multiplication of the prions in lymphoreticular and other peripheral tissues early after infection, but it is invasion of the CNS that results in the typical clinical effects. The basis for the pathogenic consequences of abnormal PrP deposition has not been clarified. Diseased brain tissue is characterized by accumulation of abnormal PrP in the form of amyloid fibrils in cytoplasmic vesicles of neurons (see Figure 34.2), and in some cases, in the form of extracellular amyloid plaques. There is, in addition, extensive vacuolation within neurons, neuronal loss, and astroglial proliferation. The extensive destruction results in the characteristic spongiform appearance of the gray matter in histologic sections. [Note: Whereas the TSE amyloid plaques are morphologically similar to those of Alzheimer's disease, the PrP gene is located on a different chromosome than is the gene for the Alzheimer amyloid-β-protein precursor, and there is no nucleotide or amino acid homology between the two.]

D. Clinical significance

The transmissible spongiform encephalopathies are a group of progressive, ultimately fatal, neurodegenerative diseases affecting humans, and a number of animal species. The disease process is fundamentally the same in all TSEs, but their clinical manifestations and histopathologies differ. The TSEs also share some similarities with conventional infectious diseases, but their differences are striking (Figure 34.4).

1. **Molecular basis of the inherited TSEs:** In each of the inherited TSEs, specific, single amino acid substitutions, or insertions of nucleotide repeat sequences, are found in the PrP gene. These are thought to increase greatly (10^6-fold) the probability of transition to the infectious conformation. In the spontaneously occurring, sporadic disease (that is, with no known exposure to infectious material and no inheritance of a mutated PrP gene) it is proposed that the altered folding occurs randomly with very low probability; however, once formed, the abnormal PrP acquires both the ability to "multiply," as well as the properties of an infectious agent. It has been recognized, however, that certain amino acid substitutions at one specific site increase susceptibility to infection.

2. **Major symptoms:** All TSEs involve deposition of the PrP protein, and in the inherited forms, each PrP mutation is associated with a characteristic clinical phenotype. For example, the most prominent features of CJD are a rapidly progressive dementia and behavioral disturbances, ending in death within one year, whereas in GSS, ataxia is the more prominent feature, with death resulting in two to six years. FFI, also fatal within one year, has the additional symptom of uncontrollable insomnia. Although there is some difference in age of onset, all human TSEs (with the exception of the BSE-associated nvCJD) occur relatively late in life, most typically between the ages of forty and sixty years.

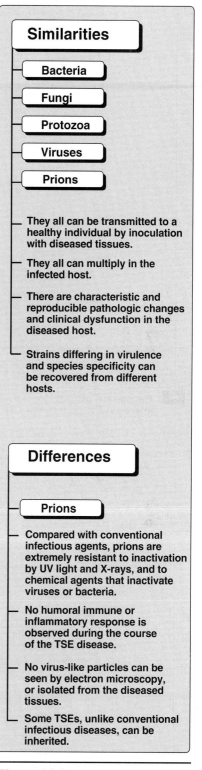

Figure 34.4
Similarities and differences between conventional and unconventional agents. TSE = Transmissible spongiform encephalopathies.

E. Laboratory identification

A presumptive diagnosis can be made on clinical grounds, but there is some overlap with other dementing illnesses. Routine laboratory tests of serum and CSF are generally normal. However, a protein released by CNS tissue damaged by any of a variety of causes is present, and in the presence of appropriate clinical signs, can be diagnostic for CJD. An additional diagnostic technique exploits the relative resistance of infectious prions to proteolytic degradation. In this method, a proteolytic digestion step degrades the normal PrP, and the remaining infectious prions are detected by immunologic techniques. The presence of infectious PrPs in peripheral lymphatic tissues provides specimens for analysis without the need for brain biopsy. Currently, however, the definitive diagnosis of these diseases is by postmortem histopathologic examination of brain sections.

F. Treatment and prevention

The TSEs are invariably fatal, and no treatment is currently available that can alter this outcome. The unusually high resistance of the infectivity to most disinfecting agents makes prevention of transmission by the usual infection control procedures ineffective. Current recommendations for decontamination of a CJD brain specimen are autoclaving at 132°C, plus immersion in either undiluted sodium hypochlorite or 1N sodium hydroxide. With respect to preventing possible transfer of BSE to humans, all animals showing signs of illness are destroyed, and preparation of animal feed from internal organs of potentially infected animals has ceased. A number of countries have prohibited importation of beef in an attempt to prevent introduction of the disease into either the domestic animal or human populations.

Study Questions

Choose the ONE correct answer

34.1 A patient dying with symptoms of Creutzfeldt-Jacob disease is postulated to have acquired this disease from eating beef contaminated with the agent of bovine spongiform encephalopathy. If this hypothesis were correct, the most likely finding in the patient would be:

A. circulating antibodies specific for bovine CNS antigens.

B. DNA copies of the bovine infectious agent integrated into chromosomes of the patient's diseased CNS tissues.

C. cytotoxic T lymphocytes directed against CNS-specific antigens found in both cattle and humans.

D. amyloid deposits that have the bovine rather than the human amino acid sequences.

E. lack of any bovine-specific protein or nucleic acid, or an immune response.

Correct answer = E. A and C: An important characteristic of the prion diseases is that there is no unique immune response to either the prion or to CNS antigens. B: A second distinguishing feature of these agents is the absence of a detectable nucleic acid genome. D: The amyloid deposits found in these diseases are composed of the diseased host's proteins, and not of proteins from the source of the infection.

34.2 The agent(s) of the transmissible spongiform encephalopathies are similar to conventional infectious agents in all of the following respects EXCEPT:

A. they multiply in the infected host.

B. the disease can be transmitted from an infected individual to a recipient.

C. there are characteristic and reproducible pathologic changes and clinical manifestations.

D. the infected host responds with the production of specific antibodies.

E. strains with different host specificity and virulence can be recovered from different hosts.

Correct answer = D. A unique characteristic of the prion diseases is that there is no immune response, and also no inflammatory reaction in the diseased tissue. This is the consequence of the fact that the agent is a modified normal host protein, and therefore does not stimulate an immune response.

Summary of Clinically Important Microorganisms

35

I. OVERVIEW

Although all of the microorganisms presented in this volume have clinical significance, some play a more critical role than do others in the pathology of disease in the United States. This chapter presents a summary of these particularly important microorganisms, using icons to aid the reader in retaining the morphology and classification of the microorganisms. The classifications of bacteria and viruses continues to be presented in pie charts, in which each segment represents a general class of microorganisms (Figure 35.1A and B). One section of the bacterial pie chart is labeled "Other," and represents any of several microorganisms specifically covered in different chapters. At the top of each box in which a new organism is introduced in this summary chapter, a "pie wedge" is pulled out with an arrow pointing to it. This indicates the general group of bacteria or viruses to which the organism belongs, according to the definitions in Figure 35.1A or B. The name in large type above the arrow in the **bacteria** section is the name of the **genus** to which the organism(s) listed below the arrow belong (exceptions will be noted in the text). In the **virus** section, the names in large type above the arrow refer to the **family** of which the individual viruses listed below the arrow are members. [Note: Only the bacteria and viruses that are summarized in this chapter are listed below the arrows. Additional organisms belonging to the same genus or family are described in the body of the text.] The order of the microorganisms in this chapter is presented alphabetically in Figure 35.2.

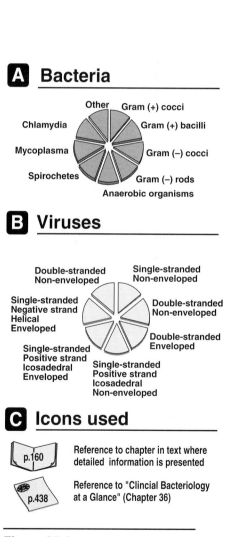

A Bacteria

Other
Gram (+) cocci
Chlamydia
Gram (+) bacilli
Mycoplasma
Gram (–) cocci
Spirochetes
Gram (–) rods
Anaerobic organisms

B Viruses

Double-stranded Non-enveloped
Single-stranded Non-enveloped
Single-stranded Negative strand Helical Enveloped
Double-stranded Non-enveloped
Double-stranded Enveloped
Single-stranded Positive strand Icosadedral Enveloped
Single-stranded Positive strand Icosadedral Non-enveloped

C Icons used

p.160 — Reference to chapter in text where detailed information is presented

p.438 — Reference to "Clincial Bacteriology at a Glance" (Chapter 36)

Figure 35.1
Representations of medically important bacteria and viruses; summary of icons used in this chapter.

Lippincott's Illustrated Reviews: Microbiology,
by William A. Strohl, Harriet Rouse, Bruce D. Fisher.
Lippincott, Williams & Wilkins, Baltimore, MD © 2001

BACTERIA

VIRUSES

FIGURE 35.2
Alphabetical listing of microorganisms summarized in this chapter. Page numbers refer to location in this chapter.

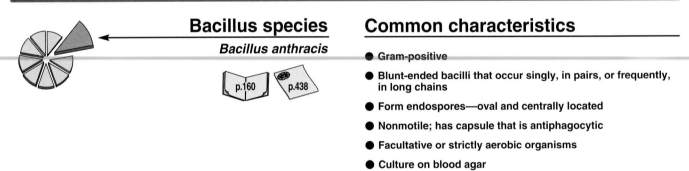

BACTERIA

Bacillus species

Bacillus anthracis

p.160   p.438

Common characteristics

● **Gram-positive**

● **Blunt-ended bacilli that occur singly, in pairs, or frequently, in long chains**

● **Form endospores—oval and centrally located**

● **Nonmotile; has capsule that is antiphagocytic**

● **Facultative or strictly aerobic organisms**

● **Culture on blood agar**

Pathogenesis/Clinical Significance

B. anthracis infects primarily domestic herbivores such as sheep, goats, and horses. Infection usually occurs through contact with infected animal products or spore-contaminated dust that is inoculated through incidental skin abrasions or is inhaled. *B. anthracis* spores are highly resistant to physical and chemical agents, and may remain viable for many years in contaminated pastures or animal materials. *B. anthracis* produces two plasmid-coded exotoxins: **edema factor**, which causes elevation of intracellular cAMP leading to severe edema, and **lethal factor**, which causes additional adverse effects. The *B. anthracis* capsule is essential for full virulence.

● **Cutaneous anthrax**

Upon introduction of organisms or spores that germinate, a papule develops. It rapidly evolves into a painless, black, severely swollen "malignant

[*B. anthrasis* is is continued on the next page]

Treatment and Prevention

● **Treatment:** *B. anthracis* is sensitive to penicillin, doxycycline and ciprofloxacin. However, these antibiotics are effective in cutaneous anthrax only when administered early in the course of the infection.

● **Prevention:** Because of the resistance of endospores to chemical disinfectants, autoclaving is the only reliable means of decontamination. A cell-free vaccine is available for workers in high-risk occupations.

Laboratory Identification

● Cultured on blood agar, *B. anthracis* forms large, grayish, nonhemolytic colonies with irregular borders.

● A direct immunofluorescence assay aids in the identification of the organism.

Bacillus anthracis (continued)

Pathogenesis/Clinical Significance	Treatment and Prevention	Laboratory Identification

pustule", which eventually crusts over. The organisms may invade regional lymph nodes, and then the general circulation, leading to a fatal septicemia. The overall mortality rate in untreated cutaneous anthrax is about twenty percent.

● **Pulmonary anthrax ("wool-sorter's disease")**

Caused by inhalation of spores, this disease is characterized by progressive hemorrhagic pneumonia and lymphadenitis (inflammation of the lymph nodes), and has a mortality rate approaching 100 percent if untreated.

● **Gastrointestinal form of anthrax**

This unusual form of anthrax is caused by ingestion of spores, for example, by eating raw or inadequately cooked meat containing *B. anthracis* spores. This is the portal of entry commonly seen in animals.

Bordetella species

Bordetella pertussis

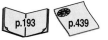

p.193   p.439

Common characteristics

● **Gram-negative**

● **Small coccobacilli that grow singly or in pairs**

● **Encapsulated**

● **Aerobic**

● **Culture on Regan-Lowe agar**

Pathogenesis/Clinical Significance	Treatment and Prevention	Laboratory Identification

B. pertussis is transmitted primarily by droplets spread by coughing. The organism survives only briefly in the environment. *B. pertussis* binds to ciliated epithelium in the upper respiratory tract. There the bacteria produce a variety of toxins and other virulence factors that interfere with ciliary activity, eventually causing the death of these cells.

● **Pertussis ("whooping cough")**

The incubation period for this disease ranges from one to three weeks. The disease can be divided into two phases: 1) the **catarrhal phase**, which begins with relatively nonspecific symptoms, and then progresses to include a dry, nonproductive cough; and 2) the **paroxysmal phase**, in which the cough worsens, causing paroxysms of coughing followed by a "whoop" as the patient inspires rapidly. Large amounts of mucus are typically produced. During the three-to-four week convalescent period, secondary complications, such as encephalopathy, seizures, and/or pneumonia, may occur.

● **Treatment:** Erythromycin is the drug of choice for *B. pertussis* infections, both as chemotherapy and as chemoprophylaxis for household contacts. Trimethoprim-sulfamethoxazole is an alternative choice for erythromycin treatment failures.

● **Prevention:** Two forms of vaccine are currently available (one of killed whole cells, and one that is acellular, containing purified *B. pertussis* proteins). Both are formulated in combination with diphtheria and tetanus toxoids.

● *B. pertussis* from nasopharyngeal samples can be cultured on selective agar such as Regan-Lowe medium, where the organism produces pinpoint, hemolytic colonies.

● More rapid diagnosis may be accomplished using a direct fluorescent antibody test to detect *B. pertussis* in smears of nasopharyngeal specimens.

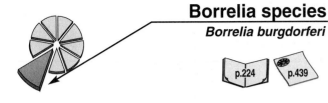

Borrelia species
Borrelia burgdorferi

p.224   p.439

Common characteristics

- Gram-negative, but some stain poorly, and need to be visualized by other means
- Long, slender, flexible, spiral- or corkscrew-shaped rods
- Organisms are highly motile
- Difficult and time-consuming to culture

Pathogenesis/Clinical Significance	Treatment and Prevention	Laboratory Identification

B. burgdorferi is transmitted to humans by the bite of a small tick (genus *Ixodes*), which must feed for at least 24 hours to deliver an infectious dose. Deer, mice, other rodents, and birds serve as reservoirs for the spirochete. The organism is not spread from human to human.

- **Lyme disease**

  The first stage of the disease begins 3 to 22 days after a tick bite, with a characteristic red, circular rash with a clear center (erythema chronicum migrans) appearing at the site of the bite. Flu-like symptoms can accompany the rash. The organism spreads via the lymph or blood to musculoskeletal sites, the skin, central nervous system, heart, and other organs. Weeks to months after the initial symptoms, the second stage of the disease begins with symptoms such as arthritis, arthralgia, cardiac complications, and neurologic complications such as meningitis. The third stage begins months to years later, with chronic arthritis and progressive central nervous system disease.

- **Treatment:** Cephalosporins, amoxicillin, or doxycycline are useful in treating the early stages of Lyme disease. If arthritic symptoms have already appeared, longer courses of antibiotics are used.
- **Prevention:** A ninety percent effective vaccine is currently available. The best prevention is wearing clothing that limits skin exposure to ticks, and using insect repellent.

- Samples of blood can be treated with Giemsa or Wright stain to visualize the large, loosely coiled *B. burgdorferi* when present.
- The polymerase chain reaction used to assist in detection of *B. burgdorferi* in body fluids provides the most definitive test.
- *B. burgdorferi* infection can be diagnosed serologically, but the number of false positives can outnumber the true positives.

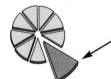

Brucella species
Brucella abortus
Brucella canis
Brucella melitensis
Brucella suis

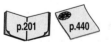

p.201   p.440

Common characteristics

- Gram-negative
- Small coccobacilli, arranged singly or in pairs
- Unencapsulated
- Aerobic, intracellular parasites
- Culture on blood agar

Pathogenesis/Clinical Significance	Treatment and Prevention	Laboratory Identification

Brucellosis is a chronic, lifelong infection in animals. Organisms localize in reproductive organs (male and female), and are shed in large numbers, for example, in milk and urine. Transmission to humans usually occurs either through direct contact with infected animal tissues or ingestion of unpasteurized milk or milk products. Human-to-human transmission is rare.

Brucellae typically enter the body through cuts in the skin or through the GI tract. They are transported via the lymphatic system to the regional lymph nodes, where they survive and multiply within host phagocytes. They are then carried by the blood to organs that are involved in the reticuloendothelial system, including the liver, spleen, kidneys, bone marrow, and other lymph nodes. Lipopolysaccharide is the major virulence factor.

- **Brucellosis (undulant fever)**

  Symptoms of brucellosis are nonspecific and flu-like (malaise, fever, sweats, anorexia and GI symptoms, headache, and back pains), and may also include depression. Untreated patients may develop an undulating pattern of fever. Brucellosis may involve any of a variety of organ systems, including the GI tract, and the skeletal, neurologic, cardiovascular, and pulmonary systems.

- **Treatment:** Combination therapy involving doxycycline and either streptomycin or gentamicin is recommended for brucellosis. Prolonged treatment (for example, six weeks) is generally necessary to prevent relapse and to reduce the incidence of complications.

- A detailed history is often crucial because of the nonspecific symptoms.
- The organism can be cultured from blood and other body fluids, or from tissue specimens, but isolation of the organism is difficult and time consuming.
- Serologic tests for agglutinating antibodies are diagnostically useful. Titers greater than 1:160 and rising are considered indicative of brucella infection.

Campylobacter species

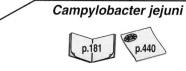

Campylobacter jejuni

p.181   p.440

Common characteristics

- **Gram-negative**
- **Curved, spiral, or S-shaped rods**
- **Single, polar flagellum results in characteristic darting motion**
- **Microaerophilic**
- **Do not ferment carbohydrates**
- **Culture on selective medium (blood agar containing antibiotics to inhibit growth of other fecal flora)**

Pathogenesis/Clinical Significance

C. jejuni is widely distributed in nature, existing as part of the normal flora of many different vertebrate species, including both mammals and fowl, wild and domestic. Transmission is via the fecal/oral route through direct contact, or exposure to contaminated meat (especially poultry) or to contaminated water.

C. jejuni infects the intestine, where it can cause ulcerative, inflammatory lesions in the jejunum, ileum, or colon. Although cytotoxins and enterotoxins have been identified, the role of these molecules in disease has not been established.

- **Acute enteritis**

  C. jejuni is the leading cause of food-borne disease in the United States. Symptoms may be both systemic (fever, headache, myalgia) and intestinal (abdominal cramping and diarrhea, which may or may not be bloody). *C. jejuni* is a cause of both traveler's diarrhea and pseudoappendicitis. Rare complications include septic abortion, reactive arthritis, and Guillain-Barre syndrome.

Treatment and Prevention

- **Treatment:** Diarrhea should be treated symptomatically (fluid and electrolyte replacement). If disease is severe, ciprofloxacin is the drug of choice.
- **Prevention:** No vaccine or preventive drug is available. Good hygiene, avoiding contaminated water, pasteurizing milk and milk products, and thoroughly cooking potentially contaminated food (for example, poultry) is important in prevention of infection.

Laboratory Identification

- Presumptive diagnosis can be made on the basis of finding curved organisms with rapid, darting motility in a wet mount of feces.

Chlamydia species

Chlamydia pneumoniae
Chlamydia psittaci
Chlamydia trachomatis

Common characteristics

- **Not routinely stained with Gram stain**
- **Small, round to ovoid organisms**
- **Envelope consists of two lipid bilayers**
- **Obligate intracellular parasites, the organisms replicate in endocytic vacuoles, creating characteristic cytoplasmic inclusion bodies**

Chlamydia pneumoniae 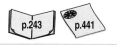 p.243 p.441

Pathogenesis/Clinical Significance

C. pneumoniae is generally transmitted by respiratory droplets. The chlamydia are energy parasites, and require exogenous ATP and NAD$^+$ for growth. They acquire these compounds by replicating inside host cells.

- **Community-acquired respiratory infection**

  C. pneumoniae is a significant cause of respiratory infections worldwide, causing pharyngitis, laryngitis, bronchitis, and interstitial pneumonia. Epidemic outbreaks have been reported.

Treatment and Prevention

- **Treatment:** Doxycycline and erythromycin are the drugs of choice.
- **Prevention:** No vaccine or preventive drug is available.

Laboratory Identification

- Neither serologic tests nor recovery by culturing is routinely available.

[CHLAMYDIA SPECIES ARE CONTINUED ON THE NEXT PAGE]

Chlamydia psittaci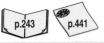

Pathogenesis/Clinical Significance	Treatment and Prevention	Laboratory Identification
● Psittacosis (ornithosis) This is a zoonotic disease transmitted to humans by inhalation of dust contaminated with respiratory secretions or feces of infected birds (such as parrots). *C. psittaci* infection of humans targets the respiratory tract, causing a dry cough, flu-like symptoms, and pulmonary infiltrates. Enlargement of the liver and spleen frequently occurs.	**● Treatment:** Tetracycline and doxycycline are the drugs of choice. Erythromycin therapy is the alternative treatment, but may be less efficacious in severe cases.	● Demonstration of a rise in antibody titer, using either complement fixation or indirect immunofluorescence tests, can aid in diagnosis.

Chlamydia trachomatis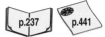

Pathogenesis/Clinical Significance	Treatment and Prevention	Laboratory Identification
● Nongonococcal urethritis (NGU) *C. trachomatis* is the major causal agent of NGU, which is the most common sexually transmitted bacterial disease in the United States. It is transmitted by personal contact, and affects both sexes. Repeated or chronic exposure to *C. trachomatis* can lead to sterility and ectopic pregnancy. Women may develop **pelvic inflammatory disease (PID).** **● Trachoma** *C. trachomatis* causes eye infections (**chronic keratoconjunctivitis**) with symptoms that range from simple irritation of the eye to blindness. This disease is widely prevalent in developing countries. It is transmitted by personal contact with infected humans or contaminated surfaces, and by flies. **● Inclusion conjunctivitis of the newborn (ICN)** Infants born to mothers infected with *C. trachomatis* can become infected during passage through the birth canal. This can lead to an acute, purulent conjunctivitis that is usually self-healing. **● Lymphogranuloma venereum (LGV)** *C. trachomatis* causes LGV, an invasive, sexually transmitted disease that is uncommon in the United States, but is endemic in Asia, Africa, and South America. LGV is characterized by transient papules on the external genitalia, followed in one to two months by painful swelling of inguinal and perirectal lymph nodes. Regional lymphatic drainage can become blocked.	**● Treatment:** Azithromycin, erythromycin, and tetracyclines such as doxycycline are useful in treating chlamydial infections. [Note: Erythromycin is used for young children and pregnant women.] **● Prevention:** No vaccine is available. Erythromycin or silver nitrate in ointment or eyedrops is applied prophylactically to newborns' eyes, especially those at risk. Proper precautions should be taken during sexual contact to prevent transmission of NGU.	● Microscopic examination of infected cells stained with direct fluorescent antibodies reveals characteristic cellular cytoplasmic inclusions. ● Nucleic acid hybridization using a DNA probe for chlamydial ribosomal RNA genes can detect *C. trachomatis* with a high degree of sensitivity. ● An enzymatic immunoassay that detects chlamydial lipopolysaccharides is also available.

Clostridia species

Clostridium botulinum
Clostridium difficile
Clostridium perfringens
Clostridium tetani

Common characteristics

● **Gram-positive**

● **Large, blunt-ended rods that produce endospores**

● **Most species are motile**

● **Obligate anaerobe**

● **Culture anaerobically on blood agar**

Clostridium botulinum

Pathogenesis/Clinical Significance	Treatment and Prevention	Laboratory Identification
C. botulinum is found in soil and aquatic sediments. Its spores contaminate vegetables, meat, and fish. *C. botulinum* exotoxin inhibits the release of acetylcholine at the neuromuscular junctions, preventing contraction and causing flaccid paralysis. **● Botulism (food poisoning) and floppy baby syndrome** Caused by ingestion of exotoxin, leading to flaccid paralysis, vomiting, and diarrhea. Death can occur due to respiratory paralysis. *C. botulinum* colonizes the large intestine, producing exotoxin that is slowly absorbed. Lethargy, poor muscle tone, and constipation result.	**● Treatment:** Antitoxin (horse antiserum) that neutralizes unbound botulinum toxin should be administered as soon as possible in suspected botulinal intoxication. **● Prevention:** Proper food preservation techniques prevent the production of the clostridial exotoxin.	● *C. botulinum* toxin can be detected in food, intestinal contents, or serum by mouse inoculation with or without neutralizing antiserum. ● The organism can be cultured and identified by standard anaerobic methods.

[CLOSTRIDIA SPECIES ARE CONTINUED ON THE NEXT PAGE]

Clostridium difficile

Pathogenesis/Clinical Significance	Treatment and Prevention	Laboratory Identification
C. difficile is found as a normal but minor component of the flora of the large intestine. Its spores can contaminate indoor as well as outdoor environments. *C. difficile* can overgrow in the colon of an individual on antibiotics that deplete the normal flora. *C. difficile* enterotoxin A causes excessive fluid secretion and an inflammatory response in the colon. Toxin B is a cytotoxin that disrupts protein synthesis, causing lysis of host cells. **• Pseudomembranous colitis** Caused by toxins A and B, this condition is characterized by watery, explosive diarrhea and pseudomembrane formation in the colon.	**•Treatment:** Discontinue the predisposing drug, and replace fluids and electrolytes. *C. difficile* is resistant to many antibiotics. Oral administration of vancomycin or metronidazole may be added in severe cases. **• Prevention:** No vaccine or preventive drug is available.	• The enterotoxin can be detected in stool samples using the ELISA test for exotoxins A and B. • The presence of a pseudomembrane in the colon can be detected by endoscopy.

Clostridium perfringens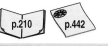

Pathogenesis/Clinical Significance	Treatment and Prevention	Laboratory Identification
C. perfringens is part of the normal flora of the vagina and gastrointestinal tract. Its spores are found in soil. *C. perfringens* alpha toxin is a phospholipase C (lecithinase) that causes lysis of endothelial and blood cells. The bacterium produces at least eleven additional exotoxins that have hemolytic or other cytotoxic and necrotic effects. **• Myonecrosis (gas gangrene)** Spores germinate in open wounds such as those caused by GI tract surgery, burns, puncture wounds, war wounds, etc., and produce cytotoxic factors. Fermentation of tissue carbohydrates causes formation of gas bubbles. As the disease progresses, increased capillary permeability leads to exotoxins being carried by the circulation from the damaged tissues to other organs, resulting in systemic effects such as shock, renal failure, and intravascular hemolysis. Untreated myonecrosis is uniformly fatal. **• Acute food poisoning** This condition is caused by the generation of spores in improperly cooked food, resulting in the production of enterotoxin that disrupts ion transport in the lower portion of the small intestine. This causes loss of fluid and intracellular proteins. **• Anaerobic cellulitis** This is clostridial infection of connective tissue in which bacterial growth spreads rapidly along fascial planes.	**• Treatment of gas gangrene:** Immediate treatment and wound debridement or amputation, and exposure of the wound to hyperbaric oxygen are important mechanisms for treating the infection. High doses of penicillin G or doxycycline should be administered. **• Treatment of food poisoning:** Clostridial food poisoning is usually self-limiting and requires only supportive care. **• Prevention:** No vaccine or preventive drug is available. Prevention of food poisoning is a matter of appropriate food handling practices.	• When specimens from diseased tissue are Gram stained, large, gram-positive rods are observed. • When cultured anaerobically on blood agar, *C. perfringens* produces a unique double-zone of β-hemolysis. • Other diagnostic biochemical tests are available that measure such characteristics as sugar fermentation and organic acid production.

Clostridium tetani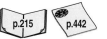

Pathogenesis/Clinical Significance	Treatment and Prevention	Laboratory Identification
C. tetani spores are common in soil. *C. tetani* exotoxin, tetanospasmin, binds irreversibly, penetrating neurons and blocking neurotransmitter release at inhibitory synapses. This causes severe, prolonged muscle spasms. **• Tetanus ("lockjaw")** Caused by *C. tetani* spores infecting a puncture wound, a severe burn, postsurgical incision, etc. In the early stages, the jaw muscles are affected, so that the mouth cannot open (**trismus** or "lockjaw"). Gradually, other voluntary muscles become involved. Death is usually the result of paralysis of the chest muscles, leading to respiratory failure.	**• Treatment:** Preferred treatment is with human hyperimmune (tetanus immune) globulin. Alternative treatment is with horse antitoxin. Sedatives and muscle relaxants are administered, and proper ventilation should be maintained. *C. tetani* is sensitive to penicillin. **• Prevention:** Inactivated tetanus toxoid (formalin-inactivated toxin) is given as part of the DPT vaccine (D=diphtheria toxoid; P=pertussis antigen).	• Diagnosis is based on clinical findings, because laboratory identification is difficult (*C. tetani* is difficult to culture, and frequently, few organisms can be isolated from infected tissue).

Corynebacterium species

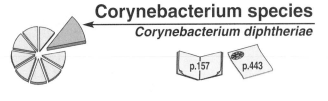

Corynebacterium diphtheriae

p.157   p.443

Common characteristics

- Gram-positive; stain unevenly
- Small, slender, pleomorphic rods that form characteristic clumps that look like Chinese characters or a picket fence
- Nonmotile and unencapsulated
- Most species are facultative anaerobes
- Culture aerobically on selective medium such as Tinsdale agar

Pathogenesis/Clinical Significance

C. diphtheriae is found on the skin, and in the nose, throat, and nasopharynx of carriers and patients with diphtheria. The organism is spread primarily by respiratory droplets.

Diphtheria is caused by the local and systemic effects of a single exotoxin that inhibits eukaryotic protein synthesis. This toxin inactivates eukaryotic polypeptide chain elongation factor EF-2 by ADP-ribosylation, thus terminating protein synthesis. [Note: The structural gene for the toxin is coded for by a bacteriophage; only those strains of *C. diphtheriae* that are lysogenic for this phage can produce toxin and are therefore virulent.]

- **Diphtheria**

  This life-threatening disease begins as a local infection, usually of the throat. The infection produces a distinctive thick, grayish, adherent exudate (called a pseudomembrane) that is composed of cell debris from the mucosa, and inflammatory products. The exudate coats the throat and may extend into the nasal passages or respiratory tract where it sometimes obstructs the airways, leading to suffocation. Generalized symptoms are due to dissemination of the toxin. Although all human cells are sensitive to diphtheria toxin, major clinical effects involve the heart (myocarditis may lead to congestive heart failure and permanent heart damage) and peripheral nerves (neuritis of cranial nerves and paralysis of muscle groups such as those that control movement of the palate or the eye).

Treatment and Prevention

- **Treatment:** A single dose of horse serum antitoxin inactivates any circulating toxin, although it does not affect toxin that is already bound to a cell-surface receptor. [Note: Serum sickness caused by a reaction to the horse protein may cause complications.] Eradication of the organism is accomplished with any of several antibiotics, such as erythromycin or penicillin.

- **Prevention:** Immunization with toxoid, usually administered in the DPT triple vaccine (together with tetanus toxoid and pertussis antigens) should be started in infancy. Booster injections of diphtheria toxoid (with tetanus toxoid) should be given at approximately ten-year intervals throughout life.

Laboratory Identification

- The initial diagnosis and decision to treat for diphtheria must be made based on clinical observation, because no reliable, rapid laboratory test is available.

- *C. diphtheriae* can be cultured on selective media such as Tinsdale agar, which contains potassium tellurite, an inhibitor of other respiratory flora. The organism can then be tested for toxin production using an immunologic precipitin reaction.

Enterococcus species

Enterococcus faecalis
Enterococcus faecium

p.154   p.443

Common characteristics

- Gram-positive
- Round to ovoid in shape, occurring in pairs or chains
- α- or nonhemolytic colonies
- Catalase-negative
- Grow in 6.5 percent NaCl; culture on bile-esculin agar

Pathogenesis/Clinical Significance

Enterococcus faecalis and *Enterococcus faecium* are part of the normal fecal flora.

- **Nosocomial infections:** Enterococci are frequent causes of such infections—especially in intensive care units. Under conditions where host resistance is lowered, or where the integrity of the gastrointestinal or genitourinary tract has been disrupted, enterococci can spread to normally sterile sites, causing urinary tract infections, bacteremia/sepsis, subacute bacterial endocarditis, biliary tract infection, or intra-abdominal abscesses.

Treatment and Prevention

- **Treatment:** A combination of a penicillin and an aminoglycoside, or the glycopeptide vancomycin is used to treat enterococcal infections. Newer antibiotics, such as the combination of quinupristin and dalfopristin, are used to threat vancmycin-resistant infections.

- **Prevention:** No vaccine is available against enterococci. Careful attention to hand washing and other cleanliness measures among hospital personnel can significantly decrease the incidence of nosocomail infections.

Laboratory Identification

- Enterococci are distinguished from the non-Group D streptococci by their ability to survive in 6.5 percent sodium chloride. They can also hydrolyze the polysaccharide esculin in the presence of bile.

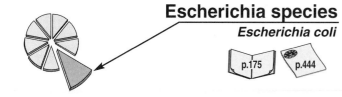

Escherichia species

Escherichia coli

p.175 p.444

Common characteristics

- Gram-negative
- Short rods
- Facultative anaerobe
- Ferments glucose and a wide range of carbohydrates
- Catalase-positive, oxidase-negative
- Culture on MacConkey agar

Pathogenesis/Clinical Significance

E. coli is part of the normal flora in the colon of humans and other animals, but can be pathogenic both within and outside the gastrointestinal tract. *E. coli* species possess three types of antigens, O, K, and H. Pili facilitate the attachment of the bacterium to human epithelial surfaces. Diseases caused by *E. coli* can be gastrointestinal and/or extraintestinal.

• Urinary tract infections (UTI)

E. coli is the most common cause of UTIs, especially in women. Symptoms include dysuria, urinary frequency, hematuria, and pyuria.

• Diarrhea

Several categories of diarrhea are caused by different strains of *E. coli*. Among the most prevalent are the following:

Enterotoxigenic *E. coli* (ETEC): This organism is a common cause of "traveler's diarrhea" in developing countries. It infects only humans, with transmission occurring through food and water contaminated with human waste, or by person-to-person contact. ETEC colonizes the small intestine, and in a process mediated by an enterotoxin that stimulates increased cAMP production, causes prolonged hypersecretion of chloride ions and water while inhibiting the reabsorption of sodium. The gut becomes full of fluid, resulting in significant watery diarrhea over a period of several days.

Enteropathogenic *E. coli* (EPEC): This organism is an important cause of diarrhea in infants, especially in developing countries. The newborn becomes infected during birth or *in utero*. EPEC attaches to mucosal cells in the small intestine, causing destruction of microvilli and development of characteristic lesions. Watery diarrhea results, which may become chronic.

Enterohemorrhagic *E. coli* (EHEC): EHEC binds to cells in the large intestine, and produces an exotoxin (**verotoxin**) that destroys microvilli, causing a severe form of copious, bloody diarrhea (**hemorrhagic colitis**) and acute renal failure (**hemolytic uremic syndrome**). Serotype O157:H7 is the most common strain of *E. coli* that produces verotoxin. The primary reservoir of EHEC is cattle. Therefore the possibility of infection can be greatly decreased by thoroughly cooking ground beef and pasteurizing milk.

• Meningitis in infants

E. coli and group B streptococci are the leading causes of neonatal meningitis. Newborns lack IgM, and therefore are particularly susceptible to *E. coli* sepsis, which can result in the organism's being carried to the brain.

Treatment and Prevention

- **Treatment for UTIs:** Trimethoprim-sulfamethoxazole or a fluoroquinolone, such as ciprofloxacin, are the drugs of choice. [Note: Isolated microorganisms must be tested for antibiotic sensitivity because multiple drug resistance, carried by transmissible plasmids, is common.]

- **Treatment for meningitis:** The combination of a cephalosporin, such as cefotaxime, plus gentamicin is usually recommended.

- **Treatment for diarrhea:** Antibiotics cited above shorten the duration of the disease. Patients with diarrhea must be rehydrated and their electrolytes replaced.

- **Prevention:** No vaccine or preventive drug is available. Diarrhea can be prevented by taking precautions in food and water consumption. Spread of infection between people can be controlled by hand washing, disinfection, etc.

Laboratory Identification

- *E. coli* can be cultured on differential medium such as MacConkey agar.

- Carbohydrate fermentation patterns are observed, for example, most strains of *E. coli* ferment lactose, produce gas during glucose fermentation, and show a positive test for mannitol fermentation.

Francisella species
Francisella tularensis

p.202   p.445

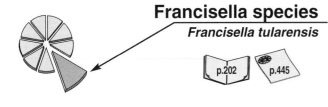

Common characteristics

● **Gram-negative**

● **Small, pleomorphic coccobacillus with a lipid-rich capsule**

● **Facultative intracellular parasite**

● **Strict aerobe**

● **Primarily pathogen of animals**

● **Rarely cultured**

Pathogenesis/Clinical Significance

The host range of *F. tularensis* is broad, and includes wild and domestic mammals, birds, and house pets. A number of biting or blood-sucking arthropods serve as vectors. Transmission is thus by contact with infected animal tissues, contaminated water, or an arthropod bite. Tularemia is an occupational risk for veterinarians, hunters and trappers, domestic livestock workers, and meat handlers.

F. tularensis is an intracellular parasite that can survive and multiply within host macrophages as well as in other cells. After cutaneous inoculation, *F. tularensis* multiplies locally, producing a papule that ulcerates after several days. Organisms spread from the local lesion to the regional lymph nodes, where they cause enlarged, tender nodes that may suppurate. From the lymph nodes, the organisms spread via the lymphatic system to various organs and tissues, including lungs, liver, spleen, kidneys, and the CNS.

● **Tularemia**

Tularemia varies in severity from mild to fulminant and fatal. Onset of symptoms is usually abrupt. The most common symptoms are flu-like (chills, fever, headache, malaise, anorexia, and fatigue), although respiratory and gastrointestinal symptoms may also occur. Ulcers may result from contact with animal products or from insect bites (ulceroglandular tularemia). Lymphadenopathy is characteristic.

Treatment and Prevention

● **Treatment:** The drug of choice for treatment of tularemia is streptomycin or, as an alternate, gentamicin.

● **Prevention:** Avoiding insect vectors and taking precautions when handling wild animals or animal products are the best means of prevention of *F. tularensis* infection.

Laboratory Identification

● Clinical presentation and history consistent with possible exposure is of primary importance in the diagnosis of tularemia. Confirmation of the clinical diagnosis is most commonly made serologically.

● The organism is rarely cultured.

Haemophilus species
Haemophilus influenzae

p.191   p.445

Common characteristics

● **Gram-negative**

● **Pleomorphic in shape, ranging from small coccobacilli to long slender filaments**

● **Obligate parasite, requiring hemin and NAD⁺ for growth**

● **Culture on chocolate agar containing hemin and NAD⁺**

Pathogenesis/Clinical Significance

H. influenzae is a normal resident of the human upper respiratory tract, and may also colonize the conjunctiva and genital tract. Transmission is by respiratory droplets.

H. influenzae may be unencapsulated, or may produce a capsule (capsular type b is associated with the most serious, invasive disease). After attaching to and colonizing the respiratory mucosa, the infection can become systemic, with bacteria spreading via the blood to the central nervous system.

● **Bacterial meningitis**

H. influenzae is a leading cause of bacterial meningitis, especially in infants and very young children.

[*H. INFLUENZAE* IS CONTINUED ON THE NEXT PAGE]

Treatment and Prevention

● **Treatment:** Antibiotic sensitivity testing should be done to determine appropriate antibiotic. Generally, a third-generation cephalosporin such as cefotaxime or ceftriaxone is effective in the treatment of meningitis. The combination of ampicillin plus sulbactam is also used.

● **Prevention:** A conjugated vaccine against *H. influenzae* capsular polysaccharide type b (Hib) is administered to infants. Rifampin is given prophylactically.

Laboratory Identification

● *H. influenzae* can be cultured on chocolate agar containing hemin (factor X) and NAD⁺ (factor V).

● Capsular swelling (quellung reaction) can be observed, and the capsule can be identified by immunofluorescent staining.

● Capsular antigen can also be detected in CSF or other body fluids using immunologic techniques.

Haemophilus influenzae (continued)

Pathogenesis/Clinical Significance	Treatment and Prevention	Laboratory Identification

● **Upper respiratory tract infections**

H. influenzae is a major cause of otitis media, sinusitis, and epiglottitis, primarily in children.

● **Pneumonia**

This organism causes pneumonia, particularly of the elderly or immuno-compromised individuals.

Helicobacter species
Helicobacter pylori

p.187 p.446

Common characteristics

● **Gram-negative**

● **Curved or spiral rods**

● **Multiple polar flagella give the organism rapid, corkscrew motility**

● **Urease-positive**

● **Culture on selective medium containing antibiotics to inhibit growth of other fecal flora**

Pathogenesis/Clinical Significance	Treatment and Prevention	Laboratory Identification

H. pylori is unusual in its ability to colonize the stomach, whose low pH normally protects against bacterial infection. Transmission is thought to be from person to person (the organism has not been isolated from food or water). Untreated, infections tend to be chronic and life-long.

H. pylori colonizes gastric mucosal cells in the stomach, surviving in the mucous layer that coats the epithelium. The organism is noninvasive, but recruits and activates inflammatory cells, thus causing a chronic inflammation of the mucosa. *H. pylori* secretes urease, producing ammonium ions that neutralize stomach acid in the vicinity of the organism, thus favoring bacterial multiplication. Ammonia can damage the gastric mucosa, and may also potentiate the effects of a cytotoxin produced by *H. pylori*.

● **Acute gastritis**

Initial infection with *H. pylori* results in decreased mucous production, and leads to acute gastritis. Both **duodenal ulcers** and **gastric ulcers** are closely correlated with infection by *H. pylori*. The organism appears to be a risk factor for development of **gastric carcinoma** and **gastric B-cell lymphoma**.

● **Treatment:** Elimination of *H. pylori* requires combination therapy with two or more antimicrobials due to rapid appearance of resistant strains. A typical regimen includes tetracycline plus metronidazole plus bismuth salts.

● **Prevention:** No vaccine or preventive drug is available.

● Characteristic corkscrew movement can be seen in smears of biopsied gastric mucosa.

● Urease-positivity can be measured by a breath test (radioactively labeled urea is cleaved by bacterial enzyme, releasing radioactive CO_2 in expired breath).

● Serologic tests are available, including ELISA for serum antibodies to *H. pylori*.

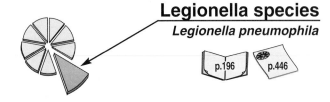

Legionella species
Legionella pneumophila

p.196   p.446

Common characteristics

- **Gram-negative (faintly staining)**
- **Slender rod in nature; coccobacillary in clinical material**
- **Facultative, intracellular parasite**
- **Organisms are unencapsulated with monotrichous flagella**
- **Culture on specialized medium**

Pathogenesis/Clinical Significance

L. pneumophila's normal habitats are water and soil, and the organism can colonize cooling towers, humidifiers, air conditioners, and water distribution systems. The organism is chlorine tolerant, and thus survives water treatment procedures.

Infections generally result from inhalation of aerosolized organisms. The resulting pathology is therefore initially confined primarily to the respiratory tract. Macrophages phagocytose the *L. pneumophila*, but the phagosome fails to fuse with a lysosome. Instead, the organisms multiply within this protected environment until the cell ruptures, releasing increased numbers of infectious bacteria.

● Legionnaires' disease

This is an acute lobar pneumonia with multisystem symptoms. Predisposing factors include immunocompromise, pulmonary compromise (due, for example, to heavy smoking or chronic lung disease), and debilitation brought on by excessive alcohol consumption, age, or surgery. Pneumonia (associated with a cough that is only slightly productive) is the predominant symptom. Watery, nonbloody diarrhea occurs in 25 to 50 percent of cases. Nausea, vomiting, and neurologic symptoms may also occur.

● Pontiac fever

This is an influenza-like illness that characteristically infects otherwise healthy individuals. Recovery is usually complete within one week.

Treatment and Prevention

- **Treatment:** Macrolides, such as erythromycin or azithromycin, are the drugs of choice for legionnaire's disease. Fluoroquinolones are also effective. No specific therapy is required for Pontiac fever.

- **Prevention:** No vaccine or preventive drug is available. Measures such as flushing the water supply with extremely hot water decrease the chance of contamination.

Laboratory Identification

- Culture *L. pneumophila* from respiratory secretions using buffered charcoal yeast extract enriched with L-cysteine, iron, and α-ketoglutarate.

- Serologic tests include a direct fluorescent antibody test and a radioimmunoassay for *L. pneumophila* antigen in the urine.

- Hybridization with *L. pneumophila* ribosomal RNA using a DNA probe is also available.

Leptospira species
Leptospira interrogans

p.227   p.447

Common characteristics

- **Gram-negative, but stains poorly, and needs to be visualized by other means**
- **Long, very slender, flexible, spiral- or corkscrew-shaped rods**
- **Highly motile**
- **Culture on specialized medium**

Pathogenesis/Clinical Significance

A number of wild and domestic animals serve as reservoirs for *L. interrogans*. Transmission to humans occurs following ingestion of food or water contaminated, for example, by animal urine containing the spirochete. These organisms can survive for several weeks in stagnant water, but are sensitive to drying.

● Leptospirosis

Different strains of *L. interrogans* are found worldwide, and cause leptospirosis, known under various local names such as **infectious jaundice**, **marsh fever**, **Weil's disease**, and **swineherd's disease**. Fever occurs about one to two weeks after infection, and *L. interrogans* is present in the blood. The organisms next infect various organs, particularly the liver and kidneys, resulting in jaundice, hemorrhage, and tissue necrosis. Large numbers of leptospira are shed into the urine by the diseased kidneys. The second phase of the disease involves a rise in IgM antibody titer accompanied by aseptic meningitis. Hepatitis frequently occurs.

Treatment and Prevention

- **Treatment:** Penicillin G or a tetracycline such as doxycycline are used during early stages of the infection.

- **Prevention:** No vaccine is available. Doxycycline is effective prophylactically. Prevention of exposure to contaminated water, and rodent control, can both help decrease the chance of infection.

Laboratory Identification

- *L. interrogans* does not stain well. However, the organisms can sometimes be observed in a fresh blood smear by dark-field microscopy.

- *L. interrogans* can be detected by serologic agglutination tests.

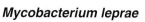

Listeria species

Listeria monocytogenes

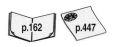

p.162   p.447

Common characteristics

- Gram-positive, staining darkly
- Slender, short rods, sometimes occurring as diplobacilli or in short chains
- Intracellular parasites
- Catalase-positive
- Distinctive tumbling motility in liquid medium
- Grow facultatively on a variety of enriched media

Pathogenesis/Clinical Significance

Listeria species are widespread among animals in nature. Infections with the pathogenic *L. monocytogenes* may occur as sporadic cases or in small epidemics, and are usually food-borne (dairy products, ground meats, and poultry).

L. monocytogenes is a facultative, intracellular parasite. It attaches to and enters a variety of mammalian cells by phagocytosis. Once inside the cell, it escapes from the phagocytic vacuole by producing a membrane-damaging toxin, **listeriolysin**. *Listeria* grows in the cytosol, and stimulates changes in cell function that facilitate its direct passage from cell to cell.

- **Listeriosis**

  Septicemia and meningitis are the most commonly reported forms of listeria infection. The organism can be transmitted from an infected mother to her newborn (listeria is a relatively common cause of newborn meningitis), or to the fetus, initiating abortion. Immunocompromised individuals, especially those with defects in cellular immunity, are susceptible to serious, generalized infections.

Treatment and Prevention

- **Treatment:** A variety of antibiotics have been successfully used to treat *L. monocytogenes* infections, including ampicillin or trimethoprim plus sulfamethoxazole.
- **Prevention:** No vaccine is available against *L. monocytogenes*. Prevention of *Listeria* infections can be accomplished by proper food preparation and handling.

Laboratory Identification

- *L. monocytogenes* can be isolated from blood, cerebrospinal fluid, and other clinical specimens.
- On blood agar, the organism produces a small colony surrounded by a narrow zone of β hemolysis.
- *Listeria* species can be distinguished by morphology, positive motility, and the production of catalase.

Mycobacterium species

Mycobacterium leprae
Mycobacterium tuberculosis

Common characteristics

- Not colored by Gram stain due to lipid-rich cell walls
- Long, slender, nonmotile rods
- Aerobic
- Resistant to drying
- Culture *M. tuberculosis* on specialized medium such as Lowenstein-Jensen agar; *M. leprae* does not grow in culture

Mycobacterium leprae

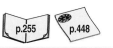

p.255   p.448

Pathogenesis/Clinical Significance

M. leprae has low infectivity. It is transmitted from human to human through prolonged contact, for example between exudates of a leprosy patient's skin lesions, and the abraded skin of another individual. No *M. leprae* toxins or virulence factors are known.

- **Hansen's disease (leprosy)**

  Leprosy is a chronic granulomatous condition of peripheral nerves and skin. There are two clinical forms: **tuberculoid leprosy**, in which destructive lesions due to the host's cell-mediated immune response occur as large macular plaques in cooler body tissues such as skin (especially nose and outer ears), testicles, and in superficial nerve endings; and **lepromatous leprosy**, in which the cell-mediated immune response is severely depressed, and the disease becomes slow but progressive, with large numbers of organisms in the lesions and blood.

Treatment and Prevention

- **Treatment for tuberculoid form:** Dapsone plus rifampin.
- **Treatment for lepromatous form:** Clofazamine. Both forms require long-term antibiotic treatment.
- **Prevention:** No preventive drug is available. Vaccination with BCG shows some protective effects in leprosy.

Laboratory Identification

- **Tuberculous leprosy:** Organisms in clinical samples are very rare; diagnosis relies on clinical findings and the histology of biopsy material.
- **Lepromatous leprosy:** Acid-fast stains of skin scrapings from nasal mucosa or other infected areas can show the presence of *M. leprae*.

Mycobacterium tuberculosis

p.246   p.448

Pathogenesis/Clinical Significance

M. tuberculosis survives and grows in host macrophages, where it can remain viable but quiescent for decades. Immunosuppression can lead to reactivation. *M. tuberculosis* produces no demonstrable endo- or exotoxins.

Tuberculosis is the principal chronic bacterial disease in humans, and is the leading cause worldwide of death from infection. Transmission is by aerosol droplets produced by coughing, and depends on crowded conditions and poor ventilation.

- **Tuberculosis:**

  Tubercles (productive granulomatous lesions) form in the lung following infection by *M. tuberculosis*. Their formation is mediated by the host immune response. The lesion may arrest and become fibrotic and calcified, or it can break down, resulting in spread of the infection via the lymph and bloodstream. *M. tuberculosis* can seed different tissues, causing, for example, chronic pneumonitis, tuberculous osteomyelitis, or tuberculous meningitis. If active tubercles develop throughout the body, this serious condition is known as miliary (disseminated) tuberculosis.

Treatment and Prevention

- **Treatment:** A long course of combined antibiotic treatment (six months or more) with isoniazid, ethambutol, streptomycin, and/or pyrazinamide (these drugs are usually used in mixtures) is required for a cure.

- **Prevention:** Bacille Calmette-Guerin vaccine (BCG) is available, and is used for tuberculin-negative individuals under sustained heavy risk of infection. Isoniazid is used prophylactically, for example, for individuals who are tuberculin-positive but asymptomatic, and who need immunosuppressive therapy for other illnesses.

Laboratory Identification

- Acid-fast bacteria can be observed in clinical specimens treated with Ziehl-Neelsen stain.

- Nucleic acid probes can be used to detect *M. tuberculosis* DNA that has been amplified by PCR.

- The organism can be cultured on specialized media such as Lowenstein-Jensen agar.

Mycoplasma species

Mycoplasma pneumoniae

p.230   p.448

Common characteristics

- Not seen with Gram stain because it lacks peptidoglycan cell walls

- Plastic, pleomorphic shape (neither rods nor cocci)

- Three-layer (trilaminar) cell membrane contains sterols

- Colonies may have "fried egg" appearance

- Rarely cultured for diagnostic purposes

Pathogenesis/Clinical Significance

M. pneumoniae is found as part of the normal flora of the human mouth and and genitourinary tract. It is transmitted by respiratory droplets.

M. pneumoniae has a membrane-associated cytoadhesin (P1) that binds to ciliated bronchial epithelial cells, and inhibits ciliary action. This results in an inflammatory response in bronchial tissues. *M. pneumoniae* produces no exo- or endotoxins.

- **Primary atypical pneumonia:**

  This disease of the lower respiratory tract is the best-known form of *M. pneumoniae* infection. It is also referred to as "walking pneumonia" because the signs and symptoms may be minimal, and the patient usually remains ambulatory throughout the illness. *M. pneumoniae* infection also causes bronchitis, pharyngitis, and nonpurulent otitis media. The highest incidence of disease occurs in older children and young adults (six to twenty years old).

Treatment and Prevention

- **Treatment:** Doxycycline and erythromycin are the drugs of choice.

Laboratory Identification

- Serologic tests such as complement fixation antibodies to *M. pneumoniae* are the most widely used procedures for establishing an identification of primary atypical pneumonia.

- *M. pneumoniae* is difficult and expensive to culture.

- Commercially available DNA probes can be used to detect *M. pneumoniae* RNA in sputum specimens.

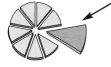

Neisseria species

Neisseria gonorrhoeae
Neisseria meningitidis

Common characteristics

- ● Gram-negative
- ● Kidney bean–shaped diplococci
- ● Piliated
- ● Oxidase-positive
- ● Aerobic
- ● Culture on Thayer-Martin agar

Neisseria gonorrhoeae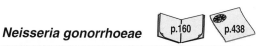

Pathogenesis/Clinical Significance

The normal habitat of *N. gonorrhoeae* is the human genital tract. It is usually transmitted during sexual contact, but can also be transmitted during the passage of a baby through an infected birth canal.

N. gonorrhoeae is highly sensitive to dehydration, and is unencapsulated. Bacterial proteins (pili and outer membrane proteins) enhance the attachment of the bacterium to host epithelial and mucosal cell surfaces, such as those of the urethra, rectum, cervix, pharynx, or conjunctiva, followed by colonization. Pilin confers resistance to phagocytosis, and an IgA protease protects against opsonization; pili and the IgA protease are the organisms' most important virulence factors.

- ● **Gonorrhea**

  Gonorrhea is a very commonly reported infectious disease in the United States. In males, symptoms include urethritis, purulent discharge, and pain during urination. In females, infection is usually localized to the endocervix, often causing a purulent vaginal discharge. If the woman's disease progresses to the uterus, **gonococcal salpingitis** (which may lead to tubal scarring and infertility), **pelvic inflammatory disease** (PID), and fibrosis can occur. Alternatively, the infection may be asymptomatic.

- ● **Ophthalmia neonatorum**

  This is a purulent conjunctivitis acquired by a newborn during passage through the birth canal of a mother infected with gonococcus. If untreated, acute conjunctivitis can lead to blindness.

- ● **Septic arthritis**

  Blood-borne (disseminated) *N. gonorrhoeae* are the most common cause of infectious arthritis in sexually active adults.

Treatment and Prevention

- ● **Treatment for uncomplicated gonorrhea:** Ceftriaxone is currently the antibiotic of choice. A tetracycline, such as doxycycline, is added when *Chlamydia* is a suspected co-pathogen. Spectinomycin is used for resistant organisms, and in patients allergic to cephalosporins.

- ● **Treatment for ophthalmia neonatorum:** Tetracycline or erythromycin is instilled into newborns' eyes to eradicate both *N. gonorrhoeae* and *Chlamydia trachomatis* (if present).

- ● **Prevention:** No vaccine or preventive drug is available. Newborns whose eyes are at risk for infection with *N. gonorrhoeae* are treated prophylactically with tetracycline or erythromycin. Taking precautions during sex (that is, using condoms) can prevent transmission of the disease.

Laboratory Identification

- ● Gram-negative diplococci are visible within neutrophils in urethral exudates.

- ● Oxidase-positive cultures grow on Thayer-Martin agar under increased oxygen tension.

- ● *N. gonorrhoeae* ferments glucose but not maltose.

Neisseria meningitidis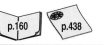

Pathogenesis/Clinical Significance

N. meningitidis is one of the most frequent causes of meningitis. Transmission is via respiratory droplets, and pili allow the attachment of *N. meningitidis* to the nasopharyngeal mucosa.

The meningococcal polysaccharide capsule is antiphagocytic, and is therefore the most important virulence factor aiding in maintenance of the infection. *N. meningitidis* also makes IgA protease (see *N. gonorrhoeae*).

[*N. MENINGITIDIS* IS CONTINUED ON THE NEXT PAGE]

Treatment and Prevention

- ● **Treatment:** Penicillin G, cefotaxime, and ceftriaxone are the drugs of choice.

Laboratory Identification

- ● Under the light microscope, *N. meningitidis* obtained from CSF appear as gram-negative diplococci, often in association with polymorphonuclear leukocytes.

Neisseria meningitidis (continued)

Pathogenesis/Clinical Significance	Treatment and Prevention	Laboratory Identification

● Meningitis

The epithelial lining of the nasopharynx normally serves as a barrier to bacteria. If meningococci penetrate that barrier and enter the blood stream they rapidly multiply, causing **meningococcemia**. This septicemia can result in intravascular coagulation, circulatory collapse, and potentially fatal shock (for which the bacterial endotoxin is largely responsible). If *N. meningitidis* crosses the blood-brain barrier it can infect the meninges, causing an acute inflammatory response that results in a purulent **meningitis**. The initial fever and malaise can rapidly evolve into severe headache, rigid neck, vomiting, and sensitivity to bright light. Coma can occur within a few hours.

● Waterhouse-Friderichsen syndrome

This syndrome is an acute, fulminating meningococcal septicemia seen mainly in very young children. It is associated with adrenal hemorrhage.

● **Prevention:** A capsular vaccine for serogroups A and C is very effective, and is used routinely by the military or during an outbreak of meningococcal serogroup A or C in the civilian population. Unfortunately, the polysaccharide of serogroup B does not elicit an effective immune response.

● **Prophylaxis:** Rifampin can be used to treat family members or other close associates of an infected individual.

● *N. meningitidis* can be cultured on chocolate agar.

● The organism is oxidase-positive, and ferments glucose and maltose in an atmosphere of five percent CO_2.

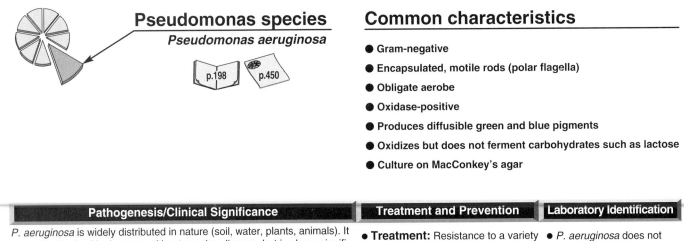

Pseudomonas species
Pseudomonas aeruginosa

p.198   p.450

Common characteristics

- ● **Gram-negative**
- ● **Encapsulated, motile rods (polar flagella)**
- ● **Obligate aerobe**
- ● **Oxidase-positive**
- ● **Produces diffusible green and blue pigments**
- ● **Oxidizes but does not ferment carbohydrates such as lactose**
- ● **Culture on MacConkey's agar**

Pathogenesis/Clinical Significance	Treatment and Prevention	Laboratory Identification

P. aeruginosa is widely distributed in nature (soil, water, plants, animals). It may colonize healthy humans without causing disease, but is also a significant opportunistic pathogen, and a major cause of nosocomial infections. *P. aeruginosa* is regularly a cause of nosocomial pneumonia, nosocomial infections of the urinary tract, surgical sites, severe burns, and of infections of patients with cystic fibrosis, or who are undergoing either chemotherapy for neoplastic diseases or antibiotic therapy for other infections. *P. aeruginosa* can grow in distilled water, laboratory hot water baths, hot tubs, wet IV tubing, and other water-containing vessels. This explains why the organism is responsible for so many nosocomial infections.

P. aeruginosa disease begins with attachment and colonization of host tissue. Virtually any tissue/organ may be affected. Pili mediate adherence, and extracellular proteases, cytotoxin, hemolysins, and pyocyanin promote tissue damage and local invasion and dissemination of the organism. Systemic disease is promoted by an antiphagocytic capsule, and endo- and exotoxins.

● Localized infections:

Localized *P. aeruginosa* infections may occur in the eye, ear, skin, urinary tract, respiratory tract, gastrointestinal tract, and central nervous system. In most cases, localized infections have the potential to lead to disseminated infection.

● Systemic infection

The gastrointestinal tract is a particularly common site for penetration. The resulting systemic infections may include bacteremia, secondary pneumonia, bone and joint infections, endocarditis, and infections of the skin/soft tissue or central nervous system.

● **Treatment:** Resistance to a variety of antibiotics is common in this species, therefore antimicrobial therapy often requires a combination of bactericidal antibiotics such as an aminoglycoside and an antipseudomonal β-lactam.

● **Prevention:** No vaccine or preventive drug is available. Prevention of burn wound infection requires the use of topical silver sulfadizine.

● *P. aeruginosa* does not ferment lactose, and is oxidase positive.

● *P. aeruginosa* produces colorless colonies on MacConkey agar. Cultured organisms produce blue (pyocyanin) and fluorescent green (pyoverdin) pigments.

Rickettsia species
Rickettsia rickettsii

p.259   p.450

Common characteristics

- Gram-negative, but stain poorly
- Small, rod-like or coccobacillary in shape
- Grow only inside living host cells
- Transmitted by infected tick
- Not routinely cultured because of obligate intracellularity

Pathogenesis/Clinical Significance

R. rickettsii is transmitted to humans by the bite of an infected wood or dog tick. It parasitizes endothelial cells lining the capillaries throughout the circulatory system, ultimately killing the host cell. This results in the formation of focal thrombi in various organs including the skin. A variety of small hemorrhages and hemodynamic disturbances create the symptoms of illness.

- **Rocky Mountain spotted fever**

  This disease is characterized by high fever, malaise, and a prominent rash that begins on the palms and soles, and then spreads to cover the body. The rash can progress from macular to petechial or frankly hemorrhagic. Untreated, infection can lead to myocardial or renal failure. The disease occurs most frequently in children and teenagers, but mortality rates are highest (five to thirty percent) among individuals older than forty years of age.

Treatment and Prevention

- **Treatment:** Doxycycline and chloramphenicol are the drugs of choice for *R. rickettsii* infections, provided the drugs are administered early in the illness. Because the principal diagnostic methods await the demonstration of seroconversion, a decision to treat must be made on clinical grounds, together with a history or suspicion of contact with a tick.

- **Prevention:** No antirickettsial vaccine is licensed in the United States, and no preventive drug is available. Prevention depends on vector control, wearing proper clothing that minimizes bare skin, and immediate removal of attached ticks.

Laboratory Identification

- Serologic procedures rely on the demonstration of a rickettsia-specific antibody response during the course of infection.

- Indirect fluorescent antibody tests using rickettsia-specific antibodies are available, primarily in reference laboratories.

Salmonella species
Salmonella typhi
Salmonella typhimurium

Salmonella typhi

p.179   p.451

Common characteristics

- Gram-negative rods
- Facultative anaerobes
- Ferment glucose and a wide range of carbohydrates, but most strains of salmonella do not ferment lactose
- Catalase-positive, oxidase-negative
- Culture on MacConkey agar

Pathogenesis/Clinical Significance

S. typhi is transmitted between humans, without animal or fowl reservoirs. Infection is via the oral/fecal route, generally through food or water contaminated by human feces. Young children and the elderly are particularly susceptible to *Salmonella* infections, as are individuals in crowded institutions or living conditions.

S. typhi causes disease by attaching to and invading macrophages of the intestinal lymphoid tissue (Peyer's patches). The bacteria replicate rapidly within these cells, and eventually spread to the reticuloendothelial system (including both liver and spleen, which become enlarged), and potentially to the gall bladder.

- **Enteric (typhoid) fever**

  This is a severe, life-threatening systemic illness, characterized by fever and, frequently, by abdominal symptoms. About thirty percent of patients have a faint, maculopapular rash on the trunk (termed "rose spots"). After one to three weeks of incubation, *S. typhi* can enter the blood, the resulting bacteremia causing fever, headache, malaise, and bloody diarrhea. Bacterial endotoxin can cause encephalopathy, myocarditis, or intravascular coagulation. Perforations of the intestine can lead to hemorrhage. Some infected individuals may become chronic carriers for periods as long as years due to persistent residual infection of the gallbladder. Public food handlers or health care deliverers who are carriers can present a serious public health problem (remember "Typhoid Mary"!).

Treatment and Prevention

- **Treatment:** Ceftriaxone and fluoroquinolones such as ciprofloxacin are the first-line drugs of choice.

- **Prevention:** A vaccine is available, but less than seventy percent of those given the vaccine are protected. Prevention requires maintaining proper hygiene and cooking food thoroughly.

Laboratory Identification

- *S. typhi* can be isolated from blood, feces, bone marrow, urine, or tissue from rose spots.

- *S. typhi* can be cultured on MacConkey agar, where it produces colorless, non–lactose-fermenting colonies.

- Serologic tests for antibodies against O antigen in patient's serum also aid in the diagnosis.

Salmonella typhimurium
p.179 p.451

Pathogenesis/Clinical Significance	Treatment and Prevention	Laboratory Identification

S. typhimurium (and other *Salmonella* species that cause enterocolitis) reside in the gastrointestinal tracts of humans, other animals, and fowl. They are transmitted through contaminated food products, or via the oral/fecal route.

- **Enterocolitis (formerly gastroenteritis, foodpoisoning)**

  Contaminated poultry products including eggs are the primary vehicle for infection of humans by *S. typhimurium*, although raw milk and pets such as turtles also transmit the disease. Salmonella adhere to and invade enterocytes of both the small and large intestine, causing a profound inflammatory response. Within 10 to 48 hours after ingestion, nausea, vomiting, abdominal cramps, and diarrhea ensue. Diarrhea usually ends spontaneously within a week.

- **Treatment:** Fluid and electrolyte replacement are important if diarrhea is severe. Antibiotics are not normally used except in immunocompromised individuals to prevent systemic spread of the infection.

- **Prevention:** No vaccine or preventive drug is available. Prevention is accomplished by proper sewage disposal, correct handling of food, and good personal hygiene.

- Organisms isolated from stool samples produce colorless colonies on MacConkey agar.

Shigella species
Shigella sonnei

p.183 p.451

Common characteristics

- **Gram-negative rods**
- **Facultative anaerobes**
- **Ferment glucose and a wide range of carbohydrates, but most strains of salmonella do not ferment lactose**
- **Catalase-positive, oxidase-negative**
- **Culture on Hektoen agar**

Pathogenesis/Clinical Significance	Treatment and Prevention	Laboratory Identification

S. sonnei is typically spread from person to person, with contaminated stools serving as a major source of organisms. Flies and contaminated food or water can also transmit the disease. The organism has a low infectious dose (less than 200 viable organisms are sufficient to cause disease). Therefore secondary cases within a household are common, particularly under conditions of crowding and/or poor sanitation.

S. sonnei invades and destroys the mucosa of the large intestine, but rarely penetrates to the deeper intestinal layers. The organism produces an exotoxin (**Shiga toxin**) with enterotoxic and cytotoxic properties.

- **Bacillary dysentery (shigellosis)**

  This disease is characterized by diarrhea with blood, mucus, and painful abdominal cramping. The disease is generally most severe in the very young and elderly, and among malnourished individuals, in whom shigellosis may lead to severe dehydration and even death.

- **Treatment:** Antibiotics such as ciprofloxacin or azithromycin can reduce the duration of illness and the period of shedding organisms, but usage is controversial because of widespread antibiotic resistance.

- **Prevention:** Protection of the water and food supplies and personal hygiene are crucial for preventing *Shigella* infections. Vaccine development is currently experimental.

- During acute illness, organisms can be cultured from stools using Hektoen agar or other media specific for intestinal pathogens.

Staphylococcus species

Staphylococcus aureus

Staphylococcus epidermidis

Staphylococcus saprophyticus

Common characteristics

● **Gram-positive, staining darkly**

● **Round cocci tending to occur in bunches like grapes**

● **True facultative anaerobic organisms**

● **Cultured on enriched media containing broth and/or blood**

Staphylococcus aureus 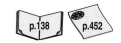 p.138 p.452

Pathogenesis/Clinical Significance	Treatment and Prevention	Laboratory Identification

S. aureus is part of the normal flora of certain mucous membranes (for example, the anterior nares, vagina), and of the skin. It is also, however, the most virulent of the staphylococci.

Infection occurs during penetration of the skin (for example, due to a wound, or during surgery), typically resulting in an abscess. Subsequent disease can be caused by the actual infection, by toxins in the absence of infection (toxinosis), or by a combination of infection and intoxication. Important *S. aureus* virulence factors include: 1) cell wall virulence factors that can promote binding to mucosal cells and exert antiopsonic (and therefore antiphagocytic) effects; 2) cytolytic exotoxins (including hemolysins); 3) superantigen exotoxins, including enterotoxins (which cause food poisoning), toxic shock syndrome toxin, and exfoliative toxin (which causes scalded skin syndrome in children, and also bullous impetigo). The most common diseases caused by *S. aureus* are the following.

● Localized skin infections

These include 1) small, superficial abscesses involving sweat or sebaceous glands, or hair follicles (for example, the common **sty**); 2) subcutaneous abscesses (**furuncles** or **boils**) that form around foreign bodies such as splinters; and 3) larger, deeper infections (**carbuncles**) that can lead to bacteremia.

● Diffuse skin infection–impetigo (pyoderma)

This is a superficial, spreading, crusty skin lesion generally seen in children.

● Deep, localized infections

S. aureus is the most common cause of acute and chronic infection of the bone marrow (**osteomyelitis**), and also the most common cause of arthritis resulting from acute infection of the joint space ("**septic joint**").

● Other infections

S. aureus can cause **acute endocarditis**, **septicemia**, and severe, **necrotizing pneumonia**. [Note: *S. aureus* is one of the most common causes of hospital-acquired (nosocomial) infections. Progression to septicemia is often a terminal event.]

● Toxinoses

Toxic shock syndrome is caused by strains of *S. aureus* that produce a specific, absorbable toxin. The syndrome results in high fever, rash, vomiting, diarrhea, hypotension, and multiorgan involvement (especially GI, renal, and/or hepatic damage). Staphylococcal **gastroenteritis** is caused by ingestion of food contaminated with toxin produced by *S. aureus*. **Scalded skin syndrome** (mild cases are sometimes called **bullous impetigo**) involves the appearance of superficial bullae resulting from the action of an exfoliative toxin that attacks the intercellular adhesive of the stratum granulosum, causing marked epithelial desquamation.

[STAPHYLOCOCCUS SPECIES ARE CONTINUED ON THE NEXT PAGE]

● **Treatment:** Serious *S. aureus* infections require aggressive treatment, including incision and drainage of localized lesions as well as systemic antibiotics. Acquired antibiotic resistance determinants are frequently present, complicating the choice of drug. For example, nearly all *S. aureus* isolates are resistant to penicillin G, and methicillin-resistant *S. aureus* (MRSA) are becoming prevalent in hospital isolates. Nafcillin and oxacillin have replaced penicillin G because they are β-lactamase resistant. Vancomycin is also used to treat MRSA, but strains resistant to this drug are emerging.

● **Prevention:** No vaccine or preventive drug is available. Infection control procedures such as barrier precautions, washing of hands, and disinfection of fomites are important in the control of nosocomial *S. aureus* epidemics.

● *S. aureus* stains strongly positive with Gram stain, and cells appear in grape-like clusters.

● *S. aureus* is catalase- and coagulase-positive.

● *S. aureus* forms deep yellow, hemolytic colonies on enriched media.

Staphylococcus epidermidis   p.143 p.452

Pathogenesis/Clinical Significance	Treatment and Prevention	Laboratory Identification
S. epidermidis is part of the normal flora of the skin and anterior nares. ● **Important cause of infections from prosthetic implants** Surgical implants, such as heart valves and catheters, are easily infected by *S. epidermidis*. Cell envelope factors that facilitate attachment to plastic surfaces act as virulence factors.	● **Treatment:** Acquired drug resistance by *S. epidermidis* is even more frequent than by *S. aureus*. Vancomycin sensitivity remains the rule, but vancomycin-resistant isolates have been reported. ● **Prevention:** No vaccine or preventive drug is available.	● *S. epidermidis* stains strongly positive with Gram stain. The cocci appear in grape-like clusters. ● The organism produces white, nonhemolytic colonies on enriched agar. It is coagulase-negative, and novobiocin-sensitive.

Staphylococcus saprophyticus p.143 p.452

Pathogenesis/Clinical Significance	Treatment and Prevention	Laboratory Identification
S. saprophyticus is part of the normal vaginal flora. ● **Cystitis in women** *S. saprophyticus* is a frequent cause of cystitis in women. [Note: A urinary coagulase-negative staphylococcus is often presumed to be *S. saprophyticus*; novobiocin resistance can be used for confirmation.]	● **Treatment:** *S. saprophyticus* tends to be sensitive to most antibiotics, even penicillin G. ● **Prevention:** No vaccine or preventive drug is available.	● *S. saprophyticus* stains strongly positive with Gram stain. The cocci appear in grape-like clusters. ● The organism produces white, nonhemolytic colonies on enriched agar. It is coagulase-negative and novobiocin-sensitive.

Streptococcus species

Streptococcus agalactiae
Streptococcus pneumoniae
Streptococcus pyogenes

Common characteristics

● **Gram-positive**

● **Ovoid to spherical in shape, occurring as pairs or chains**

● **Nonmotile, catalase-negative**

● **Most are facultative anaerobes, but grow fermentatively even in the presence of oxygen**

● **Culture on blood agar**

Streptococcus agalactiae 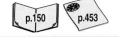 p.150 p.453

Pathogenesis/Clinical Significance	Treatment and Prevention	Laboratory Identification
S. agalactiae is a group B streptococcus. It is found normally in the vaginocervical tract of female carriers, and the urethral mucous membranes of male carriers, as well as in the GI tract (especially the rectum). Transmission occurs from an infected mother to her infant at birth, and venereally among adults. *S. agalactiae's* polysaccharide capsule is antiphagocytic, which allows the bacterium to infect tissue and induce an inflammatory response. ● **Meningitis and septicemia in neonates** Infection occurs as the infant traverses the birth canal. *S. agalactiae* is a leading cause of these syndromes in neonates, with a high mortality rate. ● **Infections of adults** *S. agalactiae* is an occasional cause of endometritis in postpartum women, and of septicemia or pneumonia in individuals with impaired immune systems.	● **Treatment:** All isolates remain sensitive to penicillin G and ampicillin, which are still the antibiotics of choice. In life-threatening infections, an aminoglycoside can be added to the regimen. ● **Prevention:** No vaccine or preventive drug is available.	● Samples of blood, cervical swabs, sputum, or spinal fluid can be cultured on blood agar. Group B streptococci are β-hemolytic, with larger colonies and less hemolysis than group A streptococci. ● *S. agalactiae* can hydrolyze sodium hippurate, and is catalase-negative.

[STREPTOCOCCUS SPECIES ARE CONTINUED ON THE NEXT PAGE]

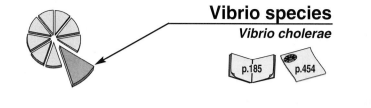

Vibrio species
Vibrio cholerae

p.185   p.454

Common characteristics

- Gram-negative
- Short, curved, rod-shaped
- Rapidly motile due to single polar flagellum
- Facultative anaerobes
- Growth of many vibrio strains requires or is stimulated by NaCl
- Culture on blood or MacConkey agar

Pathogenesis/Clinical Significance

V. cholerae is transmitted by contaminated water and food. There are no known animal reservoirs, nor animal or arthropod vectors. Outbreaks of *V. cholerae* infection have been associated with raw or undercooked seafood harvested from contaminated waters.

Following ingestion, *V. cholerae* infects the small intestine. Adhesion factors are important for colonization and virulence. The organism is noninvasive, and causes disease through the action of an enterotoxin (**cholera toxin**) that causes the activation of adenylate cyclase by ADP-ribosylation. This initiates an outpouring of fluid into the intestine.

- ### Cholera
  Full-blown cholera is characterized by massive loss of fluid and electrolytes from the body. After an incubation period ranging from hours to a few days, profuse watery diarrhea (**rice-water stools**) begins. Untreated, the death from shock may occur in hours to days, with the death rate exceeding fifty percent.

Treatment and Prevention

- **Treatment:** Replacement of fluids and electrolytes is crucial in preventing shock, and does not require bacteriologic diagnosis. Antibiotics such as doxycycline can shorten the duration of diarrhea and excretion of the organism.

- **Prevention:** Public health measures that reduce fecal contamination of water supplies and food, and adequate cooking of foods, can minimize transmission.

Laboratory Identification

- *V. cholerae* from a stool sample grows on standard, nonselective media such as blood and MacConkey agars. Thiosulfate-citrate-bile salts-sucrose (TCBS) medium can enhance isolation.

- *V. cholerae* is oxidase-positive.

Yersinia species
Yersinia pestis

p.205   p.454

Common characteristics

- Gram-negative
- Small rod that stains bipolarly
- Nonmotile, encapsulated
- Culture on MacConkey or CIN (selective) agar

Pathogenesis/Clinical Significance

Y. pestis is endemic in a variety of mammals, both urban and sylvatic, and is distributed worldwide. Infection is transmitted by fleas, which serve to maintain the infection within the animal reservoir. Humans are generally accidental and dead-end hosts. The organism can also be transmitted by ingestion of contaminated animal tissues, or via the respiratory route.

Organisms are carried by the lymphatic system from the site of inoculation to regional lymph nodes, where they are ingested by phagocytes. *Y. pestis* multiplies in these cells. Hematogenous spread of bacteria to other organs or tissues may occur, resulting in hemorrhagic lesions at these sites.

- ### Bubonic (septicemic) plague
  The incubation period (from flea bite to development of symptoms) is generally two to eight days. Onset of nonspecific symptoms, such as high fever, chills, headache, myalgia, and weakness that proceeds to prostration, is characteristically sudden. Within a short time, the characteristic, painful **buboes** develop—typically in the groin, but they may also occur in axillae or on the neck. Blood pressure drops, potentially leading to septic shock and death.

- ### Pneumonic plague
  If plague bacilli reach the lungs, they cause a purulent pneumonia that is highly contagious, and, if untreated, is rapidly fatal.

Treatment and Prevention

- **Treatment:** Streptomycin is the drug of choice; gentamicin and tetracycline are acceptable alternatives. Because of the potential for overwhelming septicemia, rapid institution of antibiotic therapy is crucial. Supportive therapy is essential for patients with signs of shock.

- **Prevention:** A formalin-killed vaccine is available for those at high risk of acquiring plague. For individuals in enzootic areas, efforts to minimize exposure to rodents and fleas is important.

Laboratory Identification

- Laboratory identification can be made by a gram-stained smear, and culture of an aspirate from a bubo (or sputum in the case of pneumonic plague).

- The organism grows on both MacConkey and blood agars, although colonies grow somewhat more slowly than do those of other Enterobacteriaceae.

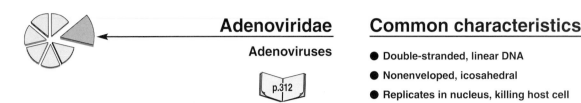

VIRUSES

Adenoviridae

Adenoviruses

p.312

Common characteristics

● Double-stranded, linear DNA

● Nonenveloped, icosahedral

● Replicates in nucleus, killing host cell

Pathogenesis/Clinical Significance

The site of the clinical syndrome caused by adenovirus infection is generally related to the mode of virus transmission. Adenoviruses are primarily agents of respiratory disease, and are transmitted via the respiratory route. Those associated specifically with gastrointestinal disease are transmitted by the fecal-oral route, whereas ocular infections are transmitted by virus-contaminated hands, ophthalmologic instruments, or swimming pools.

● **Respiratory tract diseases**

The most common manifestation of adenovirus infection of infants and young children is **acute febrile pharyngitis**, characterized by a cough, sore throat, nasal congestion, and fever. Acute respiratory disease occurs primarily in epidemics among new military recruits, and is facilitated by fatigue and crowded conditions. These syndromes may progress to true viral pneumonia, which in infants has a mortality rate of about ten percent.

● **Ocular diseases**

If both the respiratory tract and the eyes are involved, the syndrome is referred to as **pharyngoconjunctival fever**. A similar follicular conjunctivitis may occur as a separate, self-limiting disease. A more serious infection is **epidemic keratoconjunctivitis** in which the corneal epithelium is also involved, and which may be followed by corneal opacity lasting several years. The epidemic nature of this disease arises in part from transmission by improperly sterilized ophthalmologic instruments.

● **Gastrointestinal diseases**

Most of the human adenoviruses multiply in the GI tract, and can be found in stools. However, these are generally asymptomatic infections. Two serotypes have been associated specifically with **infantile gastroenteritis**, and have been estimated to account for five to fifteen percent of all viral diarrheal disease in children.

Treatment and Prevention

● **Treatment:** No antiviral agents are currently available for treating adenovirus infections.

● **Prevention:** A live, attenuated adenovirus vaccine is used to prevent epidemic respiratory disease in the military population. Although not known to be associated with human malignancies, the oncogenicity of the adenoviruses in experimental animals has inhibited the use of adenovirus vaccines on a wider scale.

Laboratory Identification

● Isolation of virus for identification is not done on a routine basis, but may be desirable in cases of epidemic disease, or a nosocomial outbreak, especially in the nursery.

● Identification of the adenovirus serotype can be done by neutralization or hemagglutination inhibition using type-specific antisera.

● Enteric adenoviruses are detected by direct test of stool specimens by ELISA.

Picornaviridae

Coxsackievirus
Hepatitis A virus (p.426)
Poliovirus (p.434)

Common characteristics

● Positive-strand, single-stranded, nonsegmented RNA genome

● Non-enveloped, icosahedral

● Genomic RNAs serve as messenger RNAs and are infectious

● Virions do not contain any enzymes

[COXSACKIEVIRUS IS CONTINUED ON THE NEXT PAGE]

Coxsackievirus p.349

Pathogenesis/Clinical Significance	Treatment and Prevention	Laboratory Identification
Coxsackieviruses are members of the genus Enterovirus. Individuals are infected with coxsackieviruses by ingestion of contaminated food or water, or inhalation of aerosols containing the virus. These viruses are stable in the low pH of the stomach, replicate in the GI tract, and are excreted in the stool (fecal-oral route). Coxsackieviruses also replicate in the oropharynx. They are carried by the blood to peripheral tissues, including the heart and central nervous system.	• **Treatment:** No antiviral agents or vaccines are currently available for treating coxsackievirus infections.	• Viruses can be isolated and cultured from the stool or from various target organs. • Evidence of infection can also be obtained by demonstration of a rise in antibody titer.

• Coxsackievirus infections

These give rise to a large variety of clinical syndromes including upper respiratory infections, meningitis, gastroenteritis, herpangina (intense swelling of the throat), pleurisy, pericarditis, myocarditis, and myositis.

Herpesviridae

Epstein-Barr virus
Herpes simplex virus, Type 1 (p.428)
Herpes simplex virus, Type 2 (p.428)
Human cytomegalovirus (p.429)
Human herpesvirus, Type 8 (p.430)
Varicella-zoster virus (p.436)

Common characteristics

● **Linear, double-stranded DNA genome**

● **Replicate in the nucleus**

● **Envelope contains antigenic, species-specific glycoproteins**

● **In the tegument between the envelope and capsid are a number of virus-coded enzymes and transcription factors essential for initiation of the infectious cycle**

● **All herpesviruses can enter a latent state following primary infection, to be reactivated at a later time**

Epstein-Barr virus p.331

Pathogenesis/Clinical Significance	Treatment and Prevention	Laboratory Identification
Most transmission of Epstein-Barr virus (EBV) occurs by intimate contact with saliva that contains virus. EBV replicates in mucosal epithelium. The virus then spreads to the lymph nodes, where it infects B cells. EBV next travels via the blood to other organs, particularly targeting liver and spleen. The B cell infection is an abortive one, leading to B cell proliferation, accompanied by nonspecific increases in total IgM, IgG, and IgA.	• **Treatment:** Although acyclovir inhibits EBV replication, none of the antiherpes drugs have been effective in modifying the course or severity of IM due to EBV, or in preventing development of EBV-related B cell malignancies. • **Prevention:** No vaccine or preventive drug is available.	• The classic diagnostic test for EBV-associated mononucleosis is detection of heterophile antibodies that agglutinate sheep and horse red blood cells. • Serologic tests, such as immunofluorescence reactions or ELISA to detect antibodies specific for viral proteins, are used to evaluate the stage of disease. • Detection of EBV DNA or RNA by hybridization, or of viral antigens using immunohistochemical techniques, can be done with cell homogenates.

• Infectious mononucleosis (IM)

The "atypical lymphocytosis" characteristic of infectious mononucleosis is caused by the active cytotoxic T cell response to the EBV antigens expressed by infected B cells. The typical IM syndrome appears after an incubation period of four to seven weeks, and includes pharyngitis, lymphadenopathy, and fever. Headache and malaise often precede and accompany the disease, which may last several weeks. Throughout life, healthy EBV carriers continue to have episodes of asymptomatic virus shedding.

• Association with Burkitt's lymphoma and other human neoplastic diseases

EBV infection has been found to be associated with Burkitt's lymphoma, nasopharyngeal carcinoma, and Hodgkin's disease. The exact role played by the EBV in these diseases is not clear.

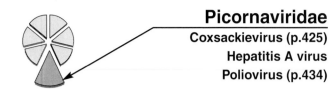

Picornaviridae

Coxsackievirus (p.425)
Hepatitis A virus
Poliovirus (p.434)

Common characteristics

● Positive-strand, single-stranded, nonsegmented RNA genome

● Non-enveloped, icosahedral

● Genomic RNAs serve as messenger RNAs and are infectious

● Virions do not contain any enzymes

Hepatitis A virus   p.352

Pathogenesis/Clinical Significance	Treatment and Prevention	Laboratory Identification

Hepatitis A virus (HAV) is a member of the genus hepatovirus. It is the most common cause of viral hepatitis in the United States. Transmission is by the fecal-oral route, and the virus is shed in the feces. For example, a common mode of transmission of the virus is through eating uncooked shellfish harvested from sewage-contaminated water. Transmission via blood (similar to HBV transmission) is rare.

● **Hepatitis A ("infectious hepatitis")**

HAV infections are most commonly seen among children, especially those living in crowded accomodations such as summer camps. The main site of replication is the hepatocyte, where infection results in severe cytopathology, and liver function is severely impaired. The prognosis for patients with HAV is generally very favorable, and development of persistent infection and chronic hepatitis is uncommon.

● **Treatment:** Immune globulin is used as postexposure prophylaxis. No antiviral agents are currently available for treating HAV infections.

● **Prevention:** Vaccines prepared from whole virus inactivated with formaldehyde are now available. Immune globulin has been used for many years, mainly as postexposure prophylaxis. Prevention of HAV infection requires taking measures to avoid fecal contamination of food and water.

● HAV grows poorly in tissue culture.

● Evidence of infection can be gained by the demonstration of a rise in antibody titer.

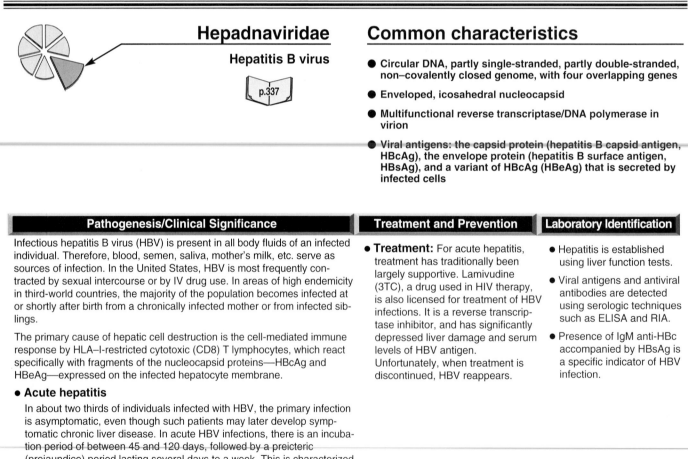

Hepadnaviridae

Hepatitis B virus

p.337

Common characteristics

● Circular DNA, partly single-stranded, partly double-stranded, non–covalently closed genome, with four overlapping genes

● Enveloped, icosahedral nucleocapsid

● Multifunctional reverse transcriptase/DNA polymerase in virion

● Viral antigens: the capsid protein (hepatitis B capsid antigen, HBcAg), the envelope protein (hepatitis B surface antigen, HBsAg), and a variant of HBcAg (HBeAg) that is secreted by infected cells

Pathogenesis/Clinical Significance	Treatment and Prevention	Laboratory Identification

Infectious hepatitis B virus (HBV) is present in all body fluids of an infected individual. Therefore, blood, semen, saliva, mother's milk, etc. serve as sources of infection. In the United States, HBV is most frequently contracted by sexual intercourse or by IV drug use. In areas of high endemicity in third-world countries, the majority of the population becomes infected at or shortly after birth from a chronically infected mother or from infected siblings.

The primary cause of hepatic cell destruction is the cell-mediated immune response by HLA–I-restricted cytotoxic (CD8) T lymphocytes, which react specifically with fragments of the nucleocapsid proteins—HBcAg and HBeAg—expressed on the infected hepatocyte membrane.

● **Acute hepatitis**

In about two thirds of individuals infected with HBV, the primary infection is asymptomatic, even though such patients may later develop symptomatic chronic liver disease. In acute HBV infections, there is an incubation period of between 45 and 120 days, followed by a preicteric (prejaundice) period lasting several days to a week. This is characterized by mild fever, malaise, anorexia, myalgia, and nausea. The acute, icteric

● **Treatment:** For acute hepatitis, treatment has traditionally been largely supportive. Lamivudine (3TC), a drug used in HIV therapy, is also licensed for treatment of HBV infections. It is a reverse transcriptase inhibitor, and has significantly depressed liver damage and serum levels of HBV antigen. Unfortunately, when treatment is discontinued, HBV reappears.

● Hepatitis is established using liver function tests.

● Viral antigens and antiviral antibodies are detected using serologic techniques such as ELISA and RIA.

● Presence of IgM anti-HBc accompanied by HBsAg is a specific indicator of HBV infection.

[HEPATITIS B IS CONTINUED ON THE NEXT PAGE]

Hepatitis B virus (cont.)

Pathogenesis/Clinical Significance	Treatment and Prevention	Laboratory Identification

phase then follows, and lasts for one to two months. It is during this phase that dark urine, due to bilirubinuria and jaundice, are evident. There usually is also an enlarged and tender liver. During the acute phase, large quantities of viral antigens, nucleic acids, and antiviral antibodies appear in the blood. In eighty to ninety percent of adults, a convalescent period of several more months is followed by complete recovery. Following resolution of the acute disease (or asymptomatic infection), about two to ten percent of adults, and over eighty percent of infants, remain chronically infected.

● **Fulminant hepatitis**

In one to two percent of acute symptomatic cases, much more extensive necrosis of the liver occurs during the initial acute illness. This is accompanied by high fever, abdominal pain, and eventual renal dysfunction, coma, seizures, and, in about eight percent of cases, death.

● **Primary hepatocellular carcinomas (HCC; hepatomas)**

HCC is one of the major causes of death due to malignancy worldwide. Approximately eighty percent of HCCs occur in chronically HBV-infected individuals. However, the mechanisms relating HBV infection and HCC are not understood. Clinically, a patient with HCC exhibits weight loss, right upper-quandrant pain, fever, and intestinal bleeding.

● **Prevention:** A vaccine is available that is constructed against the HBsAg. It is recommended as one of the routine infant immunizations, and also for adults in health care professions, or with life-styles that present a high risk of infection. Hepatitis B immunoglobulin is prepared from the blood of donors having a high titer of anti-HBs antibody. It provides passive immunization for individuals accidentally exposed to HBV, and for infants born to women who are HBV-positive.

Flaviviridae

Hepatitis C viruses

p.356

Common characteristics

● **Positive-strand, single-stranded, nonsegmented RNA genome**
● **Enveloped, icosahedral nucleocapsid**
● **Genomic RNAs serve as messenger RNAs and are infectious**
● **Virions do not contain any enzymes**

Pathogenesis/Clinical Significance	Treatment and Prevention	Laboratory Identification

Hepatitis C viruses (HCV) have in the past been the primary cause of non-A, non-B, transfusion-associated hepatitis. Tests to screen blood for HCV have been available for several years, so that HCV as a cause of transfusion-associated hepatitis is now unusual. This group of viruses is quite heterogeneous, and can be divided into several types. Transmission is via blood—through transfusion, intravenous drug use, and renal dialysis treatment. In addition, there is evidence of sexual transmission, as well as transmission from mother to child.

● **Hepatitis C**

HCV replication occurs in the hepatocyte, and probably also in mononuclear cells (lymphocytes and macrophages). Destruction of liver cells may result both from a direct effect of viral replication, and from the host immune response. The majority of infections with HCV are subclinical, but about 25 percent of infected individuals present with acute hepatitis including jaundice. More important, a significant proportion of infections progress to a chronic hepatitis and cirrhosis. Some of these individuals go on to develop hepatocellular carcinoma many years after the primary infection. Concomitant chronic infection with HBV results in more severe disease.

● **Treatment:** Treatment of patients with chronic hepatitis with α-interferon is sometimes of benefit, but in most cases, only for the period during which the patient is receiving the interferon. Chronic hepatitis caused by HCV that results in severe liver damage may be an indication for a liver transplant.

● **Prevention:** No vaccine or preventive drug is available at this time.

● A specific diagnosis can be made by demonstration of antibodies that react with a combination of recombinant viral proteins.

● Sensitive tests are also now available for detection of viral RNA, for example, by polymerase chain reaction (PCR) amplification of reverse-transcribed HCV cDNA.

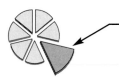

Herpesviridae

Epstein-Barr virus (p.425)
Herpes simplex virus, Type 1
Herpes simplex virus, Type 2
Human cytomegalovirus
Human herpesvirus, Type 8
Varicella-zoster virus (p.436)

Common characteristics

● **Enveloped DNA viruses**

● **Linear, double-stranded DNA genome**

● **Herpesviruses replicate in the nucleus**

● **Envelope contains antigenic, species-specific glycoproteins**

● **In the tegument between the envelope and capsid are a number of virus-coded enzymes and transcription factors essential for initiation of the infectious cycle**

● **All herpesviruses can enter a latent state following primary infection, to be reactivated at a later time**

Herpes simplex virus, type 1   p.319

Pathogenesis/Clinical Significance	Treatment and Prevention	Laboratory Identification

Herpes simplex virus type 1 (HSV-1) has a relatively rapid, cytocidal growth cycle. HSV-1 establishes latency in trigeminal ganglia after oropharyngeal infection. Transmission of HSV-1 is by direct contact with virus-containing secretions (usually saliva), or with lesions on mucosal surfaces.

● **Primary HSV-1 infections**

The virus multiplies in the nuclei of epithelial cells on the mucosal surface onto which it has been inoculated—most frequently, that of the oropharyngeal region. Vesicles or shallow ulcers containing infectious HSV-1 are produced, primarily in the oropharynx. These cause sore throat, fever, gingivitis, and anorexia. The most common symptomatic HSV-1 infections of the upper body are **gingivostomatitis** in young children, and **tonsillitis** and **pharyngitis** in adults. Infection of the eye by HSV-1 can cause severe **keratoconjuctivitis**. [Note: HSV-1 infections of the eye are the second most common cause of corneal blindness in the United States (after trauma).] If HSV-1 infection spreads to the CNS, frequently fatal **encephalitis** can occur. In immunocompetent individuals, HSV-1 infection remains localized due to cytotoxic T cells that recognize HSV-specific antigens on the surface of infected cells, and kills them before progeny virus has been produced.

● **Latent HSV-1 infections**

A life-long latent infection is usually established in the trigeminal ganglia as a result of entry of infectious virions into sensory neurons that end at the site of infection. Recurrent HSV-1 infections may be asymptomatic, but result in viral shedding in secretions. If symptoms occur, they usually include **herpes labialis** (formation of "**cold sores**" or "**fever blisters**") around the lips.

● **Treatment:** Herpesviruses encode considerably more enzymatic activities and regulatory functions than do viruses with smaller genomic size. A number of these activities duplicate the functions of cell enzymes, but because they are virus-specific, they provide excellent targets for anti-viral agents that are relatively non-toxic for the cell. Acycloguanosine (acyclovir) is selectively effective against HSV because it becomes an active inhibitor only after initially being phosphorylated by the HSV-coded thymidine kinase. The drug cannot cure a latent infection, but can minimize or prevent recurrences. Other inhibitors active against HSV DNA synthesis include famciclovir, foscarnet, and topically applied penciclovir.

● **Prevention:** No vaccine or preventive drug is available.

● Cell tissue culture inoculated with a sample of vesicle scraping, fluid, or genital swab shows gross cytopathic changes in several days; individual infected cells can be detected within 24 hours by use of immunofluorescence or immunoperoxidase staining with antibodies against viral early proteins.

● Viral DNA (amplified by PCR) can be detected in clinical samples, including CSF in patients with HSV encephalitis.

Herpes simplex virus, type 2   p.319

Pathogenesis/Clinical Significance	Treatment and Prevention	Laboratory Identification

Herpes simplex virus, type 2 (HSV-2) has a relatively rapid, cytocidal growth cycle. HSV-2 establishes latency in sacral or lumbar ganglia. Transmission of HSV-2 generally occurs by sexual contact, or by infection of a newborn during birth.

● **Primary HSV-2 infections**

Primary genital tract lesions are similar to those of the oropharynx caused by HSV-1, but the majority of these infections are asymptomatic. When symptomatic, local symptoms such as pain and itching, and systemic symptoms of fever, malaise, and myalgias may be more severe than those that accompany primary oral cavity infections.

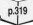

● **Treatment:** Acycloguanosine (acyclovir) is selectively effective against HSV because it becomes an active inhibitor only after initially being phosphorylated by the HSV-coded thymidine kinase. The drug cannot cure a latent infection, but can minimize or prevent recurrences. Other inhibitors active against HSV DNA synthesis include famciclovir, foscarnet, cidofovir, and topically applied penciclovir.

● Cell tissue culture inoculated with a sample of vesicle scraping, fluid, or genital swab shows gross cytopathic changes in several days; individual infected cells can be detected within 24 hours by use of immunofluorescence or immunoperoxidase staining with antibodies against viral early proteins.

[HERPES SIMPLEX VIRUS, TYPE 2 IS CONTINUED ON THE NEXT PAGE]

Herpes simplex virus, type 2 (cont.)

Pathogenesis/Clinical Significance	Treatment and Prevention	Laboratory Identification

• Primary HSV-2 infections (cont.)

Vesiculoulcerative lesions on the female's vulva, cervix, and vagina or the male's penis can be very painful. Neonatal herpes is contracted by the baby during birth. If untreated, a disseminated infection results, often involving the CNS, leading to a high mortality rate. [Note: Infection in utero appears to occur only rarely.]

• Latent HSV-2 infections

HSV-2 remains latent in the sacral ganglia. Reactivation of HSV-2 genital infection occurs frequently, and may be asymptomatic. However, the infected individual sheds virus during the reactivation period regardless of symptoms, and can transmit the virus to a sexual partner during that period.

• **Prevention:** No vaccine or preventive drug is available. Prevention of HSV transmission is enhanced by avoidance of contact with potential virus-shedding lesions and by safe sexual practices. Neonatal HSV can be prevented by delivery via cesarean section.

• Viral DNA (amplified by PCR) can be detected in clinical samples, including CSF in patients with HSV encephalitis.

Human cytomegalovirus p.326

Pathogenesis/Clinical Significance	Treatment and Prevention	Laboratory Identification

Human cytomegalovirus (HCMV) is transmitted by infected individuals through their tears, urine, saliva, semen or vaginal secretions, and breast milk. HCMV can also cross the placenta.

HCMV replicates initially in epithelial cells of the respiratory and GI tracts, followed by viremia and infection of all organs of the body. In symptomatic cases, kidney tubule epithelium, liver, and CNS, in addition to the respiratory and GI tracts, are most commonly affected. HCMV has a relatively slow replication cycle, with the formation of characteristic multinucleated giant cells, thus the name "cytomegalo-". Latency is established in nonneural tissues, primarily lymphoreticular cells, and glandular tissues.

• HCMV infectious mononucleosis

Whereas most HCMV infections occur in childhood, primary infection as an adult may result in a mononucleosis syndrome that is clinically identical to that caused by Epstein-Barr virus. It is estimated that about eight percent of infectious mononucleosis (IM) cases are due to HCMV. The major distinguishing feature of HCMV IM is the absence of the heterophile antibodies that characterize IM caused by EBV.

• Cytomegalic inclusion disease

HCMV is the most common intrauterine virus infection. Of infants born to women experiencing their first HCMV infection during pregnancy, 35 to 50 percent will become infected, of which 10 percent will be symptomatic. The severity of the latter, referred to as cytomegalic inclusion disease, ranges from fetal death to various degrees of damage to liver, spleen, blood-forming organs, and components of the nervous system (a common cause of hearing loss and mental retardation).

• HCMV infection of immunosuppressed transplant recipients

Such individuals are multiply at risk from 1) HCMV present in the tissue being transplanted, 2) virus carried in leukocytes in the associated blood transfusions, and 3) reactivation of endogenous latent virus. The resulting infection can cause destruction of GI tract tissues, hepatitis, and pneumonia, the latter being a major cause of death in bone marrow transplant recipients.

• HCMV infection of AIDS patients

Invasive opportunistic HCMV infections are common in AIDS patients. These become increasingly important as CD4+ lymphocyte counts and immune competence decline. Any organ systems can be affected, but pneumonia, and blindness due to HCMV retinitis, are especially common. Encephalitis and dementia, esophagitis, enterocolitis, and gastritis are other significant problems.

• **Treatment:** Treatment of HCMV infections is indicated primarily in immunocompromised patients. Acyclovir is ineffective because HCMV lacks a thymidine kinase. Ganciclovir is used for invasive infections of transplant recipients and AIDS patients. Cidofovir is used for ganciclovir-resistant mutants. Foscarnet can be used in combination with ganciclovir, or as an alternate treatment when resistant mutants appear.

• **Prevention:** No vaccine or preventive drug is available.

• Serologic diagnosis using ELISA techniques can distinguish primary from recurrent infection, by demonstrating either IgG seroconversion, or the presence of HCMV-specific IgM.

• Determination of the presence and amount of viral DNA or proteins in white blood cells is used to evaluate invasive disease.

• Presence of extracellular virus in urine or saliva may simply be due to an asymptomatic recurrence.

Human herpesvirus, type 8 p.334

Pathogenesis/Clinical Significance

Genome analysis of a virus recovered from cells of Kaposi's sarcoma revealed it to be a member of the human herpes family, human herpesvirus type 8 (HHV-8), also called Kaposi's sarcoma-associated herpes virus (KSHV). In contrast to the other human herpesviruses, HHV-8 infection appears to be relatively infrequent in the normal, healthy population.

• Kaposi's sarcoma

The virus has been detected in over ninety percent of patients with Kaposi's sarcoma, and in several other types of vascular tumors and lymphomas found in AIDS patients. Antibodies to HHV-8 antigens are found primarily in the populations that are at risk for HIV infection, suggesting that at least one route for transmission is exchange of body fluids.

Treatment and Prevention

● **Treatment:** Various drugs are currently being evaluated for use against HHV-8/Kaposi's sarcoma.

● **Prevention:** No vaccine or preventive drug is available.

Laboratory Identification

● DNA hybridization following PCR amplification of viral DNA isolated from clinical samples can be used to provide a definitive diagnosis.

● Antibody status of the infected individual can be determined serologically.

Retroviridae

Human Immunodeficiency Virus

p.359

Common characteristics

● **Single-stranded, positive sense, linear RNA—two copies per virion (diploid)**

● **Viral envelope contains glycoprotein that undergoes antigenic variation**

● **Virion contains reverse transcriptase**

Pathogenesis/Clinical Significance

Human immunodeficiency virus (HIV) is a nononcogenic retrovirus. Transmission occurs mainly by one of three routes: 1) sexually (it is present in both semen and vaginal secretions); 2) with blood or blood products (whole blood, plasma, clotting factors, and cellular fractions of blood by transfusion, or by inoculation with HIV-contaminated needles); and 3) perinatally (either transplacentally, during passage through the birth canal, or in breast feeding).

The specific HIV cell surface receptor is the CD4 molecule, located primarily on helper T cells. HIV enters the cell by fusion of the virus envelope with the plasma membrane. Reverse transcription takes place in the cytoplasm, with the viral RNA-dependent reverse transcriptase first synthesizing a DNA-RNA hybrid molecule, then degrading the parental RNA while replacing it with a second strand of DNA. The resulting linear molecule of double-stranded DNA is the provirus. It is transported to the nucleus and is randomly inserted into the host chromosome by viral enzymes. The integrated DNA is translated into viral mRNAs that code for viral proteins, and also will be packaged into progeny virus. Assembled virions bud through the plasma membrane. Production of virus is a continuous process, eventually killing the host cell.

• Human immunodeficiency virus infection

Several weeks after the initial infection, one third to two thirds of individuals experience symptoms similar to those of infectious mononucleosis, during which there is a very high level of virus replication in CD4+ cells. Lymph nodes become infected, which are the sites of virus persistence during the asymptomatic period. The acute phase viremia resolves into a clinically asymptomatic or "latent" period lasting from months to many years. This period is characterized by persistent generalized lymphadenopathy, diarrhea, and weight loss.

Treatment and Prevention

● **Treatment:** Inhibitors of viral reverse transcriptase include both nucleoside and non-nucleoside reverse transcriptase inhibitors. They prevent the establishment of HIV infection. Inhibitors of the viral protease delay the production of progeny virus. Administering combinations of these drugs delays the appearance of resistant mutants, therefore three or four drugs are given at the same time. This is referred to as "highly active antiretroviral therapy" or HAART.

● **Prevention:** No vaccine is available. Perinatal transmission can be reduced with zidovudine (AZT) therapy of the pregnant woman, followed by several weeks of AZT to the newborn. Prevention can be achieved by screening blood and tissues prior to transfusion or transplant, using condoms during sexual intercourse, and strict adherence to the universal precautions by health care workers

Laboratory Identification

● Amplification of viral RNA or DNA proviruses by the PCR technique is the most sensitive method for detection of virus in blood or tissue specimens.

● For purposes of screening the blood supply, ELISA testing for the p24 (CA) antigen in serum can detect infection about a week earlier than tests for antibody.

● For screening individuals, the ELISA procedure is also used to detect antibodies in serum; any positive results must be confirmed using the Western blot technique.

[HUMAN IMMUNODEFICIENCY VIRUS IS CONTINUED ON THE NEXT PAGE]

Human immunodeficiency virus (cont.)

Pathogenesis/Clinical Significance	Treatment and Prevention	Laboratory Identification

● **Acquired immunodeficiency syndrome (AIDS):**

The progression from asymptomatic infection to AIDS occurs as a continuum of progressive clinical states. The number of infected CD4+ cells decreases, and T cell precursors in the lymphoid organs are infected and killled, so the capacity to generate new CD4+ cells is gradually lost. Cells of the monocyte/macrophage lineage are also infected, and transport the virus into other organs, including the brain. When the CD4+ count falls below 200/μl, and increasingly frequent and serious opportunistic infections appear, the syndrome is defined as AIDS.

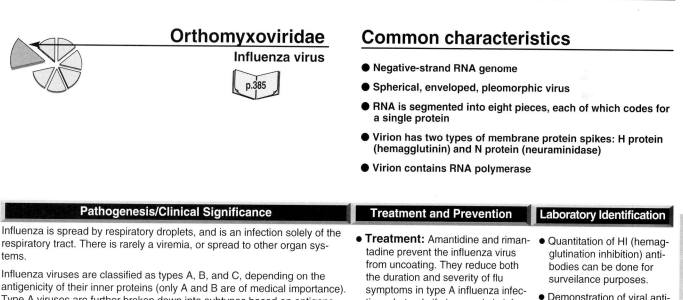

Orthomyxoviridae

Influenza virus

p.385

Common characteristics

● **Negative-strand RNA genome**

● **Spherical, enveloped, pleomorphic virus**

● **RNA is segmented into eight pieces, each of which codes for a single protein**

● **Virion has two types of membrane protein spikes: H protein (hemagglutinin) and N protein (neuraminidase)**

● **Virion contains RNA polymerase**

Pathogenesis/Clinical Significance	Treatment and Prevention	Laboratory Identification

Influenza is spread by respiratory droplets, and is an infection solely of the respiratory tract. There is rarely a viremia, or spread to other organ systems.

Influenza viruses are classified as types A, B, and C, depending on the antigenicity of their inner proteins (only A and B are of medical importance). Type A viruses are further broken down into subtypes based on antigens associated with the outer viral proteins, H and N. Influenza viruses have shown marked variation over the years in their antigenic properties, specifically of the H and N proteins. This variation is due primarily to antigenic shift.

● **Influenza (the "flu")**

Following inhalation of influenza virus particles, respiratory epithelial cells are destroyed by the host immune response, specifically, cytotoxic T cells. Typically, influenza has an acute onset characterized by chills, followed by a high fever, muscle aches, and extreme drowsiness. The disease runs its course in four to five days, after which there is a gradual recovery. The most serious problems, such as pneumonia, occur in the very young, the elderly, and people with chronic cardiac or pulmonary disease, or who are immunodeficient.

● **Reye's syndrome**

This is a rare and serious complication of viral infections in children, especially in those who have had chicken pox or influenza. Aspirin used to lower the virus-induced fever may contribute to the appearance of this syndrome. Therefore, acetaminophen is usually recommended for fevers of unknown origin in children.

● **Treatment:** Amantidine and rimantadine prevent the influenza virus from uncoating. They reduce both the duration and severity of flu symptoms in type A influenza infections, but only if given early in infection. Influenza viruses readily develop resistance to these compounds. Zanamivir and oseltamivir are newer drugs that inhibit viral neuraminidase—an enzyme required for release of virus from infected cells.

● **Prevention:** A vaccine consisting of formalin-inactivated influenza virus is available. It is of critical importance that the vaccine contain the specific subtypes of influenza virus present in the population that year. Given before the onset of symptoms, amantidine and rimantidine can also prevent disease, and are useful for treating high-risk groups.

● Quantitation of HI (hemagglutination inhibition) antibodies can be done for surveillance purposes.

● Demonstration of viral antigens in respiratory tract secretions is a more rapid method for diagnosis of influenza infection.

Paramyxoviridae

Measles virus

Mumps virus

Parainfluenza virus (p.433)

Respiratory syncytial virus (p.435)

Common characteristics

● **Nonsegmented, negative-strand RNA**

● **Spherical, enveloped viruses**

● **Some contain RNA polymerase in their virions**

● **Envelope contains F (for fusion) protein that allows virus to enter cells via a fusion process, rather than by receptor-mediated endocytosis**

Measles virus   p.382

Pathogenesis/Clinical Significance	Treatment and Prevention	Laboratory Identification
Measles virus is transmitted by sneeze- or cough-produced respiratory droplets. The virus is extremely infectious, and almost all infected individuals develop a clinical illness. ● **Measles** Measles virus replicates initially in the respiratory epithelium, and then in various lymphoid organs. Classic measles begins with a prodromal period of fever, upper respiratory tract symptoms, and conjunctivitis. Two to three days later, Koplik spots develop in the mouth and throat, and a generalized macular rash appears, beginning at the head and traveling slowly to the lower extremities. Soon after the rash appears, the patient is no longer infectious. A rare complication occurring within two weeks after the onset of the rash is **postinfectious encephalomyelitis** —an autoimmune disease. Children are particularly susceptible, especially those weakened by other diseases or hunger.	● **Treatment:** No antiviral drugs are available for measles. ● **Prevention:** A live, attenuated measles vaccine is available; it is usually administered in the form of the measles-mumps-rubella (MMR) vaccine.	● Demonstration of an increase in the titer of antiviral antibodies can be used in the diagnosis of measles.

Mumps virus   p.382

Pathogenesis/Clinical Significance	Treatment and Prevention	Laboratory Identification
Mumps virus is spread by respiratory droplets. ● **Mumps** Although about one third of infections are subclinical, the classic clinical presentation and diagnosis center on infection and swelling of the salivary glands, primarily the parotid glands. However, mumps virus can enter the bloodstream, causing widespread infection. This may involve not only salivary glands, but also the pancreas, CNS, and testes. Male sterility occasionally occurs, due to bilateral infection of the testes (orchitis).	● **Treatment:** No antiviral drugs are available for mumps. ● **Prevention:** A live, attenuated vaccine is available; it is usually administered in the form of the measles-mumps-rubella (MMR) vaccine.	● Virus may be recoverable from saliva, blood, CSF, or urine, and can be cultured. ● Serologic tests detect antiviral antibody in the blood.

Papovaviridae

Papillomavirus

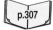
p.307

Common characteristics

- Double-stranded, circular DNA
- Nonenveloped, icosahedral
- Over seventy types of human papilloma viruses currently recognized

Pathogenesis/Clinical Significance

Transmission of human papillomavirus (HPV) infection requires direct contact with infected individuals or contaminated surfaces. All human papillomaviruses induce **hyperplastic epithelial lesions**; they infect either cutaneous (keratinizing) or mucosal (squamous) epithelium. The HPVs within each of these tissue-specific groups have varying potentials to cause malignancies. There are: 1) a small number of virus types that produce lesions having a high risk of progression to malignancy, such as in the case of **cervical carcinoma**; 2) other virus types produce mucosal lesions that progress to malignancy with lower frequency, causing, for example, **anogenital warts** (**condyloma acuminatum**, a common sexually transmitted disease) and **laryngeal papillomas** (the most common benign epithelial tumors of the larynx); 3) in those individuals with a genetic predisposition for the inability to control the spread of warts, some virus types cause multiple cutaneous warts that do not regress, but spread to many body sites (**epidermodysplasia verruciformis**)—these lesions give rise with high frequency to **squamous cell carcinomas** several years after initial appearance of the original warts; and 4) still other virus types that are associated only with benign lesions, for example, **common**, **flat**, and **plantar warts**.

Treatment and Prevention

- **Treatment:** Cutaneous warts generally require surgical removal or destruction of the wart tissue with liquid nitrogen, laser vaporization, or cytotoxic chemicals. Interferon, given orally, is effective in causing regression of laryngeal papillomas. When injected directly into genital warts, interferon is effective in about half of the patients. Cidofovir is also effective as a topical application.

- **Prevention:** The primary means of prevention is avoidance of contact with wart tissue. In the case of genital tract warts, procedures for prevention of sexually transmitted diseases should be employed, but are not always effective.

Laboratory Identification

- Diagnosis of cutaneous warts generally involves no more than visual inspection.

- Typing of human papillomavirus is done either by immunoassays for viral antigens, or by DNA hybridization.

- Human papillomavirus cannot be cultured in the laboratory.

Paramyxoviridae

Measles virus (p.432)
Mumps virus (p.432)
Parainfluenza virus
Respiratory syncytial virus (p.435)

Common characteristics

- Nonsegmented, negative-strand RNA
- Spherical, enveloped viruses
- Some contain RNA polymerase in their virions
- Envelope contains F (fusion) protein that allows virus to enter cells via a fusion process, rather than by receptor-mediated endocytosis

Parainfluenza virus p.382

Pathogenesis/Clinical Significance

There are four clinically important human parainfluenza viruses (hPIV), designated hPIV types 1 to 4. They are called "parainfluenza" because individuals may present with influenza-like symptoms, and like influenza, have both hemagglutinating and neuraminidase activity. (Unlike influenza, these activities are not subject to antigenic shift.)

Infection by these viruses is spread by respiratory droplets, and is confined to the respiratory tract.

- **Respiratory tract infections**

  Parainfluenza viruses cause **croup**, **pneumonia**, and **bronchiolitis**, mainly in infants and children. They are also a cause of the "**common cold**" in individuals of all ages.

Treatment and Prevention

- **Treatment:** No antiviral drugs are recommended for these infections. Symptoms can be treated as necessary.

- **Prevention:** No vaccine or preventive drug is available.

Laboratory Identification

- Serologic tests for antibody to the virus can aid in the diagnosis of parainfluenza virus infection.

Picornaviridae
Coxsackievirus (p.425)
Hepatitis A virus (p.426)
Poliovirus

Common characteristics

- Positive-strand, single-stranded, nonsegmented RNA genome
- Non-enveloped, icosahedral
- Genomic RNAs serve as messenger RNAs and are infectious
- Virions do not contain any enzymes

Poliovirus   p.349

Pathogenesis/Clinical Significance	Treatment and Prevention	Laboratory Identification

Poliovirus is a member of the genus Enterovirus. Individuals are infected with poliovirus by ingestion of contaminated food or water. Enteroviruses are stable in the low pH of the stomach, replicate in the GI tract, and are excreted in the stool (fecal-oral route). After replicating in the oropharynx and intestinal tract lymphoid tissue, poliovirus can enter the bloodstream and spread to the central nervous system.

- **Poliomyelitis**

  The great majority of poliovirus infections are asymptomatic. The classic presentation in those poliovirus-infected individuals who become ill is that of **flaccid paralysis**, most often affecting the lower limbs. This is due to viral replication in, and destruction of, the lower motor neurons in the anterior horn of the spinal cord. **Respiratory paralysis** may also occur, following infection of the brain stem.

- **Treatment:** No antiviral agents are currently available for treating poliovirus infections.
- **Prevention:** A killed poliovirus vaccine (Salk) that is injected, and a live, attenuated poliovirus vaccine (Sabin) that is given orally are available, and have led to the elimination of wild-type polio from Western Europe, Japan, and the Americas. The few cases that occur in the United States are either brought from other countries, or are caused by vaccine strains of virus that have reverted to a virulent form.

- Poliovirus can be isolated and cultured from the stool or cerebral spinal fluid.
- Evidence of infection can also be obtained by demonstration of a rise in antibody titer.

Rhabdoviridae
Rabies virus   p.379

Common characteristics

- Negative-strand, single-stranded, non-segmented RNA genome
- Enveloped, helical nucleocapsid
- Virus is bullet-shaped
- Virion contains RNA-dependent RNA polymerase

Pathogenesis/Clinical Significance	Treatment and Prevention	Laboratory Identification

Rabies virus is a member of the genus Lyssavirus. A wide variety of wildlife, such as raccoons, skunks, squirrels, foxes, and bats, provide a reservoir for the virus. In developing countries, domestic dogs and cats also constitute an important reservoir for rabies. Humans are usually infected by the bite of an animal, but in some cases, infection is via an aerosol, for example, of droppings from infected bats.

- **Rabies**

  Following inoculation, the virus may replicate locally, but then travels via the axoplasm of peripheral neurons to the brain, where it replicates primarily in the gray matter. From the brain, the rabies virus can travel along autonomic nerves, leading to infection of the lungs, kidney, adrenal medulla, and salivary glands. The incubation period is extremely variable, but generally lasts one to eight weeks. Symptoms of the infection include hallucinations, seizures, weakness, mental dysfunction, paralysis, coma, and finally death from a fatal encephalitis with neuronal degeneration of the brain and spinal cord. Once symptoms begin, death is inevitable. Many, but not all, patients show the classic rabid sign of hydrophobia—a painful inability to swallow liquids, leading to avoidance.

- **Treatment:** Once an individual has clinical symptoms of rabies there is no effective treatment.
- **Prevention:** Preexposure prophylaxis, which is indicated for individuals at high risk (for example, veterinarians) consists of administration of a killed virus vaccine. In the United States, this is generally the human diploid cell vaccine (HDCV). Postexposure prophylaxis is instituted after an animal bite or exposure to an animal suspected of being rabid. It consists of both passive immunization with antirabies immunoglobulin and active immunization with HDCV.

- Diagnosis rests on a history of exposure and signs and symptoms characteristic of rabies. However, a reliable history of exposure is often not obtainable, and the initial clinical presentation may vary. Therefore, a clinical diagnosis may be difficult.
- Postmortem, characteristic cytoplasmic inclusions (Negri bodies) may be seen in regions of the brain such as the hippocampus.

Paramyxoviridae

Measles virus (p.432)
Mumps virus (p.432)
Parainfluenza virus (p.433)
Respiratory syncytial virus

Common characteristics

● Nonsegmented, negative-strand RNA

● Spherical, enveloped viruses

● Some contain RNA polymerase in their virions

● Envelope contains F (for fusion) protein that allows virus to enter cells via a fusion process, rather than by receptor-mediated endocytosis

Respiratory syncytial virus

p.382

Pathogenesis/Clinical Significance

Respiratory syncytial virus (RSV) is transmitted by respiratory droplets, or by contaminated hands carrying the virus to the nose or mouth. Repeated infections are common.

● **Respiratory tract infections**

RSV is the major viral respiratory tract pathogen in the pediatric population, and the most important cause of **bronchiolitis** in infants. It may also cause **pneumonia** in young children, an **influenza-like syndrome** in adults, and **severe bronchitis with pneumonia** in the elderly. RSV does not spread systemically.

Treatment and Prevention

● **Treatment:** The only specific treatment for RSV infection is ribavirin, administered by aerosol, and this is only of moderate benefit.

● **Prevention:** No vaccine or preventive drug is available. Spread of infection between people can be controlled by hand washing and avoiding others with the infection.

Laboratory Identification

● Demonstration of an increase in the titer of antiviral antibodies or demonstration of viral antigens in respiratory secretions can provide a definitive diagnosis of RSV infection.

Togaviridae

Rubella virus

p.354

Common characteristics

● Positive-strand, single-stranded, nonsegmented RNA genome

● Enveloped, icosahedral nucleocapsid

● Genomic RNAs serve as messenger RNAs and are infectious

● Virions do not contain any enzymes

Pathogenesis/Clinical Significance

Rubella virus is a member of the genus rubivirus. The virus is transmitted via respiratory secretions from an infected individual.

● **German measles**

This is a very mild clinical syndrome (not to be confused with rubeola, caused by the measles virus). The infection is characterized by a generalized maculopapular rash, and occipital lymphadenopathy. In most cases, these symptoms may be hardly noticeable, and the infection remains subclinical.

● **Congenital rubella**

The major clinical significance of rubella is that when a pregnant woman is infected with the virus, there can be significant damage to the developing fetus, especially in the first trimester. This damage can include congenital heart disease, cataracts, hepatitis, or abnormalities related to the CNS, such as mental retardation, motor dysfunction, and deafness.

Treatment and Prevention

● **Treatment:** No antiviral drugs are presently in use.

● **Prevention:** Fetal damage due to rubella infection is preventable by use of the live, attenuated rubella vaccine that is included with the routine childhood vaccinations. This vaccine is effective, has few complications, and ensures that when women reach childbearing age, they are immune to rubella infection. The vaccine should not be given to women who are already pregnant or to immunocompromised patients, including very young babies.

Laboratory Identification

● A diagnosis of rubella infection can be made by measuring a rise in antibody titer.

● Pregnant women with anti-rubella IgM antibody are presumed to have been recently exposed to the virus.

Herpesvirideae

Epstein-Barr virus (p.425)
Herpes simplex virus, Type 1 (p.428)
Herpes simplex virus, Type 2 (p.428)
Human cytomegalovirus (p.429)
Human herpesvirus, Type 8 (p.430)
Varicella-zoster virus

Common characteristics

- Enveloped DNA viruses
- Linear, double-stranded DNA genome
- Herpesviruses replicate in the nucleus
- Envelope contains antigenic, species-specific glycoproteins
- In the tegument between the envelope and capsid are a number of virus-coded enzymes and transcription factors essential for initiation of the infectious cycle
- All herpesviruses can enter a latent state following primary infection, to be reactivated at a later time

Varicella-zoster virus p.324

Pathogenesis/Clinical Significance	Treatment and Prevention	Laboratory Identification

Pathogenesis/Clinical Significance

Varicella-zoster virus (VZV) has a relatively rapid, cytocidal growth cycle, and establishes latency in sensory nerve ganglia.

Transmission of VZV is usually via respiratory droplets, which results in initial infection of the respiratory mucosa, followed by spread to the regional lymph nodes. From there, progeny virus enters the bloodstream, undergoes a second round of multiplication in cells of the liver and spleen, and is disseminated throughout the body by infected mononuclear leukocytes.

• Varicella ("chickenpox")

Following infection of a normal, healthy child, the first symptoms include fever, malaise, headache, and abdominal pain. Next is appearance of the virus-containing vesicles ("pox") characteristic of the disease. These begin on the scalp, face, or trunk about 10 to 23 days after exposure, causing severe itching, and then proceed to the extremities and mucous membranes, such as the oropharynx, conjunctiva, and vagina. The infected individual is contagious from one to two days before appearance of the vesicles. Varicella is more serious in adults and immunocompromised patients, potentially causing pneumonia, fulminant hepatic failure, and varicella encephalitis. Fetal infection during pregnancy is uncommon, but can result in multiple developmental anomalies.

• Zoster ("shingles")

Due to the disseminated nature of the primary infection, latency is established in multiple sensory ganglia, the trigeminal and dorsal root ganglia being most common. On reactivation, there is substantial multiplication and horizontal spread of virus among the cells in the ganglion. Viral destruction of sensory ganglia leads to the pain associated with acute zoster. Debilitating postherpetic neuralgia and abnormal sensory phenomena may last as long as several months. The likelihood of reactivation increases with age and with depressed cellular immune competence.

Treatment and Prevention

- **Treatment for varicella:** Varicella in normal children does not require treatment. Treatment of primary varicella in immunocompromised patients, adults, and neonates is warranted by the severity of the disease. Acyclovir has been the drug of choice. Newer drugs—famciclovir and valacyclovir—have greater activity against VZV.

- **Treatment for zoster:** Oral acyclovir reduces the time course and acute pain of zoster, but has little or no effect on the subsequent postherpetic neuralgia. Famciclovir, given early in the acute phase of zoster, decreases acute pain and the time to resolution of lesions, and also shortens the duration of postherpetic pain.

- **Prevention:** A live, attenuated vaccine is recommended as one of the routine childhood vaccines. It is also indicated for nonimmune adults who are at risk of contagion. Varicella-zoster immune globulin can protect neonates and immunocompromised individuals who have been exposed to chickenpox or zoster lesion fluid.

Laboratory Identification

- Cell tissue culture inoculated with a sample of vesicle fluid shows gross cytopathic changes in several days; individual infected cells can be detected within 24 hours by use of immunofluorescence or immunoperoxidase staining with antibodies against viral early proteins.

- More rapid diagnosis can be made by reacting epithelial cells scraped from the base of vesicles with the stains described above, or doing in situ hybridization with VZV-specific DNA probes.

Clinical Bacteriology at a Glance

36

This chapter presents a brief summary of clinically important bacteria, using color to aid the reader in remembering their morphologies, classifications, clinical significance, and the therapies of choice. The classification of infectious organisms is again presented in a pie chart in which each segment represents a general class of microorganisms (Figure 36.1A). [Note: One section of the pie chart is labeled "Other", and represents any of several bacteria specifically covered in different chapters. The chapter(s) in which these organisms are discussed is/are shown in parentheses next to the type of organism.] In a similar way, the antimicrobial drug(s) that are generally used to treat microbial infections have been organized into a vertical bar chart (Figure 36.1B). In each summary section, the classification of the microorganism and the drug(s) of choice are highlighted. The order of the microorganisms in this chapter mirrors that of their sequence in Chapter 35, and is presented alphabetically in Figure 36.2.]

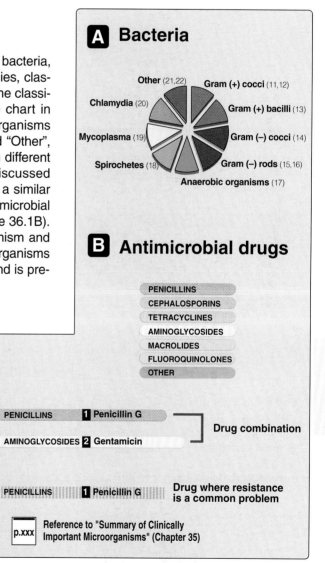

A Bacteria

Other (21,22)
Chlamydia (20)
Mycoplasma (19)
Spirochetes (18)
Gram (+) cocci (11,12)
Gram (+) bacilli (13)
Gram (–) cocci (14)
Gram (–) rods (15,16)
Anaerobic organisms (17)

B Antimicrobial drugs

PENICILLINS
CEPHALOSPORINS
TETRACYCLINES
AMINOGLYCOSIDES
MACROLIDES
FLUOROQUINOLONES
OTHER

C Key to symbols

DRUG FAMILIES	SPECIFIC DRUGS	
PENICILLINS	**1** Penicillin G	Drug of choice
PENICILLINS	**2** Penicillin G	Alternate drug
PENICILLINS	**1** Penicillin G	One of several first line drugs
PENICILLINS	**2** Penicillin G	One of several alternate drugs

p.xxx Reference to chapter in text where detailed information is presented

PENICILLINS **1** Penicillin G
AMINOGLYCOSIDES **2** Gentamicin
Drug combination

PENICILLINS **1** Penicillin G Drug where resistance is a common problem

p.xxx Reference to "Summary of Clinically Important Microorganisms" (Chapter 35)

Figure 36.1
A. Color-coded representation of medically important microorganisms. [Numbers refer to the chapter(s) where the organisms are discussed.] B. Color-coded representation of commonly used antimicrobial drugs.
C. Key to symbols used in this chapter.

Lippincott's Illustrated Reviews: Microbiology,
by William A. Strohl, Harriet Rouse, Bruce D. Fisher.
Lippincott, Williams & Wilkins, Baltimore, MD © 2001

BACTERIA

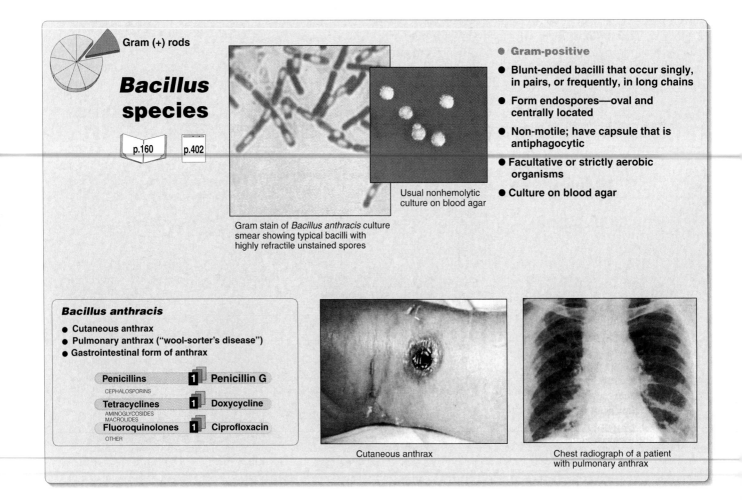

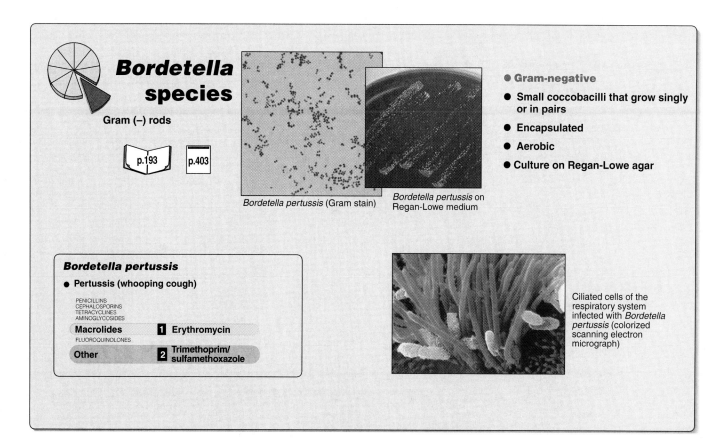

Bordetella species

Gram (–) rods

p.193 p.403

Bordetella pertussis (Gram stain)

Bordetella pertussis on Regan-Lowe medium

- Gram-negative
- Small coccobacilli that grow singly or in pairs
- Encapsulated
- Aerobic
- Culture on Regan-Lowe agar

Bordetella pertussis

- Pertussis (whooping cough)

PENICILLINS
CEPHALOSPORINS
TETRACYCLINES
AMINOGLYCOSIDES

Macrolides	**1** Erythromycin

FLUOROQUINOLONES

Other	**2** Trimethoprim/ sulfamethoxazole

Ciliated cells of the respiratory system infected with *Bordetella pertussis* (colorized scanning electron micrograph)

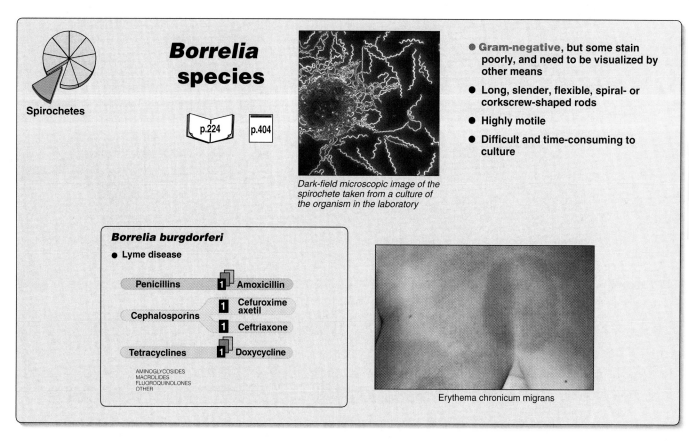

Borrelia species

Spirochetes

p.224 p.404

Dark-field microscopic image of the spirochete taken from a culture of the organism in the laboratory

- Gram-negative, but some stain poorly, and need to be visualized by other means
- Long, slender, flexible, spiral- or corkscrew-shaped rods
- Highly motile
- Difficult and time-consuming to culture

Borrelia burgdorferi

- Lyme disease

Penicillins	**1** Amoxicillin
Cephalosporins	**1** Cefuroxime axetil
	1 Ceftriaxone
Tetracyclines	**1** Doxycycline

AMINOGLYCOSIDES
MACROLIDES
FLUOROQUINOLONES
OTHER

Erythema chronicum migrans

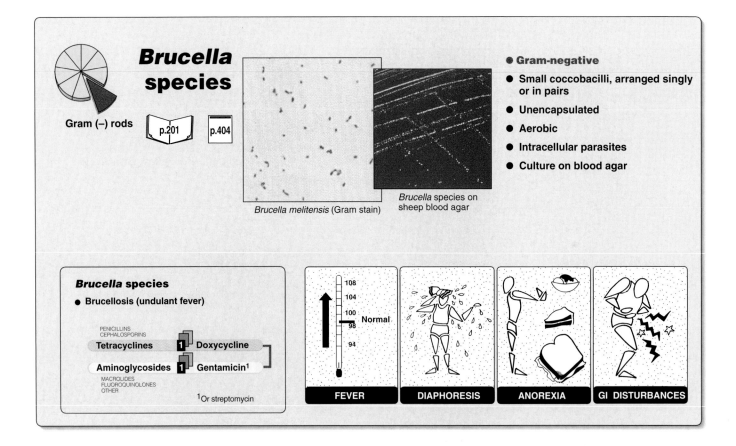

Brucella species

Gram (–) rods

p.201   p.404

Brucella melitensis (Gram stain)

Brucella species on sheep blood agar

- Gram-negative
- Small coccobacilli, arranged singly or in pairs
- Unencapsulated
- Aerobic
- Intracellular parasites
- Culture on blood agar

Brucella species

- Brucellosis (undulant fever)

PENICILLINS
CEPHALOSPORINS
Tetracyclines   **1** Doxycycline
Aminoglycosides **1** Gentamicin[1]
MACROLIDES
FLUOROQUINOLONES
OTHER
                 [1]Or streptomycin

FEVER   DIAPHORESIS   ANOREXIA   GI DISTURBANCES

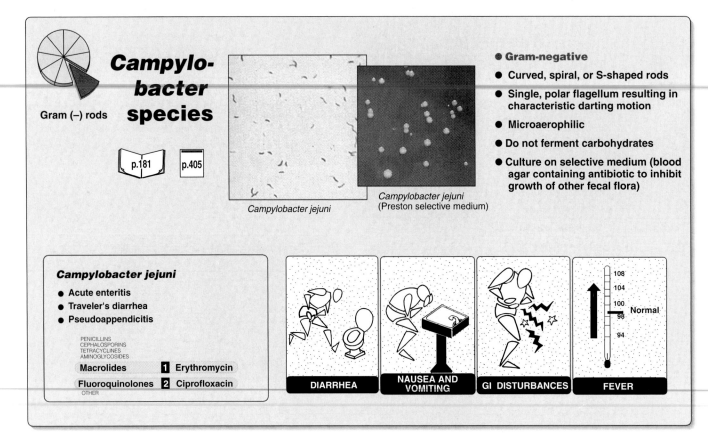

Campylo- bacter species

Gram (–) rods

p.181   p.405

Campylobacter jejuni

Campylobacter jejuni (Preston selective medium)

- Gram-negative
- Curved, spiral, or S-shaped rods
- Single, polar flagellum resulting in characteristic darting motion
- Microaerophilic
- Do not ferment carbohydrates
- Culture on selective medium (blood agar containing antibiotic to inhibit growth of other fecal flora)

Campylobacter jejuni

- Acute enteritis
- Traveler's diarrhea
- Pseudoappendicitis

PENICILLINS
CEPHALOSPORINS
TETRACYCLINES
AMINOGLYCOSIDES
Macrolides   **1** Erythromycin
Fluoroquinolones **2** Ciprofloxacin
OTHER

DIARRHEA   NAUSEA AND VOMITING   GI DISTURBANCES   FEVER

Chlamydia species

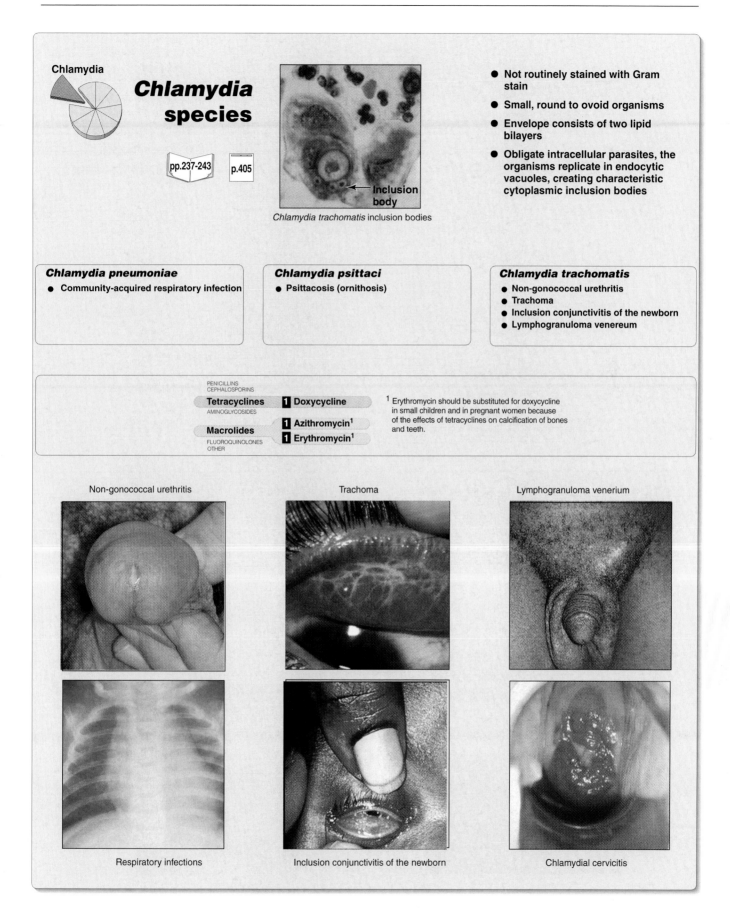

Chlamydia

pp.237-243 p.405

Chlamydia trachomatis inclusion bodies

- Not routinely stained with Gram stain
- Small, round to ovoid organisms
- Envelope consists of two lipid bilayers
- Obligate intracellular parasites, the organisms replicate in endocytic vacuoles, creating characteristic cytoplasmic inclusion bodies

Chlamydia pneumoniae
- Community-acquired respiratory infection

Chlamydia psittaci
- Psittacosis (ornithosis)

Chlamydia trachomatis
- Non-gonococcal urethritis
- Trachoma
- Inclusion conjunctivitis of the newborn
- Lymphogranuloma venereum

PENICILLINS
CEPHALOSPORINS
Tetracyclines 1 Doxycycline
AMINOGLYCOSIDES
Macrolides 1 Azithromycin[1]
FLUOROQUINOLONES 1 Erythromycin[1]
OTHER

[1] Erythromycin should be substituted for doxycycline in small children and in pregnant women because of the effects of tetracyclines on calcification of bones and teeth.

Non-gonococcal urethritis

Trachoma

Lymphogranuloma venerium

Respiratory infections

Inclusion conjunctivitis of the newborn

Chlamydial cervicitis

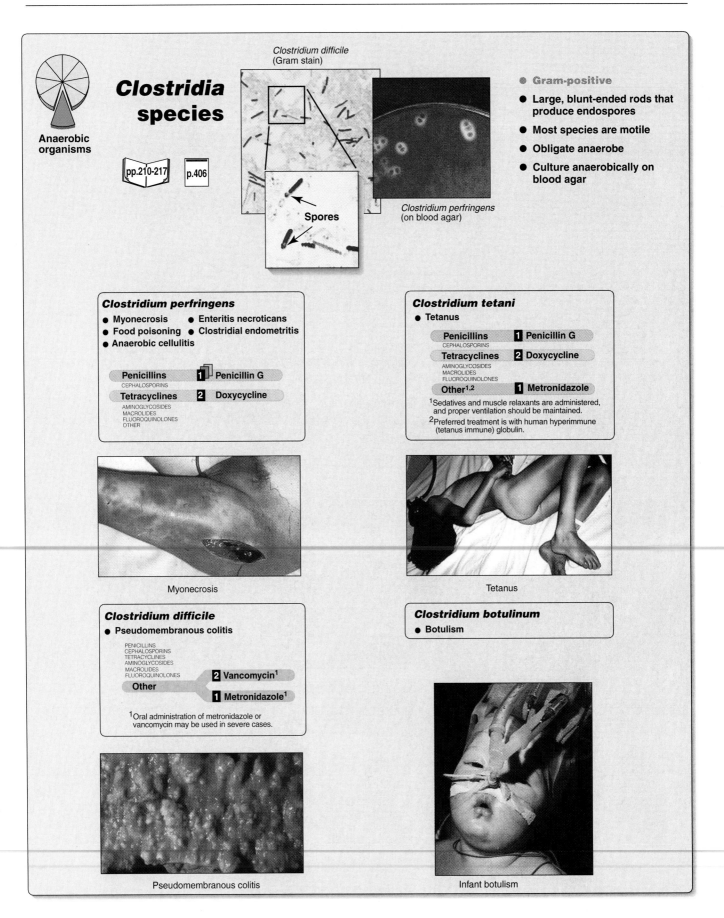

Anaerobic organisms

Clostridia species

pp.210-217   p.406

Clostridium difficile (Gram stain)

Spores

Clostridium perfringens (on blood agar)

- Gram-positive
- Large, blunt-ended rods that produce endospores
- Most species are motile
- Obligate anaerobe
- Culture anaerobically on blood agar

Clostridium perfringens

- Myonecrosis
- Food poisoning
- Anaerobic cellulitis
- Enteritis necroticans
- Clostridial endometritis

Penicillins CEPHALOSPORINS	**1** Penicillin G
Tetracyclines	**2** Doxycycline

AMINOGLYCOSIDES
MACROLIDES
FLUOROQUINOLONES
OTHER

Myonecrosis

Clostridium tetani

- Tetanus

Penicillins CEPHALOSPORINS	**1** Penicillin G
Tetracyclines AMINOGLYCOSIDES MACROLIDES FLUOROQUINOLONES	**2** Doxycycline
Other[1,2]	**1** Metronidazole

[1]Sedatives and muscle relaxants are administered, and proper ventilation should be maintained.
[2]Preferred treatment is with human hyperimmune (tetanus immune) globulin.

Tetanus

Clostridium difficile

- Pseudomembranous colitis

PENICILLINS
CEPHALOSPORINS
TETRACYCLINES
AMINOGLYCOSIDES
MACROLIDES
FLUOROQUINOLONES

Other   **2** Vancomycin[1]
             1 Metronidazole[1]

[1]Oral administration of metronidazole or vancomycin may be used in severe cases.

Pseudomembranous colitis

Clostridium botulinum

- Botulism

Infant botulism

Corynebacteria species

Gram (+) rods

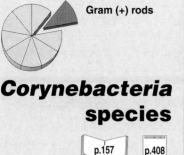

p.157 p.408

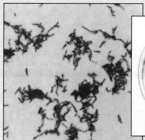

Corynebacterium diphtheriae Gram stain

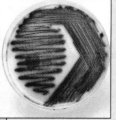

Corynebacterium diphtheriae grown on tellurite blood medium

- Gram-positive; stain unevenly
- Small, slender, pleomorphic rods that form characteristic clumps that look like Chinese characters or a picket fence
- Nonmotile and unencapsulated
- Most species are facultative anaerobes
- Culture aerobically on selective medium, such as Tinsdale agar containing tellurite (an inhibitor of the other respiratory flora).

Corynebacterium diphtheriae

- Diphtheria[1]

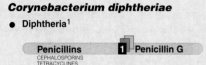

Penicillins	[1] Penicillin G
CEPHALOSPORINS TETRACYCLINES AMINOGLYCOSIDES	
Macrolides	[1] Erythromycin
FLUOROQUINOLONES OTHER	

[1]Treatment of diphtheria requires prompt neutralization of toxin, followed by eradication of the organism. A single dose of horse serum antitoxin inactivates any circulating toxin, although it does not affect toxin that is already bound to a cell-surface receptor.

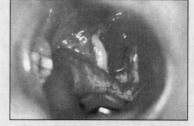

Corynebacterium diphtheriae infection of the throat. Gross swelling congestion of the whole pharyngeal and tonsillar area with a gray exudate covering the tonsil.

Enterococcus species

Gram (+) cocci

p.154 p.408

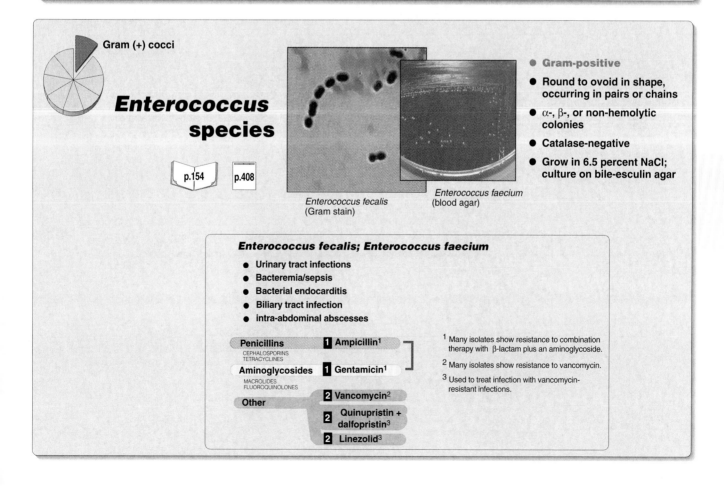

Enterococcus fecalis (Gram stain)

Enterococcus faecium (blood agar)

- Gram-positive
- Round to ovoid in shape, occurring in pairs or chains
- α-, β-, or non-hemolytic colonies
- Catalase-negative
- Grow in 6.5 percent NaCl; culture on bile-esculin agar

Enterococcus fecalis; Enterococcus faecium

- Urinary tract infections
- Bacteremia/sepsis
- Bacterial endocarditis
- Biliary tract infection
- intra-abdominal abscesses

Penicillins	[1] Ampicillin[1]
CEPHALOSPORINS TETRACYCLINES	
Aminoglycosides	[1] Gentamicin[1]
MACROLIDES FLUOROQUINOLONES	
Other	[2] Vancomycin[2]
	[2] Quinupristin + dalfopristin[3]
	[2] Linezolid[3]

[1] Many isolates show resistance to combination therapy with β-lactam plus an aminoglycoside.

[2] Many isolates show resistance to vancomycin.

[3] Used to treat infection with vancomycin-resistant infections.

Escherichia species

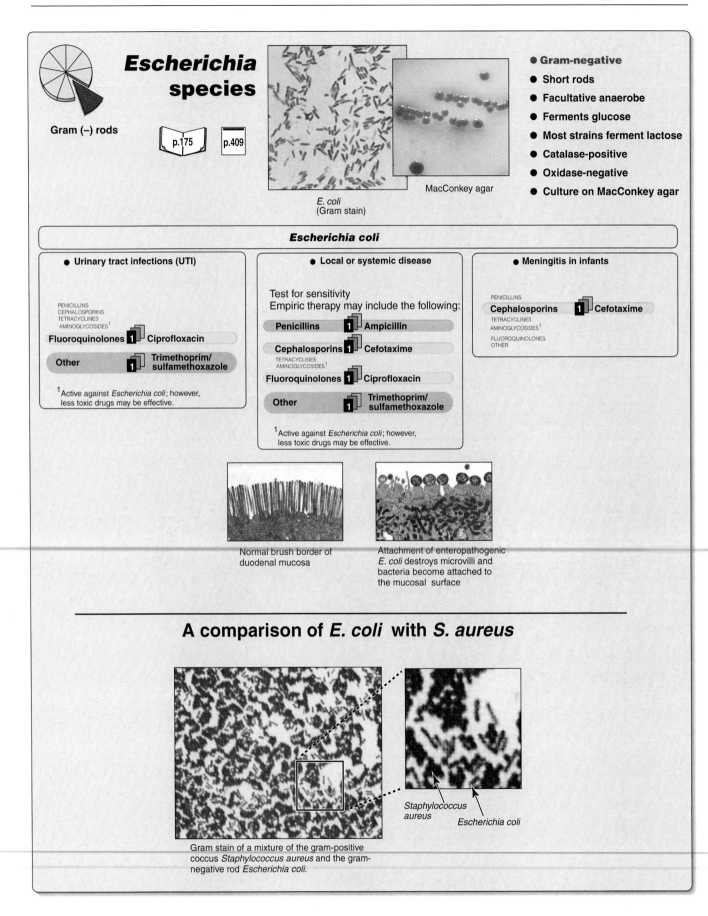

Gram (–) rods

p.175 p.409

E. coli
(Gram stain)

MacConkey agar

- **Gram-negative**
- **Short rods**
- **Facultative anaerobe**
- **Ferments glucose**
- **Most strains ferment lactose**
- **Catalase-positive**
- **Oxidase-negative**
- **Culture on MacConkey agar**

Escherichia coli

● Urinary tract infections (UTI)

PENICILLINS
CEPHALOSPORINS
TETRACYCLINES
AMINOGLYCOSIDES[1]

Fluoroquinolones 1 — **Ciprofloxacin**

Other 1 — **Trimethoprim/sulfamethoxazole**

[1]Active against *Escherichia coli*; however, less toxic drugs may be effective.

● Local or systemic disease

Test for sensitivity
Empiric therapy may include the following:

Penicillins 1 — **Ampicillin**

Cephalosporins 1 — **Cefotaxime**

TETRACYCLINES
AMINOGLYCOSIDES[1]

Fluoroquinolones 1 — **Ciprofloxacin**

Other 1 — **Trimethoprim/sulfamethoxazole**

[1]Active against *Escherichia coli*; however, less toxic drugs may be effective.

● Meningitis in infants

PENICILLINS
Cephalosporins 1 — **Cefotaxime**
TETRACYCLINES
AMINOGLYCOSIDES[1]
FLUOROQUINOLONES
OTHER

Normal brush border of
duodenal mucosa

Attachment of enteropathogenic
E. coli destroys microvilli and
bacteria become attached to
the mucosal surface

A comparison of *E. coli* with *S. aureus*

*Staphylococcus
aureus*

Escherichia coli

Gram stain of a mixture of the gram-positive
coccus *Staphylococcus aureus* and the gram-
negative rod *Escherichia coli*.

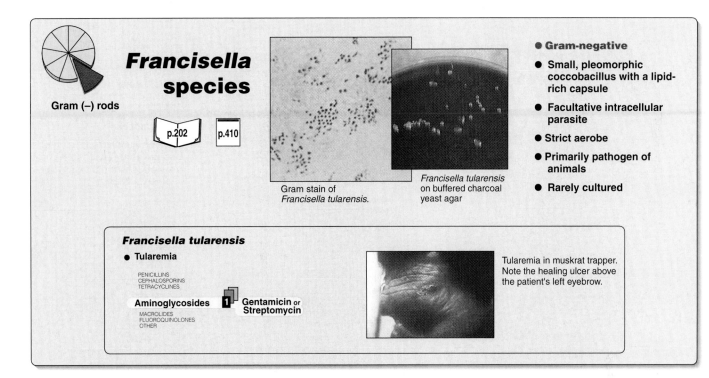

Francisella species

Gram (−) rods

p.202 | p.410

Gram stain of *Francisella tularensis.*

Francisella tularensis on buffered charcoal yeast agar

- **Gram-negative**
- Small, pleomorphic coccobacillus with a lipid-rich capsule
- Facultative intracellular parasite
- Strict aerobe
- Primarily pathogen of animals
- Rarely cultured

Francisella tularensis
- Tularemia

PENICILLINS
CEPHALOSPORINS
TETRACYCLINES

Aminoglycosides 1 **Gentamicin** or **Streptomycin**

MACROLIDES
FLUOROQUINOLONES
OTHER

Tularemia in muskrat trapper. Note the healing ulcer above the patient's left eyebrow.

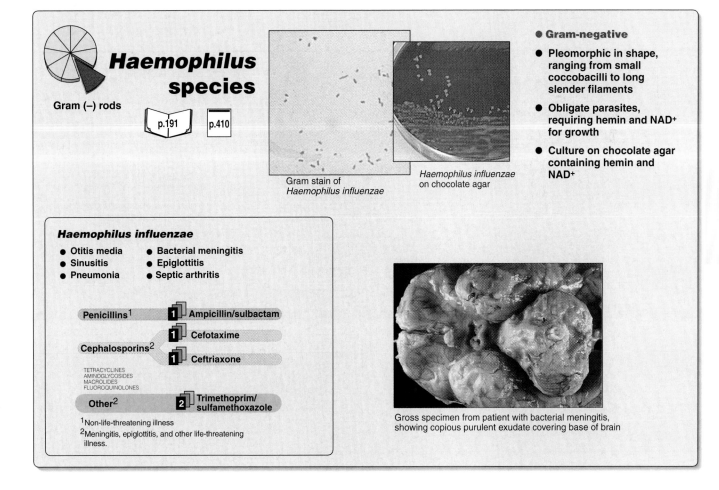

Haemophilus species

Gram (−) rods

p.191 | p.410

Gram stain of *Haemophilus influenzae*

Haemophilus influenzae on chocolate agar

- **Gram-negative**
- Pleomorphic in shape, ranging from small coccobacilli to long slender filaments
- Obligate parasites, requiring hemin and NAD+ for growth
- Culture on chocolate agar containing hemin and NAD+

Haemophilus influenzae
- Otitis media
- Sinusitis
- Pneumonia
- Bacterial meningitis
- Epiglottitis
- Septic arthritis

Penicillins[1] 1 **Ampicillin/sulbactam**

Cephalosporins[2] 1 **Cefotaxime**
1 **Ceftriaxone**

TETRACYCLINES
AMINOGLYCOSIDES
MACROLIDES
FLUOROQUINOLONES

Other[2] 2 **Trimethoprim/sulfamethoxazole**

[1]Non-life-threatening illness
[2]Meningitis, epiglottitis, and other life-threatening illness.

Gross specimen from patient with bacterial meningitis, showing copious purulent exudate covering base of brain

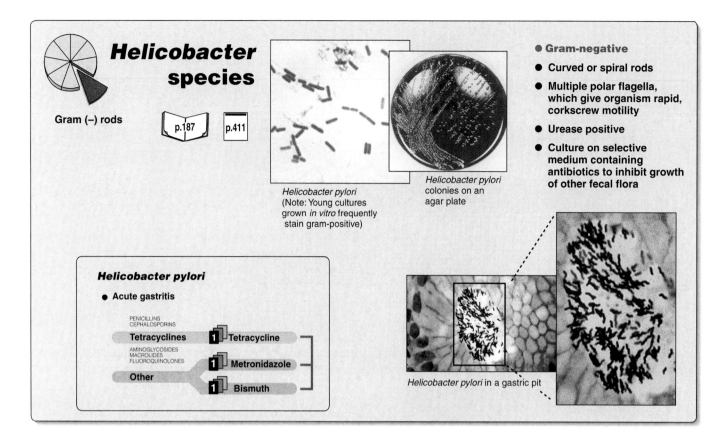

Helicobacter species

Gram (–) rods   p.187   p.411

Helicobacter pylori (Note: Young cultures grown *in vitro* frequently stain gram-positive)

Helicobacter pylori colonies on an agar plate

- **Gram-negative**
- Curved or spiral rods
- Multiple polar flagella, which give organism rapid, corkscrew motility
- Urease positive
- Culture on selective medium containing antibiotics to inhibit growth of other fecal flora

Helicobacter pylori

- Acute gastritis

PENICILLINS
CEPHALOSPORINS
Tetracyclines   1 Tetracycline
AMINOGLYCOSIDES
MACROLIDES
FLUOROQUINOLONES   1 Metronidazole
Other   1 Bismuth

Helicobacter pylori in a gastric pit

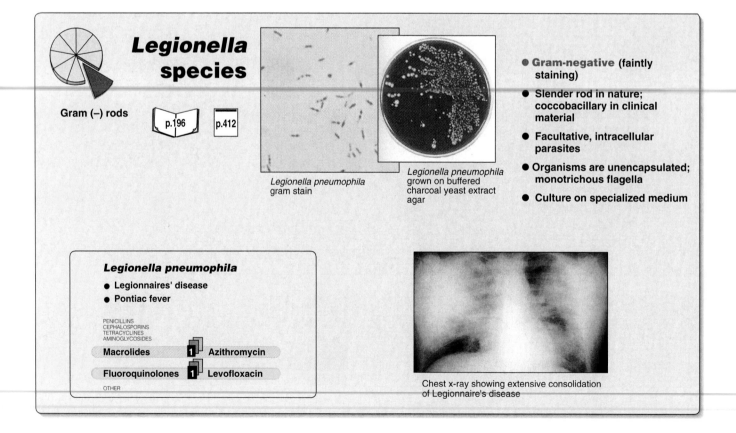

Legionella species

Gram (–) rods   p.196   p.412

Legionella pneumophila gram stain

Legionella pneumophila grown on buffered charcoal yeast extract agar

- **Gram-negative** (faintly staining)
- Slender rod in nature; coccobacillary in clinical material
- Facultative, intracellular parasites
- Organisms are unencapsulated; monotrichous flagella
- Culture on specialized medium

Legionella pneumophila

- Legionnaires' disease
- Pontiac fever

PENICILLINS
CEPHALOSPORINS
TETRACYCLINES
AMINOGLYCOSIDES
Macrolides   1 Azithromycin
Fluoroquinolones   1 Levofloxacin
OTHER

Chest x-ray showing extensive consolidation of Legionnaire's disease

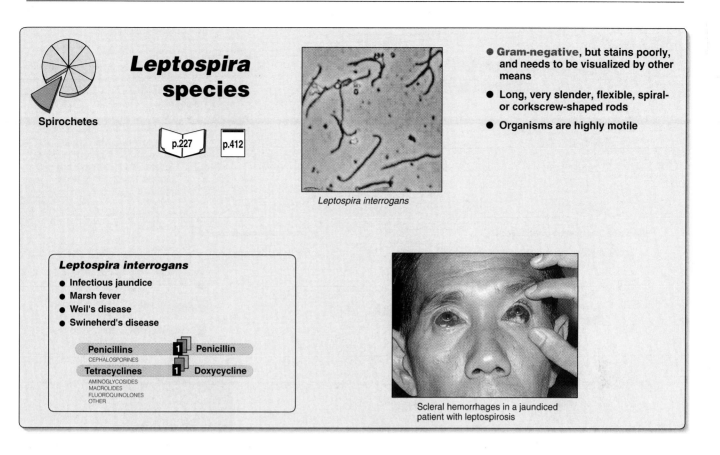

Leptospira species

Spirochetes

p.227   p.412

Leptospira interrogans

- **Gram-negative**, but stains poorly, and needs to be visualized by other means
- Long, very slender, flexible, spiral- or corkscrew-shaped rods
- Organisms are highly motile

Leptospira interrogans
- Infectious jaundice
- Marsh fever
- Weil's disease
- Swineherd's disease

Penicillins	**1** Penicillin
CEPHALOSPORINES	
Tetracyclines	**1** Doxycycline
AMINOGLYCOSIDES MACROLIDES FLUOROQUINOLONES OTHER	

Scleral hemorrhages in a jaundiced patient with leptospirosis

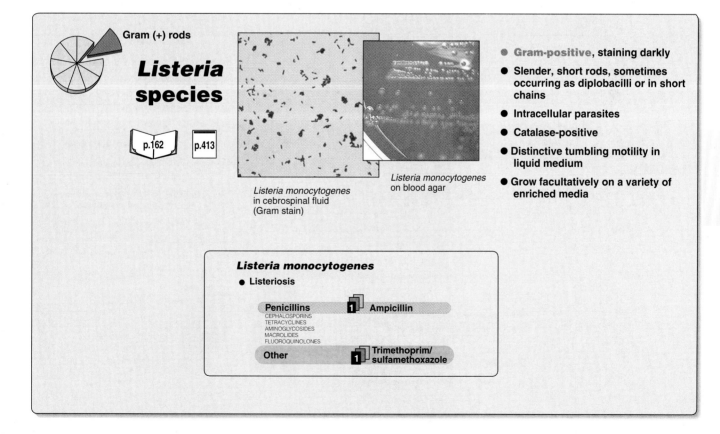

Listeria species

Gram (+) rods

p.162   p.413

Listeria monocytogenes in cebrospinal fluid (Gram stain)

Listeria monocytogenes on blood agar

- **Gram-positive**, staining darkly
- Slender, short rods, sometimes occurring as diplobacilli or in short chains
- Intracellular parasites
- Catalase-positive
- Distinctive tumbling motility in liquid medium
- Grow facultatively on a variety of enriched media

Listeria monocytogenes
- Listeriosis

Penicillins	**1** Ampicillin
CEPHALOSPORINS TETRACYCLINES AMINOGLYCOSIDES MACROLIDES FLUOROQUINOLONES	
Other	**1** Trimethoprim/ sulfamethoxazole

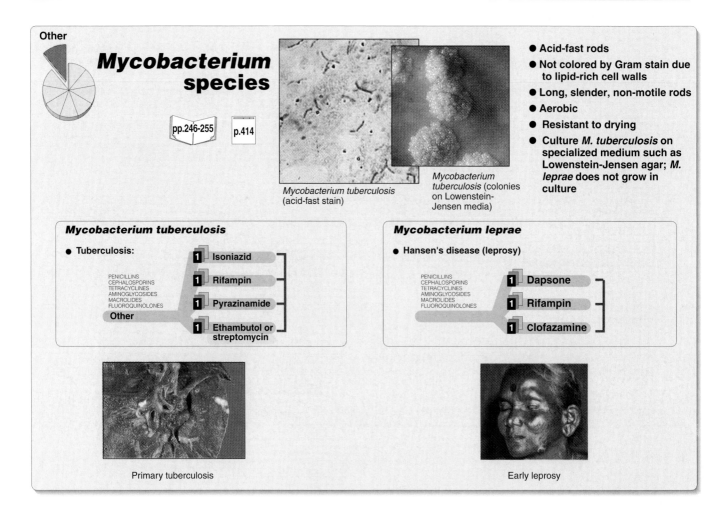

Other

Mycobacterium species

pp.246-255   p.414

Mycobacterium tuberculosis
(acid-fast stain)

Mycobacterium tuberculosis (colonies on Lowenstein-Jensen media)

- Acid-fast rods
- Not colored by Gram stain due to lipid-rich cell walls
- Long, slender, non-motile rods
- Aerobic
- Resistant to drying
- Culture *M. tuberculosis* on specialized medium such as Lowenstein-Jensen agar; *M. leprae* does not grow in culture

Mycobacterium tuberculosis

- Tuberculosis:

PENICILLINS
CEPHALOSPORINS
TETRACYCLINES
AMINOGLYCOSIDES
MACROLIDES
FLUOROQUINOLONES
Other

- **1** Isoniazid
- **1** Rifampin
- **1** Pyrazinamide
- **1** Ethambutol or streptomycin

Mycobacterium leprae

- Hansen's disease (leprosy)

PENICILLINS
CEPHALOSPORINS
TETRACYCLINES
AMINOGLYCOSIDES
MACROLIDES
FLUOROQUINOLONES

- **1** Dapsone
- **1** Rifampin
- **1** Clofazamine

Primary tuberculosis

Early leprosy

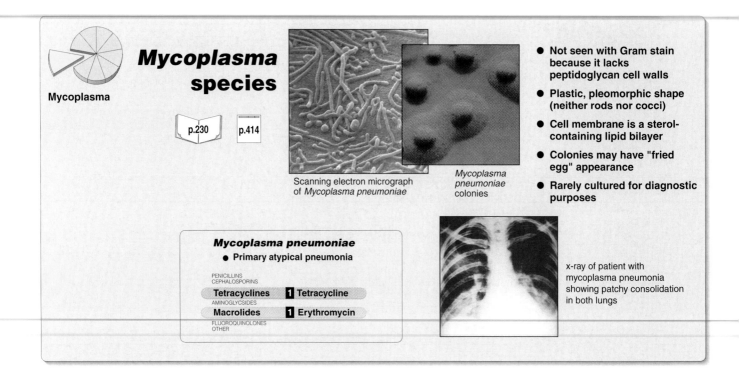

Mycoplasma

Mycoplasma species

p.230   p.414

Scanning electron micrograph of *Mycoplasma pneumoniae*

Mycoplasma pneumoniae colonies

- Not seen with Gram stain because it lacks peptidoglycan cell walls
- Plastic, pleomorphic shape (neither rods nor cocci)
- Cell membrane is a sterol-containing lipid bilayer
- Colonies may have "fried egg" appearance
- Rarely cultured for diagnostic purposes

Mycoplasma pneumoniae

- Primary atypical pneumonia

PENICILLINS
CEPHALOSPORINS
Tetracyclines   **1** Tetracycline
AMINOGLYCSIDES
Macrolides   **1** Erythromycin
FLUOROQUINOLONES
OTHER

x-ray of patient with mycoplasma pneumonia showing patchy consolidation in both lungs

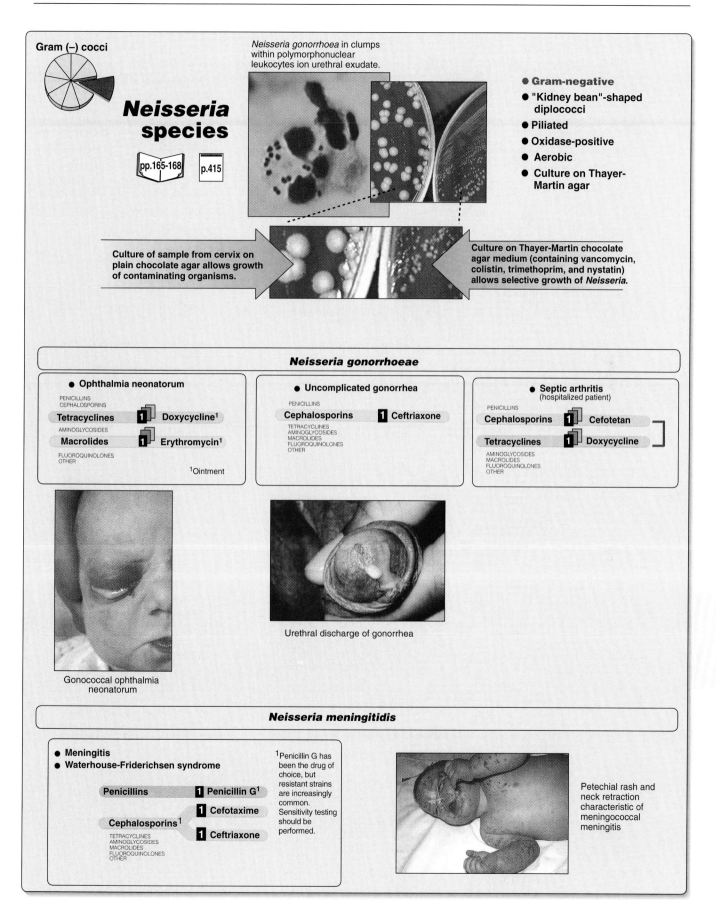

Gram (–) cocci

Neisseria species

pp.165-168   p.415

Neisseria gonorrhoea in clumps within polymorphonuclear leukocytes ion urethral exudate.

- **Gram-negative**
- "Kidney bean"-shaped diplococci
- Piliated
- Oxidase-positive
- Aerobic
- Culture on Thayer-Martin agar

Culture of sample from cervix on plain chocolate agar allows growth of contaminating organisms.

Culture on Thayer-Martin chocolate agar medium (containing vancomycin, colistin, trimethoprim, and nystatin) allows selective growth of *Neisseria*.

Neisseria gonorrhoeae

- **Ophthalmia neonatorum**

PENICILLINS
CEPHALOSPORINS
Tetracyclines 1 Doxycycline[1]
AMINOGLYCOSIDES
Macrolides 1 Erythromycin[1]
FLUOROQUINOLONES
OTHER
[1]Ointment

- **Uncomplicated gonorrhea**

PENICILLINS
Cephalosporins 1 Ceftriaxone
TETRACYCLINES
AMINOGLYCOSIDES
MACROLIDES
FLUOROQUINOLONES
OTHER

- **Septic arthritis**
(hospitalized patient)

PENICILLINS
Cephalosporins 1 Cefotetan
Tetracyclines 1 Doxycycline
AMINOGLYCOSIDES
MACROLIDES
FLUOROQUINOLONES
OTHER

Gonococcal ophthalmia neonatorum

Urethral discharge of gonorrhea

Neisseria meningitidis

- **Meningitis**
- **Waterhouse-Friderichsen syndrome**

Penicillins 1 Penicillin G[1]
Cephalosporins[1] 1 Cefotaxime
  1 Ceftriaxone
TETRACYCLINES
AMINOGLYCOSIDES
MACROLIDES
FLUOROQUINOLONES
OTHER

[1]Penicillin G has been the drug of choice, but resistant strains are increasingly common. Sensitivity testing should be performed.

Petechial rash and neck retraction characteristic of meningococcal meningitis

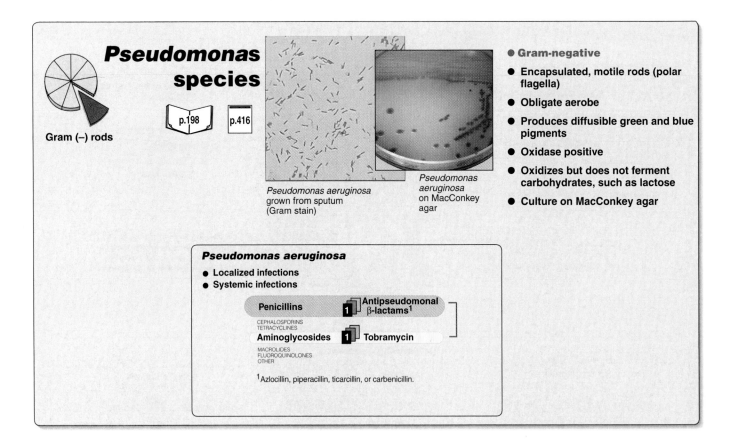

Pseudomonas species

Gram (–) rods

p.198　　p.416

Pseudomonas aeruginosa grown from sputum (Gram stain)

Pseudomonas aeruginosa on MacConkey agar

- **Gram-negative**
- Encapsulated, motile rods (polar flagella)
- Obligate aerobe
- Produces diffusible green and blue pigments
- Oxidase positive
- Oxidizes but does not ferment carbohydrates, such as lactose
- Culture on MacConkey agar

Pseudomonas aeruginosa
- Localized infections
- Systemic infections

Penicillins　　1　Antipseudomonal β-lactams[1]

CEPHALOSPORINS
TETRACYCLINES
Aminoglycosides　　1　Tobramycin

MACROLIDES
FLUOROQUINOLONES
OTHER

[1] Azlocillin, piperacillin, ticarcillin, or carbenicillin.

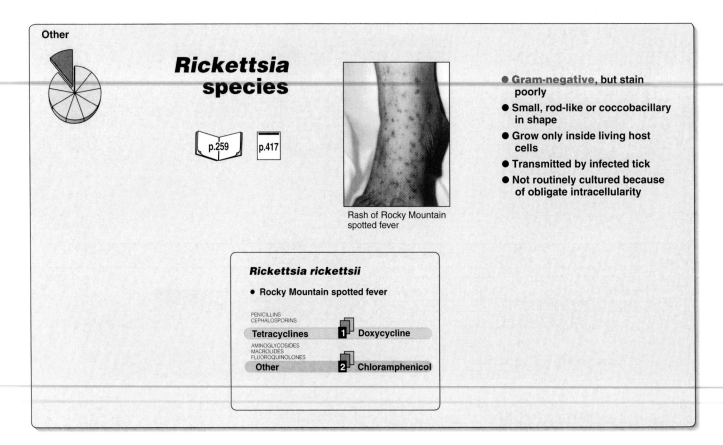

Other

Rickettsia species

p.259　　p.417

Rash of Rocky Mountain spotted fever

- **Gram-negative**, but stain poorly
- Small, rod-like or coccobacillary in shape
- Grow only inside living host cells
- Transmitted by infected tick
- Not routinely cultured because of obligate intracellularity

Rickettsia rickettsii
- Rocky Mountain spotted fever

PENICILLINS
CEPHALOSPORINS
Tetracyclines　　1　Doxycycline

AMINOGLYCOSIDES
MACROLIDES
FLUOROQUINOLONES
Other　　2　Chloramphenicol

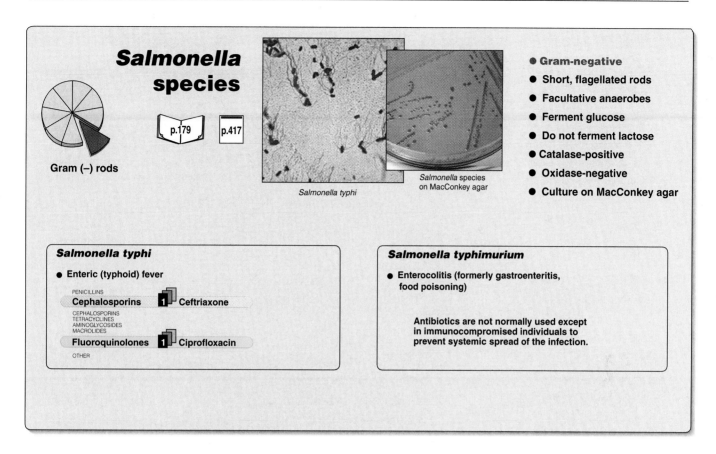

Salmonella species

Gram (–) rods

p.179   p.417

Salmonella typhi

Salmonella species on MacConkey agar

- **Gram-negative**
- Short, flagellated rods
- Facultative anaerobes
- Ferment glucose
- Do not ferment lactose
- Catalase-positive
- Oxidase-negative
- Culture on MacConkey agar

Salmonella typhi

- Enteric (typhoid) fever

PENICILLINS
Cephalosporins 1 Ceftriaxone
CEPHALOSPORINS
TETRACYCLINES
AMINOGLYCOSIDES
MACROLIDES
Fluoroquinolones 1 Ciprofloxacin
OTHER

Salmonella typhimurium

- Enterocolitis (formerly gastroenteritis, food poisoning)

Antibiotics are not normally used except in immunocompromised individuals to prevent systemic spread of the infection.

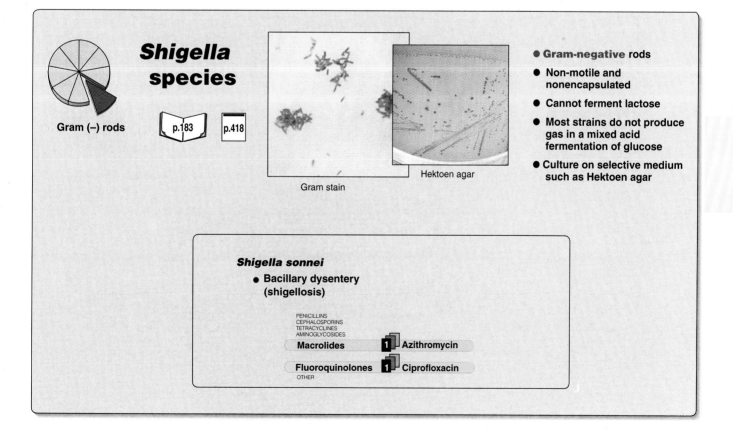

Shigella species

Gram (–) rods

p.183   p.418

Gram stain

Hektoen agar

- **Gram-negative rods**
- Non-motile and nonencapsulated
- Cannot ferment lactose
- Most strains do not produce gas in a mixed acid fermentation of glucose
- Culture on selective medium such as Hektoen agar

Shigella sonnei

- Bacillary dysentery (shigellosis)

PENICILLINS
CEPHALOSPORINS
TETRACYCLINES
AMINOGLYCOSIDES
Macrolides 1 Azithromycin
Fluoroquinolones 1 Ciprofloxacin
OTHER

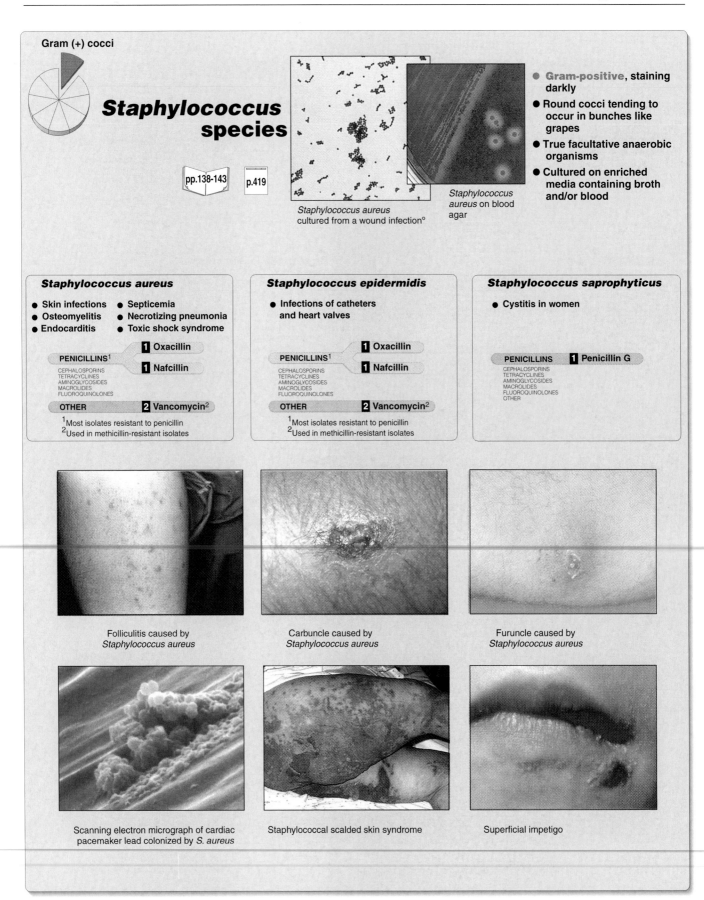

Gram (+) cocci

Staphylococcus species

pp.138-143   p.419

Staphylococcus aureus cultured from a wound infection°

Staphylococcus aureus on blood agar

- **Gram-positive**, staining darkly
- Round cocci tending to occur in bunches like grapes
- True facultative anaerobic organisms
- Cultured on enriched media containing broth and/or blood

Staphylococcus aureus

- Skin infections
- Osteomyelitis
- Endocarditis
- Septicemia
- Necrotizing pneumonia
- Toxic shock syndrome

PENICILLINS[1]
1 Oxacillin
1 Nafcillin

CEPHALOSPORINS
TETRACYCLINES
AMINOGLYCOSIDES
MACROLIDES
FLUOROQUINOLONES

OTHER
2 Vancomycin[2]

[1] Most isolates resistant to penicillin
[2] Used in methicillin-resistant isolates

Staphylococcus epidermidis

- Infections of catheters and heart valves

PENICILLINS[1]
1 Oxacillin
1 Nafcillin

CEPHALOSPORINS
TETRACYCLINES
AMINOGLYCOSIDES
MACROLIDES
FLUOROQUINOLONES

OTHER
2 Vancomycin[2]

[1] Most isolates resistant to penicillin
[2] Used in methicillin-resistant isolates

Staphylococcus saprophyticus

- Cystitis in women

PENICILLINS
1 Penicillin G

CEPHALOSPORINS
TETRACYCLINES
AMINOGLYCOSIDES
MACROLIDES
FLUOROQUINOLONES
OTHER

Folliculitis caused by *Staphylococcus aureus*

Carbuncle caused by *Staphylococcus aureus*

Furuncle caused by *Staphylococcus aureus*

Scanning electron micrograph of cardiac pacemaker lead colonized by *S. aureus*

Staphylococcal scalded skin syndrome

Superficial impetigo

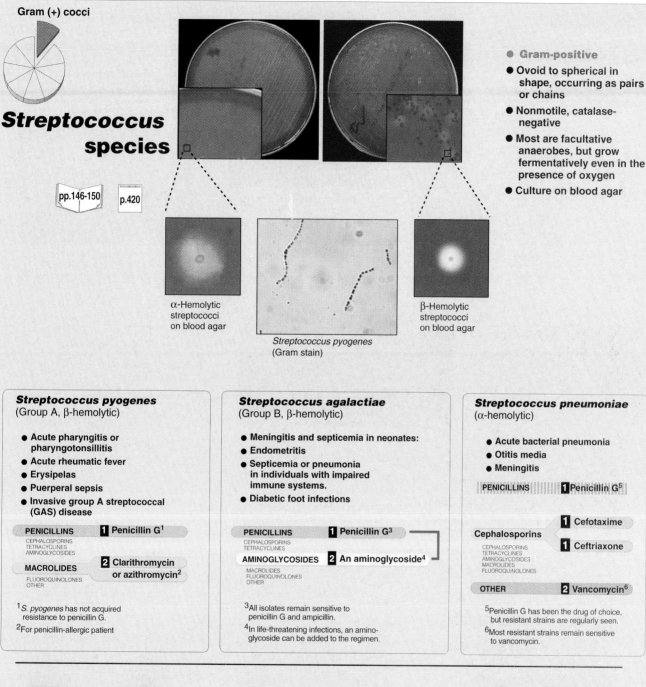

Gram (+) cocci

Streptococcus species

pp.146-150 p.420

- **Gram-positive**
- Ovoid to spherical in shape, occurring as pairs or chains
- Nonmotile, catalase-negative
- Most are facultative anaerobes, but grow fermentatively even in the presence of oxygen
- Culture on blood agar

α-Hemolytic streptococci on blood agar

Streptococcus pyogenes (Gram stain)

β-Hemolytic streptococci on blood agar

Streptococcus pyogenes
(Group A, β-hemolytic)

- Acute pharyngitis or pharyngotonsillitis
- Acute rheumatic fever
- Erysipelas
- Puerperal sepsis
- Invasive group A streptococcal (GAS) disease

PENICILLINS	**1** Penicillin G[1]
CEPHALOSPORINS TETRACYCLINES AMINOGLYCOSIDES	
MACROLIDES	**2** Clarithromycin or azithromycin[2]
FLUOROQUINOLONES OTHER	

[1] *S. pyogenes* has not acquired resistance to penicillin G.

[2] For penicillin-allergic patient

Streptococcus agalactiae
(Group B, β-hemolytic)

- Meningitis and septicemia in neonates:
- Endometritis
- Septicemia or pneumonia in individuals with impaired immune systems.
- Diabetic foot infections

PENICILLINS	**1** Penicillin G[3]
CEPHALOSPORINS TETRACYCLINES	
AMINOGLYCOSIDES	**2** An aminoglycoside[4]
MACROLIDES FLUOROQUINOLONES OTHER	

[3] All isolates remain sensitive to penicillin G and ampicillin.

[4] In life-threatening infections, an aminoglycoside can be added to the regimen.

Streptococcus pneumoniae
(α-hemolytic)

- Acute bacterial pneumonia
- Otitis media
- Meningitis

| PENICILLINS | **1** Penicillin G[5] |

Cephalosporins **1** Cefotaxime

1 Ceftriaxone

| CEPHALOSPORINS TETRACYCLINES AMINOGLYCOSIDES MACROLIDES FLUOROQUINOLONES | |

| OTHER | **2** Vancomycin[6] |

[5] Penicillin G has been the drug of choice, but resistant strains are regularly seen.

[6] Most resistant strains remain sensitive to vancomycin.

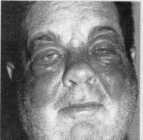

Facial erysipelas

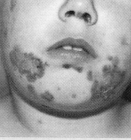

Impetigo

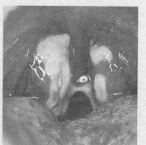

Streptococcal pharyngitis

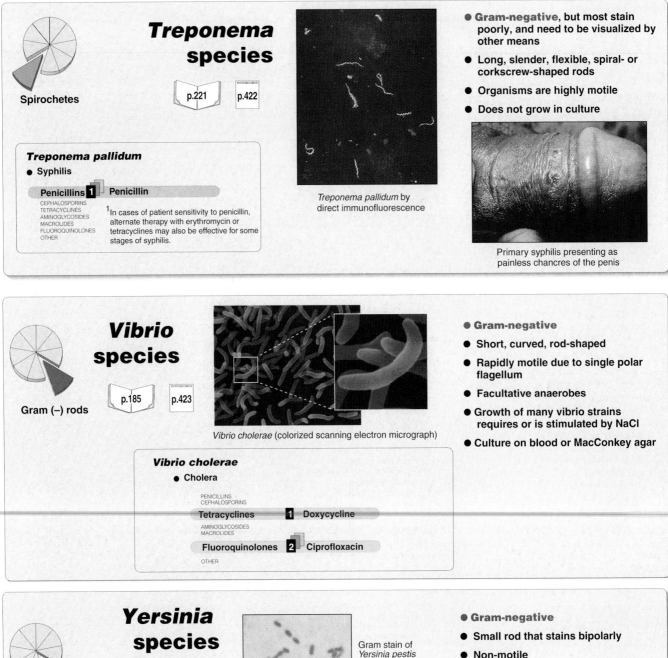

Treponema species

Spirochetes

p.221   p.422

- **Gram-negative**, but most stain poorly, and need to be visualized by other means
- Long, slender, flexible, spiral- or corkscrew-shaped rods
- Organisms are highly motile
- Does not grow in culture

Treponema pallidum by direct immunofluorescence

Primary syphilis presenting as painless chancres of the penis

Treponema pallidum
- Syphilis

Penicillins **1** — Penicillin

CEPHALOSPORINS
TETRACYCLINES
AMINOGLYCOSIDES
MACROLIDES
FLUOROQUINOLONES
OTHER

[1] In cases of patient sensitivity to penicillin, alternate therapy with erythromycin or tetracyclines may also be effective for some stages of syphilis.

Vibrio species

Gram (–) rods

p.185   p.423

Vibrio cholerae (colorized scanning electron micrograph)

- **Gram-negative**
- Short, curved, rod-shaped
- Rapidly motile due to single polar flagellum
- Facultative anaerobes
- Growth of many vibrio strains requires or is stimulated by NaCl
- Culture on blood or MacConkey agar

Vibrio cholerae
- Cholera

PENICILLINS
CEPHALOSPORINS

Tetracyclines **1** — Doxycycline

AMINOGLYCOSIDES
MACROLIDES

Fluoroquinolones **2** — Ciprofloxacin

OTHER

Yersinia species

Gram (–) rods

p.205   p.423

Gram stain of *Yersinia pestis*

- **Gram-negative**
- Small rod that stains bipolarly
- Non-motile
- Encapsulated
- Culture on blood or CIN (selective) agar

Yersinia pestis
- Bubonic (septicemic) plague
- Pneumonic plague

PENICILLINS
CEPHALOSPORINS
TETRACYCLINES

Aminoglycosides **1** — Streptomycin

MACROLIDES
FLUOROQUINOLONES
OTHER

Microbiology Made Manageable

37

I. ORGANIZING THE MICROORGANISMS AND DRUGS

Trying to assimilate the names and characteristics of and the specific drug therapies for pathogenic organisms can be an overwhelming experience unless the flood of information is organized into logical groupings. In addition, it is helpful if these relationships can be visualized, using a consistent color-coding system. To this end, the authors have adopted several graphic formats that are used throughout this book. For example, as introduced in Chapter 1, the **antimicrobial drugs** that are commonly used to treat bacterial infections have been organized into seven groups, and are represented here as colored bars (Figure 37.1A). [Note: One bar is labeled "Other," and represents any of several drugs not represented by the other bars.] **Bacteria** have been organized into nine groups based on Gram stain, morphology, and biochemical and other characteristics. Each group is represented by a colored wedge of a pie chart (Figure 37.1B), for example, the green wedge represents the spirochetes. [Note: One section of the bacterial pie chart is labeled "Other," and represents any of several microorganisms that are not encompassed by other pie segments.] **Viral pathogens** have likewise been organized into seven group-

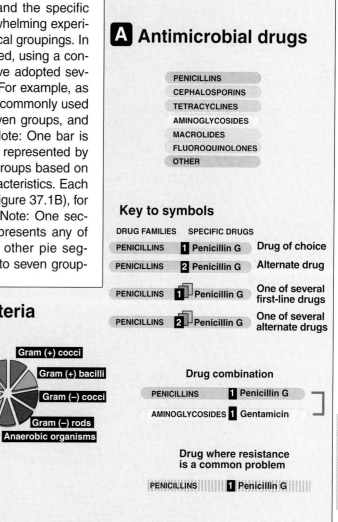

Figure 37.1
A. Color-coded representation of classes of commonly used antimicrobial drugs. B. Bacteria organized into nine groups based on Gram stain, morphology, and biochemical and other characteristics. C. Viruses organized into seven groups based on the nature of their genome, symmetry of organization, and the presence or absence of a lipid envelope.

Lippincott's Illustrated Reviews: Microbiology,
by William A. Strohl, Harriet Rouse, Bruce D. Fisher.
Lippincott, Williams & Wilkins, Baltimore, MD © 2001

ings based on the nature of their genome, symmetry of organization, and the presence or absence of a lipid envelope (Figure 37.1C). In Chapters 11 through 34, single "slices" of each pie were examined independently, with the organisms discussed listed in the first figure of each chapter. In this chapter, all of the bacteria and viruses discussed in this text are presented on two summary pie charts (Figures 37.2 and 37.3). To provide an additional tool for easy location of microorganisms, bacteria and viruses discussed in this book are also listed alphabetically, with a color citation indicating where the pathogen is located in the pie chart, and a page number indicating where in the text the primary discussion of each organism begins.The two pie charts and their associated lists can be used much in the same way as the white and yellow pages in a telephone directory. If you are interested in a particular pathogen, you can locate the name of the microorganism in the alphabetic listing of the organisms. Conversely, if you are interested in a group of related pathogens, such an anaerobic bacteria, you can locate the group at the center of the graph; from there you can identify closely related organisms. Finally, a summary of **recommended drugs for selected microorganisms**, also using color-coding as a visual aid, is shown in Figure 37.4 and 37.5.

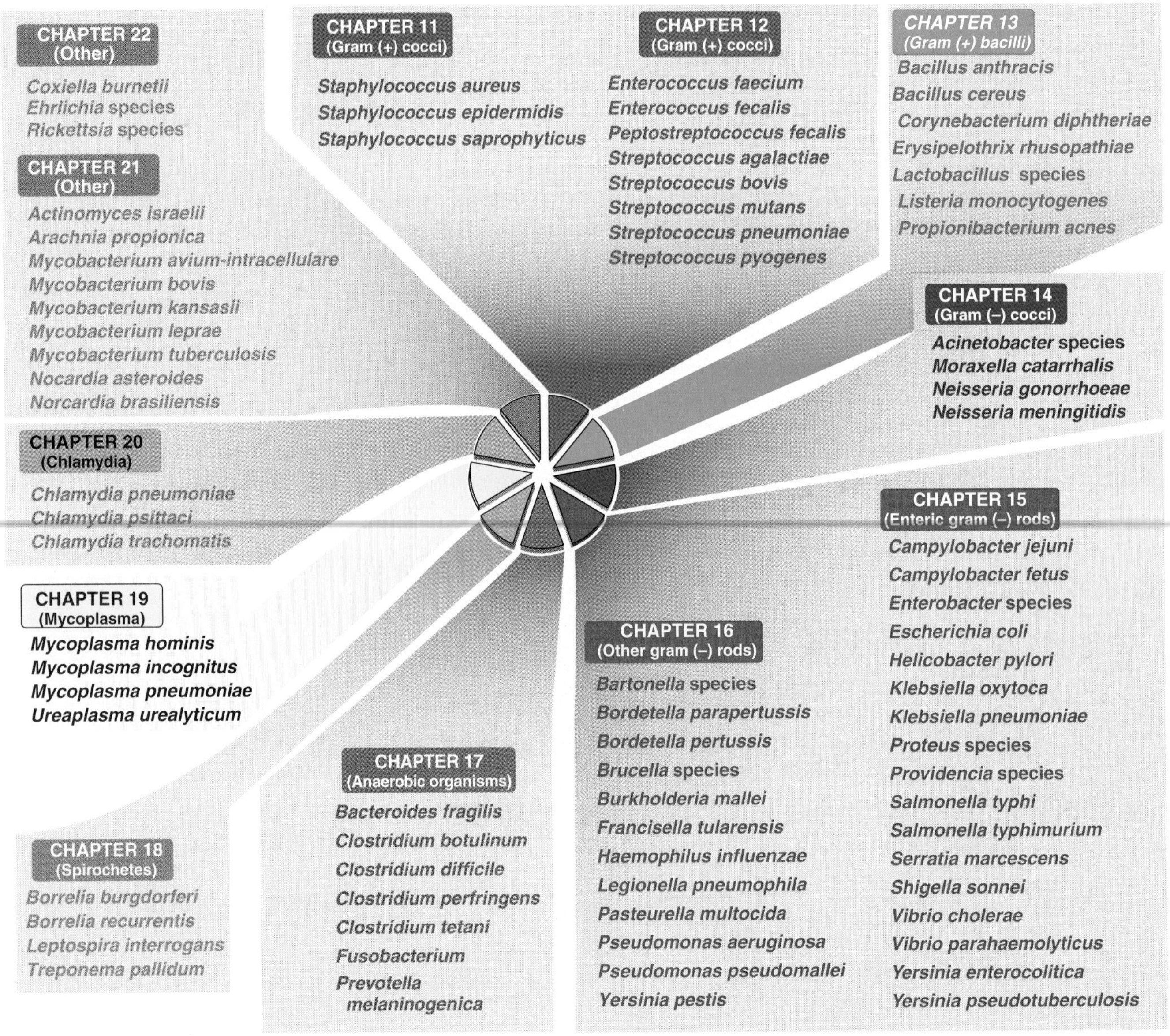

CHAPTER 22
(Other)

Coxiella burnetii
Ehrlichia species
Rickettsia species

CHAPTER 21
(Other)

Actinomyces israelii
Arachnia propionica
Mycobacterium avium-intracellulare
Mycobacterium bovis
Mycobacterium kansasii
Mycobacterium leprae
Mycobacterium tuberculosis
Nocardia asteroides
Norcardia brasiliensis

CHAPTER 20
(Chlamydia)

Chlamydia pneumoniae
Chlamydia psittaci
Chlamydia trachomatis

CHAPTER 19
(Mycoplasma)

Mycoplasma hominis
Mycoplasma incognitus
Mycoplasma pneumoniae
Ureaplasma urealyticum

CHAPTER 18
(Spirochetes)

Borrelia burgdorferi
Borrelia recurrentis
Leptospira interrogans
Treponema pallidum

CHAPTER 11
(Gram (+) cocci)

Staphylococcus aureus
Staphylococcus epidermidis
Staphylococcus saprophyticus

CHAPTER 12
(Gram (+) cocci)

Enterococcus faecium
Enterococcus fecalis
Peptostreptococcus fecalis
Streptococcus agalactiae
Streptococcus bovis
Streptococcus mutans
Streptococcus pneumoniae
Streptococcus pyogenes

CHAPTER 13
(Gram (+) bacilli)

Bacillus anthracis
Bacillus cereus
Corynebacterium diphtheriae
Erysipelothrix rhusopathiae
Lactobacillus species
Listeria monocytogenes
Propionibacterium acnes

CHAPTER 14
(Gram (–) cocci)

Acinetobacter species
Moraxella catarrhalis
Neisseria gonorrhoeae
Neisseria meningitidis

CHAPTER 15
(Enteric gram (–) rods)

Campylobacter jejuni
Campylobacter fetus
Enterobacter species
Escherichia coli
Helicobacter pylori
Klebsiella oxytoca
Klebsiella pneumoniae
Proteus species
Providencia species
Salmonella typhi
Salmonella typhimurium
Serratia marcescens
Shigella sonnei
Vibrio cholerae
Vibrio parahaemolyticus
Yersinia enterocolitica
Yersinia pseudotuberculosis

CHAPTER 16
(Other gram (–) rods)

Bartonella species
Bordetella parapertussis
Bordetella pertussis
Brucella species
Burkholderia mallei
Francisella tularensis
Haemophilus influenzae
Legionella pneumophila
Pasteurella multocida
Pseudomonas aeruginosa
Pseudomonas pseudomallei
Yersinia pestis

CHAPTER 17
(Anaerobic organisms)

Bacteroides fragilis
Clostridium botulinum
Clostridium difficile
Clostridium perfringens
Clostridium tetani
Fusobacterium
Prevotella melaninogenica

Figure 37.2
Medically important bacteria discussed in this book, organized into similar groups based on morphology, biochemistry, and/or staining properties.

Acinetobacter (p. 173)

Actinomyces israelii (p. 256)

Arachnia propionica (p. 256)

Ⓢ *Bacillus anthracis* (p. 160)

Bacillus cereus (p. 162)

Bacteroides fragilis (p. 219)

Bartonella species (p. 193)

Bordetella parapertussis (p. 193)

Ⓢ *Bordetella pertussis* (p. 193)

Ⓢ *Borrelia burgdorferi* (p. 224)

Borrelia recurrentis (p. 226)

Ⓢ *Brucella* species (p. 201)

Burkholderia mallei (p. 200)

Campylobacter fetus (p. 181)

Ⓢ *Campylobacter jejuni* (p. 181)

Ⓢ *Chlamydia pneumoniae* (p. 243)

Ⓢ *Chlamydia psittaci* (p. 243)

Ⓢ *Chlamydia trachomatis* (p. 237)

Ⓢ *Clostridium botulinum* (p. 213)

Ⓢ *Clostridium difficile* (p. 217)

Ⓢ *Clostridium perfringens* (p. 210)

Ⓢ *Clostridium tetani* (p. 215)

Ⓢ *Corynebacterium diphtheriae* (p. 157)

Corynebacterium ulcerans (p. 160)

Coxiella burnetii (p. 263)

Ehrlichia species (p. 262)

Enterobacter species (p. 189)

Ⓢ *Enterococcus faecium* (p. 154)

Ⓢ *Enterococcus fecalis* (p. 154)

Erysipelothrix rhusopathiae (p. 163)

Ⓢ *Escherichia coli* (p. 175)

Ⓢ *Francisella tularensis* (p. 202)

Fusobacterium (p. 219)

Ⓢ *Haemophilus influenzae* (p. 191)

Ⓢ *Helicobacter pylori* (p. 187)

Klebsiella oxytoca (p. 186)

Ⓢ *Klebsiella pneumoniae* (p. 189)

Lactobacillus species (p. 163)

Ⓢ *Legionella pneumophila* (p. 196)

Leptospira interrogans (p. 227)

Ⓢ *Listeria monocytogenes* (p. 162)

Moraxella catarrhalis (p. 173)

Mycobacterium avium-intracellulare (p. 254)

Mycobacterium bovis (p. 253)

Mycobacterium kansasii (p. 254)

Ⓢ *Mycobacterium leprae* (p. 255)

Ⓢ *Mycobacterium tuberculosis* (p. 246)

Mycoplasma hominis (p. 232)

Mycoplasma incognitus (p. 232)

Ⓢ *Mycoplasma pneumoniae* (p. 230)

Ⓢ *Neisseria gonorrhoeae* (p. 165)

Ⓢ *Neisseria meningitidis* (p. 168)

Nocardia asteroides (p. 257)

Nocardia brasiliensis (p. 257)

Pasteurella multocida (p. 204)

Peptostreptococcus (p. 155)

Prevotella melaninogenica (p. 219)

Propionibacterium acnes (p.163)

Proteus species (p. 189)

Providencia species (p. 189)

Ⓢ *Pseudomonas aeruginosa* (p. 198)

Pseudomonas pseudomallei (p. 200)

Ⓢ *Rickettsia* species (p. 259)

Ⓢ *Salmonella typhi* (p. 179)

Ⓢ *Salmonella typhimurium* (p. 179)

Serratia marcescens (p. 189)

Shigella sonnei (p. 183)

Ⓢ *Staphylococcus aureus* (p. 138)

Ⓢ *Staphylococcus epidermidis* (p. 143)

Ⓢ *Staphylococcus saprophyticus* (p. 143)

Ⓢ *Streptococcus agalactiae* (p. 150)

Streptococcus bovis (p. 155)

Streptococcus mutans (p. 1555)

Ⓢ *Streptococcus pneumoniae* (p. 150)

Ⓢ *Streptococcus pyogenes* (p. 146)

Ⓢ *Treponema pallidum* (p. 221)

Ureaplasma urealyticum (p. 232)

Ⓢ *Vibrio cholerae* (p. 185)

Ⓢ *Vibrio parahaemolyticus* (p. 186)

Yersinia enterocolitica (p. 186)

Yersinia pestis (p. 205)

Ⓢ *Yersinia pseudo-tuberculosis* (p. 186)

Figure 37.2 (continued)

[Note: Page numbers indicate where detailed information about the organism is presented. The symbol Ⓢ indicates that the bacterium is summarized in Chapter 35.]

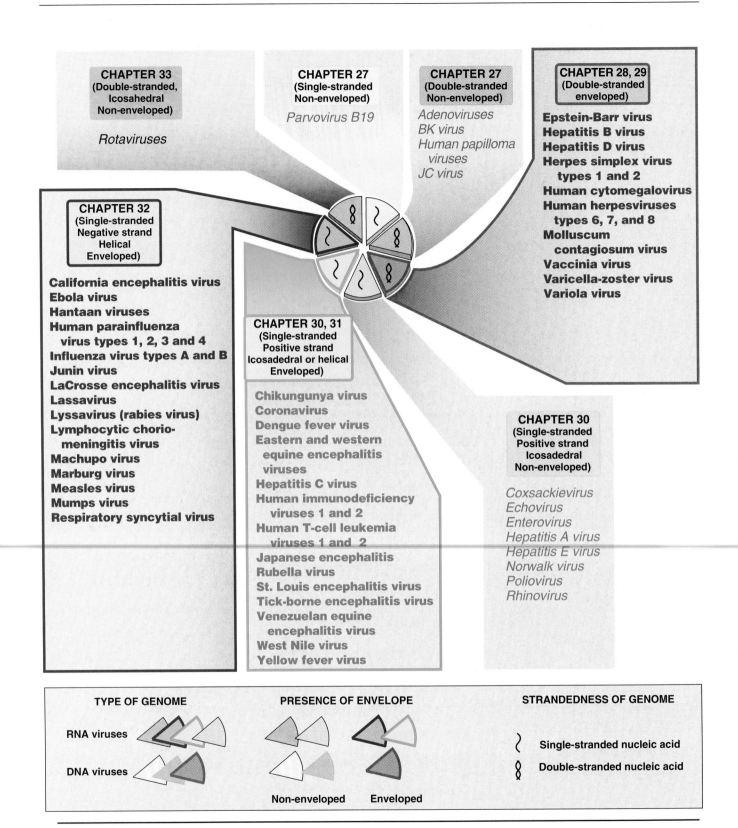

Figure 37.3
Medically important viruses discussed in this book, organized into similar groups based on the nature of the genome, symmetry of organization, and the presence or absence of a lipid envelope.

Ⓢ *Adenoviruses* (p. 312)

BK virus (p. 311)

California encephalitis virus (p. 391)

Chikungunya virus (p. 353)

Coronavirus (p. 357)

Ⓢ *Coxsackievirus* (p. 349)

Dengue fever virus (p. 354)

Eastern and western equine
   encephalitis viruses (p. 353)

Ebola virus (p. 390)

Echovirus (p. 349)

Enterovirus (p. 349)

Ⓢ **Epstein-Barr virus** (p. 331)

Hantaan viruses (p. 391)

Ⓢ *Hepatitis A virus* (p. 352)

Ⓢ **Hepatitis B virus** (p. 337)

Ⓢ **Hepatitis C virus** (p. 356)

Hepatitis D virus (p. 345)

Hepatitis E virus (p. 357)

Ⓢ **Herpes simplex virus types 1 and 2** (p. 319)

Ⓢ **Human cytomegalovirus** (p. 326)

Human herpesviruses types 6, 7 (p. 329)

Ⓢ **Human herpesviruses type 8** (p. 334)

Ⓢ **Human immunodeficiency viruses 1 and 2** (p. 359)

Ⓢ *Human papilloma viruses* (p. 307)

Ⓢ **Human parainfluenza
   virus types 1, 2, 3 and 4** (p. 382)

**Human T-cell leukemia
   viruses 1 and 2** (p. 376)

Ⓢ **Influenza virus types A and B** (p. 385)

Japanese encephalitis (p. 354)

JC virus (p. 311)

Junin virus (p. 391)

LaCrosse encephalitis virus (p. 391)

Lassavirus (p. 391)

Ⓢ **Lyssavirus (rabies virus)** (p. 379)

Lymphocytic choriomeningitis virus (p. 391)

Machupo virus (p. 391)

Marburg virus (p. 390)

Ⓢ **Measles virus** (p. 382)

Molluscum contagiosum virus (p. 334)

Ⓢ **Mumps virus** (p. 382)

Norwalk virus (p. 357)

Parvovirus B19 (p. 314)

Ⓢ *Poliovirus* (p. 349)

Rhinovirus (p. 352)

Ⓢ **Respiratory syncytial virus** (p. 382)

Rotaviruses (p. 393)

Ⓢ **Rubella virus** (p. 354)

St. Louis encephalitis virus (p. 354)

Tick-borne encephalitis virus (p. 354)

Vaccinia virus (p. 334)

Ⓢ **Varicella-zoster virus** (p. 324)

Variola virus (p. 334)

Venezuelan equine encephalitis virus (p. 353)

West Nile virus (p. 354)

Yellow fever virus (p. 354)

Figure 37.3 (continued)
[Note: Page numbers in parentheses indicate where detailed information about the virus is presented].
The symbol Ⓢ indicates that the virus is summarized in Chapter 35. Enveloped viruses are printed in **bold.**

	PENICILLINS	CEPHALOSPORINS	TETRACYCLINES	AMINOGLYCOSIDES
Gram (+) cocci			**Gram (+) cocci**	
Staphylococcus aureus[1]	1 Oxacillin 1 Nafcillin			
Staphylococcus epidermidis	1 Oxacillin 1 Nafcillin			
Streptococcus agalactiae	1 Penicillin G			1 An aminoglycoside[4]
Streptococcus pneumoniae	Penicillin G[5]	1 Cefotaxime 1 Ceftriaxone		
Streptococcus pyogenes	1 Penicillin G[3]			
Enterococcus species	1 Penicillin G[15]			1 An aminoglycoside[15]
Gram (+) bacilli			**Gram (+) bacilli**	
Bacillus anthracis	1 Penicillin G		1 Doxycycline	
Corynebacterium diphtheriae	2 Penicillin G			
Listeria monocytogenes	1 Ampicillin			
Gram (−) cocci			**Gram (−) cocci**	
Neisseria gonorrhoeae	Penicillin G[9]	1 Ceftriaxone		
Neisseria meningitidis	1 Penicillin G[10]	1 Cefotaxime 1 Ceftriaxone		
Enteric Gram (−) rods			**Enteric Gram (−) rods**	
Campylobacter jejuni				
Escherichia coli	1 Ampicillin[7]	1 Cefotaxime		
Helicobacter pylori			1 Tetracycline	
Salmonella typhi		1 Ceftriaxone		
Shigella sonnei	1 Ampicillin			
Other Gram (−) rods			**Other Gram (−) rods**	
Bordetella pertussis				
Brucella species			1 Doxycycline	1 Gentamicin or streptomycin
Francisella tularensis				1 Gentamicin
Haemophilus influenzae	1 Ampicillin/sulbactam[11]	1 Cefotaxime[12] 1 Ceftriaxone[12]		
Legionella pneumophila				
Pseudomonas aeruginosa	1 Antipseudomonal β-lactams[13]			1 Tobramycin
Yersonia pestis			1 Doxycycline	1 Streptomycin

Figure 37.4

Some antimicrobial agents useful in treating infections due to selected clinically important pathogens.
See pp. 462–463 for explanations of the footnotes.

MACROLIDES	FLUOROQUINOLONES	OTHER		
Gram (+) cocci		**Gram (+) cocci**		
		[2] Vancomycin[2]		
		[2] Vancomycin[2]		
[2] Clarithromycin or Azithromycin[8]				
		[2] Vancomycin[6]		
[■] Clarithromycin or Azithromycin[8]				
		[2] Vancomycin[16]	[2] Quinupristin + dalfopristin[17]	[2] Linezolid[18]
Gram (+) bacilli		**Gram (+) bacilli**		
	[1] Ciprofloxacin			
[1] Erythromycin				
		[1] Trimethoprim/ sulfamethoxazole		
Gram (–) cocci		**Gram (–) cocci**		
Enteric Gram (–) rods		**Enteric Gram (–) rods**		
[1] Erythromycin	[2] Ciprofloxacin			
	[1] Ciprofloxacin	[1] Trimethoprim/ sulfamethoxazole		
		[1] Omeprazole[18]	[1] Metronidazole	[1] Bismuth
	[1] Ciprofloxacin			
	[1] Ciprofloxacin			
Other Gram (–) rods		**Other Gram (–) rods**		
[1] Erythromycin		[2] Trimethoprim/ sulfamethoxazole		
		[1] Trimethoprim/ sulfamethoxazole		
[1] Azithromycin	[1] Levofloxacin			

Figure 37.4 (continued)

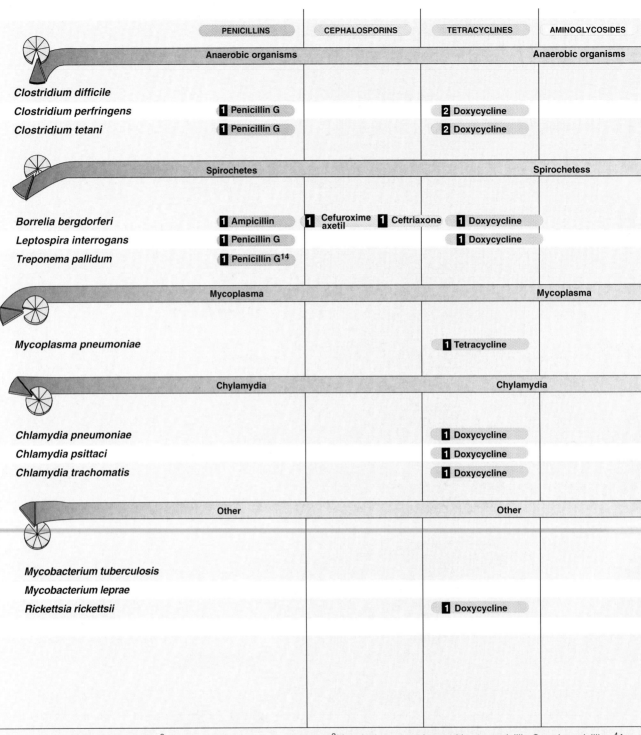

	PENICILLINS	CEPHALOSPORINS		TETRACYCLINES	AMINOGLYCOSIDES
Anaerobic organisms					**Anaerobic organisms**
Clostridium difficile					
Clostridium perfringens	1 Penicillin G			2 Doxycycline	
Clostridium tetani	1 Penicillin G			2 Doxycycline	
Spirochetes					**Spirochetess**
Borrelia bergdorferi	1 Ampicillin	1 Cefuroxime axetil	1 Ceftriaxone	1 Doxycycline	
Leptospira interrogans	1 Penicillin G			1 Doxycycline	
Treponema pallidum	1 Penicillin G[14]				
Mycoplasma					**Mycoplasma**
Mycoplasma pneumoniae				1 Tetracycline	
Chylamydia					**Chylamydia**
Chlamydia pneumoniae				1 Doxycycline	
Chlamydia psittaci				1 Doxycycline	
Chlamydia trachomatis				1 Doxycycline	
Other					**Other**
Mycobacterium tuberculosis					
Mycobacterium leprae					
Rickettsia rickettsii				1 Doxycycline	

[1]Most isolates resistant to penicillin. [2]Used in methicillin-resistant isolates. [3]Most isolates remain sensitive to penicillin G and ampicillin. [4]An aminoglycoside is added to therapy in life-threatehing infections. [5]Penicillin G has been the drug of choice, but resistant strains are regularly seen. [6]Most resistant strains remain sensitive to vancomycin; use of this antibiotic (in combination with cefotaxime or ceftriaxone) should be reserved for the critically ill patient, for example, children with meningitis possibly caused by *S. pneumoniae*. [7]*Escherichia coli* often shows significant resistance to antimicrobial agents, particularly to ampicillin. Ampicillin/clavulanate or ampicillin/sulbactam are alternates. Sensitivity testing is an essential part of therapy.

Figure 37.4 (continued)
Some antimicrobial agents useful in treating infections due to clinically important pathogens.

MACROLIDES	FLUOROQUINOLONES	OTHER
Anaerobic organisms		**Anaerobic organisms**
		2 Vancomycin **1** Metronidazole
		1 Metronidazole
Spirochetes		**Spirochetes**
Mycoplasma		**Mycoplasma**
1 Erythromycin		
Chylamydia		**Chylamydia**
1 Azithromycin		
1 Azithromycin		
1 Azithromycin		
Other		**Other**
	1 Isoniazid **1** Rifampin **1** Pyrazinamide **1** Ethambutol or streptomycin	
	1 Dapsone **1** Rifampin **1** Clofazimine	
	1 Chloramphenicol	

[8]For penicillin-allergic patients. [9] Resistance to penicillin G is common. [10]Penicillin G has been the drug of choice, but resistant strains are increasingly common. Sensitivity testing should be performed. [11]Non-life threatening illness. [12]Meningitis, epiglottitis and other life threatening illnesses. [13]Piperacillin, ticarcillin, ticarcillin + clavulanic acid, or piperacillin + taxobactam. [14]In cases of patient sensitivity to penicillin, alternate therapy with erythromycin or tetracylines is also effective, but penicillin is by far the drug of choice. [15]Many isolates show resistance to combination therapy with β-lactam plus an aminoglycoside. [16]Many isolates show resistance to vancomycin. [17]Used to treat infection with vancomycin resistant infections.[18]Omeprazole is a proton-pump inhibitor.

Figure 37.4 (continued)

	BASE ANALOGUES	PHOSPHATE ANALOGUE	PYROPHOSPHATE ANALOGUE	OTHER
Double-stranded, enveloped DNA viruses				
Hepatitis B virus				Lamivudine + Interferon-α
Herpes simplex types 1 and 2	Acyclovir Valacyclovir Ganciclovir	Cidofovir	Foscarnet	Famciclovir Penciclovir (topical)
Human cytomegalovirus	Ganciclovir	Cidofovir	Foscarnet	
Varicella virus	Acyclovir Valacyclovir			Famciclovir

	NUCLEOSIDE REVERSE TRANSCRIPTASE INHIBITORS	NON-NUCLEOSIDE REVERSE TRANSCRIPTASE INHIBITORS	PROTEASE INHIBITORS	OTHER
Single-stranded, positive strand, enveloped RNA viruses				
Human immunodeficiency virus	Abacavir sulfate Didanosine Lamivudine Stavudine Zalcitabine Zidovudine	Delavirdine Efavirenz Nevirapine	Amprenavir Indinavir sulfate Lopinavir Nelfinavir mesylate Ritonavir Saquinavir	
Hepatitis C virus				Ribavirin + Interferon-α

	NEURAMINIDASE INHIBITORS		OTHER	
Single-stranded, negative strand, enveloped RNA viruses				
Influenza virus types A	Oseltamivir Zanamivir		Amantadine Rimantidine	

Figure 37.5

Summary of therapeutic applications of selected antiviral agents.

Illustrated Case Studies

38

I. OVERVIEW

These extended case studies complement the basic information presented in Chapters 1 to 34. They reinforce basic principles of clinical microbiology, such as the role of a Gram stain, and the patient's history in instituting effective antimicrobial therapy—concepts useful in answering examination questions, and in the clinics. Most of the cases provide clinical information obtained from a single patient; a few cases describe a composite of typical features derived from several patients.

Case 1: Man with necrosis of the great toe

This 63-year-old man with a long history of diabetes mellitus was seen in consultation because of an abrupt deterioration in his clinical status. He was admitted to the hospital for treatment of an ulcer, which had been present on his left great toe for several months. Figure 38.1 shows a typical example of perforating ulcer in a diabetic man.

Because of the inability of medical therapy (multiple courses of oral antibiotics) to resolve the ulcer, he underwent amputation of his left leg below the knee. On the first postoperative day he developed a temperature of 101°F,

and on the second postoperative day he became disoriented and his temperature reached 105.2°F. His amputation stump was mottled with many areas of purplish discoloration, and the most distal areas were quite obviously necrotic (dead). Crepitus (the sensation of displacing gas when an area is pressed with the fingers) was palpable up to his patella. An X-ray of the left lower extremity showed gas in the soft tissues, extending beyond the knee to the area of the distal femur. A Gram stain of a swab from the necrotic tissue is shown in Figure 38.2.

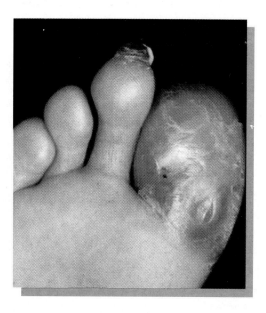

Figure 38.1
Perforating ulcer of the great toe.

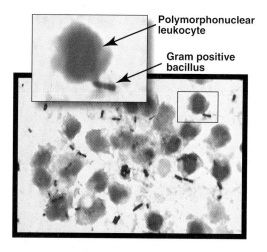

Polymorphonuclear leukocyte

Gram positive bacillus

Figure 38.2
Gram stain of material swabbed from deep within a crepitant area. There are numerous polymorphonuclear leukocytes, and many large gram-positive bacilli, as well as a few gram-negative bacilli and cocci.

Lippincott's Illustrated Reviews: Microbiology,
by William A. Strohl, Harriet Rouse, Bruce D. Fisher.
Lippincott, Williams & Wilkins, Baltimore, MD © 2001

38.1 Based on the morphology of the gram-positive organisms, their most likely identification is:

    A. *Streptococcus pyogenes.*

    B. *Escherichia coli.*

    C. *Actinomyces israelii.*

    D. *Clostridium perfringens.*

    E. *Staphylococcus aureus.*

> Correct answer = **D** (*Clostridium perfringens*), which is a rather large, gram-positive bacillus. **A** (*Streptococcus pyogenes*) cannot be correct because it is a gram-positive coccus, not a bacillus. **B** (*Escherichia coli*) is incorrect because it is a gram-negative rod, not gram-positive. **C** (*Actinomyces israelii*) is, in fact a gram-positive bacillus, but it is thin to the point of being described as filamentous, and characteristically branched, and therefore, is essentially impossible to mistake for a *Clostridium*. **E** (*Staphylococcus aureus*) is gram-positive, but a coccus, not a bacillus.

The patient was treated with massive intravenous doses of aqueous penicillin G, together with intravenous gentamicin. He underwent an above-knee amputation of his leg and, after a very stormy period of hectic fever and hypotension, he began to improve. Cultures from deep within his necrotic amputation stump grew *Clostridium perfringens* and *Pseudomonas aeruginosa*. Throughout his course his hemoglobin, which was tested repeatedly while he was very ill, remained stable.

Discussion: This patient had *Clostridium perfringens* gas gangrene, one of the dreaded complications that may follow lower extremity amputation in diabetics. Diabetics sometimes require amputation of part or all of a lower extremity because the blood supply to these limbs is reduced by accelerated atherosclerosis, which occludes blood vessels. The resulting dead or dying tissue has very low oxygen tension, which greatly favors the growth of anaerobes. *Clostridium perfringens* colonizes the area around the anus, and may extend onto the lower extremities. If the amputation is low enough it may leave behind tissue whose blood supply is compromised to the point that oxygen tension in the remaining stump favors the growth of anaerobes. The elaboration, by *Clostridium perfringens*, of large amounts of gas that are not absorbed by the tissues allows the clostridial organisms to spread along fascial planes, which are separated by the pressure of the gas as the clostridium grows. Thus the gas acts as a "virulence factor", which makes this organism quite ferocious.

The reason that the physicians were worried about the stability of the patient's hemoglobin is that another virulence factor of *Clostridium perfringens* is an exotoxin (the α-toxin) with lecithinase activity. Since red blood cell membranes are rich in lecithin, this toxin, which is secreted by the bacteria directly into the bloodstream, destroys red blood cell membranes, causing cells to lyse. Patients who die of overwhelming *Clostridium perfringens*

infection may have sufficient red blood cells destroyed so rapidly that the resulting anemia is itself fatal.

For those who might have wondered what the *Pseudomonas aeruginosa* was doing in the wound, it probably got there by being selected out by the antibiotics that the patient received prior to his surgery, during the attempts at treating his ulcer medically. Antibiotics exert great pressure on the microbial flora of the skin and bowel. Less resistant organisms on his skin and in his bowel were replaced by those, such as *Pseudomonas aeruginosa*, which could withstand many antibiotics. Anaerobic infections tend to be mixed with facultative anaerobic and aerobic bacteria, as this one was.

Case 2: Adult conjunctivitis

This 15-year-old boy was admitted because of pain and redness of his left eye, which had lasted for four days. He had always been well. Four days prior to medical evaluation he awoke with pain in his left eye, accompanied by a thick yellow discharge of the conjunctiva. He saw an ophthalmologist, who obtained a culture of the yellow discharge, and prescribed tobramycin ophthalmic antibiotic drops, which the patient began to use the same day.

The patient's eye remained severely inflamed after four days of treatment with eye drops (Figure 38.3). The conjunctiva was very swollen and injected (the blood vessels were very dilated). At a follow-up visit on the fourth day of treatment, the patient reported minimal improvement in his symptoms. The culture taken at the first visit had grown a gram-negative diplococcus that fermented only glucose.

A swab of the yellow discharge from this patient's eye would have the appearance of Figure 38.4 on Gram stain, with numerous polymorphonuclear leukocytes, several con-

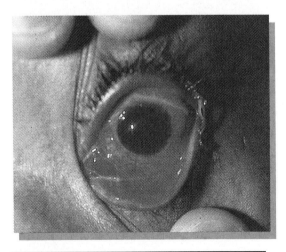

Figure 38.3
Inflamed eye of patient.

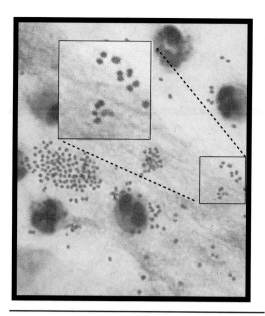

Figure 38.4
Gram-stain of discharge from eye.

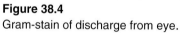

...taining kidney bean–shaped, gram-negative diplococci whose longer dimension is side-by-side with that of its mate in the pair.

38.2 Based on the morphology and fermentation characteristics of the organism that grew in the culture, the most likely etiology of this eye infection is:

A. *Escherichia coli.*

B. *Neisseria gonorrhoeae* (gonococcus).

C. *Neisseria meningitidis* (meningococcus).

D. *Streptococcus pneumoniae* (pneumococcus).

E. *Staphylococcus aureus.*

The correct answer is **B** (*Neisseria gonorrhoeae*). It is a gram-negative diplococcus whose only sugar fermentation is glucose, and it is known to cause serious ocular infections when it is placed directly in the eye (see below). **A** (*Escherichia coli*) is incorrect because *Escherichia coli*, while gram-negative, is a bacillus and not a coccus. **C** (*Neisseria meningitidis*) is not acceptable because, although it is a gram-negative diplococcus, it ferments both maltose *and* glucose, eliminating it from consideration based on the information available. **D** (*Streptococcus pneumoniae*) is wrong because it is a gram-*positive* diplococcus and not a gram-*negative* diplococcus. **E** (*Staphylococcus aureus*) is incorrect because it is a gram-*positive* coccus and is characteristically arranged in clusters, not in pairs.

The patient was treated with ceftriaxone, and his eye cleared dramatically. At the time of his second visit to the ophthalmologist he was asked whether he had had any genital symptoms. He related that he had had a purulent (full of pus) discharge from his penis for several days before the onset of his ocular symptoms. He wasn't sure whether his current female sexual partner had been having any vaginal discharge.

38.3 The most likely source from which this organism entered the patient's eye is:

A. his unwashed hands after touching a toilet seat.

B. his unwashed hands after touching his penis.

C. kissing his girlfriend's cheek.

D. a public swimming pool.

E. a dry cotton towel that he used to dry his face.

The correct answer is **B** (his penis). *Neisseria gonorrhoeae* most commonly causes urethritis (inflamed urethra) in males, and it is most probable that this patient inadvertently rubbed his eyes with his hands after contaminating them with material from his penis. **A** is unlikely because gonococci do not survive very well on inanimate objects (fomites) and, although many an unfaithful husband or boyfriend would like his partner to believe that toilet seats are good sources of acquiring gonorrhea, it just doesn't happen that way. **C** (his girlfriend's cheek) is very unlikely because facial skin is seldom involved with gonorrhea and he would have had to rub his eye directly on an infectious lesion to get *Neisseria gonorrhoeae* into it. **D** (a swimming pool) is very unlikely because of the dilution effect of the water in a pool and the probable inhibition of the growth of gonococci, which are very fastidious, by chlorine or other antibacterial substances in a public swimming pool. **E** is incorrect because *Neisseria gonorrhoeae* is very susceptible to drying and because cotton contains fatty acids that actually inhibit this organism. In fact, it is recommended that swabs which are used to obtain material for gonococcal cultures **not** be made of cotton. In addition, the environmental fragility of the gonococcus is such that it is important that specimens for gonococcal culture be transferred promptly from the patient either to the definitive culture plate or to a reliable transfer medium until they can be inoculated onto culture plates. This is especially true for a specimen taken from an eye, because other fastidious organisms, such as haemophilus species, may cause conjunctivitis that is clinically indistinguishable from that caused by *Neisseria gonorrhoeae.*

Discussion: This patient had adult gonococcal conjunctivitis. In this syndrome the gonococcus is carried from a genital discharge to the patient's own eye by his or her hands. In newborns who acquire gonococcal eye infections by passing through the uterine cervix and vagina of mothers with active gonorrhea, the syndrome is called "ophthalmia neonatorum." Topical therapy with antibiotic drops is inadequate to treat gonococcal conjunctivitis, an infection that requires therapy with a systemically administered (for example, intravenous or intramuscular) antibiotic. If proper treatment is not given, the organism may invade more deeply into the eye, causing it to rupture. If this patient's urethritis had been treated earlier, his ocular infection might have been prevented. Figure 38.5 summarizes the chronology of the case.

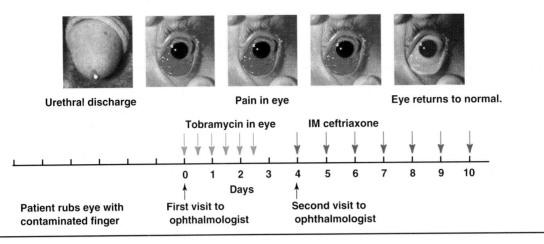

Urethral discharge   Pain in eye   Eye returns to normal.

Figure 38.5
Summary of case.

Case 3: Gas within a bulla

This 60-year-old woman was seen in consultation because of a skin lesion and fever that had been present for 24 hours. She had been in failing health for many years because of chronic active hepatitis. Recently, because of progression of liver disease, oral prednisone at a dose of 60 mg daily had been begun. The day prior to admission to the hospital she developed fever and chills, and she was admitted for intravenous antibiotics. When she arrived at the hospital, she complained of pain in her right knee and thigh.

Physical examination revealed a stuporous woman (unresponsive to verbal stimuli, barely responsive to painful stimuli). The temperature was 100°F. Remarkable findings, in addition to her mental status, included edema of the right thigh and leg, and areas of erythema (redness due to tiny dilated blood vessels in the skin) of both thighs and legs. On the medial aspect of the right lower extremity, proximal and distal to the knee, there was an area of purpura (hemorrhage into the skin, Figure 38.6). Within this area there were bullae (large blisters), one of which was filled with red fluid. At the top of the fluid in this bulla there floated many tiny bubbles. (Figure 38.7) There was marked asterixis of the hands (a flapping tremor indicative of metabolic encephalopathy that, in a stuporous patient, can be elicited by holding the wrists in slight extension).

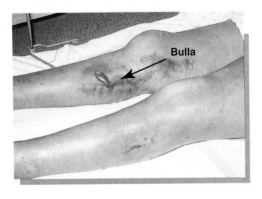

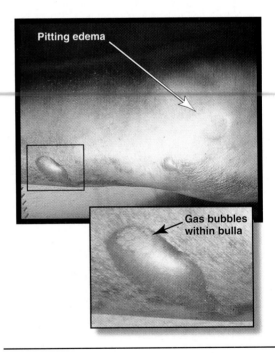

Figure 38.6
There is erythema of the thighs and legs and a patch of purpura proximal and distal to the right knee. Within the more distal purpuric area there is a bulla.

Figure 38.7
Close-up of the area in Figure 38.6, showing the bulla with bubbles above highlight from the flash. To the right in the figure is a depression caused by thumb pressure, illustrating the presence of pitting edema.

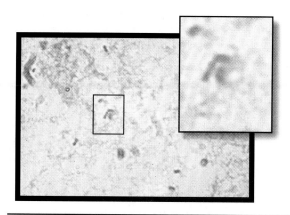

Figure 38.8
The Gram stain of the bulla fluid shows gram-negative organisms, probably rods. The shorter-appearing forms probably represent rods seen at an angle, from their ends.

Because of the presence of a cellulitis with purpura, and a bulla with cherry-red fluid and gas, a presumptive diagnosis of *Clostridium perfringens* sepsis was made, with the plan being to treat the patient with very high doses of penicillin G. However, Gram stain of the fluid aspirated from the bulla revealed the appearance seen in Figure 38.8.

38.4   The organism seen in this Gram stain is most likely to be:

    A. *Clostridium perfringens*
    B. *Streptococcus pyogenes*
    C. *Escherichia coli*
    D. *Neisseria meningitidis*
    E. *Lactobacillus casei*

> The correct answer is **C** (*Escherichia coli*), which is the only gram-negative rod on the list. **A** (*Clostridium perfringens*) is associated with gas-forming infections and bullae filled with red fluid, but it is a gram-positive rod. Skin infections due to **B** (*Streptococcus pyogenes*) may also form bullae, some even with reddish fluid. But *Streptococcus pyogenes* is a gram-positive coccus, not a gram-negative rod. **D** (*Neisseria meningitidis*) is a gram-negative organism associated with purpuric skin lesions, but it is a coccus (usually seen in pairs) and not a rod. **E** (*Lactobacillus casei*) is a gram-positive rod that is seldom involved in invasive disease.

To the surprise of the consultant, this patient did not have a clostridial infection. *Escherichia coli* alone grew from blood cultures and from the bulla fluid. It turned out to be susceptible to all the antibiotics against which it was tested, including ampicillin and gentamicin, but this information was not available for 48 hours. She was empirically treated with ampicillin, clindamycin, and gentamicin, beginning as soon as the results of the Gram stain were available. However, the morning after the initial consultation visit, in spite of treatment with two drugs effective against her *E. coli*, she died in hepatic failure.

Discussion: This patient illustrates many important clinico-microbiologic points. First, many organisms may cause similar-appearing clinical lesions, so that as much hard microbiological data as possible must be collected prior to treatment. This allows assessment of the efficacy of therapy on grounds that may go beyond clinical responses (such as reduction of fever). The Gram stain was the initial tip that, despite the clinical appearance of the lesion, this was not a gram-positive anaerobic process but a gram-negative process, allowing optimal antibiotic selection within minutes of assessment of the patient. Second, this patient reminds us that not all gas-forming infections are due to the notorious clostridial genus. Gas is produced by the metabolism of a wide variety of microorganisms of quite varied morphologies. With *E. coli*, gas does not accumulate as it does with clostridial species because the gas produced by *E. coli* is mainly carbon dioxide, which is absorbed by the tissues almost as fast as it is produced by the microorganism. Culture is necessary for speciation and to allow antibiotic susceptibility testing. Finally, the patient died even though she was treated quite promptly with the right drugs. It was reassuring to have cultures that proved the *in vitro* efficacy of her antibiotic regimen. It is probable that her underlying liver disease was so advanced that this episode of sepsis caused her to go into irreversible hepatic coma. In addition, the steroid therapy may have interfered with her ability to fight off any infection. Although her physicians were dismayed at her death, they could feel confident that she did not die because of inadequate antibiotic therapy or incorrect antibiotic choices. The appropriateness of the initial antibiotic regimen resulted from the clinical-microbiologic correlation of the lesion and the Gram stain.

Case 4: Man with a rash

This 25-year-old man was admitted to the hospital for shortness of breath, which had been present for one day. He had been well until three days before admission, in mid-June, when he developed sneezing, and a runny and stuffy nose. The next day he noted a non-productive cough. Red blotches were observed on his face the following day, at which time the patient began to complain of retro-orbital headache and feverishness. One day later there was more rash on his face, and it had spread to his arms and trunk. Progressive malaise and shortness of breath prompted hospital admission.

There had been no known tick exposure. At age three months the patient's mother was told that an illness with rash, which the patient had, was measles. He had never received a dose of measles vaccine.

38.5 The illness in the differential diagnosis that prompted the question about tick exposure is:

    A. Dengue fever.

    B. Measles (rubeola).

    C. German measles (rubella).

    D. Meningococcemia.

    E. Rocky Mountain spotted fever.

> The correct answer is **E** (Rocky Mountain spotted fever), which is the only tick-borne disease on this list. This patient's rash made the physician of record think of Rocky Mountain spotted fever, especially because it occurred in June, when ticks are quite active in many areas of the United States. (See below for further elaboration on this point.) **A** (Dengue fever) is, in fact, a disease carried by an arthropod vector, but the vector of dengue fever is a mosquito and not a tick. **B** (measles), **C** (German measles), and **D** (meningococcemia) are not vector-borne, but are transmitted by inhalation of contagious material that may be breathed out by an infected individual into ambient air, a simpler and rather more direct mode of transmission.

On physical examination the temperature was 100°F, the pulse 84 beats per minute, and the respirations mildly labored at a rate of 22 per minute. (Normal respiratory rate is somewhere between 14 and 18. It takes real work to breathe at 22 per minute, and this is often quite obvious when you look at a patient, for which reason the respirations are described as "labored.") The skin was warm and dry. The face was completely erythematous (red, but

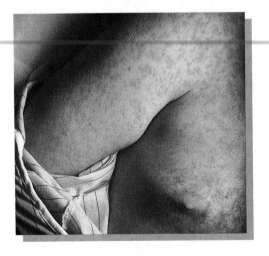

Figure 38.9
There is an extensive erythematous maculopapular rash covering the trunk and extremities. Not shown in this figure are the patient's face, on which the lesions were so confluent that his entire face was erythematous, and the back, which had many large confluent areas of erythema.

blanching upon pressure) and there was an erythematous maculopapular (flat spots and raised bumps) rash on the trunk and extremities (Figure 38.9), with large confluent areas on the back. Similar lesions were present on the palms. There were shotty (the size of shot (ammunition for a shot gun)) anterior cervical and supraclavicular lymph nodes. The conjunctivae were hyperemic (too red, from dilated blood vessels) along the outer margins of the lids. The throat was extremely hyperemic. The buccal mucosa contained several raised white spots, each the size of a grain of salt, opposite the lower molars. The chest was resonant and clear. The remainder of the physical examination was unremarkable.

The white blood cell count was 3100/µl (lower than the lower limit of normal, which in many laboratories is 4000/µl), with a differential of 70% polymorphonuclear leukocytes, 22% band forms, 7% lymphocytes, 1% monocytes. (These results are very suggestive of a viral infection.) The partial pressure of oxygen in arterial blood, with the patient breathing air enriched to make its oxygen content 24%, was 110 mm Hg (abnormally low, for such a high percentage of oxygen in inspired air at sea level). The chest film revealed interstitial infiltrates (not involving the actual alveolar spaces, but mainly the interalveolar septa) in both lower lobes.

Because of clinical suspicions raised by the history and physical examination, antibodies against rubeola virus were measured, with the following results:

Complement fixation	Hemagglutination inhibition
Hospital day three	
<1: 8	1:20
Ten days later	
1:64	1:80

Using acute and convalescent phase sera for a retrospective immunologic diagnosis, the presence of at least a fourfold rise in these antibodies is considered conclusive proof that the illness, which is clinically compatible with measles, was, in fact, measles, and not one of its late spring/early summer mimics, such as Rocky Mountain spotted fever, an enterovirus infection, or early meningococcemia.

38.6 The clinical clues that would make the consultant consider measles prominently in the differential diagnosis included all of the following EXCEPT:

    A. the pattern of spread of the rash.

    B. the presence of the white spots on the buccal mucosa.

    C. the appearance of the illness in June.

    D. the interstitial pneumonia.

    E. the relatively low total white blood cell count.

The correct answer is **C** (appearance of the illness in June). Unlike many vector-borne illnesses, measles in the United States is a disease of cooler weather, quite typically the winter. While it is not impossible to see measles in June (after all, this patient got it in June), it is not among the data that would heighten suspicion that an illness is measles. The other answers are incorrect because they are data that do heighten the suspicion of measles: **A** (the pattern of spread of the rash) is very typical of the way in which measles evolves on the skin, that is, from the face to the trunk and extremities, in contrast to Rocky Mountain spotted fever, which classically begins at the periphery (wrists and ankles) and spreads centripetally; **B** (the white spots on the buccal mucosa) were Koplik's spots, an enanthem (mucosal rash) that is felt to be pathognomonic (distinctly characteristic) of measles; **D** (interstitial pneumonia), while nonspecific, is quite compatible with an illness such as measles, which characteristically causes an interstitial "giant cell" pneumonia, interfering with the transport of oxygen across the alveolar septa into the pulmonary capillaries; **E** (the relatively low white blood cell count) is also what is expected in many viral illnesses, including measles.

Discussion: This patient had serologically proven measles at age 25. He somehow had escaped laws requiring measles immunization for entry into school, perhaps because he was thought to have had actual measles in infancy. Whether he actually had measles at age three months will never be known with certainty, but it is unlikely. Because of the very high degree of immunity to measles in adults of his mother's age, the presence of specific maternal antimeasles antibody, crossing the placenta into his circulation, should have protected him from measles for many months after his birth. On the other hand, if he did actually have measles at age three months, it is unlikely that he would have acquired durable immunity to this virus, owing to the immaturity of the immune system in so young an infant.

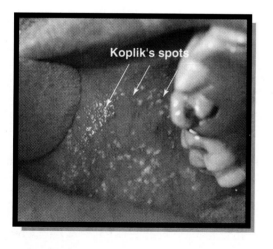

Figure 38.10
Koplik's spots.

However, this patient had Koplik's spots (Figure 38.10). In the setting of a compatible febrile illness with rash, Koplik's spots are very good evidence of measles. Serologic evidence was obtained because, at the time of his illness, in his state of residence, the measles situation was unstable, and the State Health Department was very interested in unassailable proof that a suspicious illness was, in fact, measles. Whereas viral cultures could have been obtained, serologic evidence was used to prove the etiology of this patient's illness, for reasons of convenience and cost. This is a common practice for documenting the viral etiology of diseases in the clinical setting.

This lucky patient gradually improved, and was discharged from the hospital. Many individuals with measles, especially adults and very young children, suffer severe illness with measles, often with serious immediate complications (such as bacterial pneumonia) and long-term sequelae that involve the central nervous system.

Case 5: Woman with cough

This 39-year-old woman was admitted with fever and cough, which had been present for several days. She had daily cough productive of green sputum (indicating the presence of inflammatory cells, most probably polymorphonuclear leukocytes), and was treated with inhaled bronchodilators for what was believed to be asthma. The patient had a long history of productive cough (cough yielding sputum) and in 1976, invasive studies documented bronchiectasis (a condition in which inflammation has caused permanent dilation of the walls of bronchi). She was treated with antibiotics, and had no further physician contact until 1982, when she developed pneumonia. This resolved with antibiotics.

In 1991 (two years prior to the current admission) she again developed pneumonia. Noninvasive studies, including computerized tomographic (CT) scan of the chest, confirmed bronchiectasis of the left lower lobe and lingula. The patient's physicians believed that there was also bronchiectasis elsewhere in the lungs. With antibiotics this pneumonia resolved, and for several months prior to this admission she took cefaclor, an oral second-generation cephalosporin, one out of every four weeks. This was changed to azithromycin (a macrolide with antimicrobial spectrum broader than that of erythromycin). Shortly before admission, because of increasing fever and productive cough, the antimicrobial regimen was again changed, this time to trimethoprim-sulfamethoxazole. Her symptoms became worse, and she agreed to be admitted to the hospital. There was no exposure to dusts, fumes, danders, or toxins. A parrot was the only house pet.

38.7 Pets are sometimes important sources of infection to their owners. The organism that is most closely associated with parrots is:

    A. *Pasteurella multocida.*

    B. *Mycobacterium marinum.*

    C. *Francisella tularensis.*

    D. *Chlamydia psittaci.*

    E. *Coxiella burnetii.*

> The correct answer is **D** (*Chlamydia psittaci*). This organism, which does not grow in ordinary culture media, is closely associated with many types of birds, not only the "psittacine" birds (parrots, parakeets) from which it gets its specific name. The birds need not appear ill to be capable of transmitting *C. psittaci* to humans. The other choices are all associated with animals or their environments, but not birds. **A** (*Pasteurella multocida*) is found in the mouths of animals, especially cats and dogs, and is a gram-negative rod. **B** (*Mycobacterium marinum*) is an acid-fast bacillus that infects traumatic wounds that are sustained in salt or brackish water. **C** (*Francisella tularensis*) is classically associated with handling freshly killed rabbits, although it has also been acquired from other mammals. **E** (*Coxiella burnetii*) is categorized with the *Rickettsiae* and causes Q fever, an infection that may occur after exposure to livestock (for example, parturient sheep).

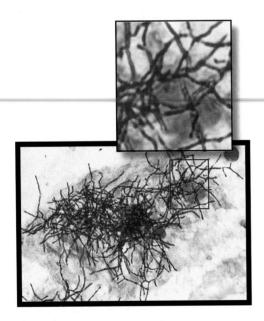

Figure 38.11
Gram stain of sputum shows many filamentous, branched gram-positive rods. Their fine caliber and the prominent presence of branching are important distinguishing morphologic characteristics.

The patient's temperature was 103°F. She was alert and in no distress. Examination of the chest revealed it to be normally resonant throughout, with diffuse coarse wheezes (musical sounds indicating constriction of bronchi and consistent with, but not diagnostic of, asthma). There was mild clubbing of the fingers and toes (bulbous swellings of the distal digits seen in patients with a variety of chronic illnesses, especially those involving the lungs).

The chest film revealed right lower lobe pneumonia. Gram stain of expectorated sputum revealed many filamentous, branched gram-positive rods. (Figure 38.11) These failed to grow in cultures but had grown, aerobically, from sputum cultured in 1991.

38.8 From this Gram stain, the possible genera into which the organism fits include:

    A. *Candida.*

    B. *Nocardia.*

    C. *Clostridium.*

    D. *Actinomyces.*

    E. *Pseudomonas.*

> Both **B** (*Nocardia*) and **D** (*Actinomyces*) are correct answers, as both are gram-positive filamentous rods with prominent branching. Their fine, threadlike (filamentous) diameter distinguishes them immediately from the much larger fungal genera, such as **A** (*Candida*). Multiple overlapping pseudohyphae of *Candida* species may appear to be branches, but their much larger size makes their identity as fungi, and not bacteria, quite evident. **C** (*Clostridium*) is, indeed, a gram-positive rod, but it is not branched, and its width is much greater than that of *Nocardia* or *Actinomyces*. **E** (*Pseudomonas*) can't be correct for many reasons, the most important of which is that it is a gram-negative rod.

The patient was treated with high doses of trimethoprim-sulfamethoxazole, intravenously at first. It was then given orally, because of the decrease in her temperature and marked improvement in her cough. Subsequent Gram stains of her sputum showed near-disappearance of the filamentous gram-positive rods (that had been identified as *Nocardia asteroides* in 1991).

Discussion: The *Nocardia* had probably never been eradicated from her lungs in 1991, and had most likely smoldered there until it finally reached a quantity adequate to cause symptoms and radiographic changes of pneumonia. The absence of treatment effective against *Nocardia*, after resolution of the 1991 pneumonia, made this very likely to occur. Bronchiectasis made this patient's mucociliary clearance mechanisms ineffective, allowing persistence of bacteria in areas that are normally sterile. *Nocardia* may be quite tenacious under these circumstances, making it necessary to maintain this patient, probably for years, on a regimen that will at least suppress the organism to levels that do not make her ill.

It should be noted that expectorated sputum is not usually cultured for anaerobes, since there would be contamination of the sputum with mouth flora, heavy in anaerobes, on its way from lungs to collection container. Documentation of an anaerobe, such as *Actinomyces*, as the cause of a lung lesion requires that the specimen be obtained without passing through the mouth. One way to do this is to pass a needle through the chest wall, under CT scan guidance, directly into the lesion. This was never done to this patient, whose filamentous branched gram-positive rod did not grow in sputum obtained during this episode of pneumonia. It was, after all, not cultured anaerobically, so that *Actinomyces*, if present, would not have grown. But her physicians felt confident that *Nocardia* was the culprit, for two reasons: 1) *Nocardia* was what had been in her sputum previously, and 2) there was a clear response to trimethoprim-sulfamethoxazole, which would not be expected to have a significant effect on *Actinomyces*. Unfortunately, not every organism that causes disease, including *Nocardia*, will be successfully grown in cultures every time. That (and the rapid availability of the presumptive answer) is why Gram stain is such an important tool in the clinical application of microbiology.

Case 6: Woman with swollen wrist

This 25-year-old woman was admitted because of swelling and pain of her left wrist of ten days' duration. She had always been well. Twelve days before admission she was bitten on the left hand by her pet cat. Two days later she developed pain, redness, and swelling of her hand, and her physician treated her with oral cloxacillin (a penicillin derivative, active against *Staphylococcus aureus* and *Streptococcus pyogenes*, with the ability to withstand staphylococcal β-lactamase). After transient improvement

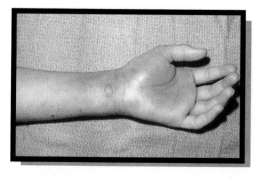

Figure 38.12
The thenar eminence is swollen and the patient is able to flex and extend her wrist and fingers only minimally, due to pain. This photo was taken just prior to removal of wrist joint fluid from a point within the circle on the volar aspect of the wrist.

in her symptoms and signs of inflammation, she became worse, so that by the time of admission she was unable to close her fingers or move her wrist. In addition, she noted evening fevers as high as 100.2°F.

On physical examination her temperature was 99.7°F. The left wrist and thenar eminence were erythematous (red, but with blanching of the redness on pressure, indicating dilation of cutaneous blood vessels—the "rubor" of the classic signs of inflammation). There was markedly reduced range of motion, both extension and flexion, of the fingers. Extension and flexion of the wrist were limited to just a few degrees. The patient's wrist and hand are shown in Figure 38.12.

The white blood cell count was 13,000/μL, with a marked increase in the percentage of immature granulocytes (the "left shift" of an acute inflammatory process). Gram stain of the wrist fluid, which was cloudy when aspirated, revealed sheets of polymorphonuclear leukocytes and many gram-negative rods (Figure 38.13).

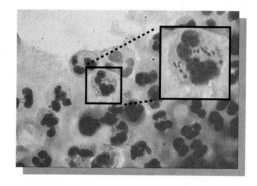

Figure 38.13
Gram stain of wrist fluid. There are innumerable ("sheets") polymorphonuclear leukocytes, and many gram-negative rods.

38.9 From among the following, the gram-negative rod that is most commonly associated with cat bites is:

    A. *Pasteurella multocida*.

    B. *Bartonella henselae*.

    C. *Streptobacillus moniliformis*.

    D. *Streptococcus pyogenes*.

    E. *Lactobacillus casei*.

The correct answer is **A** (*Pasteurella multocida*), a gram-negative rod that frequents the mouths of some animals, particularly cats, but also dogs. The extreme sharpness of feline teeth causes enormous pressure at the site of the puncture during a bite, allowing inoculation of the organism deep into tissues. **B** (*Bartonella henselae*) is incorrect, although it is a gram-negative rod associated with exposure to cats. In immunocompetent hosts, the principal condition caused by this organism, which is carried mainly on the paws of cats, is cat scratch disease, whose name implies transmission by cat scratches not cat bites. **C** (*Streptobacillus moniliformis*) is also a gram-negative rod, pleomorphic, which is most commonly acquired by the bite or scratch of rats or mice. While it may be carried—and transmitted—by carnivores that prey on these rodents, it is less characteristically associated with cat-induced injuries than with rat or mouse exposure. The simplest reason that **D** (*Streptococcus pyogenes*) is wrong is that it is a gram-positive coccus, not a gram-negative rod. Likewise, **E** (*Lactobacillus casei*) cannot be a correct answer because it is a gram-positive rod, and not gram-negative.

Culture of the wrist joint fluid yielded *Pasteurella multocida* and *Pseudomonas aeruginosa*. The patient underwent open debridement of her wrist, which showed extensive damage of the joint space and tendons in the vicinity of the joint space. With intravenous penicillin G (aimed at the *Pasteurella multocida*) and gentamicin (aimed at the *Pseudomonas aeruginosa*), together with intensive physical therapy, she had complete recovery of flexion and extension of her wrist and fingers.

Discussion: *Pasteurella multocida* is a notorious cause of infection induced by animal bites, especially those of cats. It has a propensity to invade osteoarticular tissues, which are often very near to the point at which the animal bites. Serious illness has occurred in newborns who have been licked by the family cat, presumably due to inoculation of *Pasteurella multocida* onto the infant, and invasion of the bloodstream because of the immaturity of the neonatal immune system. It is important to make the clinical association of animals and *Pasteurella multocida*, since this organism is resistant to a number of antibiotics, yet sensitive to penicillin G, which ordinarily would not be used to treat infection due to most gram-negative rods.

Case 7: Man with endophthalmitis

This 66-year-old man with non–insulin-dependent diabetes mellitus had been feeling well until one week earlier. At that time he noted the sudden onset of shaking chills lasting about 20 minutes, associated with low back pain that radiated into the medial aspect of both thighs. These episodes occurred several times over the next few days. About two days after the onset of these chills he developed pain, swelling, and erythema (redness that blanches with pressure, due to dilation of superficial blood vessels as part of the inflammatory response (rubor)) of his left hand. The next day he noted a "black spot" obscuring his vision on his right eye, progressing over the next day to complete loss of vision in his right eye. His ophthalmologist found a hypopyon (collection of pus in the anterior chamber) and treated him with a subconjunctival injection of gentamicin (an aminoglycoside antibiotic) 80 mg, methylprednisolone (a glucocorticoid anti-inflammatory agent) 40 mg, topical gentamicin, and atropine (an anticholinergic to keep the pupil dilated) eye drops. The patient's diabetes had been well controlled with chlorpropamide (a sulfonylurea oral

hypoglycemic agent) and diet. There was no history of trauma to the eye.

The pain in his back and his left hand became worse the next day, and the following day, because the hypopyon was much worse, the ophthalmologist admitted the patient to the hospital. The anterior chamber was opaque (Figure 38.14) and the intraocular pressure was increased.

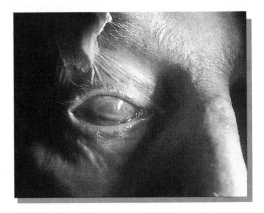

Figure 38.14
The patient's right eye at the time of admission to the hospital. The cornea is cloudy and there is a collection of white blood cells (hypopyon) behind it in the anterior chamber.

Physical examination revealed the temperature to be 97.8°F, the pulse regular at 90 beats per minute, and the blood pressure 160/90 mm Hg. The cornea of the right eye was opaque, with a dense hypopyon along its lower half. The retina could not be visualized behind this hypopyon. The left hand revealed erythema, swelling, warmth, tenderness, and very decreased range of motion of the third, fourth, and fifth metacarpo-phalangeal (MCP) joints (Figure 38.15). There was a small, healing laceration of the left shin.

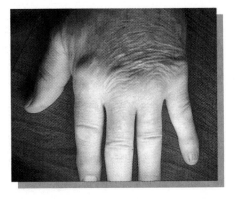

Figure 38.15
The patient's left hand at the time of admission to the hospital. The lateral three MCP joints are swollen, with erythema especially visible over the fourth MCP joint.

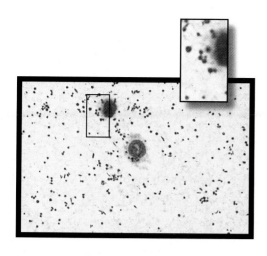

Figure 38.16

Gram stain of the anterior chamber fluid taken at the time of admission to the hospital. There are polymorphonuclear leukocytes and many gram-positive cocci, some distorted to an elongated shape.

The white blood cell (WBC) count was 16,500/μl (normal 5,000 to 10,000), with 78% polymorphonuclear leukocytes, 20% band forms, and 2 lymphocytes (a "left shift" toward immature granulocytes, consistent with an acute inflammatory process). Gram stain of fluid aspirated from the anterior chamber of the right eye (Figure 38.16) revealed many polymorphonuclear leukocytes and large numbers of gram-positive cocci, some irregular in shape (a reflection of partial efficacy of the injected gentamicin, which was injuring these organisms without killing them). Blood cultures taken at the time of hospitalization yielded gram-positive cocci in long chains (Figure 38.17) that were identified as *Streptococcus agalactiae*. The same organism grew from cultures of the anterior chamber fluid.

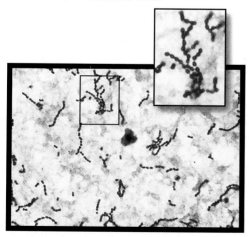

Figure 38.17

Gram stain of organisms grown from blood cultures. These are gram-positive cocci in chains, consistent with a member of the species *Streptococcus*.

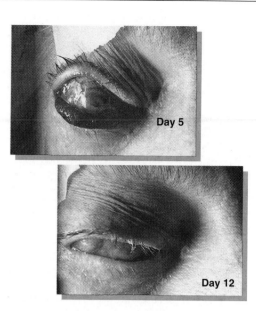

Figure 38.18

Top panel: The patient's right eye after 5 days of intravenous penicillin G, showing persistence of the hypopyon and intense chemosis (edema of the conjunctiva itself, which has swelled to the point that it is hanging over the lower eyelid). Bottom panel: The patient's right eye after 10 days of intravenous penicillin G, with resolution of the chemosis, but persistence of corneal opacification.

38.10 *Streptococcus agalactiae* is also known by its Lancefield group which is:

A. Group A

B. Group B

C. Group C

D. Group D

E. Group G

The correct answer is **B** (Group B). Since *Streptococcus agalactiae* is in Group B, all of the other choices are incorrect.

This patient went on to have a stormy course, with intense pain in his eye, where the inflammation increased for several days before it started to improve (Figure 38.18).

He was found on further study to have infective endocarditis (an infection of a heart valve, with growths of bacteria, called "vegetations," which may break off into the arterial circulation). He thus had "showers" of bacteria-laden material in his arterial tree, explaining his low back pain, the acute arthritis of his left hand, and the very active infection of his eye. The "portal of entry" of this bacterial infection was most probably the laceration of his shin. Diabetics are more likely to harbor *Streptococcus agalactiae* on their skin, especially on the lower extremities. Because his diabetes impaired his ability to contain a localized infection, he was more prone to having the bacteria that contaminated the laceration invade his bloodstream, from which some of them colonized a heart valve and, from there, further seeded tissues with end-artery circulation (eye, hand, vertebral column). He was treated with a total of six weeks of intravenous aqueous penicillin G, 4 million units every 4 hours, and he eventually got better, but the vision in his right eye was permanently lost.

Case 8: Man with fever and paraplegia

This 32-year-old man complained of fever and myalgias (muscle pain) for one week. He had always been in good health. In late July he visited a grassy area of rural New Jersey. Two days later he developed diarrhea, fever, malaise (a general feeling of not being well), and a rash. He saw a physician three days after the onset of these symptoms and, because of elevated serum transaminase levels, was told he had hepatitis. The diarrhea had stopped, and he now complained of headache, primarily frontal and retro-orbital (over and behind the eyes).

There was no travel outside New Jersey, and there was no history of injecting drug use, multiple sexual partners, or homosexual contact.

On examination he was well-developed, well-nourished, and comfortable. His temperature was 103.5°F, his pulse 120 beats per minute (a rapid heart rate consistent with his fever). The conjunctivae were injected (bloodshot), and the

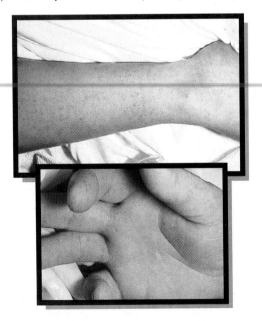

Figure 38.19

Top: The patient's ankle, showing numerous tiny cutaneous hemorrhages (petechiae). Bottom: The patient's right hand. There is edema to the extent that he cannot flex his fingers beyond the point shown in this photo.

pharynx slightly more red than normal. A diffuse, confluent, erythematous macular rash covered the back and chest (red, but blanching when pressed (erythematous) and not raised above the level of surrounding skin (macular)). The liver was slightly enlarged, with a total span measuring 13 cm. Its edge was tender (painful to the touch of the examiner). The muscles of the patient's arms and legs were also tender. Numerous petechiae were present on the extremities, as shown in Figure 38.19. His hands were edematous, preventing him from closing them into a fist (see Figure 38.19).

The hemoglobin was 13.4 g/dl (slightly less than the lower limit of normal of 14), the white blood cell (WBC) count 13,500/μl (normal 5,000 to 10,000), with 68% polymorphonuclear leukocytes, 20% band forms, 7% lymphocytes, and 5% monocytes. (A high total WBC with increased percentage of immature granulocytes indicates an acute inflammatory process.) The platelet count was 91,000/μl (normal 140,000 to 400,000). Serum aspartate aminotransferase (AST) was 273 (normal up to 40), and serum alanine aminotransferase (ALT) was 198 (normal up to 45). (The abnormal transaminases are consistent with an inflammatory process of the liver.) The chest film was normal. Blood cultures drawn at the time of admission to the hospital were ultimately sterile.

Because of the season during which this illness occurred, and because of its involvement of several systems (skin, muscles, liver, alimentary canal), the physicians caring for this man suspected Rocky Mountain spotted fever and began therapy with doxycycline (a long-acting tetracycline). One day after institution of this treatment, he became paraplegic and stuporous, recovering, with physical therapy, over the next several weeks. The doxycycline was continued for a total of ten days.

38.11 The diagnosis of Rocky Mountain spotted fever is ordinarily confirmed by which of the following tests:

    A. blood cultures.

    B. Weil-Felix ("febrile") agglutinins.

    C. antibodies against *Rickettsia rickettsii*.

    D. antibodies against *Rickettsia prowazekii*.

    E. antibodies against *Salmonella typhi*.

The correct answer is **C** (antibodies against *Rickettsia rickettsii*). *R. rickettsii* is the microbial etiology of Rocky Mountain spotted fever. **A** (blood cultures) is incorrect. In clinical practice, because rickettsiae are obligate intracellular pathogens, ordinary liquid blood culture media, which are cell-free, cannot support their growth. In addition, laboratory accidents that have resulted in aerosolization of rickettsial cultures have caused fatalities, and most clinical laboratories are unwilling to work with these organisms in culture. **B** (Weil-Felix ("febrile") agglutinins), which are antibodies directed against Proteus OX-19 and OX-2 antigens, are not specific enough, cross-reacting with antigens of other rickettsial species. Thus B is wrong.

D (antibodies against *Rickettsia prowazekii*) is not correct because *R. prowazekii* is the etiology of epidemic typhus, not Rocky Mountain spotted fever. **E** (antibodies against *Salmonella typhi*) is incorrect because *S. typhi* is one of the etiologies of enteric fever, not Rocky Mountain spotted fever. The name "typhoid" fever may make one think about a possible relationship to a rickettsia species that causes "typhus" but the two should never be confused.

Complement-fixing antibody titers against *Rickettsia rickettsii* were positive at a dilution of 1:32 on day 10 of illness and 1:128 three weeks later. This four-fold rise in specific antibody confirms that the illness that this young man suffered was Rocky Mountain spotted fever.

Discussion: There is much about this patient's story that is very typical of Rocky Mountain spotted fever, and therefore very instructive. He became ill at the height of the summer, when ticks are most active. He spent time in a grassy area of a state which is well within the range of *Dermacentor variabilis*, the dog tick, which is a competent vector of *R. rickettsii*. The cell that *R. rickettsii* infects is the vascular endothelial lining cell. Thus it makes sense that Rocky Mountain spotted fever involves many different organ systems (which all have a blood supply), and causes the kind of leakiness of blood vessels that leads to edema and petechial hemorrhages. The vascular injury, together with certain immune-mediated events, may result in disseminated intravascular coagulation, consuming platelets and leading to the low platelet count that was seen in this patient. Any tissue can be involved, but the skin and central nervous system seem to be preferred targets of *R. rickettsii*, explaining the extent of his rash and the complication of paraplegia.

The onset of paraplegia after appropriate therapy was begun warrants special comment. In addition to causing blood vessels to leak, vasculitis may also result in occlusion of blood vessels. It is probable that, prior to the administration of the doxycycline, infection of this patient's spinal cord vessels had progressed to the point that spinal cord ischemia (impaired blood supply) was inevitable, causing injury and even death of enough motor neurons to lead to paraplegia. One of the reasons that Rocky Mountain spotted fever is such a frightening disease is its potential to cause infarction of tissue.

Case 9: Woman with fever

This 28-year-old woman developed fever the day after the birth of her second child. She had always been well and had emigrated to the United States from India seven years earlier. Her first pregnancy, four years later, resulted in a healthy baby girl, who was well at home throughout the patient's second pregnancy. The patient was admitted to the hospital in active labor at the term (that is, after the full nine months) of her second pregnancy. Vaginal examination revealed amniotic fluid stained with meconium, and so the patient was taken to the operating room for emergency cesarean section. (Meconium is fetal feces, and when it is present in the amniotic fluid prior to birth, it indicates that the baby is in enough distress to warrant quick delivery.) Prior to the administration of anesthesia, labor had progressed to the point that a healthy, full-term female infant was delivered vaginally.

The mother developed a temperature of 102°F on the first postpartum (after delivery) day. She was treated with oral ampicillin 500 mg every 6 hours. Temperature maxima of 101 to 102°F continued. She complained of mild headache and a sense of chilliness each evening, when her temperature reached its maximum. (This is not unusual in patients with fever.)

Further questioning at the time of the consultant's visit indicated that the patient is a vegetarian and had, during the week prior to parturition, consumed several meals consisting of pizza with extra Mexican-style cheese. Her three-year-old daughter had had otitis media (a middle ear infection) two weeks before the patient went into labor, but was well at home at the time the patient was admitted to the obstetric unit.

Physical examination done in the early afternoon of the third postpartum day revealed an alert woman in no distress. The temperature was 99°F. The general physical examination was within normal limits. The uterus was enlarged as expected following a delivery. The lochia (the normal bloody vaginal discharge that follows the birth of a baby) was normal in amount and appearance and did not have a foul smell.

The blood count was within normal limits, as was the chest film. Blood cultures, taken at the onset of fever, yielded a gram-positive bacillus, morphologically identical to that shown in Figure 38.20. Aerobic subculture on blood agar yielded colonies that were β-hemolytic. Further subculture revealed the organism to be motile.

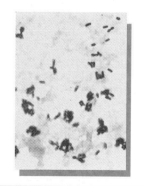

Figure 38.20
Gram stain of blood culture shows gram-positive diphtheroid-like rods, many of which are at angles to one another. The material in the background is debris from the red cells in the blood inoculated into the liquid blood culture medium.

38.12 The most likely etiology of this patient's bacteremia is:

    A. *Streptococcus pyogenes.*

    B. *Escherichia coli.*

    C. *Propionibacterium acnes.*

    D. *Clostridium perfringens.*

    E. *Listeria monocytogenes.*

> The correct answer is **E** (*Listeria monocytogenes*). It is a gram-positive rod that may easily be mistaken for a diphtheroid. However, its β hemolysis and motility distinguish it from diphtheroids, which are much less likely to be hemolytic, and are nonmotile. Whereas **A** (*Streptococcus pyogenes*) and **B** (*Escherichia coli*) may cause postpartum bacteremia, both are incorrect answers to the question, because *Streptococcus pyogenes* is a gram-positive *coccus* and not a bacillus and *Escherichia coli*, while a bacillus, is gram-*negative* and not gram-positive. Although **D** (*Clostridium perfringens*) is a gram-positive bacillus, it is a wrong answer because it is anaerobic, and would be most unlikely to grow in aerobic subculture. The absence of a foul smell from the lochia, while not entirely ruling out anaerobic infection, lessens the probability that anaerobes are present.

The organism that grew from the cultures was *Listeria monocytogenes*. Ampicillin was continued, but the route was changed from oral to intravenous, and the dose raised to 3 g every 6 hours. (The reason is that high blood levels of ampicillin are required to eradicate a bacteremia due to an organism susceptible to this drug. Such high blood levels could not be achieved with oral administration of ampicillin.) Fever resolved rapidly, and the remainder of the postpartum course was uneventful for the patient. However, her baby became quite ill on its second day of life, and had to be transferred to a neonatal intensive care unit, requiring assisted ventilation for several days. Blood cultures from the baby grew out the same gram-positive bacillus. After much intensive care and many days of antibiotics, the baby also recovered.

Discussion: This patient had perinatal listeriosis. *Listeria monocytogenes* is an especially important pathogen among immunocompromised individuals, pregnant women, and newborns. The portal by which *Listeria monocytogenes* entered the mother's bloodstream was shown by cultures of her lochia to be her genital tract. It is probably from there that it entered the baby as well. The most likely source from which she acquired *Listeria monocytogenes* was the cheese on her pizza. While *Listeria monocytogenes* is present in a number of different foods, dairy products are among the most important sources of food-borne listeriosis. The association is so strong that pregnant women, especially in the third trimester, and immunocompromised individuals are advised not to eat soft cheeses. Because of its superficial resemblance to commensal diphtheroids, it is easy to miss *Listeria monocytogenes* in cultures. The combination of β-hemolysis and the motility it exhibits in special agar tubes when cultured at 20 to 25°C serve to distinguish this important pathogen from nonpathogenic look-alikes, allowing appropriate treatment of patients and rewarding vigilance in the clinical laboratory.

Case 10: Man in coma

This 52-year-old man was found unresponsive at home on the day of admission. He had had a long history of alcoholism, complicated by a seizure disorder. For several days prior to admission he had been drinking heavily. He was found by relatives at home, unresponsive, with continuous epileptiform movements. (He did not regain consciousness between seizures.) In the Emergency Room his temperature was 105°F. His neck was stiff. Chest examination suggested pneumonia involving the upper and middle lobes of the right lung. A chest X-ray was taken (Figure 38.21). There was no response to verbal stimuli. (He was in a coma.)

Because of the fever and unconsciousness, lumbar puncture was done promptly to examine the cerebrospinal fluid (CSF). The CSF was very cloudy. There were 561 WBC/μl (98% polymorphonuclear leukocytes (PMNs)). The protein concentration was 380 mg/dl, the glucose concentration 5 mg/dl. (These findings are typical for acute bacterial meningitis.)

38.13 The test that will yield the most rapidly available information about the presumptive bacterial cause of this patient's infection is:

    A. blood culture.

    B. CSF culture.

    C. CSF Gram stain.

    D. urine culture.

    E. sputum Gram stain.

> The correct answer is **C** (the CSF Gram stain). Although the Gram stain does not tell the exact genus and species of an organism, it narrows down the choices so that an intelligent guess regarding the probable microbial etiology is possible, considering the morphology and the overall clinical situation. Since the Gram stain takes only minutes to perform, precious time is saved in initiating therapy that is as specific as possible. **A** (blood culture) and **B** (CSF culture) are both wrong answers because of the time required for visible growth to appear in cultures, and the additional time required to identify organisms that do grow. Also, sometimes organisms may be so fastidious that they do not grow easily, further increasing the time it takes to identify them. **D** is wrong because the site of the clinically evident infection is not the urinary tract. **E** is wrong primarily because it may be difficult to obtain reliable sputum from an unconscious patient, resulting in unnecessary delays. Also, in patients whose infection involves the meninges, regardless of the source, defining the central nervous system process takes priority over most other diagnostic considerations and is most likely to lead to the most specific possibility because of the absence of "normal" resident flora in the CSF.

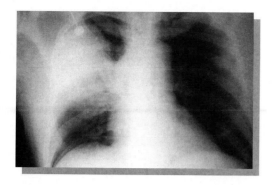

Figure 38.21
Chest film. The white areas are "liquid density" and the black areas are "air density." The central shadow represents the patient's heart. The wedge-shaped white areas on the left are the radiographic appearance of pneumonia involving the middle and upper lobes of the right lung.

Gram stain of the cerebrospinal fluid showed scant PMNs, and very large numbers of gram-positive cocci in pairs (Figure 38.22). The chest film confirmed pneumonia of the right upper and middle lobes. The peripheral WBC count was 4,700/ml (73 percent PMNs, 19 percent bands). (For a patient with this degree of illness due to infection, this WBC count is unusually low, and reflects his inability to mount appropriate defenses against his infection.)

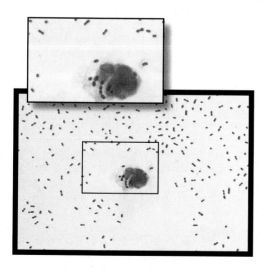

Figure 38.22
Gram stain of the sediment of this patient's cerebrospinal fluid, showing a single polymorphonuclear leukocyte and large numbers of gram-positive cocci in pairs.

38.14 In this patient with lobar pneumonia and CSF that has a heavy concentration of gram-positive cocci in pairs (diplococci), the most likely microbial etiology of his infections is:

A. *Neisseria meningitidis.*
B. *Staphylococcus haemolyticus.*
C. *Streptococcus pneumoniae.*
D. *Listeria monocytogenes.*
E. *Cryptococcus neoformans.*

The correct answer is **C** (*Streptococcus pneumoniae*), which is a gram-positive coccus that often occurs in pairs and is a notorious cause of community-acquired pneumonia, especially in heavy alcohol users. It has a propensity to invade the central nervous system, causing meningitis. **A** (*Neisseria meningitidis*) is incorrect because it is a gram-negative diplococcus, albeit an important cause of meningitis in adults. **B** (*Staphylococcus haemolyticus*) is wrong because this organism, indeed a gram-positive coccus, is not likely to be arrayed in pairs, but rather in clusters. Moreover, it is not often associated with lung infections, or with meningitis unless there is an antecedent break in the meninges, as with surgery or trauma. **D** (*Listeria monocytogenes*) is wrong because the organism is a gram-positive bacillus and not a coccus, although it is a well-known cause of meningitis, especially in heavy alcohol users. **E** (*Cryptococcus neoformans*) is wrong because, in spite of its name, it is not a coccus but a yeast, which is considerably larger than a coccus. (*Cryptococcus*, by the way, appears gram-positive in Gram stains, and can cause both pneumonia and meningitis, but you would never mistake it for a bacterium, both because of its size and because it has the morphologic property of budding.)

Penicillin (which when this patient was treated, was the drug of choice for *Streptococcus pneumoniae* infections) in very high doses was given within minutes of the lumbar puncture. The patient never regained consciousness, continuing to have seizures almost constantly for the next two days, despite aggressive anticonvulsant treatment. His heart rate slowed and his blood pressure became immeasurably low. Resuscitation attempts failed and he was pronounced dead on his third hospital day.

An α-hemolytic, gram-positive coccus, morphologically identical to the organism that was seen in the CSF Gram stain, grew from cultures of blood and CSF. It was identified as *Streptococcus pneumoniae*.

Discussion: *Streptococcus pneumoniae*, commonly known as the pneumococcus, is the most frequent cause of meningitis in adults, and usually enters the bloodstream (and from there the central nervous system) via the lungs. Occasionally, even with the most intensive supportive care and the earliest possible specific antimicrobial treatment, patients with pneumococcal infections die. This patient was at a particular disadvantage because his heavy alcohol use diminished his ability to fight many types of infection by reducing the capacity of his bone marrow to mount a response of the types of cells, polymorphonuclear leuko-

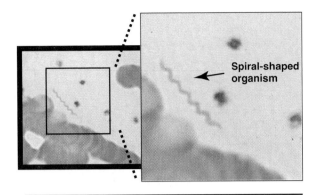

Figure 38.23

Wright stain of this patient's peripheral blood smear, revealing a spiral-shaped organism among (but not within) the circulating blood cells.

cytes, needed to engulf pneumococci and destroy them. The relatively small number of PMNs in his CSF were unable to keep up with the rapid proliferation of pneumococci in his subarachnoid space (where the CSF is located). Ordinarily, when CSF is cloudy in meningitis, it is because of a large number of PMNs in it. This patient's CSF was cloudy more from the massive numbers of pneumococci it contained. (Note: When this patient was seen, penicillin-resistant pneumococci were very rare; nowadays, empiric therapy would be vancomycin.)

Case 11: Man with recurrent fever

This 21-year-old male university student had fever intermittently for several weeks. The patient had always been well, and was a varsity football player at an East Coast university. Shortly after the end of the school year he spent six weeks in North Carolina at an encampment on a military base. During this time he recalled multiple tick bites. He personally removed a number of ticks that had been embedded in his skin. He spent the remainder of the summer at his family's home in eastern Washington, and at their summer cabin in Idaho. After several weeks in the West, he developed fever as high as 105°F, accompanied by headache, myalgias (muscle pains), arthralgias (joint pains), nausea, and occasional vomiting. After five days his symptoms abated and he felt well. Ten days after the resolution of these symptoms he had them again, but they were less severe and only lasted about two days. Ten days after the second febrile illness he had a third, similar episode that also resolved after about two days.

He returned to his university at the end of the summer, and about two weeks after his last febrile episode, he again developed fever, this time mild, and accompanied by generalized malaise. When he was examined his temperature was 98°F, and his pulse 72 beats per minute. His physical examination was completely within normal limits except that his spleen tip was palpable about 4 cm below his left costal margin with deep inspiration. His hemoglobin concentration was 12.6 g/dl (lower limit of normal 14), his white blood cell

count was normal at 4500/µl, his platelet count 135,000/µl (lower limit of normal 140,000). An incidental observation was made by the laboratory technician who examined the patient's peripheral blood smear for the blood count. What was seen is shown in Figure 38.23.

38.15 Which of the following tick-borne infections is compatible with the microbial morphology shown in Figure 38.23.

    A. Rocky Mountain spotted fever (*Rickettsia rickettsii*)

    B. Colorado tick fever (*Coltivirus*)

    C. Ehrlichiosis (*Ehrlichia* species)

    D. Relapsing fever (*Borrelia* species)

    E. Babesiosis (*Babesia microti*)

The correct answer is **D** (relapsing fever), which is caused by a spirochetal organism of the genus *Borrelia*. Spirochetes do not appear on Gram stain but those that cause relapsing fever may be seen in Wright stain smears of peripheral blood. **A** (Rocky Mountain spotted fever) is incorrect because *Rickettsiae* are not visible with ordinary stains, and they do not have the spiral morphology seen in Figure 38.23. **B** (Colorado tick fever) is a wrong answer because viruses are generally too small to be seen with light microscopy. Pathologic changes that some viruses cause (for example, inclusion bodies) are visible with light microscopy, but the virus itself is not. **C** (Ehrlichiosis) is not caused by a spirochete. The abnormality that it creates is seen in circulating leukocytes and, because of its fancied resemblance to a mulberry, is called a morula. **E** (Babesiosis) also is not caused by a spirochete. The etiologic agent, a protozoan that resembles malarial forms, may, however, be seen in Wright stain preparations of peripheral blood.

The patient was treated with doxycycline 200 mg per day for ten days. Shortly after his first dose of doxycycline he had severe fever and chills. He subsequently felt better and recovered completely. Of note is the fact that six of his family members, who also spent time at the home in Idaho, also had an illness characterized by recurrent episodes of fever and other constitutional symptoms.

Discussion: This young man had a very typical case of relapsing fever, an illness that is transmitted by lice or ticks. Ticks are responsible for endemic disease. Those ticks that transmit *Borrelia* species that cause relapsing fever prefer humid environments and altitudes of 1500 to 6000 feet. Although this patient remembered tick bites in North Carolina, it is probable that he acquired relapsing fever in Idaho, since several family members who were with him in Idaho, and not North Carolina, had a similar illness. Tick-borne disease is generally not as severe as disease spread by lice, probably because of species differences in virulence among borreliae. Slightly fewer than half the people with tick-borne relapsing fever have an enlarged spleen. The symptoms are nonspecific, although the relapsing course may suggest the diagnosis. However, other tick-borne diseases, such as malaria and babesiosis, may present with similarly nonspecific symptomatology that may occur in episodes. Several tick-borne diseases may have characteristic manifestations visible in peripheral blood smears. The need to pay attention to findings seen in peripheral blood is well illustrated by this patient.

His apparent exacerbation of symptoms with the initial treatment is also typical of relapsing fever (and a few other spirochetal diseases). Rapid lysis of spirochetes causes endotoxin release and the attendant symptoms, which may be severe, including fever, chills, hypotension, and leukopenia. This "Jarisch-Herxheimer" reaction is clinically similar to an exaggeration of the febrile episodes observed with untreated disease.

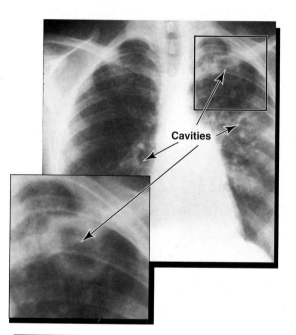

Figure 38.24
The chest film revealed infiltrates in both lungs, with two cavities in the left upper lobe and probably another in the right lung.

Case 12: Woman from Ecuador with cough

This 23-year-old woman had been having pain in her left anterior and posterior chest for one month. A native of Ecuador, the patient had been in the United States for 4 years, and had always been well. Two months prior to the current visit, she developed cough productive of whitish sputum, worse in the early morning. There was no attendant shortness of breath, and she had not noted any particular odor of the sputum. She had not had hemoptysis (the coughing up of blood). About one month after the onset of the cough, she began to have intermittent pleuritic (worse with coughing or deep breathing) left chest pain. In the one-and-one-half months leading up to the current visit, she had noted increasing fatigue and weight loss of ten pounds, but no loss of appetite. There was no history of fever or night sweats.

The patient had never injected drugs. She had had a total of two sexual partners, her last sexual contact having occurred two years earlier.

The physical examination revealed a well developed, well nourished young woman in no distress, with a temperature of 98°F, a pulse of 98 beats per minute, respiratory rate of 18 per minute, and blood pressure 102/60. There was no significant lymphadenopathy (no swollen lymph nodes). The chest revealed fine crackles in the suprascapular areas bilaterally, greater on the left than on the right. (There was probably fluid in the alveoli of the upper lobes.) The left upper lobe area was dull to percussion. (There was probably enough fluid in at least most of the alveoli in this area to cause the lungs to seem solidified ("consolidated") on the physical examination.) The remainder of the physical examination was unremarkable. The patient's chest film (Figure 38.24) shows infiltrates of both upper lobes, with at least two cavities in the left upper lobe and a probable cavity of the right lung (arrows).

38.16 Because of the history of productive cough and weight loss in a woman from South America, with cavitary pulmonary infiltrates seen on the chest film, the physicians caring for this patient suspected tuberculosis. Which of the following studies will give the most rapid presumptive support to the diagnosis of active pulmonary tuberculosis?

A. Tuberculin (PPD) skin test

B. Sputum culture for acid-fast bacilli (AFB)

C. Sputum Gram stain

D. Sputum acid-fast stain

E. Sputum assay for *Mycobacterium tuberculosis* by polymerase chain reaction (PCR)

The correct answer is **D** (sputum acid-fast stain), which takes just minutes to perform and, when positive in a compatible clinical setting (which this patient certainly provides), is very strong presumptive evidence of active tuberculosis. **A** (PPD skin test) is not correct because a positive tuberculin reaction indicates infection with tuberculosis, but not necessarily active disease. **B** (sputum culture for AFB) is incorrect because cultures may take up to 6-8 weeks to yield growth of organisms. Cultures are important to confirm the diagnosis of tuberculosis, and to provide an isolate whose susceptibility to antituberculous drugs can be tested, but sputum cultures do not contribute to rapid presumptive diagnosis. **C** (sputum Gram stain) is incorrect because tubercle bacilli (and other AFB) are not visualized with Gram stain. **E** (PCR assay of sputum) takes several hours and is not usually available in ordinary community-based clinical laboratories. When it is positive (see below) it is very helpful, but at the present time, it is not practical for use with expectorated sputum.

The physicians caring for this patient obtained sputum for AFB stain and culture. The AFB stain (Figure 38.25) showed large numbers of acid-fast bacilli, some of which had the typical beaded appearance of *Mycobacterium tuberculosis*.

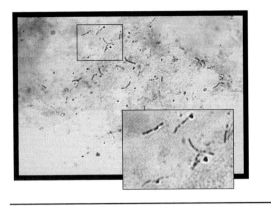

Figure 38.25
Acid-fast stain of this patient's sputum, showing many acid-fast bacilli. Beaded appearance of several of the AFB (inset) is characteristic, although not definitively diagnostic, of *Mycobacterium tuberculosis*.

38.17 The "classic" solid medium that is used to cultivate *Mycobacterium* species is:

A. Sabouraud agar.

B. Lowenstein-Jensen medium.

C. MacConkey agar.

D. Thayer-Martin medium.

E. sheep blood agar.

The correct answer is **B** (Lowenstein-Jensen medium), an egg-based solid medium that supports the growth of *Mycobacterium* species, including *M. tuberculosis*. **A** (Sabouraud agar) is used to cultivate fungi, not AFB. **C** (MacConkey agar) is a medium that is selective for gram-negative bacilli, not AFB. **D** (Thayer-Martin medium) is chocolate agar to which certain antibiotics have been added, and is a medium selective for *Neisseria gonorrhoeae* in specimens taken from non-sterile sites, such as genital secretions. **E** (sheep blood agar) is a general-purpose medium for bacteria that does not support the growth of *Mycobacteria*.

This patient's sputum was cultured in a liquid medium that produced fluorescence in the presence of actively respiring *Mycobacteria*, allowing growth to be detected in nine days. The presence of *Mycobacterium tuberculosis* in this culture was confirmed by DNA probe. The organism was later found to be susceptible to all antituberculous medications tested. On the basis of the positive AFB stain of her sputum, the patient was treated with isoniazid, rifampin, pyrazinamide, and ethambutol. She gained weight and stopped coughing shortly after the onset of treatment. She continued to respond very well to her treatment. Laboratory studies later confirmed that she was **not** co-infected with human immunodeficiency virus (HIV).

Discussion: One could hardly ask for a more classical presentation of pulmonary tuberculosis. The patient comes from an area of high endemicity for tuberculosis, and the constellation of weight loss, productive cough, and cavitary pulmonary infiltrates is extremely characteristic of tuberculosis. (Note: If she had had fever and night sweats, her presentation would have been "classic.") Although it is possible that she acquired tuberculosis after coming to the United States, it is likely that her active disease represents recrudescence (reactivation) of an infection that she acquired many years earlier. Sound cell-mediated immunity (CMI) has been found to be of great importance in containing tuberculous infection. It is not surprising, therefore, that tuberculosis is one of the infections that is especially severe in patients whose CMI is impaired by HIV infection. The association between active TB and HIV disease is so strong that the presence of active TB is felt to be a reason to look for concomitant HIV infection. That is why this patient was tested for HIV.

Case 13: Woman with headache

This 68-year-old, right-handed woman was admitted to the hospital because of headaches that began about one month earlier.

She was in good general health. About one month prior to admission she developed progressively severe headaches and vertigo (a sensation that her environment was spinning around her). Shortly after the onset of these complaints, she noted photophobia (discomfort from light, to the extent that room lighting caused her eyes to hurt). The photophobia increased to the point that she had to wear sunglasses to cope with Christmas tree lights indoors. She was observed by her family to become increasingly lethargic (drowsy) and forgetful, prompting her hospitalization.

Physical examination revealed a lethargic woman who was oriented to person and place but not to time. (She knew her name and where she was, but not the month or the year or that Christmas and New Year's Day had just passed.) The temperature was 98.9°F. There was moderate resistance to anterior flexion of her neck beyond 60°. The lungs had crackles at both bases (consistent, in this instance, with findings described below in the chest X-ray). Neurologic examination revealed pain when her straightened legs were raised beyond 45° (evidence, with the resistance to neck flexion, that there was at least moderate inflammation of the meninges). In addition, when reaching for objects with her hands, she consistently over-reached and missed them ("past-pointing," indicative of cerebellar dysfunction). This latter finding was worse on the left than on the right.

Computerized tomography of the head revealed only mild cerebral atrophy (shrinkage—probably age-related). Because of the signs of meningeal irritation, a lumbar puncture was performed shortly after admission to the hospital.

The peripheral white blood cell count was 11,800/μl (normal between 5000 and 10,000), with 83 percent polymorphonuclear leukocytes, 9 percent band forms, 4 percent lymphocytes, and 4 percent monocytes (a slight increase in immature granulocytes, suggesting an acute inflammatory process somewhere within the patient). The chest X-ray revealed diffuse interstitial infiltrates of both lower lobes (that is, increased fluid in the septa separating very minute air spaces).

The cerebrospinal fluid (CSF) obtained during the lumbar puncture was clear and colorless, with a total white blood cell count of 18/μl (normal up to 4), with 75 percent polymorphonuclear leukocytes and 25 percent lymphocytes. (Polymorphonuclear leukocytes are never normally present in CSF.) The CSF glucose was 28 mg/dl with simultaneous blood glucose of 119 mg/dl. (The blood glucose was within normal limits; but CSF glucose considerably less than 50 percent of blood glucose suggests that a viable microorganism is present in the subarachnoid space.) The CSF protein concentration was 58 mg/dl (very slightly above the upper limit of normal for this patient's age).

While performing the white blood cell count on the CSF, an alert laboratory technician observed structures that did not resemble white blood cells. A sample of CSF was centrifuged and the sediment resuspended in India ink. Under the microscope, in dramatic relief among the India ink particles, were the organisms shown in Figure 38.26.

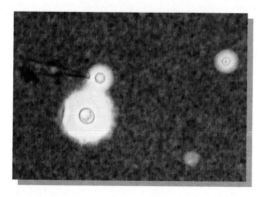

Figure 38.26
India ink preparation of CSF. A cell and its clear zone appears to be separating from a larger, similar cell. This process, called "budding," is characteristic of yeast cells. The clear zone surrounding the cells is actually a polysaccharide capsule displacing the India ink particles.

38.18   The most likely etiology of this patient's meningitis is:

    A. *Streptococcus pneumoniae.*

    B. *Candida albicans.*

    C. *Histoplasma capsulatum.*

    D. *Clostridium perfringens.*

    E. *Cryptococcus neoformans.*

The correct answer is **E** (*Cryptococcus neoformans*). It is a yeast that reproduces by budding and is characterized by a polysaccharide capsule. The presence of the polysaccharide capsule is very helpful for rapid diagnosis in microscopic examination of clinical specimens such as CSF. The capsule may appear gram-negative, and the yeast cell itself gram-positive, in Gram stains. But India ink very dramatically brings the capsule into view under the microscope. **A** (*Streptococcus pneumoniae*) is incorrect because, being a bacterium, it is much smaller than yeast and it does not manifest budding. *S. pneumoniae* progeny are the same size as its parent cell. It also does not display its polysaccharide capsule in ordinary preparations. **B** (*Candida albicans*) is a yeast that manifests budding but it is not encapsulated. Hence this cannot be a correct answer. **C** (*Histoplasma capsulatum*) is incorrect for the same reason—it does not display a polysaccharide capsule in clinical specimens. **D** (*Clostridium perfringens*) is incorrect because, while larger in size than many bacteria, it is still much smaller than a yeast cell. Also, clostridia are not encapsulated and are not round, as are yeast cells.

The organism that grew from cultures of CSF and blood was *Cryptococcus neoformans*. Despite very aggressive therapy with amphotericin B, both intravenously and instilled directly into a lateral cerebral ventricle, the patient followed a relentless downhill course and died on the eighth day of treatment. Autopsy confirmed severe meningitis due to *Cryptococcus neoformans*.

Discussion: Invasive disease due to this organism is strongly suggestive of a defect in cell-mediated immunity, and its presence in this patient caused the clinicians caring for her to suspect that she had a malignant lymphoma. (This patient was treated in the early 1980s, prior to the emergence of human immunodeficiency virus (HIV) as a significant cause of severely impaired cell-mediated immunity. Moreover, she had none of the known risk factors that might lead to HIV infection.) In addition to the cryptococcal disease itself, autopsy revealed a clinically inapparent malignant lymphoma that was limited to the patient's urinary bladder and fallopian tubes.

The lymphoma did not cause this patient's death the way many cancerous tumors do, that is, by causing failure of a vital organ. Instead, the profound defect in cell-mediated immunity that accompanies lymphomas (as well as a number of other clinical entities) created in this patient a predisposition to infection with an organism whose progression she could not resist. As *Cryptococcus neoformans* often does, it attacked her central nervous system preferentially. By the time this infection created clinical symptoms of headache, photophobia, and vertigo, it had passed the point of reversibility, and caused her death.

It is characteristic of malignancies that are accompanied by an immune defect that death is the result of an overwhelming infection. By correlating the immune defect with the underlying disease, one may often anticipate the complicating infection, and intervene in time to enjoy a favorable clinical outcome. Or, as with this patient, the presence of an opportunistic infection (one that takes particular advantage of individuals with an immune compromise) may herald the clinical onset of an immune-compromising disease. It is therefore quite important to be able to match an organism with the list of illnesses associated with the corresponding immune defect.

Case 14: Hematuria in an Egyptian-born man

This 34-year-old man had always enjoyed good health. Several months before this visit he began to notice gross hematuria (he could see blood in his urine). The hematuria was unaccompanied by fever, pain, or burning on urination or by any increased sense of urgency to void. He had not had unexplained weight loss.

Born in Cairo, Egypt, he spent his childhood summers on his grandparents' farm in the Nile Delta. He recalled swimming in the Nile twice, the last time when he was in his early 20s. He finished college in Egypt and was well enough to complete military service there. His only infirmity was loss of vision in his right eye since childhood, for reasons unknown to the patient. He had not been back to Egypt since entering the United States ten years before the onset of the hematuria. He was working as a computer technician. There was no history of exposure to toxins either at work or during recreational activities.

The physical examination was completely within normal limits, except for a red opacity of the lens of the right eye, which was blind. His hemoglobin, 13.5 g/dl, was just below the lower limit of normal of 14. The rest of the laboratory studies were all normal.

Because of concern that the hematuria might herald a malignancy, the patient underwent fiberoptic cystoscopy (an examination that directly visualizes the inside of the urinary bladder). A mass was noted in the fundus of the bladder, biopsy of which is shown in Figure 38.27.

38.19 The part of the history that is most specifically connected with the diagnosis of infection with *Schistosoma haematobium* is which of the following?

  A. The presence of gross hematuria
  B. The patient's origin in Egypt
  C. Swimming in the Nile
  D. Concurrent blindness
  E. The mild anemia (hemoglobin 13.5 g/dl)

The correct answer is **C** (swimming in the Nile). *Schistosoma haematobium* is a fluke that requires a very specific snail to complete its life cycle. This snail is found only in certain bodies of water in Africa, most notably the Nile River. **A** (gross hematuria) is a symptom that results from the propensity of *S. haematobium* to invade bladder veins, where adult flukes lay their eggs. However, gross hematuria may occur with many conditions, and thus is not as specifically connected with *S. haematobium* infec-

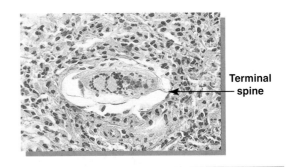

Figure 38.27
Biopsy of the urinary bladder shows areas of inflammation, within many of which are structures such as this one, an ovum with a terminal spine. The presence of this spine at the end of the ovum (a "terminal" spine) identifies the ovum as that of *Schistosoma haematobium*.

tion as is exposure to the snail vector caused by swimming in the Nile. **B** (being from Egypt) is of itself not enough to suspect schistosomiasis, since Egyptians who have not swum in water that is infested with the specific snail vector are not at risk of acquiring this parasite. **D** (blindness) is part of another parasitic infection associated with fresh water, onchocerciasis ("River blindness"). The roundworm *Onchocerca volvulus* is transmitted to humans by the bite of the black fly, which frequents the fresh water rapids of certain rivers, including some in Africa. **E** (anemia) is part of many disease processes and so is not necessarily a hint to the diagnosis of *S. haematobium* infection.

A person from the Nile Valley who has gross hematuria should be suspected of having infection with *S. haematobium* regardless of what other diagnoses may need to be entertained by the rest of the history. The fluke's life cycle illustrates why this is true. Infected humans inevitably excrete *S. haematobium* eggs in their urine, which finds its way into the water. Once thus excreted, these eggs develop into a very motile form called a miracidium that "homes in" on the intermediate host, which is a snail. In the snail, the fluke metamorphoses into a form called a cercaria, which swims freely in the water, waiting to penetrate the intact skin of a person who may be swimming or wading in this water. Once in the human, *S. haematobium* develops into adults, which migrate to the veins of the vesical plexus around the bladder. The female lays eggs, which create an inflammatory response that leads to bleeding, which is perceived by the infected individual as gross hematuria. The passage of these eggs, in urine, into water inhabited by the correct species of snail, completes the life cycle.

This patient was treated with praziquantel, a potent drug that is effective against a number of helminths, including schistosoma species. His hematuria resolved, and repeat cystoscopy revealed resolution of the infective process. He was warned not to swim in the Nile if he should return to Egypt.

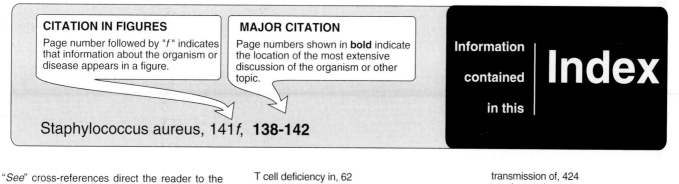

"*See*" cross-references direct the reader to the synonymous term. "*See also*" cross-references direct the reader to related topics. [Note: Positional and configurational designations in chemical names (for example, "3-", "α-", "N-", "D-") are ignored in alphabetizing.]

Figure Sources

Fig. 2.1: Peters, G., Gray, E. D., and Johnson, G. M. in Bisno, A. L. and Waldvogel, F. A. *Infections Associated with Indwelling Medical Devices.* American Society for Microbiology, 1989. Fig. 1, p. 62.

Fig. 4.1 Meridian Diagnostics, Inc, Cincinnati, Ohio.

Fig. 4.1: Forbes, B. A., Sahm, D. I. F., and Weissfeld, A. S. *Baily & Scott's Diagnostic Microbiology.* Mosby, Inc. 1988. Fig. 14-11, p. 200.

Fig. 4.4: Wistreich, G. *Microbiology Perspectives: A Photographic Survey of the Microbial World.* Prentice-Hall, Inc. 1999. Fig. 193, p. 86.

Fig. 4.6: Bottone, E. J., Girolami, R., and Stamm, J. M., *Schneierson's Atlas of Diagnostic Microbiology,* Ninth Edition, Abbott Laboratories, 1984, p. 49.

Fig. 4.7: Becton-Dickinson Microbiology Systems.

Fig. 4.8: Mahon, C. R. and Manuselis, G., *Textbook of Diagnostic Microbiology,* W. B. Saunders Company, 1995. Fig. 9-2A, p. 310.

Fig. 4.9: Alexander, S. K. and Strete, D. *Microbiology: A Photographic Atlas for the Laboratory.* Benjamin Cummings, 2001. Fig. 5.6, p. 71.

Fig. 4.9: Cappuccino, J. G. and Sherman, N., *Microbiology: A Laboratory Manual,* Fourth Edition, Benjamin/Cummings Publishing Company, Inc, 1996. Color plate 28.

Fig. 4.9: de la Maza, L. M., Pezzlo, M. T. and Baron, E. J., *Color Atlas of Diagnostic Microbiology,* Mosby, *1997.* Fig. 8-16, p. 61.

Fig. 4.9: Forbes, B. A., Sahm, D. I. F., and Weissfeld, A. S. *Baily & Scott's Diagnostic Microbiology.* Mosby, Inc. 1988. Fig. 13.8, p. 173.

Fig. 4.9: Gillies, R.R. and Dodds, T.C., *Bacteriology Illustrated,* Third Edition, Williams and Wilkins Company, 1973, p. 41.

Fig. 4.13: Forbes, B. A., Sahm, D. I. F., and Weissfeld, A. S. *Baily & Scott's Diagnostic Microbiology.* Mosby, Inc. 1988. Fig. 15-6, p. 212.

Fig. 6.7: Swartz, R. and Holmes, C. *N Engl J Med* 333:1546 (1995).

Fig. 7.6: Janeway, C.A. and Travers, P. *Immuno-Biology,* Second Edition, Garland Publishing, Inc. 1996. Fig. 1.8, p. 1:9.

Fig. 7.7: Janeway, C.A. and Travers, P. *Immuno-Biology,* Second Edition, Garland Publishing, Inc. 1996. Fig. 1.7, p. 1:8.

Fig. 8.3: Janeway, C.A. and Travers, P. *Immuno-Biology,* Second Edition, Garland Publishing, Inc. 1996. Fig. 3.1, p. 3:3.

Fig. 8.5: Janeway, C.A. and Travers, P. *Immuno-Biology,* Second Edition, Garland Publishing, Inc. 1996. Fig. 3.26, p. 3:26.

Fig. 9.15: Lim, D. *Microbiology,* Second Edition. MCB/McGraw-Hill, 1998. Fig. 3.13, p. 55.

Fig. 11.5: p. 141: Courtesy Dr. Agrégé Mohamed Denguezli, Service de dermatologie CHU Sousse Tunisie.

Fig. 11.9: Peters, G., Gray, E. D., and Johnson, G. M. in Bisno, A. L. and Waldvogel, F. A. *Infections Associated with Indwelling Medical Devices.* American Society for Microbiology, 1989. Fig. 1, p. 62.

Fig. 12.2: Gillies, R.R. and Dodds, T.C., *Bacteriology Illustrated,* Third Edition, Williams and Wilkins Company, 1973, p. 47.

Fig. 12.4: Volk, W. A., Gebhardt, B. M., Hammarskjold, M. and Kadner, R. J., *Essentials of Microbiology,* Fifth Edition, Lippincott-Raven, Philadelphia, 1996. Fig. 24-3, p.332.

Fig. 12.6: Meltzer,D. L. and Kabongo, M. *American Family Physician,* July, 1997; pp. 145, 147.

Fig. 12.13: MacFaddin, J. F. *Biochemical Tests for Identification of Medical Bacteria.* Lippincott Williams & Wilkins, 2000. Fig. 3.1, p. 806.

Fig. 12.13 Gillies, R.R. and Dodds, T.C., *Bacteriology Illustrated,* Third Edition, Williams and Wilkins Company, 1973, p. 58.

Fig. 1213: Hart, T. and Shears, P., *Color Atlas of Medical Microbiology,* Mosby-Wolfe. 1996. Fig. 123, p. 97.

Fig. 12.17: Courtesy of Dr. Joseph Kisslo, Duke University Medical Center.

Fig. 13.2: Alexander, S. K. and Strete, D. *Microbiology: A Photographic Atlas for the Laboratory.* Benjamin Cummings, 2001. Fig. 2.7, p. 13.

Fig. 13.4: Hart, T. and Shears, P., *Color Atlas of Medical Microbiology,* Mosby-Wolfe. 1996. Plate 140, p. 107.

Fig. 13.4: Courtesy Harriet C.W. Thompson, M.S., Department of Microbiology, Immunology &, Parasitology, Louisiana State University Health Sciences Center, New Orleans, LA

Fig. 13.8: Bottone, E. J., Girolami, R., and Stamm, J. M., *Schneierson's Atlas of Diagnostic Microbiology,* Ninth Edition, Abbott Laboratories, 1984, p. 5.

Fig. 13.8: Bottone, E. J., Girolami, R., and Stamm, J. M., *Schneierson's Atlas of Diagnostic Microbiology,* Ninth Edition, Abbott Laboratories, 1984, p. 5.

Fig. 13.10: Bottone, E. J., Girolami, R., and Stamm, J. M., *Schneierson's Atlas of Diagnostic Microbiology,* Ninth Edition, Abbott Laboratories, 1984, p. 7.

Fig. 13.10: Krammer, T. T. *Comparative Pathogenic Bacteriology* (Filmstrip). W. B. Saunders Company 1972. Slide 76.

Fig. 14.2: Bottone, E. J., Girolami, R., and Stamm, J. M., *Schneierson's Atlas of Diagnostic Microbiology,* Ninth Edition, Abbott Laboratories, 1984. p. 37.

Fig. 14.2: Sherris, J. C., Editor. *Medical Microbiology,* Second Edition, Appelton & Lange, 1990. Fig. 19.3, p. 349.

Fig. 14.4: Schaechter, M., Engleberg, N. C., Eisenstein, B. I., and Medoff, G. *Mechanism of Microbial Disease,* Third Edition. Williams and Wilkins, 1998. Fig. 14.6, p. 166.

Fig. 14.5: Hoeprich, P. D., Jordan, M. C. and Ronald, A. R., *Infectious Diseases, a Treatise of Infectious Processes,* Fifth Edition, J.B. Lippincott Company, Philadelphia, 1994. Fig. 70-6, p. 681.

Fig. 14.7: Bottone, E. J., Girolami, R., and Stamm, J. M., *Schneierson's Atlas of Diagnostic Microbiology,* Ninth Edition, Abbott Laboratories, 1984. p. 37.

Fig. 14.9: Images in Clinical Medicine. *N Engl J Med,* 336:707 (1997).

Fig. 14.12: Beeching, N.J. and Nye, F.J., *Diagnostic Picture Tests in Clinical Infectious Disease,* Mosby-Wolfe, 1996. Fig. 61, p. 33.

Fig. 14.17: Hart, T. and Shears, P., *Color Atlas of Medical Microbiology,* Mosby-Wolfe. 1996. Fig. 209; p. 144.

Fig. 15.7: Volk, W. A., Benjamin, D. C., Kadner, R. J. and Parsons, J. T., *Essentials of Microbiology,* Fourth Edition, J. B. Lippincott Company,1991. Fig. 16.12, p. 250.

Fig. 15.11: Koneman, E. W., Allen, S. D., Janda, W. M., Schreckenberger, P. C. and Winn, W. C., *Color Atlas and Textbook of Diagnostic Microbiology,* Fifth

Edition, J. B. Lippincott Company, 1997. Plate 6-1A.

Fig. 15.17: Volk, W. A., Gebhardt, B. M., Hammarskjold, M. and Kadner, R. J., *Essentials of Microbiology,* Fifth Edition, Lippincott-Raven, Philadelphia, 1996. Fig. 26-5, p. 373.

Fig. 15.20: Genta, R. M. and Graham, D. Y. *N Engl J Med,* 335:250, 1996.

Fig. 16.2: Musher, D. *J. Infectious Diseases,* 149:4, 4/84.

Fig. 16.4: Quintiliani, R. and Bartlett, R. C., *Examination of the Gram-Stained Smear.* Hoffman-La Roche Inc., 1994.

Fig. 16.7: NIBSC/Science Photo Library/Photo Researcher, Inc.

Fig. 16.10: Koneman, E. W., Allen, S. D., Janda, W. M., Schreckenberger, P. C. and Winn, W. C., *Color Atlas and Textbook of Diagnostic Microbiology,* Fifth Edition, J. B. Lippincott Company, Philadelphia, 1997. Plate 8-3D.

Fig. 16.12: Leboffe, M.J. and Pierce, B. E. *A Photographic Atlas for the Microbiology Laboratory.* Morton Publishing Company. 1999. Fig. 11-23, p. 132.

Fig. 16.16: Kassirer, J. P., *Images in Clinical Medicine,* Massachusetts Medical Society, 1997. p. 203.

Fig. 16.19: Leboffe, M. J. and Pierce, B. E. *A Photographic Atlas for the Microbiology Laboratory.* Morton Publishing Company. 1999. Fig. 11-7; p. 124.

Fig. 16.22: Volk, W. A., Gebhardt, B. M., Hammarskjold, M. and Kadner, R. J., *Essentials of Microbiology,* Fifth Edition, Lippincott-Raven, Philadelphia, 1996. Fig. 27-5, p 393.

Fig. 16.23: Center for Disease Control, Atlanta.

Fig. 16.25: Hart, T. and Shears, P., *Color Atlas of Medical Microbiology,* Mosby-Wolfe. 1996. Fig. 221, p. 150.

Fig. 16.25: Krammer, T. T. *Comparative Pathogenic Bacteriology* (Filmstrip). W. B. Saunders Company 1972. Slide: 34.

Fig. 16.27: Hart, T. and Shears, P., *Color Atlas of Medical Microbiology,* Mosby-Wolfe. 1996. Fig. 190, p. 133

Fig. 16.29: Wistreich, G. *Microbiology Perspectives: A Photographic Survey of the Microbial World.* Prentice-Hall, Inc. 1999. Fig. 140, p. 63.

Fig. 17.5: Stephens, M. B. *Postgraduate Medicine,* Vol 99, No. 4, April 1996. p. 218.

Fig. 17.6: Bottone, E. J., Girolami, R., and Stamm, J. M., *Schneierson's Atlas of Diagnostic Microbiology,* Ninth Edition, Abbott Laboratories, 1984. p. 9.

Fig. 17.9: Finegold, S.M., Baron, E. J. and Wexler, H. M. *A Clinical Guide to Anaerobic Infections.* Star Publishing Company, 1992. Fig. 87, p. 85.

Fig. 17.11: Finegold, S.M., Baron, E. J. and Wexler, H. M. *A Clinical Guide to Anaerobic Infections.* Star Publishing Company, 1992. Fig. 86, p. 82.

Fig. 17.12: Courtesy of Dr. Gary E. Kaiser, The Community College of Baltimore County.

Fig. 17.13: Kelly, C. P., Pothoulakis, C. and LaMont, J. T. *N Engl J Med* 330:259 (1994).

Fig. 17.17: Finegold, S.M., Baron, E. J. and Wexler, H. M. *A Clinical Guide to Anaerobic Infections.* Star Publishing Company, 1992. Fig. 133, p. 124.

Fig. 18.3: McMilan, A. and Scott, G. R. *Sexually Transmitted Diseases.* Churchill Livingstone., 1991 Fig. 63, p. 42.

Fig. 18.4: Brown, T. J., Yen-Moore, A. and Tyring, S.

K. *Journal of the American Academy of Dermatology.* Volume 41, Number 4. October 1999. Fig. 1.

Fig. 18.4: Brown, T. J., Yen-Moore, A. and Tyring, S. K. *Journal of the American Academy of Dermatology.* Volume 41, Number 4. October 1999. Fig. 4.

Fig. 18.4: McMilan, A. and Scott, G. R. *Sexually Transmitted Diseases.* Churchill Livingstone, 1991 Fig. 63, p. 42.

Fig. 18.4: Brown, T. J., Yen-Moore, A. and Tyring, S. K. *Journal of the American Academy of Dermatology.* Volume 41, Number 4. October 1999. Fig. 8,

Fig. 18.5: McMilan, A. and Scott, G. R. *Sexually Transmitted Diseases.* Churchill Livingstone., 1991. Fig. 136, p. 92.

Fig. 18.8: American Society Microbiology (Microbelibrary.org). Jeffrey Nelson, Rush University.

Fig. 18.10: Verdon, M. E., Sigal, Leonard H., *American Family Physician.* August 1997. p. 429.

Fig. 18.10: Master, E. J. *Postgraduate Medicine*, Vol 94, No1, p. 137, July 1993.

Fig. 18.15: Volk, W. A., Benjamin, D. C., Kadner, R. J. and Parsons, J. T., *Essentials of Microbiology*, Fourth Edition, J. B.Lippincott Company,1991. Fig. 31-5, p. 490.

Fig. 19.3: Volk, W. A., Benjamin, D. C., Kadner, R. J. and Parsons, J. T., *Essentials of Microbiology*, Fourth Edition, J. B.Lippincott Company,1991. Fig. 32-2, p. 296.

Fig. 19.3: Kassirer, J. P., *Images in Clinical Medicine*, Massachusetts Medical Society, 1997. p. 38.

Fig. 20.2: Cutlip, R. C., National Animal Disease Center. United States Department of Agriculture. Agricultural Research Service.

Fig. 20.5: Courtesy of Dr. Umberto Benelli, Online Atlas of Ophthalmology

Fig. 20.6(B): McMilan, A. and Scott, G. R. *Sexually Transmitted Diseases.* Churchill Livingstone, 1991. Fig. 24, p. 18.

Fig. 20.6(C): Armstrong, D. and Cohen, J., *Infectious Diseases.* Mosby 1999. Fig. 25.9. Section 8.25.6.

Fig. 20.6(D): Courtesy of Dr. Umberto Benelli, Online Atlas of Ophthalmology

Fig. 20.6(E): Brown, T. J., Yen-Moore, A. and Tyring, S. K. *Journal of the American Academy of Dermatology.* Volume 41, Number 4. October 1999. Fig. 10

Fig. 20.6F: Hoeprich, P. D., Jordan, M. C. and Ronald, A. R., *Infectious Diseases, a Treatise of Infectious Processes*, Fifth Edition, J. B. Lippincott Company, Philadelphia, 1994. Fig. 70-6, p. 681.

Fig. 20.6(G): Brown, T. J., Yen-Moore, A. and Tyring, S. K. *Journal of the American Academy of Dermatology.* Volume 41, Number 4. October 1999. Fig. 1.

Fig. 20.6(H): Brown, T. J., Yen-Moore, A. and Tyring, S. K. *Journal of the American Academy of Dermatology.* Volume 41, Number 4. October 1999. Fig. 4.

Fig. 20.6(I): Brown, T. J., Yen-Moore, A. and Tyring, S. K. *Journal of the American Academy of Dermatology.* Volume 41, Number 4. October 1999. Fig. 8.

Fig. 20.6(K): Salkind, M. R. *A Slide Atlas of Common Diseases*, Parthenon Publishing Group, 1994. Fig. 175.

Fig. 20.6(L): Salkind, M. R. *A Slide Atlas of Common Diseases*, Parthenon Publishing Group, 1994. Fig. 183.

Fig. 20.6(M): Gillies, R. R. and Dodds, T.C.,

Bacteriology Illustrated, Third Edition, Williams and Wilkins Company, Baltimore, 1973. p.198. 59.

Fig. 20.6(N): Salkind, M. R. *A Slide Atlas of Common Diseases*, Parthenon Publishing Group, 1994. Fig. 172.

Fig. 20.6(O): Brown, T. J., Yen-Moore, A. and Tyring, S. K. *Journal of the American Academy of Dermatology.* Volume 41, Number 5. November 1999. Fig. 1.

Fig. 20.6 (P): Ordoukhanian, E. and Lane, A. T., *Postgraduate Medicine*, 101, February, p. 225, 1997.

Fig. 20.6 (Q): Kassirer, J. P., *Images in Clinical Medicine*, Massachusetts Medical Society, 1997. p. 28.

Fig. 20.6 (R): Stone, D. R. and Gorbach, S. L. *Atlas of Infectious Diseases.* W. B. Saunders Company, 2000. Fig. 6-26, p. 103.

Fig. 20.6 (S): Salkind, M. R. *A Slide Atlas of Common Diseases*, Parthenon Publishing Group, 1994. Fig. 59.

Fig. 20.6 (T): Courtesy of Dr. Umberto Benelli, Online Atlas of Ophthalmology

Fig. 20.6 (U): Copyrighted image used with permission of the authors, Virtual Hospital (TM), www.vh.org

Fig. 20.6 (V): Salkind, M. R. *A Slide Atlas of Common Diseases*, Parthenon Publishing Group, 1994. Fig. 25.

Fig. 20.6(W): Stone, D. R. and Gorbach, S. L. *Atlas of Infectious Diseases.* W. B. Saunders Company, 2000. Fig. 6-4, p. 91.

Fig. 21.2: A. M. Siegelman/Visuals Unlimited.

Fig. 21.2: Alexander, S. K. and Strete, D. *Microbiology: A Photographic Atlas for the Laboratory.* Benjamin Cummings. Fig. 2.17, p. 15.

Fig. 21.3: World Health Organization.

Fig. 21.5: Center for Disease Control, Atlanta, 1999.

Fig. 21.6: Tortora G. J., Funke, B. R. and Case C. E. *Microbiology, An Introduction.* Addison Wesley Longman, Inc. 1998. Fig. 24.10, p. 639.

Fig. 21.7: Iseman, Michael D., S/M Infectious Diseases Division. National Jewish Medical Research Center.

Fig. 21.8: WebPath, courtesy of Edward C. Klatt MD, Florida State University College of Medicine

Fig. 21.10: Talaro, K. P. and Talaro, A. *Foundations in Microbiology, 3rd Edition.* WCB/McGraw-Hill, 1999. Fig. 19.19, p. 612.

Fig. 21.10: Greer, Ken/Visuals Unlimited.

Fig. 21.12: Center for Disease Control, Atlanta.

Fig. 21.16A: Courtesy of CDC/Dr. Edwin P. Ewing, Jr.

Fig. 21.16C: Hocquelourx, L., et al. *Chest*, volume 113, number 2, February 7 1998. The American College of Chest Physicians. Fig. 1.

Fig. 21.19: Binford, C.H and Connor D.H. *Pathology of Tropical and Extraordinary Diseases: An Atlas*, Washington, D.D. 1976, Armed Forces Institute of Pathology

Fig. 22.2: Volk, W. A., Gebhardt, B. M., Hammarskjold, M. and Kadner, R. J., *Essentials of Microbiology*, Fifth Edition, Lippincott-Raven, Philadelphia, 1996. Fig. 34-1, p. 459.

Fig. 22.3: Greer, Ken/Visuals Unlimited.

Fig. 23.2(A): Larone, D. H. *Medically Important Fungi. A Guide to Identification.* Third Edition. American Society for Microbiology, 1995. p. 71.

Fig. 23.2(B): Schaf, David /Peter Arnold, Inc.

Fig. 23.3(A): Champe, S. P. and Simon, L. D. Cellular Differentiation and Tissue Formation in the Fungus

Aspergillus nidulan, in *Morphogenesis*. Edited by Rossomando, E. F. and Alexander, S. Marcel Dekker, Inc. 1992. Fig. 2.

Fig. 23.3(B): Champe, S. P. and Simon, L. D. Cellular Differentiation and Tissue Formation in the Fungus Aspergillus nidulan, in *Morphogenesis*. Edited by Rossomando, E. F. and Alexander, S. Marcel Dekker, Inc. 1992. Fig. 3.

Fig. 23.4: Volk, W. A., Gebhardt, B. M., Hammarskjold, M. and Kadner, R. J., *Essentials of Microbiology*, Fifth Edition, Lippincott-Raven, Philadelphia, 1996. Fig. 35-3, p.477.

Fig. 23.5(A): Habif, Thomas p. *Clinical Dermatology, A Color Guide to Diagnosis and Therapy.* Mosby. 1996. Fig. 13-7, p. 367.

Fig. 23.5(B): Habif, Thomas p. *Clinical Dermatology, A Color Guide to Diagnosis and Therapy.* Mosby. 1996. Fig. 13-21, p. 374.

Fig. 23.5(C): Habif, Thomas p. *Clinical Dermatology, A Color Guide to Diagnosis and Therapy.* Mosby. 1996. Fig. 13-38, p. 383.

Fig. 23.5(D): Habif, T. P. *Clinical Dermatology, A Color Guide to Diagnosis and Therapy.* Mosby. 1996. Fig. 13-16, p. 371.

Fig. 23.5 (E): Mir, M. A., *Atlas of Clinical Diagnosis*, W. J. B. Saunders Company Ltd., 1995. Fig. 10.21; p. 203.

Fig. 23.6(A): *Scientific American Medicine.* August 1998.

Fig. 23.6(B): Stone, D. R. and Gorbach, S. L. *Atlas of Infectious Diseases.* W. B. Saunders Company, 2000. Fig. 7-7 p. 122.

Fig. 23.6(C): Courtesy of Victor Newcomer.

Fig. 23.7: Rubin, E. and Farber, J. L. *Pathology*, Second Edition. J. B. Lippincott Company, 1994. Fig. 9-60, p. 419.

Fig. 23.8(A): Rubin, E. and Farber, J. L. *Pathology*, Second Edition. J. B. Lippincott Company, 1994. Fig. 9-57, p. 416.

Fig. 23.8(B): Rubin, E. and Farber, J. L. *Pathology*, Second Edition. J. B. Lippincott Company, 1994. Fig. 9-58, p. 417.

Fig. 23.8(C): Davies, S. F. and Sarosi, G. A. *Clinics in Chest Medicine.* W. W. Saunders Company.1996. 17: (4) (December). Fig. 4.

Fig. 23.8(D): Koneman and Roberts, *Practical Laboratory Mycology.* Williams and Wilkins.

Fig. 23.9: Center for Disease Control, Atlanta.

Fig. 23.10: Murray, P. R., Kobayashi, G. S., Pfaller, M. A. and Rosenthal, K. S., *Medical Microbiology, Second Edition*, Mosby, 1994. Fig. 44-3, p. 418.

Fig. 23.10: Murray, P. R., Kobayashi, G. S., Pfaller, M. A. and Rosenthal, K. S., *Medical Microbiology, Second Edition*, Mosby, St. Louis, 1994. Fig. 44-3, p. 418.

Fig. 23.11: Goldman, M., Johnson, p. C. and Sarosi, G. A.. *Clinics in Chest Medicine.* W. B. Saunders Company, 1999. Fig. 3. Volume 20, Number 3, September 1999.

Fig. 23.13: Kassirer, J. P., *Images in Clinical Medicine*, Massachusetts Medical Society, 1997. p. 44.

Fig. 23.14: Rubin, E. and Farber, J. L. *Pathology*, Second Edition. J. B. Lippincott Company, 1994. Fig. 9-51, p. 409.

Fig. 23.15: Rubin, E. and Farber, J. L. *Pathology*, Second Edition. J. B. Lippincott Company, 1994. Fig. 9-55, p. 414.

Fig. 23.16: McGee, J., Isaacson, P. G., and Wright, N. A. *Oxford Textbook of Pathology.* Oxford Press, 1992. Fig. 6.30.

Fig. 23.18: Volk, W. A., Gebhardt, B. M.,

Hammarskjold, M. and Kadner, R. J., *Essentials of Microbiology*, Fifth Edition, Lippincott-Raven, 1996. Fig. 35-18, p. 492.

Fig. 23.20: Emond, R. T. D., Rowland, H.A.K. and Welsby, P. D., *Color Atlas of Infectious Diseases*, Third Edition, Mosby-Wolfe. 1995. Fig. 339. p. 283.

Fig. 24.3: Gillies, R. R. and Dodds, T. C., *Bacteriology Illustrated*, Third Edition, Williams and Wilkins Company, 1973. p. 194.

Fig. 24.4(A): Gillies, R. R. and Dodds, T. C., *Bacteriology Illustrated*, Third Edition, Williams and Wilkins Company, 1973. p. 196.

Fig. 24.6: Gillies, R. R. and Dodds, T. C., *Bacteriology Illustrated*, Third Edition, Williams and Wilkins Company, 1973. p. 198.

Fig. 24.11: Sun, T. *Parasitic Disorders. Pathology, Diagnosis and Management*, Second Edition. Williams and Wilkins, 1999. Fig. 5.7, p. 23.

Fig. 24.13: Armed Forces Institute of Pathology.

Fig. 25.2: de la Maza, L. M., Pezzlo, M. T. and Baron, E. J., *Color Atlas of Diagnostic Microbiology, Mosby, 1997.* Fig. 15-104, p. 170.

Fig. 25.6: Kassirer, J. P., *Images in Clinical Medicine*, Massachusetts Medical Society, 1997. p. 295.

Fig. 25.9: Kassirer, J. P., *Images in Clinical Medicine*, Massachusetts Medical Society, 1997. p. 306.

Fig. 27.4(A): Ordoukhanian, E. and Lane, Alfred T., *Postgraduate Medicine*, 101, February, pp. 223-232, 1997.

Fig. 27.4(B): Ordoukhanian, E. and Lane, Alfred T., *Postgraduate Medicine*, 101, February, pp. 223-232, 1997.

Fig. 27.4(C): Ordoukhanian, E. and Lane, Alfred T., *Postgraduate Medicine*, 101, February, pp. 223-232, 1997.

Fig. 27.7: Arthur, R. R, Shah, K.V. *Papovaviridae* In: The Polyomavirues. In Lennette E.H., Halonen P., Murphy, F. A., eds. *Laboratory Diagnosis of Infectious Diseases: Principles and Practices*, vol. II, Springer-Verlag 1988: 317-332.

Fig. 27.8(B): Ginsberg, H. S. *The Adenoviruses*, Plenum Publishers,1984.

Fig. 27.8(C): Volk, W. A., Benjamin, D. C., Kadner, R. J. and Parsons, J. T., *Essentials of Microbiology*, Fourth Edition, J. B.Lippincott Company,1991. Fig. 41.4, p. 563,

Fig. 27.11: Kassirer, J. P., *Images in Clinical Medicine*, Massachusetts Medical Society, 1997, p. 19.

Fig. 28.2: Volk, W. A., Gebhardt, B. M., Hammarskjold, M. and Kadner, R. J., *Essentials of Microbiology*, Fifth Edition, Lippincott-Raven, Philadelphia, 1996. Fig. 38-4A, p. 522. lippincott book.

Fig. 28.4: Fields, B. N., Knipe, D. M. and Howley, P. M. *Virology, Third Edition*, Lippincott Williams and Wilkins, 1996. Fig 10, p. 2315.

Fig. 28.5(top): Fields, B. N., Knipe, D. M. and Howley, P. M.. *Virology, Third Edition*, Lippincott Williams and Wilkins, 1996. Fig. 13, p. 2317.

Fig. 28.5(bottom): Fields, B. N., Knipe, D. M. and Howley, P. M.. *Virology, Third Edition*, Lippincott Williams and Wilkins, 1996. Fig. 12, p. 2316.

Fig. 28.12: Habif, T. P. *Clinical Dermatology, A Color Guide to Diagnosis and Therapy*. Mosby. 1996. Fig. 12-34, p. 345.

Fig. 28.13: Stephen K., *Hospital Practice*. July 15, 1996. Fig. 2, p. 139.

Fig. 28.15: Courtesy of Joan Barenfanger, Laboratory Medicine, Memorial Medical Center,

Springfield, IL

Fig. 28.16: Ball, A. P. and Gray, J. A., *Colour Guide Infectious Diseases*, Churchill Livingstone, Edinburgh, 1992. Fig. 56, p. 40.

Fig. 28.19: Custom Medical Stock Photo.

Fig. 28.24: Murray, p. R., Kobayashi, G. S., Pfaller, M. A. and Rosenthal, K. S., *Medical Microbiology, Second Edition*, Mosby, St. Louis, 1994. Fig. 56-16, p. 589.

Fig. 28.25: WebPath, courtesy of Edward C. Klatt MD, Florida State University College of Medicine.

Fig. 28.27(A): Murray, P. R., Kobayashi, G. S., Pfaller, M. A. and Rosenthal, K. S., *Medical Microbiology, Second Edition*, Mosby, 1994. Fig. 57-1. 45, p. 596.

Fig. 28.28: Henderson, D. A., et al. *Journal American Medical Association* 281:2130, 1999.

Fig. 29.3(B): Volk, W. A., Benjamin, D. C., Kadner, R. J. and Parsons, J. T., *Essentials of Microbiology*, Fourth Edition, J. B.Lippincott Company,1991. Fig. 45-1, p. 601.

Fig. 29. 7: Murray, P. R., Kobayashi, G. S., Pfaller, M. A. and Rosenthal, K. S., *Medical Microbiology, Second Edition*, Mosby, St. Louis, 1994. Fig. 68-12, p 714.

Fig. 30.2: Volk, W. A., Benjamin, D. C., Kadner, R. J. and Parsons, J. T., *Essentials of Microbiology*, Fourth Edition, J. B. Lippincott Company,1991. Fig. 46-1, p. 608.

Fig. 30.7: Moyer, L., Warwick, M., and Mahoney, F. J. *American Family Physician*. Fig. 2, 54: (Number 1) p. 112 (1996).

Fig. 31.5: Cotras, *Robbins Pathologic Basis of Disease*, Sixth Edition, W. B. Saunders Company, 1996. Fig. 7-38.

Fig. 31.6: Talaro, K. P. and Talaro, A. *Foundations in Microbiology, 3rd Edition*. WCB/McGraw-Hill, 1999. Fig. 25.12, p.801.

Fig. 31.15: Antman, K. and Change, Y. *N Engl J Med.* 342 (number 14) 1027 (2000).

Fig. 31.16(A): Hoeprich, P. D., Jordan, M. C. and Ronald, A. R., *Infectious Diseases, a Treatise of Infectious Processes*, Fifth Edition, J.B. Lippincott Company, Philadelphia, 1994. Fig. 46-1, p. 476.

Fig. 31.16(B): Katz, D. S. and Leung, A. N. Radiology of Pneumonia. *Clinics in Chest Medicine*. Fig. 2. Volume 20. Number 3, September 1999. W. B. Saunders Company.

Fig. 31.16(C): Katz, D. S. and Leung, A. N. Radiology of Pneumonia. *Clinics in Chest Medicine*. Fig. 4. Volume 20. Number 3, September 1999. W. B. Saunders Company.

Fig. 31.16(D): Volk, W. A., Benjamin, D. C., Kadner, R. J. and Parsons, J. T., *Essentials of Microbiology*, Fourth Edition, J. B. Lippincott Company,1991. Fig. 17.11, p. 245.

Fig. 31.16(E): Goldman, M., Johnson, P. C. and Sarosi, G. A. Pneumonia: Fungal Pneumonias. *Clinics in Chest Medicine*. Volume 20, Number 3, September 1999. W. B. Saunders Company. Fig. 1.

Fig. 31.16(F): Salkind, M. R. *A Slide Atlas of Common Diseases*, Parthenon Publishing Group, 1994. Fig. 59.

Fig. 31.16(G): Stone, D. R. and Gorbach, S. L. *Atlas of Infectious Diseases*. W. B. Saunders Company, 2000. Fig. 6-17 p. 98.

Fig. 31.16-H: Emond, R. T. D., Rowland, H. A. K. and Welsby, P. D., *Color Atlas of Infectious Diseases*,

Third Edition, Mosby-Wolfe. 1995. Fig. 339. p. 283.

Fig. 31.16(J): Center for Disease Control, Atlanta.

Fig. 31.16(K): Salkind, M. R. *A Slide Atlas of Common Diseases*, Parthenon Publishing Group, 1994. Fig. 25.

Fig. 31.16(L): Salkind, M. R. *A Slide Atlas of Common Diseases*, Parthenon Publishing Group, 1994. Fig. 9.

Fig. 31.16(N): Arthur, R. R, Shah, K.V. *Papovaviridae* In: The Polyomavirues. In Lennette E.H., Halonen P., Murphy, F. A., eds. *Laboratory Diagnosis of Infectious Diseases: Principles and Practices*, Vol. II, Springer-Verlag 1988: 317-332.

Fig. 31.20: Armstrong, D. and Cohen, J., *Infectious Diseases*. Mosby 1999. Fig. 10.5, p. 8.10.4.

Fig. 31.21: Katayarma, C. Y. Li and Yam, L.T. *American Journal of Pathology*, 67:361, 1972. J. B. Lippincott Company.

Fig. 32.2(A): Fields, B. N., Knipe, D. M. and Howley, P. M.. *Virology, Third Edition*, Lippincott Williams and Wilkins, 1996. Fig. 1, p. 1140.

Fig. 32.2(B): Fields, B. N., Knipe, D. M. and Howley, P. M.. *Virology, Third Edition*, Lippincott Williams and Wilkins, 1996.

Fig. 32.4: Volk, W. A., Benjamin, D. C., Kadner, R. J. and Parsons, J. T., *Essentials of Microbiology*, Fifth Edition, J. B.Lippincott Company,1991. Fig. 49-3, p. 640.

Fig. 32.6: Center for Disease Control, Atlanta.

Fig. 32.7: Salkind, M. R. *A Slide Atlas of Common Diseases*, Parthenon Publishing Group, 1994. ISBN: 1-85070-608-5. Fig. 81.

Fig. 32.8: Mir, M. A., *Atlas of Clinical Diagnosis*, W. J. B. Saunders Company Ltd., 1995. Fig. 1.211, p. 42.

Fig. 32.10(A): Fields, B. N., Knipe, D. M. and Howley, P. M.. *Virology, Third Edition*, Lippincott Williams and Wilkins, 1996. Fig. 2, p. 1401.

Fig. 32.12: Fields, B. N., Knipe, D. M. and Howley, P. M. *Virology, Third Edition*, Lippincott Williams and Wilkins, 1996. Fig. 2, p. 1357. Photo courtesy of George Leser, Northwestern University, Evanston, Il.

Fig. 32.15: Jensen, M. M., Wright, D. N., and Robison, R. A. *Microbiology for the Health Sciences*. Prentice Hall, 1995. Fig. 33-2, p. 420.

Fig. 31.16: Treanor, J., et al. *Journal American Medical Association*, 283:1016-1024 (2000). Fig. 2, p. 1020.

Fig. 32.17: Courtesy Dr. Frederick A. Murphy, School of Veterinary Medicine, University of California, Davis.

Fig. 33.2: Kapikian, A. Z., Kim, H. W., and Wyatt, R. G. Science 185:1049-1053, 1974.

Fig. 34.2: Hart, T. and Shears, P., *Color Atlas of Medical Microbiology*, Mosby-Wolfe. 1996. Fig. 16, p. 16.

Fig. 36.2 (upper left): Bottone, E. J., Girolami, R., and Stamm, J. M., *Schneierson's Atlas of Diagnostic Microbiology*, Ninth Edition, Abbott Laboratories, 1984. p. 5.

Fig. 36.2 (upper right): Bottone, E. J., Girolami, R., and Stamm, J. M., *Schneierson's Atlas of Diagnostic Microbiology*, Ninth Edition, Abbott Laboratories, 1984. p. 5.

Fig. 36.2 (bottom): Volk, W. A., Gebhardt, B. M., Hammarskjold, M. and Kadner, R. J., *Essentials of Microbiology*, Fifth Edition, Lippincott-Raven, Philadelphia, 1996. Fig. 29-2, p. 410.

Fig. 36.3(upper left): Alexander, S. K. and Strete, D.

Microbiology: A Photographic Atlas for the Laboratory. Benjamin Cummings, 2001. Fig. 9.2, p. 123.

Fig. 36.3 (upper right): Koneman, E. W., Allen, S. D., Janda, W. M., Schreckenberger, p. C. and Winn, W. C., *Color Atlas and Textbook of Diagnostic Microbiology*, Fourth Edition, J. B. Lippincott Company, Philadelphia, 1992. Plate 7-2 E.

Fig. 36.3 (bottom): NIBSC/Science Photo Library/Photo Researcher, Inc.

Fig. 36.4 (next to bottom): American Society Microbiology (Microbelibrary.org). Jeffrey Nelson, Rush University.

Fig. 36.4 (bottom): Ledbetter, L. S., Hsu, S., and Less, J. B., *Postgraduate Medicine* 107: 51, No 4, May 1, 2000.

Fig. 36.5(left): Leboffe, M.J. and Pierce, B. E. *A Photographic Atlas for the Microbiology Laboratory.* Morton Publishing Company. 1999. Fig. 11-7, p. 124.

Fig. 36.5 (right): de la Maza, L. M., Pezzlo, M. T. and Baron, E. J., *Color Atlas of Diagnostic Microbiology, Mosby, 1997.* Fig. 9-18, p. 77.

Fig. 36.6 (left): Koneman, E. W., Allen, S. D., Janda, W. M., Schreckenberger, P. C. and Winn, W. C., *Color Atlas and Textbook of Diagnostic Microbiology*, Fourth Edition, J. B. Lippincott Company, 1992. Plate 5-1A.

Fig. 36.6 (right): Varnam, A. H. and Evans, M. G. *Foodborne Pathogens.* Mosby-Yearbook, Inc. 1991. Fig. 170, p. 228.

Fig. 36.7 (top center): Wistreich, G. *Microbiology Perspectives: A Photographic Survey of the Microbial World.* Prentice-Hall, Inc. 1999. Fig. 158-B, p. 71.

Fig. 36.7 (middle row, center): Courtesy of Dr. Umberto Benelli, Online Atlas of Ophthalmology.

Fig. 36.7 (middle row, right): Courtesy of Vanderbilt University Medical Center, Department of Emergency Medicine.

Fig. 36.7 (bottom row, left): McMillan, A. and Scott, G. R. *Sexually Transmitted Diseases.* Churchill Livingstone, 1991. Fig. 25, p. 16.

Fig. 36.7 (bottom row, middle): Courtesy of Dr. Umberto Benelli, Online Atlas of Ophthalmology.

Fig. 36.7 (bottom row, right): McMillan, A. and Scott, G. R. *Sexually Transmitted Diseases.* Churchill Livingstone, 1991. Fig. 24, p. 18.

Fig. 36.8 (top, right): Finegold, S. M. and Sutter, V. L., *Anaerobic infections.* The Upjohn Company, 1986. Fig. 60, p. 51.

Fig. 36.8 (bottom, left): Finegold, S. M., Baron, E. J. and Wexler, H. M. *A Clinical Guide to Anaerobic Infections.* Star Publishing Company, 1992. Fig. 70, p. 69.

Fig. 36.8 (bottom, center): Finegold, S. M., Baron, E. J. and Wexler, H. M. *A Clinical Guide to Anaerobic Infections.* Star Publishing Company, 1992. Fig. 86, p. 82.

Fig. 36.8 (bottom, right): Kelly, C. P., Pothoulakis, C., and LaMont, J. T. *N Engl J Med.* 330:257-262 (1994).

Fig. 36.9 (left): Alexander, S. K. and Strete, D. *Microbiology: A Photographic Atlas for the Laboratory.* Benjamin Cummings, 2001. Fig. 2.7, p. 13.

Fig. 36.9 (right): Courtesy Harriet CW Thompson, M.S., Department of Microbiology, Immunology &, Parasitology, Louisiana State University Health Sciences Center, New Orleans,

Fig. 36.9 (bottom): Farrar, W. E., Wood, M. J., Innes, J. A., Tubbs, H., *Infectious Diseases.* Second Edition, Gower Medical Publishing, 1992. Fig. 1.35. p. 1.11.

Fig. 36.11 (top, left): Atlas, R. M. *Microorganisms in our World.* Mosby, 1995, p. 41.

Fig. 36.11 (middle, left): Varnam, A. H. and Evans, M. G. *Foodborne Pathogens.* Mosby-Yearbook, Inc. 1991. Fig. 73, p. 111.

Fig. 36.11 (middle, right): Varnam, A. H. and Evans, M. G. *Foodborne Pathogens.* Mosby-Yearbook, Inc. 1991. Fig. 75, p. 111.

Fig. 36.11 (bottom, left): Alexander, S. K. and Strete, D. *Microbiology: A Photographic Atlas for the Laboratory.* Benjamin Cummings. Fig. 3.13, p. 38

Fig. 36.12 (top, left): Koneman, E. W., Allen, S. D., Janda, W. M., Schreckenberger, P. C. and Winn, W. C., *Color Atlas and Textbook of Diagnostic Microbiology*, Fifth Edition, J. B. Lippincott Company, 1997. Plate 8-3H.

Fig. 36.12 (top, right): Koneman, E. W., Allen, S. D., Janda, W. M., Schreckenberger, P. C. and Winn, W. C., *Color Atlas and Textbook of Diagnostic Microbiology*, Fourth Edition, J. B. Lippincott Company, 1992. Plate 7-2J.

Fig. 36.12 (bottom): Center for Disease Control, Atlanta.

Fig. 36.13 (left): Quintiliani, R. and Bartlett, R. C., *Examination of the Gram-Stained Smear.* Hoffman-La Roche Inc., 1994. Fig. 7.

Fig. 36.13 (bottom): Farrar, W. E., Wood, M. J., Innes, J. A., Tubbs, H., *Infectious Diseases.* Second Edition, Gower Medical Publishing, 1992. Fig. 3.3, p. 3.4.

Fig. 36.14 (top, left): Leboffe, M.J. and Pierce, B. E. *A Photographic Atlas for the Microbiology Laboratory.* Morton Publishing Company. 1999. Fig. 11-21, p. 131.

Fig. 36.14 (top, right): Xia, H.X., Kean, C.T., and O'Morain. *European J. Clin. Microbiol. & Inf. Dis.* 13: 406 (1994).

Fig. 36.14 (bottom): Genta, R. M., and Graham, D. Y. *N Engl J Med.* 335:250 (Number 4) 1996.

Fig. 36.15 (left): Leboffe, M. J. and Pierce, B. E. *A Photographic Atlas for the Microbiology Laboratory.* Morton Publishing Company. 1999. Fig. 11-23, p. 132.

Fig. 36.15 (right): Koneman, E. W., Allen, S. D., Janda, W. M., Schreckenberger, P. C. and Winn, W. C., *Color Atlas and Textbook of Diagnostic Microbiology*, Fourth Edition, J. B. Lippincott Company, 1992. Plate 8-1 E.

Fig. 36.15 (bottom): Farrar, W. E., Wood, M. J., Innes, J. A., Tubbs, H., *Infectious Diseases.* Second Edition, Gower Medical Publishing, 1992. Fig. 2.29, p. 2.11

Fig. 36.16: Wistreich, G. *Microbiology Perspectives: A Photographic Survey of the Microbial World.* Prentice-Hall, Inc. 1999. Fig. 72, p. 39.

Fig. 3616 (bottom): Farrar, W. E., Wood, M. J., Innes, J. A., Tubbs, H., *Infectious Diseases.* Second Edition, Gower Medical Publishing, 1992. Fig. 13.40., p. 13.15

Fig. 36.18 (top, left): Wistreich, G. *Microbiology Perspectives: A Photographic Survey of the Microbial World.* Prentice-Hall, Inc. 1999. Fig. 193, p. 86.

Fig. 36.18 (top, right): Center for Disease Control, Atlanta.

Fig. 36.18 (bottom, left): WebPath, courtesy of Edward C. Klatt MD, Florida State University College of Medicine.

Fig. 36.18 (bottom, right): Hogeweg, M. *Tropical Doctor* Suppl. 1, p. 15-21, 1992.

Fig. 36.19 (top, right): Michael Gabridge/Visuals Unlimited.

Fig. 36.19 (top, left): Kassirer, J. P., *Images in Clinical Medicine*, Massachusetts Medical Society,

1997, p. 38.

Fig. 36.19 (bottom): Farrar, W. E., Wood, M. J., Innes, J. A., Tubbs, H., *Infectious Diseases.* Second Edition, Gower Medical Publishing, 1992. Fig. 2.25, p. 2.8.

Fig. 36.20 (left): Bottone, E. J., Girolami, R., and Stamm, J. M., *Schneierson's Atlas of Diagnostic Microbiology*, Ninth Edition, Abbott Laboratories, 1984. p 37.

Fig. 36.20 (right): Bottone, E. J., Girolami, R., and Stamm, J. M., *Schneierson's Atlas of Diagnostic Microbiology*, Ninth Edition, Abbott Laboratories, 1984. p. 37.

Fig. 36.20 (left, center row) : McMilan, A. and Scott, G. R. *Sexually Transmitted Diseases.* Churchill Livingstone, 1991. Fig. 17, p. 12.

Fig. 36.20 (right, center row): Brown, T. J., Yen-Moore, A., and Tyring, S. K. *Journal of the American Academy of Dermatology.* Volume 41, Number 4. October 1999. Fig. 10.

Fig. 36.22: Greer, Ken/Visuals Unlimited.

Fig. 36.23: Wistreich, G. *Microbiology Perspectives: A Photographic Survey of the Microbial World.* Prentice-Hall, Inc. 1999. Fig. 131, p. 59.

Fig. 36.24 (right): Leboffe, M. J. and Pierce, B. E. *A Photographic Atlas for the Microbiology Laboratory.* Morton Publishing Company. 1999. Fig. 11-35, p.137.

Fig. 36.25 (middle row, left): Courtesy of The Canadian Infectious Diseases Society

Fig. 36.25 (middle row, center): Courtesy of Dr. John Bezzant.

Fig. 36.25 (middle row, right): Courtesy of Dr. John Bezzant.

Fig. 36.25 (bottom row, left): Costerton, J. W. and Lappin-Scott, H. M. ASM News 55 (12):653,

Fig. 36.25 (bottom row, center): Courtesy Dr. Agrégé Mohamed Denguezli, Service de dermatologie CHU Sousse Tunisie.

Fig. 36.25 (bottom row, right): Courtesy of Dr. John Bezzant.

Fig. 36.26 (top row, left): Courtesy of Dr. Donna Duckworth.

Fig. 36.26 (top row, right): Courtesy of Dr. Donna Duckworth.

Fig. 36.26 (bottom row, left): Bisno, A. L. and Stevens, D. L., *N Engl J Med.* 334: (#4), 241 (1996).

Fig. 36.26 (bottom row, middle): Peterson, P. K. and Dahl, M. V., *Dermatologic Manifestations of Infectious Diseases.* The Upjohn Company, 1982. Fig. 48-1, p. 105.

Fig. 36.26 (bottom row, right): Mir, M. A., *Atlas of Clinical Diagnosis*, W. J. B. Saunders Company Ltd., 1995. Fig. 2.103; p. 86.

Fig. 36.27 (left): McMillan, A. and Scott, G. R. *Sexually Transmitted Diseases.* Churchill Livingstone, 1991. Fig. 64, p. 42.

Fig. 36.27 (right): Brown, T. J., Yen-Moore, A. and Tyring, S. K. *Journal of the American Academy of Dermatology.* Volume 41, Number 4. October 1999. Fig. 1.

Fig. 36.28: Copyright Dennis Kunkel Microscopy, Inc.

Fig. 36.29: Leboffe, M. J. and Pierce, B. E. *A Photographic Atlas for the Microbiology Laboratory.* Morton Publishing Company. 1999. Fig. 11-44; p. 142.